MW01156717

The Handbook of Global Health Policy

Handbook of Global Policy Series

Series Editor
David Held
Master of University College and Professor of Politics and International Relations at Durham University

The *Handbook of Global Policy* series presents a comprehensive collection of the most recent scholarship and knowledge about global policy and governance. Each handbook draws together newly commissioned essays by leading scholars and is presented in a style which is sophisticated but accessible to undergraduate and advanced students, as well as scholars, practitioners, and others interested in global policy. Available in print and online, these volumes expertly assess the issues, concepts, theories, methodologies, and emerging policy proposals in the field.

Published

The Handbook of Global Climate and Environment Policy
Robert Falkner

The Handbook of Global Energy Policy
Andreas Goldthau

The Handbook of Global Companies
John Mikler

The Handbook of Global Security Policy
Mary Kaldor and Iavor Rangelov

The Handbook of Global Health Policy
Garrett Brown, Gavin Yamey, and Sarah Wamala

The Handbook of
Global Health
Policy

Edited by Garrett W. Brown,
Gavin Yamey, and Sarah Wamala

This is an essential state-of-the-art guide to global health and its associated policies. It covers an extensive range of issues including the governance, financing, and architecture of global health; the influence of evidence and politics on health policy; human and national security; trans-border threats; and human rights and partnerships. In doing so, it maps out key debates and policy structures involved in global health policy, and isolates and examines new policy initiatives.

This unique text provides a definitive source and specification of the key areas in the field; it builds upon the interdisciplinary experience of its three editors to examine the ethical and practical dimensions of new and current policy models and their effect on the future development of global health policy and global health. It also brings together an international team of authors, a significant number of whom are from low- and middle-income countries, to ensure an inclusive view of current policy debates.

The book takes a further step from earlier research – from defining and demonstrating the associations between global mechanisms and global health, to examining health policies that influence global health. The book examines each health policy topic through two different lenses: one chapter focuses on ethical/more critical questions related to that topic, while an accompanying chapter explores the more practical/empirical dimensions. In this way, the book offers a 360 degree overview of global health policy, its formulation and its implications.

WILEY
Blackwell

The Handbook of
Global Health Policy

Garrett W. Brown is Reader in the Department of Politics at the University of Sheffield, UK. He is the author of *Grounding Cosmopolitanism: From Kant to the Idea of a Cosmopolitan Constitution* (2009) and co-editor of *The Cosmopolitanism Reader* (with David Held, 2010).

Gavin Yamey leads the Evidence to Policy initiative (E2Pi), a global health policy think tank in the Global Health Group at the University of California, San Francisco, USA. He is a frequent commentator on National Public Radio, and has published over 100 articles in peer-reviewed medical journals.

Sarah Wamala is the former Director-General of the Swedish National Institute of Public Health and she is currently serving at the Swedish Ministry of Health and Social Affairs. She is also affiliated with Karolinska Institute as Professor of Health Policy and Leadership. She has published extensively, and is the editor of *Globalization and Health* (with Ichiro Kawachi, 2007).

WILEY
Blackwell

The Handbook of Global Health Policy

Edited by

Garrett W. Brown, Gavin Yamey, and Sarah Wamala

WILEY Blackwell

This edition first published 2014
© 2014 John Wiley & Sons, Ltd

Registered Office
John Wiley & Sons Ltd, The Atrium, Southern Gate, Chichester, West Sussex, PO19 8SQ, UK

Editorial Offices
350 Main Street, Malden, MA 02148-5020, USA
9600 Garsington Road, Oxford, OX4 2DQ, UK
The Atrium, Southern Gate, Chichester, West Sussex, PO19 8SQ, UK

For details of our global editorial offices, for customer services, and for information about how to apply
for permission to reuse the copyright material in this book please see our website at
www.wiley.com/wiley-blackwell.

The right of Garrett W. Brown, Gavin Yamey, and Sarah Wamala to be identified as the authors of the
editorial material in this work has been asserted in accordance with the UK Copyright, Designs and
Patents Act 1988.

All rights reserved. No part of this publication may be reproduced, stored in a retrieval system, or
transmitted, in any form or by any means, electronic, mechanical, photocopying, recording or otherwise,
except as permitted by the UK Copyright, Designs and Patents Act 1988, without the prior permission
of the publisher.

Wiley also publishes its books in a variety of electronic formats. Some content that appears in print may
not be available in electronic books.

Designations used by companies to distinguish their products are often claimed as trademarks. All brand
names and product names used in this book are trade names, service marks, trademarks or registered
trademarks of their respective owners. The publisher is not associated with any product or vendor
mentioned in this book.

Limit of Liability/Disclaimer of Warranty: While the publisher and authors have used their best efforts in
preparing this book, they make no representations or warranties with respect to the accuracy or
completeness of the contents of this book and specifically disclaim any implied warranties of
merchantability or fitness for a particular purpose. It is sold on the understanding that the publisher is
not engaged in rendering professional services and neither the publisher nor the author shall be liable for
damages arising herefrom. If professional advice or other expert assistance is required, the services of a
competent professional should be sought.

Library of Congress Cataloging-in-Publication Data

The handbook of global health policy / edited by Garrett W. Brown, Gavin Yamey,
and Sarah Wamala.
     pages cm
  Includes index.
  ISBN 978-0-470-67419-2 (hardback)
  1. World health.   2. Public health International cooperation.   3. Globalization
Health aspects.   I. Brown, Garrett Wallace, editor of compilation.   II. Gavin Yamey,
editor of compilation.   III. Wamala, Sarah P., editor of compilation.
RA441.H34 2014
362.1–dc23   2013049096

A catalogue record for this book is available from the British Library.

Cover image: Vinita Yadav, a 23-year-old Indian, holds her newborn baby girl Nargis, born on October
31, 2011. The world's population reached 7 billion on October 31, 2011 according to projections by the
United Nations. Photo © Pawan Kumar / Reuters.
Cover design by Design Deluxe.

Set in 9.5/12pt Sabon by Aptara Inc., New Delhi, India

Contents

Figures and Tables

Figures

Tables

Notes on Contributors

Ashkan Afshin is a physician and epidemiologist at the Departments of Epidemiology and Global Health and Population at Harvard School of Public Health. His research interests include population prevention of non-communicable diseases, in particular global policies related to diet and lifestyle. Dr Afshin has led several systematic reviews and meta-analyses of the effectiveness of different population interventions to improve diet and he was a key author on an American Heart Association systematic review and scientific statement related to policy measures for the prevention of cardiovascular disease.

James Arkinstall is Head of Communications at the Médecins Sans Frontières (MSF) Access Campaign. After a stint with the International HIV/AIDS Alliance and field postings with MSF in West and Central Africa, he joined the MSF Access Campaign as a campaigner on tuberculosis and pediatric HIV/AIDS in 2005. He holds degrees in International Relations, Hindi, and Farsi from the University of Cambridge and the Institut National des Langues et Civilisations Orientales in Paris.

Yibeltal Assefa is a Director for the Planning, Monitoring, and Evaluation of the Multi-sectoral HIV/AIDS response in Ethiopia. He is a medical doctor with a Master of Science in Disease Control. He used to work as a Medical Director in Humera District Hospital, Ethiopia, from 2001 to 2005. He was the National HIV/AIDS Program Manager for Ethiopia from September 2006 to December 2008. Dr Assefa was later a Director of Medical Services in the Federal Ministry of Health of Ethiopia between January 2009 and May 2010. He has been a member of a variety of advisory committees for the World Health Organization (WHO) for patients' retention in care, and the consolidated guidelines for the use of antiretroviral drugs. He is a member of the Core Group of the WHO's TB/HIV program. Dr Assefa is also a member of the Technical Evaluation Reference Group for the Global Fund to Fight AIDS, Tuberculosis and Malaria.

Manica Balasegaram is a medical doctor who trained at the University of Nottingham, United Kingdom. He received further postgraduate training in internal and emergency medicine in the United Kingdom and Australia. He joined Médecins Sans Frontières (MSF) in 2001, working as a doctor in the field in several countries in sub-Saharan Africa and southern Asia. After gaining significant research experience, Dr Balasegaram became Head of the Manson Unit – a London-based medical research and implementation arm of MSF – in 2005. He then joined MSF's partner organization Drugs for Neglected Diseases initiative (DNDi) in 2008, finishing as DNDi's Head of Leishmaniasis Clinical Development Team before joining the Access Campaign in 2012. Dr Balasegaram has worked extensively on issues around access to medicines, with a focus on tropical and neglected diseases; he has training in both public health and tropical medicine from the London School of Hygiene and Tropical Medicine. He also has substantial experience in clinical trials and drug development working as a site investigator, principal investigator, and project manager.

Amy Barnes is a Lecturer in Health Policy and Management at the School of Health and Related Research at the University of Sheffield. She works at the disciplinary interface between public health, public policy, management, development studies, and politics. Her research has focused on issues of global health governance, participation, evidence use, partnership working, and inequalities within health systems. Dr Barnes' recent work explores how aid mechanisms (the Global Fund, sectorwide approaches, and budget support) reshape health systems, the participation of African actors in global health policy, and the linkages between community participation/control and health inequalities.

Rajaie Batniji is a Resident Physician in Internal Medicine at Stanford University and a scholar affiliated with Stanford's Center on Democracy, Development, and the Rule of Law. His research examines the selection of priority diseases and countries in global health, and he is interested in global health financing and the priority-setting process of international institutions. His work has also examined social determinants of health in the Middle East. He is a co-investigator on Global Underdevelopment Action Fund projects explaining US global health financing and political causes of public health crisis. Dr Batniji received his doctorate in International Relations (DPhil) from Oxford University where he studied as a Marshall Scholar. He also earned an MD from the University of California, San Francisco School of Medicine and MA and BA (with distinction) degrees in History from Stanford University. Dr Batniji was previously based at Oxford's Global Economic Governance Program, and he has worked as a consultant to the World Health Organization.

Sonia Bhalotra is Professor of Economics, University of Essex, United Kingdom. She holds an MPhil and DPhil from Oxford and a BSc from Delhi. Her research has involved estimating causal impacts on health and survival of maternal nutrition, state health expenditure, recessions, poverty, food subsidies, war, access to antibiotics, access to clean water, fertility choices, sex-selective abortion, cultural practices, and women's political representation. She is interested in the intergenerational transmission of health, the long-term socioeconomic benefits of childhood health interventions and maternal mortality. Her research uses micro-data from across developing countries and data for America and Scandinavia in the early twentieth century when infectious disease, sanitation, and nutrition were public health issues. Professor Bhalotra has served on steering committees and scientific committees in the health domain, and was recently a member of the research subgroup of the World Health Organization Scientific Resource Group on Health Equity Analysis and Research.

Agnes Binagwaho is the Minister of Health of the Republic of Rwanda. After practicing as a pediatrician for over 15 years, Dr Binagwaho led the National AIDS Control Commission between 2002 and 2008. She then served as Permanent Secretary in the Ministry of Health until 2011. Dr Binagwaho chairs the Rwanda Pediatric Society and is a member of the Global Task Force on Expanded Access to Cancer Care and Control in Developing Countries. She serves on the editorial advisory boards of *PLOS Medicine, Lancet Global Health*, and the *Journal of Health and Human Rights*. Dr Binagwaho is a Senior Lecturer in the Department of Global Health and Social Medicine at Harvard Medical School, and Clinical Professor of Pediatrics at the Geisel School of Medicine at Dartmouth.

Garrett W. Brown is Reader in Political Theory and Global Ethics in the Department of Politics at the University of Sheffield. He is Director of the Centre for Political Theory and Global Justice and has written extensively on global ethics, international law, cosmopolitan global justice, and global health governance. He is currently co-lead on an IDRC/EQUINET research project on performance-based funding in global health and is working with the Global Health Diplomacy Network to help strengthen the role of African actors in global health policy formation. His recent publications on cosmopolitan justice include *Grounding Cosmopolitanism* (Edinburgh University Press, 2009) and *The Cosmopolitanism Reader* (Polity Press, 2011) with David Held.

Carlos Bruen is a public health researcher and a PhD candidate in the Division of Population Health Sciences, Royal College of Surgeons in Ireland. His research focuses on global health policy, systems, and governance, including the emergence and evolution of new global health initiatives, and the role of individuals, organizations, and networks in shaping health systems responses and institutional change. He has been involved in the work of the Global Health Initiatives in Africa project and the Global HIV/AIDS Initiatives Network, as well as contributing to research for multilateral, national, and nongovernmental organizations. Prior to this he was a teaching and research fellow at the University College Dublin (Equality Studies Centre), responsible for programs on global politics and development.

Ruairí Brugha is a medical doctor, public health specialist, and Professor and Head of the Department of Epidemiology and Public Health Medicine at the Royal College of Surgeons in Ireland, with 25 years' experience in international health research. This included six years in Africa in the 1980s and 1990s as a clinician, public health specialist, and researcher at the district level; and 10 years at the London School of Hygiene and Tropical Medicine, where he was Head of the Health Policy Unit 2003–2005 and editor of *Health Policy and Planning*. His research interest is primarily in health systems and policy research, especially in Africa. During the 2000s, he conducted country-level studies and published on the effects of Global Health Initiatives on country health systems. He was a member of the Global Policy Advisory Council that co-drafted the Global Code on the International Recruitment of Health Personnel and is publishing research on the health workforce and health worker migration.

Peter Byass is Professor of Global Health and Director of the Umeå Centre for Global Health Research, located at Umeå University in the north of Sweden. He also holds honorary chairs at the Universities of Aberdeen, Scotland, and Witwatersrand, South Africa. Umeå University is designated as a World Health Organization (WHO) Collaborating Centre for Verbal Autopsy, for which Peter is also Director. He has worked in health measurement across Africa and Asia for nearly 30 years, specializing more recently in cause of death determination using innovative approaches to verbal autopsy (attributing causes to deaths that are not routinely certified). He is passionate about moving from top-down towards bottom-up evidence on global health. Professor Byass currently chairs the Scientific Advisory Committee of the INDEPTH Network, and serves on a number of WHO advisory groups. He is Deputy Editor of the open-access journal *Global Health Action*.

Mike M. Callaghan is a Doctoral Fellow in Medical Anthropology at the University of Toronto. He earned his Master's degree in Anthropology from the University of Alberta, Canada, for research among the Sherpas of Nepal. His current work focuses on public-sector antiretroviral therapy in the coastal region of Namibia, where he combines qualitative and quantitative approaches to examine patient outcomes. Previously, while working with the University of Cape Town and Médecins Sans Frontières, he studied health systems in sub-Saharan Africa – particularly the challenge of human resources in HIV/AIDS testing, treatment, and care. His overarching interest is in applying anthropological perspectives to health, development, governance, and the processes of globalization. He lives in Switzerland.

Michelle Childs was Director of Policy Advocacy at the Médecins Sans Frontières Access Campaign until February 2013. Previously, she was Head of European Affairs at Knowledge Ecology International (KEI), where she worked with non-governmental organizations throughout Europe on access to medicine and access to knowledge issues, and lobbied European and United Nations institutions. She was a member of the Transatlantic Consumer Dialogue working group on intellectual property, adviser to the Stop Aids Campaign and CEO of Essential Inventions. Prior to joining KEI, Michelle was Head of Policy Research and Analysis at the Consumers' Association UK, the largest member-driven consumer group in Europe. She has also been a personal advisor to the Director General of the Office of Fair Trading UK, a consultant to the Hong Kong Telecoms Regulator, and a policy adviser to the UK Telecoms Regulator. She has also worked as a solicitor in the commercial litigation department of a London law firm handling a range of disputes. She holds a law degree LLB (Hons).

Christopher J. Coyne is the F. A. Harper Professor of Economics at George Mason University and the Associate Director of the F. A. Hayek Program for Advanced Study in Philosophy, Politics, and Economics at the Mercatus Center. He is also the co-editor of *The Review of Austrian Economics*, the co-editor of *The Independent Review*, and the book review editor of *Public Choice*. Professor Coyne is the author of *Doing Bad by Doing Good: Why Humanitarian Action Fails* (Stanford University Press, 2013), *After War: The Political Economy of Exporting Democracy* (Stanford University Press, 2007), *Media, Development and Institutional Change* (co-authored with Peter Leeson; Edward Elgar Publishing, 2009), and the editor (with Rachel Mathers) of *The Handbook on the Political Economy of War* (Edward Elgar Publishing, 2011). In addition, he has authored numerous academic articles, book chapters, and policy studies.

Veronique de Geoffroy has a Master's degree in International Humanitarian Law and has worked for a number of non-governmental organizations in emergency contexts since 1993. She is currently Director of Operations at Groupe URD (Urgence-Réhabilitation-Développement), and focuses particularly on the issues of the quality of aid, international humanitarian law, and civil/military cooperation.

Stefan Elbe is Director of the Centre for Global Health Policy at the University of Sussex and Co-Convener of the British International Studies Association Working Group on Global Health. Professor Elbe has published widely on the international politics of health, especially health security. His books include *Security and Global Health* (Polity, 2010) and *Virus Alert: Security, Governmentality and the AIDS Pandemic* (Columbia University

Press, 2010). He is currently leading a four-year project on the role of pharmaceuticals in global health security, funded by the European Research Council.

Paul Farmer is Kolokotrones University Professor and Chair of the Department of Global Health and Social Medicine at Harvard Medical School, Chief of the Division of Global Health Equity at Brigham and Women's Hospital in Boston, and co-founder of Partners In Health. He also serves as a United Nations Special Adviser to the Secretary-General on Community Based Medicine and Lessons from Haiti. Dr Farmer and his colleagues have pioneered novel community-based treatment strategies that demonstrate the delivery of high-quality healthcare in resource-poor settings. He has written extensively on health, human rights, and the consequences of social inequality, and he is a member of the Institute of Medicine of the National Academy of Sciences and of the American Academy of Arts and Sciences.

Richard G. A. Feachem directs the Global Health Group at University of California, San Francisco (UCSF) Global Health Sciences and is Professor of Global Health at UCSF and University of California, Berkeley. From 2002 to 2007, Dr Feachem served as founding Executive Director of the Global Fund to Fight AIDS, Tuberculosis and Malaria and Under-Secretary-General of the United Nations. From 1995 to 1999, he was Director for Health, Nutrition, and Population at the World Bank. Previously (1989–1995), he was Dean of the London School of Hygiene and Tropical Medicine. Professor Feachem holds a Doctor of Science degree in Medicine from the University of London, and a PhD in Environmental Health from the University of New South Wales. He has worked in international health and development for 40 years and has published extensively on public health, health policy, and development finance.

Abraham Flaxman is Assistant Professor of Global Health at the Institute for Health Metrics and Evaluation (IHME) at the University of Washington. He is the research lead for the computational algorithms research team. Dr Flaxman is the primary architect of a software tool known as DisMod-MR which IHME is using to estimate the global burden of disease. He and other researchers use the tool to fill in gaps in incomplete data on stroke, malaria, depression, and other diseases from government records and surveys and to correct inconsistencies.

Lisa Forman is the Lupina Assistant Professor in Global Health and Human Rights at the Dalla Lana School of Public Health, and Director of the Comparative Program on Health and Society at the Munk School of Global Affairs at the University of Toronto. Her research focuses on the contribution of international human rights law to remediating global health inequities, including in relation to access to medicines in low- and middle-income countries and the post-2015 health development agenda. Lisa qualified as an attorney of the High Court of South Africa, with a BA and LLB from the University of the Witwatersrand. She has published widely on the right to health, and is co-editor (with Jillian Clare Kohler) of *Access to Medicines as a Human Right: Implications for Pharmaceutical Industry Responsibility* (University of Toronto Press, 2012). Her graduate studies include a Master's degree in Human Rights Studies from Columbia University and a Doctorate of Juridical Science from the University of Toronto's Faculty of Law.

Julio Frenk has, since January 2009, been Dean of the Faculty at Harvard School of Public Health and T. and G. Angelopoulos Professor of Public Health and International Development, a joint appointment with the Harvard Kennedy School of Government. Dr Frenk served as the Minister of Health of Mexico from 2000 to 2006, where he introduced universal health coverage. He was the founding director of the National Institute of Public Health of Mexico and has also held leadership positions at the Mexican Health Foundation, the World Health Organization, and the Bill & Melinda Gates Foundation. He is a member of the US Institute of Medicine, the American Academy of Arts and Sciences, and the National Academy of Medicine of Mexico. He is the author of more than 130 articles in academic journals, as well as many books and book chapters.

Nancy Fullman is a Policy Translation Specialist at the Institute for Health Metrics and Evaluation (IHME), where she works to translate global health research into relevant, accessible, and timely materials for evidence-based policy-making and program needs. Her two main projects focus on assessing health system effectiveness and evaluating the impact of malaria control policies on child mortality. Nancy Fullman previously led communications and advocacy efforts on behalf of malaria-eliminating countries at the Global Health Group at the University of California, San Francisco (UCSF). At UCSF, her primary role was to drive the dissemination of evidence addressing the challenges posed by the final stages of malaria control and eventual elimination. She completed a fellowship at IHME from 2008 to 2011, through which she conducted research on malaria interventions and received a Master of Public Health in Health Metrics and Evaluation from the University of Washington.

Octavio Gómez-Dantés is Senior Researcher at the Center for Health Systems Research of the National Institute of Public Health of Mexico. Between 2001 and 2006 he was Director General for Performance Evaluation at the Ministry of Health of Mexico, and between 2007 and 2008 he worked as Director of Analysis and Evaluation at the CARSO Health Institute (Mexico City). His areas of academic expertise are health policy and global health. Dr Gómez-Dantés holds a medical degree from the Autonomous Metropolitan University (Mexico), and two Master's degrees, one in Public Health and the other in Health Policy and Planning, both from the Harvard School of Public Health.

François Grünewald is an engineer in agriculture science with a specialization in rural economy. He has spent 30 years working on development, emergency, and post disaster rehabilitation projects in Africa, Asia, Central Europe, and Central/Latin America, as well as at headquarter levels. He has worked with non-governmental organizations (NGOs), the United Nations, and the International Committee of the Red Cross. In 1997, he became chairman of Groupe URD (Urgence-Réhabilitation-Développement). He has written several books and articles on complex emergencies and the management of socionatural disasters. François Grunewald has been, among others, team leader of the Post Hurricane Mitch inter-NGO evaluation from 1999 to 2001, the DFID/UNICEF evaluation of the response to the Darfur crisis, the evaluation of the French response to the 2004 tsunami, the Inter-Agency Standing Committee evaluation of the International response to the crisis in the Horn of Africa and of many evaluations after the Haiti earthquake and more recently of the situations in the Sahel and Mali.

Sophie Harman is a Senior Lecturer in the School of Politics and International Relations at Queen Mary University of London. Her research interests are in the governance of global health and development, with a specific interest in HIV/AIDS, Africa, agency, and the World Bank. She has published widely in these areas in international journals and edited collections and has participated in international research projects on African agency and performance-based financing in global health. She is co-convenor of the British International Studies Association Global Health Working Group and is on the Executive Board of the International Studies Association Global Health Section. Her books include *Global*

Health Governance (2012) and *The World Bank and HIV/AIDS* (2010), and has edited the books *African Agency in International Politics* (with W. Brown, 2013), *Governing the World? Cases in Global Governance* (with D. Williams, 2013) and *Governance of HIV/AIDS: Making Participation and Accountability Count* (with F. Lisk, 2009), all published by Routledge.

Peter S. Hill is a public health physician and academic with research and teaching interests in global health governance, global health initiatives, health systems strengthening, and indigenous health. He is currently an Associate Professor at the University of Queensland, Australia. He is a principal investigator with the European Union-funded Go4Health research project examining the roles of multilateral organizations in the construction of the post-2015 sustainable development goals. He has extensive policy analysis experience, having analyzed the Cambodian health sector, and more recently managing the Evidence for Health Policy Project in Vietnam, in collaboration with the Health Strategy and Policy Institute, Hanoi School of Public Health, and Hue Medical University in Vietnam. He has three decades of research and professional experience across West Africa, Southeast Asia and the Pacific – with particular focus on Nigeria, Cambodia, Vietnam, Papua New Guinea, and Aboriginal Australia – consulting for AusAID, GIZ, the Global Fund to Fight AIDS, Tuberculosis and Malaria, and the World Health Organization.

Adam Kamradt-Scott is Senior Lecturer at the Centre for International Security Studies in the Department of Government and International Relations, University of Sydney. His research primarily focuses on the norms and practices of global health security, particularly the management of infectious diseases (e.g., SARS, pandemic influenza) and other threats to human health, biosecurity and civil-military relations, health-related multilateralism and diplomacy, and securitization theory. He has published a number of journal articles and book chapters on these themes.

Vanessa Kerry is Director of the Program in Global Public Policy and Social Change in the Department of Global Health and Social Medicine at Harvard Medical School. She is the founder and CEO of Global Health Service Corps, a non-profit organization that partners with the Peace Corps to build the capacity of developing country health systems by deploying health professionals as educators. She is also a physician at Massachusetts General Hospital and serves as the Associate Director of Partnerships and Global Initiatives at the hospital's Center for Global Health. Her academic focus is on developing essential partnerships between medicine and public and foreign policy. She is working to help highlight the impacts of political decisions on health, the need to invest in human resources for health in developing countries, and the role health can have in improving foreign assistance efforts.

Shahab Khatibzadeh is a postdoctoral fellow in the Department of Epidemiology at Harvard School of Public Health. He holds an MD from Tehran University of Medical Sciences and an MPH in Quantitative Methods from Harvard School of Public Health. Dr Khatibzadeh has led several projects in Iran focusing mainly on system and capacity building for the Iranian healthcare system through planning and policy-making efforts at organizational and national levels. His current research interests include assessing the effect of lifestyle, especially dietary habits, on non-communicable diseases. Dr Khatibzadeh's current work aims to measure the impact of dietary factors on cardiovascular disease, diabetes, and cancer at national and global levels, and to investigate dietary quality and its economic determinants among adult women globally.

Felicia M. Knaul is Associate Professor at Harvard Medical School and Director of the Harvard Global Equity Initiative and the Global Task Force on Expanded Access to Cancer Care and Control in Developing Countries. She is also Senior Economist at the Mexican Health Foundation where she leads a research group on health financing and reform. Felicia is founder and President of the Mexican non-governmental organization *Tómatelo a Pecho,* which promotes breast cancer research and advocacy initiatives. Dr Knaul's publications span topics such as cancer care and control, health system reform and financial protection, women and health, and children in poverty, and include several books and a memoir entitled *Beauty Without the Breast.* She has held senior government posts in Mexico and Colombia, worked with multilateral agencies including the World Health Organization and the World Bank, and serves on the boards of numerous organizations including the Union for International Cancer Control.

Ronald Labonté holds a Canada Research Chair in Globalization and Health Equity at the Institute of Population Health, and is Professor in the Faculty of Medicine, University of Ottawa, and in the Faculty of Health Sciences, Flinders University of South Australia. His work focuses on the health equity impacts of contemporary globalization, on which he has published extensively. From 2005 until 2008 he chaired the Globalization Knowledge Network for the World Health Organization's Commission on the Social Determinants of Health, some of whose work is published in the book *Globalization and Health: Pathways, Evidence and Policy* (Routledge, 2009). Present research interests include health equity impacts of comprehensive primary healthcare reforms, health worker migration, medical tourism, global health diplomacy, and globalization and tobacco control.

Katherine Leach-Kemon works as a Policy Translation Specialist at the Institute for Health Metrics and Evaluation (IHME), with the aim of disseminating research findings in a manner that is both accessible and useful for decision-makers worldwide. She has worked at IHME since 2008, originally as a postgraduate fellow. She has published several articles on the topic of global health financing and most recently wrote *The Global Burden of Disease: Generating Evidence, Guiding Policy* (2013). Prior to working as a Policy Translation Specialist, she worked as the Data Development Manager to raise awareness of IHME's research among employees of ministries of health and national statistics agencies and to build support for data sharing. She received her Master of Public Health from the Department of Global Health at the University of Washington in 2008.

Rafael Lozano is the Director of the Health Systems Research Center at the National Institute of Public Health, Mexico and Professor of Global Health at the Institute for Health Metrics and Evaluation (IHME) at the University of Washington. Dr Lozano is one of the core team authors of the Global Burden of Disease 2010 study and is now the Director of Latin American and Caribbean Initiatives. Prior to joining IHME he worked at the Ministry of Health in Mexico as the General Director of Health Information. Dr Lozano has also been a leading contributor to epidemiological statistics, theory, and methods, working at the World Health Organization in Geneva as Senior Epidemiologist for the Global Program on Evidence for Health Policy for three years, in addition to working at Mexico's National Institute of Public Health, as Head of the Department of Epidemiology and the Division of Epidemiological Transition. He holds an MD from Universidad Nacional Autonoma de Mexico and a Master's degree in Social Medicine from Universidad Autonoma Metropolitana in Mexico.

Renata Micha is a clinical dietitian and epidemiologist who specializes in nutritional and cardiovascular epidemiology, with a focus on diet and global chronic disease. Dr Micha received her degree in Nutrition and Dietetics from Harokopio University of Athens, Greece, and her PhD in Public Health Nutrition from King's College London, United Kingdom. She subsequently did her three-year postdoctoral training in nutritional and cardiovascular epidemiology at the Department of Epidemiology, Harvard School of Public Health, where she mainly focused on leading the work of the 2010 Global Burden of Diseases Nutrition and Chronic Diseases Expert Group. In November 2011 she joined the academic staff at the Agricultural University of Athens, and she is currently a Research Associate at the Unit of Human Nutrition, Agricultural University of Athens, and at the Department of Epidemiology, Harvard School of Public Health. Since January 2012 Dr Micha has served as the Director of the first Hellenic National Health and Nutrition Survey.

Mary Moran is Executive Director and founder of Policy Cures, an independent research group formed at the London School of Economics and Political Science in 2004, which covers all aspects of global health research and development. Dr Moran has over 20 years' experience in health policy and practice, including 10 years specializing in neglected disease policy. She is an Honorary Senior Lecturer at the London School of Hygiene and Tropical Medicine, and an Expert Adviser to the World Health Organization, Organisation of Economic Co-operation and Development, European Commission, Australian Government, the GAVI Alliance (formerly called the Global Alliance for Vaccines and Immunization), and the Wellcome Trust. Prior to forming Policy Cures, she worked for over a decade in emergency medicine; was an Australian diplomat; Director of Médecins Sans Frontières (MSF) Access to Essential Medicines Campaign in Australia; and a Europe-based policy advocate with MSF on issues relating to access to medicines for neglected patients.

Michael Moran is a Research Fellow at the Asia-Pacific Centre for Social Investment and Philanthropy at Swinburne University, Australia. He completed his PhD at the University of Melbourne, an edited version of which will appear as *Private Foundations and Development Partnerships: American Philanthropy and Global Development Agendas* (Routledge, 2014). Before completing his PhD he worked in corporate research and in advocacy in the development non-governmental organization sector. He has published articles in *Global Society*, *Third Sector Review*, and the *Asian Journal of Entrepreneurship and Sustainability* as well as several book chapters for Routledge, Sage Publishers, Palgrave MacMillan, and Wiley Blackwell.

Dariush Mozaffarian is a cardiologist and epidemiologist, Co-Director of the Program in Cardiovascular Epidemiology and Associate Professor of Medicine and Epidemiology in the Division of Cardiovascular Medicine, Brigham and Women's Hospital and Harvard Medical School, and the Department of Epidemiology, Harvard School of Public Health. Dr Mozaffarian holds a BS in Biological Sciences from Stanford, an MD from Columbia, an MPH from the University of Washington, and a Doctorate in Epidemiology from Harvard. His research focuses on the effects of lifestyle, particularly diet, on cardiovascular health and disease in the United States and globally. Dr Mozaffarian has authored or co-authored more than 200 scientific publications on lifestyle and cardiovascular health, including the influence of nutrients, foods, and diet patterns; on the global dietary burdens of chronic diseases; and on evidence-based dietary policies to address these burdens. He has served on numerous committees and advisory boards, including for the World Health Organization, United Nations Food and Agriculture Organization, and the American Heart Association.

Valbona Muzaka is Senior Lecturer in International Political Economy at King's College London, United Kingdom, and one of the editors of *New Political Economy*. Her research interests are in the area of global governance, especially of intellectual property rights (IPRs) and trade. She has authored *The Politics of Intellectual Property Rights and Access to Medicines* (Palgrave, 2011) and a number of journal articles and chapters on the political economy of IPRs. She is currently working on a Leverhulme research project on the IPR policies adopted by India and Brazil in the area of pharmaceuticals and genetic resources.

Gorik Ooms is a human rights lawyer, who graduated from the University of Leuven in 1989. During most of his professional career he worked with Médecins Sans Frontières Belgium, of which he was Executive Director from August 2004 until May 2008. In 2008, he obtained his PhD degree in Medical Sciences from Ghent University for a thesis on the right to health. In August 2008, he joined the Department of Public Health at the Institute of Tropical Medicine, Antwerp. He was appointed Global Justice Fellow at the MacMillan Center for International and Area Studies at Yale for the 2009–2010 academic year with a Fulbright Scholarship, and he continues to be a corresponding fellow there. At present, he is Postdoctoral Researcher at the Institute of Tropical Medicine, Antwerp and Adjunct Professor of Law at Georgetown, Washington, DC.

Lauren Paremoer is a faculty member of the Political Studies Department at the University of Cape Town and was awarded a Fulbright Scholarship to pursue her PhD in Political Studies at the New School for Social Research. Her research focuses on the legal and bureaucratic regimes that govern access to HIV/AIDS treatment and public healthcare in the global South, and amongst members of the African diaspora in the global North. Her work seeks to analyze the conservative and transformative potentialities of public health regimes and the management of the HIV/AIDS epidemic with respect to these communities. It is orientated around three related questions on how public health regimes and epidemic management techniques: (i) mark out the boundaries of political communities and the nature of their solidarities; (ii) legitimize the market society; and (iii) shape the subjectivity of citizens. She has also undertaken research on women's access to land and housing in South Africa and the consolidation of democracy in South Africa.

Justin Parkhurst is a Senior Lecturer in Global Health Policy at the London School of Hygiene and Tropical Medicine. He received his Master's degree in Development Studies and Doctorate in Sociology and Social Policy from the University of Oxford. He has worked at the London School of Hygiene and Tropical Medicine since 2001, often applying social science insights to key public health and development questions. He has past experience researching HIV prevention, particularly in sub-Saharan Africa and with a focus on structural approaches to HIV. More recently, his research has focused on the politics of evidence for health policy, with concern for the institutional governance mechanisms shaping the use of evidence in decision-making.

Thomas Pogge received his PhD in Philosophy from Harvard University, then went on to teach in the Columbia University Departments of Philosophy and Political Science before going to Yale University as the Leitner Professor of Philosophy and International Affairs and founding Director of the Global Justice Program. He holds part-time positions at King's College London and the Universities of Oslo and Central Lancashire. He is a member of the Norwegian Academy of Science as well as President of Academics Stand Against Poverty (ASAP), an international network aiming to enhance the impact of scholars, teachers, and students on global poverty, and of Incentives for Global Health, a team effort toward developing a complement to the pharmaceutical patent regime that would improve access to advanced medicines for the poor worldwide. His recent publications include *Politics as Usual* (Polity, 2010); *World Poverty and Human Rights* (Polity, 2008); *John Rawls: His Life and Theory of Justice* (Oxford University Press, 2007); and *Freedom from Poverty as a Human Right* (Oxford University Press and UNESCO, 2007).

Julie Knoll Rajaratnam is a Senior Monitoring and Evaluation Officer based in PATH's Seattle office. Her areas of expertise include evaluation design, health metrics, quantitative methods development, quality assurance, capacity building and training, social determinants of health, and maternal, neonatal, and child health. Dr Rajaratnam provides technical guidance to multiple projects across PATH, including the evaluation of a large-scale community mobilization effort to improve maternal and neonatal health outcomes in Uttar Pradesh, the evaluation of a Safe Motherhood advocacy effort in India, Yemen, and Uganda, and a community-based test and treat campaign for malaria elimination in Ethiopia. She is a Clinical Assistant Professor at the University of Washington and previously worked at the Institute for Health Metrics and Evaluation (IHME) in Seattle. Dr Rajaratnam holds a PhD in Population Studies from Johns Hopkins Bloomberg School of Public Health, and a BA from Macalester College.

Matt X. Richardson was most recently Director of the Department of Knowledge Development at the Swedish National Institute of Public Health. He holds a PhD in Integrative Physiology, an MSc in Health Sciences and a BSc in Neuroscience. His research began with investigating gene expression in animals in response to stressful environmental situations and continued with human physiological and behavioral adaptation to similar environments. A natural progression of this research path led to public health, where he has focused on the determinants of health at the national and international level in his work for the Swedish government. Dr Richardson has served on a number of expert panels and commissions ranging from research in the fields of nutrition, alcohol and narcotics, and mental illness to cross-sectorial partnership in public health. He continues to work in varied fields from human performance to public health policy.

Arne Ruckert is a Researcher at the University of Ottawa's Institute of Population Health, working on health equity issues in the Globalization and Health Equity Unit. His principal areas of research include the international financial institutions, international aid architecture, the financial crisis and health equity, social determinants of health, and human rights-based approaches to development and health. He has worked as an independent consultant for various development organizations and is teaching development courses in the School of Political Studies and the School of International Development and Global Studies at the University of Ottawa. He has recently edited a collection on *Post-Neoliberalism in the Americas* (Palgrave, 2009) and his research has been published widely, including in *The Lancet, Review of International Political Economy, Critical Public Health, Canadian Journal of Public Health*, and *Health Promotion International*.

Simon Rushton is a Research Fellow in the Department of Politics at the University of Sheffield, United Kingdom. He was previously a Research Fellow in the Centre for Health and International Relations at Aberystwyth University. His work focuses on international responses to HIV/AIDS and other diseases, the links between health and security, the changing architecture of global health governance, and issues surrounding health, conflict, and post-conflict reconstruction. He is co-editor of the journal *Medicine, Conflict and Survival* and an Associate Fellow of the Centre for Global Health Security at the Royal Institute of International Affairs, Chatham House. Amongst other ongoing projects, he is currently editing (with Jeremy Youde) *The Routledge Handbook of Health Security* (forthcoming, 2014).

Marco Schäferhoff is Associate Director at SEEK Development. The focus areas of his work are in global health policy and development issues. Before joining SEEK Development, Dr Schäferhoff worked as Research Fellow in the Collaborative Research Center "Governance in Areas of Limited Statehood" at the Freie Universität of Berlin. His research focus was on global health and development policies as well as on transnational actors of global politics. He was also a lecturer at the Otto Suhr Institute of Political Science at the Freie Universität of Berlin, and taught graduate and undergraduate seminars on global health governance, theories of international relations, and research methods in social sciences. Dr Schäferhoff has published a wide range of scientific contributions on international financing for health and development and transnational cooperation. He holds an advanced degree in Politics and a PhD in Political Science.

Laura A. Schmidt is a Professor of Health Policy in the School of Medicine at the University of California at San Francisco (UCSF). She holds a joint appointment in the Philip R. Lee Institute for Health Policy Studies and the Department of Anthropology, History, and Social Medicine. Dr Schmidt is also Co-Director of the Community Engagement and Health Policy Program for UCSF's Clinical and Translational Sciences Institute. She received her PhD training in sociology at UC Berkeley and while there completed doctoral coursework in public health, and also holds a Master's degree in Clinical Social Work. Dr Schmidt has dedicated her career to intervening on the social determinants of health, and to understanding how lifestyle risk factors, such as alcohol and poor diet, influence chronic disease and health inequality. The hallmarks of Dr Schmidt's substantive research and teaching are the use of mixed methods and translational approaches for evidence-based policy-making.

Matthew T. Schneider is a Technical Advisor on the Health Economics, Financing, and Policy team in the Office of HIV/AIDS at the US Agency for International Development (USAID). His role with USAID allows him to work with US government country teams, national governments, and other international donors to collect and use financial data in the strategic planning for a world with improved health. Mr Schneider received his Bachelor's and Master's degrees in Public Health from the University of California Berkeley and the University of Washington, respectively. He completed a fellowship at the Institute for Health Metrics and Evaluations at the University of Washington where he worked on the Health Financing and Impact Evaluation working groups. His background in program evaluation, financing, and econometric modeling has allowed him to be a consultant on global health policy teams and global health program monitoring systems think-tanks, foundations, and non-profit implementing institutions.

Christina Schrade is Founder and Director of SEEK Development, a consulting and policy research group dedicated to supporting human development globally. She combines expertise in strategy, organizational development, and evaluation with comprehensive knowledge of international development and health issues. Key areas of her work are the global aid architecture, innovative development financing, and public–private and results-based approaches in international development cooperation. She also brings strong sector expertise in reproductive, maternal, newborn, and child health and AIDS, tuberculosis, and malaria, and extensive experience in leading large-scale multistakeholder projects. Before founding SEEK Development, she held senior management positions at the Global Fund to Fight AIDS, Tuberculosis and Malaria. She also worked on a range private sector and international development assignments as a project manager at the consulting firm McKinsey and Company. She has taught and conducted research at various academic institutions. She holds a Master of Public Administration from Harvard University, and a Master in International Relations; she also completed formal training in business administration, negotiation, and leadership development.

Ted Schrecker is Professor of Global Health Policy at Durham University, and Adjunct Professor of Epidemiology and Community Medicine at the University of Ottawa, Canada. His academic background is in political science, and his research interests include the impacts of transnational economic integration (globalization) on population health and issues at the interface of science, ethics, law, and public policy. Professor Schrecker coordinated the knowledge network on globalization that supported the work of the World Health Organization Commission on Social Determinants of Health, and more recently edited the *Research Companion to the Globalization of Health* (Ashgate, 2012). A four-volume collection of major works in *Global Health* that he co-edited with three colleagues was published in 2011 in the Sage Library of Health and Social Welfare. He is also the author or co-author of numerous book chapters and articles on globalization and health, for journals including *Social Science and Medicine, Globalization and Health, Health Policy and Planning, Bulletin of the World Health Organization*, and *Global Public Health*.

Hugo Slim is Senior Research Fellow at the Oxford Institute for Ethics, Law, and Armed Conflict at the University of Oxford where he leads research on humanitarian ethics and the protection of civilians. Dr Slim is a Visiting Professor at the University of Oregon and Oxford Brookes University and an Associate Lecturer at the Graduate Institute in Geneva. Hugo has worked for Save the Children UK and the United Nations in Africa and the Middle East, and has been on the board of Oxfam GB and an International Advisor to the British Red Cross. He is currently on the board of the Catholic Agency for Overseas Development. He was Reader in International Humanitarianism at Oxford Brookes University 1994–2003 and Chief Scholar at the Centre for Humanitarian Dialogue in Geneva 2003–2007. Dr Slim's publications include *Essays in Humanitarian Action* (2012), *Killing Civilians: Method, Madness and Morality in War* (2007), and *Protection: A Guide for Humanitarian Agencies* (2005).

Francisco Songane is the former Minister of Health of Mozambique (2000–2004). Dr Songane has also served as the Director of the Partnership for Maternal, Newborn, and Child Health. He was the Chair of the Council on Health Research for Development/Global Forum for Health Research 2012 Steering Committee, and recently joined UNICEF as Representative in Angola. Dr Songane's public health career has involved extensive work at subnational, national, and international levels. Trained in Mozambique, the United States, and England, he was a district medical director and teacher, as well as the director of Mozambique's second largest hospital. Dr Songane's extensive involvement with the international community has included serving as Executive Committee Member and Board Member of the GAVI Alliance (formerly called the Global Alliance for Vaccines and Immunization). He was also a member of Task Force 4 of the United Nations Millennium Project (2002–2004), analyzing the practicalities of achieving the goals related to maternal and child health. Dr Songane trained as a medical doctor and obstetrician/gynecologist at the University of Eduardo Mondlane in Maputo, Mozambique as well as at St James University Hospital in Leeds, United Kingdom. Dr Songane has a Master of Public Health from Boston University and Master of Science in Financial Economics from the University of London.

Michael Stevenson is a doctoral candidate in the Global Governance Program at the University of Waterloo, Canada. His research examines the agency of the Rockefeller and Bill & Melinda Gates Foundations in the governance of global health and food security. He holds an MA in Interdisciplinary Studies from the University of British Columbia and a BA in Political Studies from Trent University. His work has been published in a variety of journals, including *Global Society* and *Third World Quarterly*. Prior to returning to academia, he worked as a Senior Policy Analyst within the British Columbia Ministry of Health Services.

Christine Straehle is Associate Professor of Ethics and Applied Ethics at the Graduate School of Public and International Affairs at the University of Ottawa. She has written on issues of global justice, health, and migration. Her latest research examines vulnerability as a concept in global justice theory. Her work has appeared in a variety of journals, such as *Bioethics, Politics, Philosophy and Economics*, and *Contemporary Political Theory*. She is the editor or co-editor of several books, including *Health Inequalities and Global Justice* (2012).

Viroj Tangcharoensathien is a senior expert in Health Economics at Thailand's Ministry of Public Health and adviser to the International Health Policy Program. He served a decade in rural health services and won the "Best Rural Doctor" award in 1986 from Thailand's Medical Association. His doctoral thesis at the London School of Hygiene and Tropical Medicine (LSHTM) received the Woodruff Medal in 1991. His work on health financing, major health reforms, and capacity strengthening in health policy and systems research was recognized when he received the Edwin Chadwick Medal from LSHTM in 2011 for contribution to the generation of evidence that improves health systems in the interests of the poor. He has published more than 100 articles in international peer-reviewed journals. He chaired the negotiation of the World Health Organization Global Code of Practice on the International Recruitment of Health Personnel, which was adopted in consensus by the World Health Assembly Resolution 63.16 in May 2010.

Nadine Voelkner is Assistant Professor in International Relations at the University of Groningen in the Netherlands and Associate Researcher at the Centre for Global Health Policy at the University of Sussex, United Kingdom. She holds an MSc and DPhil from Sussex and a BA (Hons) from the School of Oriental and African Studies, University of London. She is co-author of *Critical Security Methods: New Frameworks for Analysis* (Routledge, forthcoming) which resulted from the Economic and Social Research Council-funded International Collaboratory on Critical Methods in Security Studies. Her research has revolved around understanding the global politics of human security including the governance of health security in relation to Burmese migrant communities in Thailand. Her current work investigates the role of the medical sciences (biotechnology, synthetic genomics) and advances in medical knowledge in the medicalization of insecurity.

Jimmy Volmink is currently Dean of the Centre for Evidence-based Health Care, Stellenbosch University and Director of the SA Cochrane Centre, South African Medical Research Council. He has previously held appointments as Deputy Dean (Research) at Stellenbosch University, GlaxoWellcome Chair of Primary Health Care at the University of Cape Town, and Director of Research and Analysis at the Global Health Council in Washington, DC. After obtaining his BSc and MBChB degrees from the University of Cape Town and a DCH from the South African College of Medicine, he worked as a family doctor and district surgeon for 12 years, before obtaining a MPH degree from Harvard University and a DPhil in Epidemiology from the University of Oxford. His major research interest is the evaluation of the effects of healthcare interventions, with extensive experience in teaching evidence-based medicine and in working with clinicians and policy-makers to promote the use of research in decision-making. He serves on the advisory boards of various international health and scientific organizations, including two terms as a Council Member of the Academy of Science of South Africa and as a Guest Editor of the *British Medical Journal* Special Issue on Africa in 2005.

Sarah Wamala, BSc, MSc, PhD, is the former Director-General/Special Investigator at the Swedish Ministry of Health and Social Affairs. She is affiliated with Karolinska Institute as professor of health policy and leadership. She has served as the Director General of the Swedish National Institute of Public Health 2008–2013, and in various executive managerial positions in health systems. She was appointed as a global health care thought leader at the Center for Health Innovation, Chicago and as distinguished executive mentor by the Global Initiative for Women in Health Care and Life Sciences. She was one of the international scientific expert members of the selection panel for the British National Institute for Health Research's 5-year research program on health protection research. She is the recipient of the Knut & Alice Wallenberg's prize. She holds a PhD in Public Health Medicine from Karolinska Institute, a Master's degree in Biostatistics from Stockholm University, and a Bachelor's degree in Economics from Makerere University. Her further training includes epidemiology and health economics from Tufts University (USA), Cambridge School of Public Health (UK), and Stockholm School of Economics. She is also trained in leadership and managerial skills at Stanford University Graduate Business School (USA). She is one of the 200 prominent women in Sweden who were selected to participate in the executive program on executive board skills 2009–2010. She has published extensively and is the co-editor (with Ichiro Kawachi, Harvard School of Public Health) of the book *Globalization and Health* by Oxford University Press.

Jonathan Weigel is a PhD student in Political Economy and Government at Harvard, and a research assistant to Dr Paul Farmer in the Department of Global Health and Social Medicine at Harvard Medical School. His research interests include the long-run political economy of development, fragile states and epidemic disease, and foreign aid effectiveness. He holds a BA in Social Studies from Harvard College, and studied political theory at Cambridge University on a Harvard–Cambridge Scholarship.

Claudia R. Williamson is an Assistant Professor of Economics at Mississippi State University. Her research focuses on applied microeconomics, the political economy of development, and the effectiveness of development policies, such as foreign aid. She has authored numerous articles in refereed journals including the *Journal of Law and Economics, World Development, Journal of Comparative Economics, Public Choice,* and *Southern Economic Journal.* Claudia completed her PhD in Economics at West Virginia University in May 2008. She spent 2007–2008 at George Mason University as the F. A. Hayek Visiting Scholar in Philosophy, Politics, and Economics. She was a postdoctoral fellow at the Development Research Institute of New York University 2009–2012 and she spent 2008–2009 as an Assistant Professor of Economics at Appalachian State University. During the summer of 2007, she performed fieldwork on land titling in rural Peru.

Gavin Yamey is a physician and medical journal editor with training in public health who leads the Evidence to Policy initiative (E2Pi) in the Global Health Group at the University of California, San Francisco (UCSF). He is also an Associate Professor of Epidemiology and Biostatistics in the UCSF School of Medicine. His policy research focuses on achieving large-scale change in global health, particularly related to infectious diseases of poverty and to reproductive, maternal, newborn, and child health. He teaches master's courses in global health policy at UCSF and at the London School of Hygiene and Tropical Medicine. Dr Yamey has been an External Advisor to the World Health Organization and to TDR, the Special Program for Research and Training in Tropical Diseases. He was a member of the Lancet Commission on Investing in Health, chaired by Lawrence Summers and co-chaired by Dean Jamison, which published its final report in December 2013, and currently leads the Economics and Finance Working Group of the Lancet Commission on Global Surgery. He was assistant editor of the *BMJ*, a founding senior editor of *PLOS Medicine*, and consulting editor of *PLOS Neglected Tropical Diseases*. He is a frequent commentator on National Public Radio, and has published over 100 articles in peer-reviewed medical journals.

Jeremy Youde is an Associate Professor and department head in the Department of Political Science at the University of Minnesota Duluth (UMD). He received his BA from Grinnell College and MA and PhD from the University of Iowa. Prior to his appointment at UMD in 2008, he taught at San Diego State University and Grinnell College. His research on global health politics has appeared in journals such as *International Relations*, *International Journal*, *Social Science and Medicine*, *Health Policy and Planning*, *Contemporary Security Policy*, *Politics and the Life Sciences*, and *Global Society*. He is the author of three books: *AIDS, South Africa, and the Politics of Knowledge* (Ashgate, 2007), *Biopolitical Surveillance and Public Health in International Politics* (Palgrave Macmillan, 2010), and *Global Health Governance* (Polity, 2012).

Foreword

Global Health Policy-Making in Transition

Sir Richard G. A. Feachem

The landscape of global health – including the ways in which the international community acts to tackle shared health challenges – is undergoing rapid transitions. An epidemiological and demographic transition is well underway, in which people are living longer and are more likely to suffer from chronic, non-communicable, and disabling conditions than from acute fatal infections (Murray *et al.* 2012). Such trends in turn are related to a risk factor transition – a shift over time towards the greater prominence of behavioral risk factors, such as smoking, sedentary lifestyles, and harmful use of alcohol (Lim *et al.* 2012). This evolution in the global pattern of diseases and risks is happening against a background of profound changes in the way in which global health is financed. After a decade of very rapid growth, international finance to address global health issues, sometimes called development assistance for health, has now flatlined as a result of budget crises in most large donor countries (IHME 2012). There is widespread concern that such assistance may even decline.

Another, less noticed, transition is also occurring in the global health field, one that could have profound long-term consequences. The world is shifting from global health as a focus for development assistance from wealthy to less wealthy countries, to global health as a focus for action to achieve global public goods and to overcome "global public bads." *The Handbook of Global Health Policy* lays out an initial roadmap for the collective commitment, collective action, and collective policy-making that will lead us to a genuinely twenty-first-century approach to global health.

Reducing global poverty, and completely eliminating extreme poverty (defined as living on under US$1.25/day), is arguably the most important global public good. The era of the Millennium Development Goals will come to an end in 2015, and it is likely that the goal of "getting to zero" on extreme poverty by 2030 will be a cornerstone of the second generation of these important collective goals. For example, in February 2013, the World Bank made a commitment to work with countries towards this 2030 goal. As Jim Kim, the Bank's President, said in his address to the 66th session of the World Health Assembly in May, 2013: "for the first time, we've set an expiration date for extreme poverty" (World Bank 2013).

Improved health, in my view, should be in second place as a global public good of massive importance to humankind. There will always be lengthy and heated discussions about the precise priorities of different diseases and risks within the global public goods for health agenda. An important starting point is those causes and risks that kill poor people far more frequently than less poor people. These constitute the so-called "unfinished agenda," which is largely comprised of the high burden of avertable infectious, reproductive, maternal, newborn, and child mortality in low- and middle-income countries. A recent analysis in *The Lancet*, conducted by the Commission on Investing in Health (http://GlobalHealth2035.org, last accessed December 2013), concludes that the world has the financial and ever-improving technical resources to reduce such death rates down to universally low levels seen in rich countries by 2035 (Jamison *et al.* 2013). The world could realistically achieve a "grand convergence" in health within a generation.

There is an equally important "global public bads agenda." The leading global public bad in health is our current inability to identify, contain, or effectively respond to newly emerging viruses with pandemic potential in a way that is adequate to prevent devastating global pandemics in the future. We should be particularly worried about the emergence of new influenza viruses, and the extreme consequences of a pandemic with a new influenza virus that is both highly fatal and easily transmitted among humans. Other significant global public bads that the world is not currently equipped to deal with include the global spread of antibiotic and other drug resistance and the rapidly increasing trade in counterfeit drugs, including those for malaria (Jack 2012).

What emerges so clearly from this handbook is that achieving global public goods in health and avoiding global public bads depend on an ambitious agenda of global progress in collective decision-making and collective action. If there was a "government of the world," it would take on this challenge as a very high order of business. Without such a government, we must create surrogate and replacement governance vehicles and mechanisms to ensure continuing progress in human health and development and robust preparedness for future threats.

Increasingly, these global collective efforts will not be framed as "aid" or "development assistance" – outmoded concepts that are rooted in the aftermath of the Marshall Plan and the period of rapid decolonization. These concepts are already ill-suited for the geopolitical realities of the twenty-first century, still carrying the post-colonial taint of charity and patronizing assumptions. They must be swept away and replaced by genuine global commitments to the achievement of public goods and the avoidance of public bads in health. Such outcomes are in the collective interest of all of humankind, and will require concerted action by *all* countries in order for them to be achieved.

The Handbook of Global Health Policy points the way towards this new and very different global architecture. A striking feature of the book is that the chapters do not take a disease-specific view, nor are they focused on specific regions of the world or on specific income groups, but are instead cross-cutting in nature. In 2010, I co-authored an editorial for the *BMJ* with Gavin Yamey and Christina Schrade – an editor and an author of this book, respectively – which we titled "A moment of truth for global health" (Feachem *et al.* 2010). We argued that cross-cutting policy issues tend to be neglected for several reasons:

> There is no vigorous advocacy or lobby group for these matters. A cross cutting agenda can feel threatening to some advocates for specific health topics. From a political perspective, the agenda will hardly win votes – it will not cause ripples of excitement to run through parliaments or electorates. But if we remain stuck in our silos during this time of economic uncertainty we will miss our opportunity to fashion an overarching global health system that can effectively deliver health for all.

This handbook takes up this challenge of producing a genuinely global and cross-cutting synthesis of issues and policy. It benefits from being one in a series of handbooks on global policy, including topics such as security, governance, energy, and climate, and so is situated within a broader examination of global policy issues.

A major innovation of the book is that each topic in global health policy is viewed through multiple "lenses." One chapter on a topic, for example, may be written by an epidemiologist who examines issues such as disease burden, risk factors, and health interventions; its paired chapter may be written by an ethicist or philosopher, who examines ethical issues surrounding that topic, such as our humanitarian obligations or questions of justice and fairness. Such diversity of views is entirely fitting: the next generation of global health policy-making will be shaped not just by health professionals but by lawyers, social scientists, economists, civil society activists, sociologists, anthropologists, engineers, and others.

Indeed, the three editors (Garrett Brown, Gavin Yamey, and Sarah Wamala) and 61 other authors of this handbook come from a remarkable range of backgrounds and from countries of all income groups. Some are very senior, including three Ministers or former Ministers of Health. Others comprise a bright constellation of rising stars, who may well be the global health policy leaders of the future.

In their introduction, the editors call this handbook "a new kind of textbook that aims to capture innovations in policy across the whole spectrum from theory to practice." The book deserves to be widely read and its policy innovations discussed and debated. Such conversations can help us, as an international community, move towards a global health system that is ready to meet twenty-first-century health challenges.

References

Feachem R, Yamey G, Schrade C. 2010. A moment of truth for global health. *BMJ* 340, c2869.

IHME (Institute for Health Metrics and Evaluation). Financing Global Health 2012: The End of the Golden Age? http://www.healthmetricsandevaluation.org/publications/policy-report/financing-global-health-2012-end-golden-age (last accessed November 2013).

Jack A. 2012. Faking it. *BMJ* 345, e7836.

Jamison DT, Summers LH, Alleyne G *et al.* 2013. Global health 2035: a world converging within a generation. *Lancet* 382, 1898–955

Lim SS, Vos T, Flaxman AD, Danaei G, Shibuya K, Adair-Rohani H. 2012. A comparative risk assessment of burden of disease and injury attributable to 67 risk factors and risk factor clusters in 21 regions, 1990–2010: a systematic analysis for the Global Burden of Disease Study 2010. *Lancet* 380, 2224–60.

Murray CJ, Vos T, Lozano R, Naghavi M, Flaxman AD. 2012. Disability-adjusted life years (DALYs) for 291 diseases and injuries in 21 regions, 1990–2010: a systematic analysis for the Global Burden of Disease Study 2010. *Lancet* 380, 2197–223.

World Bank. 2013. World Bank Group President Jim Yong Kim's Speech at World Health Assembly: Poverty, Health and the Human Future. http://www.worldbank.org/en/news/speech/2013/05/21/world-bank-group-president-jim-yong-kim-speech-at-world-health-assembly (last accessed November 2013).

Acknowledgments

Assembling a book as comprehensive as *The Handbook on Global Health Policy* is not an easy task. Along the way we have received considerable help and sage advice that has increased the quality of this volume and that has made the process much less painful. To begin, we would like to thank all the contributors who authored chapters and to commend them on their quality research, dedication, timeliness, and patience with us as editors. In addition, we would like to thank the Italian National Research Council, the Centre for Political Theory and Global Justice at the University of Sheffield, the Karolinska Institute, Sweden, the Swedish National Institute of Public Health, and the Global Health Group at the University of California, San Francisco for offering various levels of institutional support that helped with the creation of this book. We would also like to thank Sir Richard Feachem, Gil Walt, Sir Michael Marmot, David Held, three anonymous reviewers, and Wiley Blackwell for their helpful comments and suggestions for how to improve this volume. Finally, huge appreciation is due to Andreas Papamichail for helping us to organize the final manuscript and for taking charge of the authors' biographies.

G. W. Brown, G. Yamey, and S. Wamala, 2014

Introduction

Garrett W. Brown, Gavin Yamey, and Sarah Wamala

Why Global Health Policy

The world has become increasingly interconnected. Because of this interdependence, humanity is presented with new and challenging collective action problems such as global poverty, a lack of global development, climate change, human and national security, nuclear proliferation, transborder infectious diseases, the globalization of disease risk factors, and global economic crisis. Traditional multilateral policy models are strained to sufficiently tackle these global problems. As a result, academics, practitioners, and politicians have increasingly called for a broadening of existing structures of global governance, global public policy formation, and global policy implementation. One such growing concern involves global health. There are new calls to find innovative ways to generate robust global health policy so as to effectively respond to some of the world's most pressing health concerns.

Because of an increased interconnection between globalization and public health, the last decade has seen growing interest in global health governance and global health more generally, including new research centers and teaching programs related to global health policy. In addition, more mainstream academic circles have started to pay closer attention to global health policy and its important place in global politics with a plethora of social science publications being generated since the turn of the millennium. Furthermore, as shown by the recent media attention to H1N1 (swine flu), H7N9 (bird flu), MERS-CoV (originally called "novel coronavirus" or nCoV) and TDR-TB (totally drug-resistant tuberculosis), global policies on how we tackle health priorities can greatly affect our everyday lives and have profound implications for the collective security of states, regions, and human beings. As is becoming increasingly clear, due to various transformations associated with globalization, it is no longer possible to speak solely in terms of domestic health policy.

The Handbook of Global Health Policy, First Edition. Edited by Garrett W. Brown, Gavin Yamey, and Sarah Wamala.
© 2014 John Wiley & Sons, Ltd. Published 2014 by John Wiley & Sons, Ltd.

In response to this growing interest, *The Handbook of Global Health Policy* presents a comprehensive overview and discussion of the field of global health policy. Unlike other books that focus more generally on global health governance or on only one particular health policy area, this book focuses directly on key new areas in the field. We have focused on policy rather than governance because policy generally relates to the creation of guidelines or principles deemed necessary to achieve specific governance outcomes. The design of these policies tends to have two key considerations involved in their formulation and which ultimately guide the practice of how issues are governed: an ethical/moral dimension regarding the decision of "who gets what and why" and more practical dimensions involving questions regarding "how, when, and where." Although these two dimensions are not mutually exclusive and most policy decisions reflect an amalgamation of the ethical and the practical, it is nevertheless fair to say that all policy must respond to these two sets of questions. It is also fair to say that the way in which policy decisions respond to these questions will have profound and lasting impacts upon people's lives. As a result, this book seeks to explore how health policy has been formulated, how these formulations are changing in innovative ways, and what moral and practical implications these new and current policy models have on the future development of global health policy and global health more generally.

The State of the World's Health

A key assertion made repeatedly throughout this book is that the adoption of the Millennium Development Goals (MDGs) in the year 2000 by 193 United Nations (UN) Member States was one of the most transformative events in modern global health policy-making. Three of these goals were specific to health – MDG 4 (reducing child mortality), MDG 5 (reducing maternal mortality), and MDG 6 (controlling HIV/AIDS and other infectious diseases) – thus putting health at the very top of the global development agenda.

As discussed by Michael Moran and Michael Stevenson in Chapter 28, the MDGs ushered in an unprecedented era of intense international health cooperation, characterized by new actors, new money, new technologies, and new forms of governance in global health. What did the MDGs era achieve in terms of changing global health outcomes, what did it neglect, and what health challenges can be anticipated in the "post-2015" era?

The period from 2000 to 2010 saw an explosive rise in development assistance for health (DAH), in which annual DAH almost tripled, from US$10.8 billion to $28.2 billion in 2010, an annualized growth rate of over 11.2% (IHME 2012). A large proportion of this new money was targeted at MDG 6, and channeled into vertical programs tackling HIV/AIDS, tuberculosis (TB), and malaria. While the role of aid in improving health outcomes remains debated, there is increasingly good evidence that such targeting of health aid towards infectious diseases had impressive pay-offs. For example, the most recent Global Burden of Disease Study 2010 (GBD 2010) found that there have been large reductions in mortality in eastern and southern sub-Saharan Africa since 2004, coinciding with the aggressive scale-up of antiretroviral therapy and malaria prevention tools such as insecticide-treated bed nets (Wang *et al.* 2012). This scale-up was mostly funded by DAH, particularly from the Global Fund to Fight AIDS, Tuberculosis and Malaria, the US President's Plan for AIDS Relief (PEPFAR), and the US President's Malaria Initiative (PMI). Such scale-up would not have been possible without strong national attention towards health. Indeed, over the last two decades many low- and middle-income countries (LMICs) instituted significant national health reforms, coupled with increased domestic spending on health (Elovainio and Evans 2013).

Important progress has been made in tackling "the big three" infectious diseases: the annual number of new HIV infections fell from 3.2 million in 2001 to 2.5 million in 2011, malaria incidence rates have fallen by 17% since 2000, and the 1990 death rate from TB is on course to be halved by 2015 (UN 2012; UNAIDS 2012). The GBD 2010 study found a decline in deaths from other infectious diseases from 1990 to 2010, particularly diseases of childhood, including diarrheal diseases, lower respiratory infections, measles, and tetanus (Lozano *et al.* 2012). Nevertheless, there will still be a major global burden of HIV, TB, malaria, and other infectious diseases after 2015.

Countdown to 2015, a multidisciplinary collaboration that tracks global progress towards MDGs 4 and 5, notes that both child and maternal mortality have fallen substantially since 1990 (Bhutta *et al.* 2010). But the rate of decline remains too slow for the 2015 MDG targets to be met (Box 1). Thus in the post-2015 era, the global health community will still be tackling an "unfinished agenda" of avertable infectious, reproductive, maternal, newborn, and child deaths in high mortality settings.

Box 1 Global Progress Towards MDGs 4 and 5

The MDG 4 target is a reduction of two thirds in the under-5 mortality rate from 1990 to 2015, while the MDG 5 target is a reduction of three quarters in the maternal mortality ratio over the same time period.

The UN Inter-agency Group for Child Mortality Estimation (2013) estimates that from 1990 to 2012, the global number of under-5 deaths fell from 12.6 million to 6.6 million, and the under-5 mortality rate fell from 90 to 48 per 1000 live births. This annual rate of reduction is, however, too slow to reach MDG 4.

The UN Maternal Mortality Estimation Inter-agency Group (2010) estimates that from 1990 to 2010 the number of maternal deaths worldwide fell from 546,000 to 287,000, and the global maternal mortality ratio fell from 400 to 210 maternal deaths per 100,000 live births. The group notes that MDG 5 is "very unlikely to be achieved by 2015, unless there are remarkable further reductions from 2011 to 2015."

Overall, there will need to be a substantial acceleration in the rate of decline of child and maternal mortality for MDGs 4 and 5 to be met.

In addition, the MDGs did nothing at all to confront the "emerging agenda" of non-communicable diseases (NCDs), which are now responsible for two thirds of all deaths worldwide (Lozano *et al.* 2012). LMICs have recently experienced a catastrophic rise in NCD incidence, and age-adjusted mortality rates for several NCDs are now higher in LMICs than in high-income countries (di Cesare *et al.* 2013). The dramatic increase in deaths from cardiovascular disease, cancers, diabetes, and chronic respiratory illnesses in LMICs is related to populations living longer and to an "epidemic" of NCD risk factors, particularly smoking, alcohol, sedentary lifestyles, and the consumption of highly processed foods (WHO 2011). The emerging agenda also includes global preparedness for future shocks, such as a new pandemic, the global rise of antibiotic resistance, and the risks posed by nuclear, biological, and chemical weapons. As of February 2014, for example, the World Health Organization (WHO) had been informed of 308 laboratory-confirmed human cases of H7N9 influenza, including 63 deaths (WHO 2014).

The global health community is thus facing an unprecedented array of global public health challenges that calls for new ways of doing business. On top of the health issues outlined above, we are also facing deep inequities between and within countries in the social determinants of health, particularly education and income, as well as the highly interrelated crises of globalization, which McMichael (2013) argues is "a syndrome, not a set of separate changes." This "syndrome" includes financial instability, global warming, environmental and ecological degradation, food insecurity, and mass migration.

A New Kind of Handbook to Guide Action on these Challenges

An intense debate is now underway on what should come next in the post-2015 era. This debate is raising some provocative questions. Should health still play an outsized role in the development agenda or is it time to give other sectors, such as climate or food security, their turn in the spotlight? Should we move beyond the successful vertical approach of the last decades, aimed at tackling specific diseases such as HIV/AIDS, TB, and malaria, and focus our attention instead on building health systems and expanding health insurance in LMICs? And, in the face of a global NCD explosion and the threat of emerging pandemics that could bring global society to a halt, what kinds of new cooperation, partnerships, and financing mechanisms are needed?

This debate is taking place upon a background of realignments in the global health order that will reshape the policy-making landscape in the coming decades. As discussed below, after a decade of rising aid for health, referred to as the "golden window" for global health (McNeil 2010), such aid has now flat-lined in the wake of the global financial crisis. As Legge and Sanders (2013) have noted, "healthcare based on donor funding is neither secure nor sustainable." While DAH is likely to play an important ongoing role in supporting health programs in the world's poorest countries, donors have begun to retreat from supporting middle-income countries (MICs), such as South Africa, India, and China (DFID 2011; Smith 2013).

On top of such "donor retreat," the aid enterprise is changing in other ways. Many countries that were aid *recipients*, such as Brazil, China, and Russia, are now themselves becoming donors, and are exploring new aid modalities that are very different from those used by traditional donors, such as emphasizing "South–South" cooperation (Walz and Ramachandran 2011). Many emerging economies, such as India and China, have invested heavily in research and development and have become the world's leading producers and suppliers of global medicines, including antibiotics and antiretrovirals (Morel *et al.* 2005). The astonishing economic growth rate of many MICs provides them the opportunity to ratchet up their own domestic health investments to achieve universal health coverage, strengthen their national health systems, and free themselves from the uncertainty and volatility inherent in aid dependence. All in all, we are witnessing "shifting spheres of influence" in global health policy (Oberth 2012).

These new threats, shifts, and transformations are prompting calls to find innovative ways to generate robust global health policies that are "fit for purpose" in tackling such complexity. *The Handbook of Global Health Policy* is a response to such calls. It is a new kind of textbook that aims to capture innovations in policy across the whole spectrum from theory to practice, organized across seven key domains of global health that make up the seven sections of the book. These domains address politics and governance (Part I); the role of scientific evidence and disease burden assessments in shaping policy (Part II); the distribution of risks and diseases (Part III); the securitization of health and the global humanitarian enterprise (Part IV); issues of financing, trade, and political economy

(Part V); the human rights and partnerships agendas (Part VI); and health in a post-globalized world (Part VII). The book aims to reflect the contemporary policy debates that are illuminating the field and to offer novel, intersectoral policy options and solutions that can help address the dizzying range of twenty-first-century global health challenges.

There are at least three ways in which this book takes an unusual approach compared with traditional treatments of global health. First, we examine each topic through multiple lenses. In particular, for most topics we commissioned paired chapters that reflect different views or approaches. One chapter is written by practitioners working at the frontline of public health, including clinicians, public health professionals, and epidemiologists, providing a practical, empirical perspective, often focused on how to achieve large-scale change. The paired chapter examines some of the key theoretical debates, dilemmas, and ethical issues surrounding that topic, including issues of justice, ethical tensions, and humanitarian obligations. For example, in Chapter 9, Ashkan Ashfin, a physician and epidemiologist at Harvard University, United States, and his colleagues examine one of the most important NCD risk factors – poor quality diet – and propose a series of sound, evidence-based dietary policies. A paired chapter (Chapter 10) by Christine Straehle, who teaches ethics at the University of Ottawa in Canada, goes beyond the "practical" dimension of addressing risk factors to explore, from an ethical standpoint, what it means to be "at risk" in global health.

We believe that this approach provides a more comprehensive picture, capturing the many complicated but interrelated policy components of global health – from practical questions concerning "how, when, and where" to the moral, ethical, and critical questions of "who, what, and why." This broad approach is in part a reflection of our diverse backgrounds as editors. Garrett Wallace Brown studies and teaches political theory, global health governance, and applied global ethics at the University of Sheffield, United Kingdom. Gavin Yamey, a physician and medical journal editor with training in public health, leads a global health policy think tank in the Global Health Group at the University of California, San Francisco, United States. Sarah Wamala studied economics at Makerere, University, Uganda, moved to Sweden as a refugee, trained in biostatics and public health served for 5 years as the Director-General of the Swedish National Institute of Public Health, and is now Director General at the Swedish Ministry of Health and Social Affairs.

Second, we sought to include academics and practitioners from the global South, who have been notably absent from many global health textbooks. The global burden of disease falls most heavily on LMICs and the exclusion of authors from these countries deprives readers from hearing the views of those closest to the problems. While there are certainly shared health problems that transcend national boundaries and that can be addressed by global solutions, these solutions will often require local adaptation, as captured in the mantra "globalize the evidence, localize the decision" (Eisenberg 2002). Authors in this handbook provide "localized" insights from countries including Ethiopia, Mexico, Mozambique, Rwanda, South Africa, and Thailand.

Third, an important feature of the book is that all authors have summarized their chapters in the form of key take home messages and actionable policy guidance. We recognize that the rich complexity of global health policy cannot be easily reduced to simple talking points. Nevertheless, we believe that encouraging authors to lay out the key themes, plus the major policy lessons, in their chapter has made this textbook highly accessible to a wide audience and has given it added educational value. Every chapter has an abstract that summarizes the contents; a box called "Key points," which gives the key messages in the form of bullet points; a box called "Key policy implications," which draws out the most important policy applications of the chapter; and a list of valuable readings on the topic (including journal articles, books, and web resources).

Breadth, diversity, accessibility, and practical value were the key principles that we adopted in editing this book. We asked authors to avoid jargon as much as possible, and to target their writing to undergraduates, postgraduates, researchers, clinicians, public health professionals, and policy-makers worldwide. Since this is a "handbook," we also prompted all authors, even those writing from an ethical or critical stance, to think about how readers might *apply* their chapter to their daily lives studying, teaching, or working in the field of global health policy. We hope that the end result is a book that will be used in print and online by, among others, junior and senior staff in ministries of health and finance, donor agencies, students, and professors preparing to teach their next class.

Five Key Themes Emerging from the Book

One interesting by-product of assembling a comprehensive book like *The Handbook of Global Health Policy* is that one begins to see a number of common themes across the chapters as well as between their related subjects. This was certainly the case with this volume and common themes around interdisciplinary research, governance mechanisms, health financing, policy foundations, and health justice started to emerge as the collection came together. In particular, there is common agreement that despite the great strides made in global health, there is still much work to be done. Across all chapters there was an overwhelming sense that the study and practice of global health is hugely complex with multifarious interconnections that transcend existing disciplinary boundaries and that require a more collaborative and interdisciplinary approach in researching and setting global health policy. Furthermore, all of the authors suggested that current governance mechanisms and financing models were generally not sufficient to meet twenty-first-century health challenges and that new innovations in how to design and operationalize effective global health policy are necessary. Lastly, there is an implicit normative consensus that the health of human beings matters and that there are compelling ethical and practical reasons to alleviate existing global health inequalities (by *normative*, we mean a moral demand that we *should* or *ought* to do something). As will be explored further below, all of the authors in *The Handbook of Global Health* are in some sense engaged with these issues and in the process are providing interesting and useful insights for how to positively reshape global health policy in the near and distant future.

Theme 1: Global Health is Increasingly Multidimensional, Requiring Innovation in Interdisciplinary and Collaborative Approaches

One key theme that emerges from this book is the idea that while some level of specialization is undoubtedly required to effectively study global health, the everyday realities of how global health is experienced renders its study inherently multidimensional, requiring an increased use of interdisciplinary and collaborative approaches. For example, Arne Ruckert and Ronald Labonté (Chapter 14) defend the analytical potential of the social determinants of health (SDH) approach. In doing so they argue that seemingly secondary elements such as education, financial regulation, and labor standards can have a huge impact upon individual health as well as the resiliency of broader health systems. As the authors state, "global health is shaped by various social factors and living conditions" and to better understand the causal pathways that "link individual SDHs to health outcomes" will also require wider socioeconomic knowledge beyond the realm of medical science and technology. Furthermore, adopting a SDH approach to health involves more than just medical and social science, since embedded within the SDH lexicon is a fundamental concern with alleviating social inequalities that lead to uneven distributions in health outcomes. As a result, Garrett Wallace Brown and Lauren Paremoer (Chapter 4) argue that ethical questions of fairness, distributive justice, and moral responsibility are inherent to the SDH approach and thus add yet another level of multidimensionality to the study of SDH and its policy directives.

The need for interdisciplinarity is furthered by Ted Schrecker (Chapter 21), when he suggests that "global finance is a public health issue, and health researchers and practitioners must acquire sufficient familiarity to participate proactively in key policy debates." Not to do so, he argues, means that "the extent to which global financial markets influence health by way of its social determinants" will remain "a neglected area of research," which will underestimate the critical pathways that "link the operation of global financial markets to adverse health effects." To substantiate his claim, Schrecker examines two key health links associated with global financial markets. He suggests that the existing structural "conditionalities" within financial markets limit the health policy options available to LMICs as well as allowing the ability for mass elite capital flight, which adversely reduces available social resources and intensifies economic inequality. In both cases, argues Schrecker, these market forces impinge upon local socioeconomic conditions and thus have a significant detrimental affect on SDH.

As Matt X. Richardson and his colleagues argue (Chapter 30), the need for interdisciplinarity is only magnified as the forces of globalization transform the scope, intensity, and effects of economic, political, technological, and medical policies for human health. The worry here, they argue, is that "globalization is a multifocal, multivariate process that affects health through increasing interconnectedness in global economic, political, and cultural realms." As the complexities of this interconnectedness grow, so will the need to develop better conceptual and methodological tools to help us understand the interrelations between globalization and global health. For Richardson and colleagues, various forces of globalization have greatly contributed to global development. However, at the same time, globalization has also amplified global inequalities as well as diminished the capacities of governments to respond to many of the negative externalities associated with global processes. These negative externalities go beyond the economic form of globalization as described by Schrecker to also include increased risks from transborder communicable infectious diseases as well as a rise of NCDs through the spread of westernized consumption patterns and urbanized lifestyles. Richardson and colleagues argue that "policies must focus on protecting the health of those on the periphery of globalization and most likely to fall ill of it, and on fine-tuning global integration such that the benefits are more evenly spread amongst populations, within and between countries." This argument about the need to protect those "on the periphery" runs implicitly or explicitly throughout all chapters in this book.

If Richardson, Schrecker, Ruckert and their co-authors are correct to suggest that the aim of global health policy should be to distribute health benefits and burdens more evenly and equitably, then global health policy is, by its very nature, more than a technical issue about "how, when, and where." Securing policy equity is also an ethical issue of determining "who get's what and why" (Brown 2012). If so, as many authors in *The Handbook on Global Health Policy* suggest, then determining key issues in global health will be largely a politically negotiated process where particular normative and practical arguments will be made in order to support why some policies are more legitimate and justified than others. In most cases, the need to have broadened understandings of these complexities and the political tools available to respond to them is a key component of effective health interventions (see Chapter 2 by Sophie Harman).

This kind of broad view is especially important, argues Hugo Slim (Chapter 18), in cases where action is needed immediately in order to respond to humanitarian crises. As he suggests, "humanitarian action is routinely steeped in the deep politics of global, national and local interests" and the normal complexities of implementing effective health policy are only accelerated by emergency situations. Slim argues for the development of a better prepared humanitarian system involving input from a multitude of key sectors that can recognize and respond to the political dynamics intrinsic to global health governance. Yet, as Slim suggests, "there is significant knowledge and expertise in humanitarian medicine in the UN agencies, national government ministries and NGOs." The main problem is that "leadership of international humanitarian operations is often weak and confused because of inter-state and inter-agency dynamics, so that combined humanitarian resources are seldom coordinated and leveraged to achieve maximum value." Slim's chapter nicely captures an idea that runs throughout this book. The study and practice of global health is complex and multidimensional with profoundly interconnected technical, political, and ethical elements that require increasingly interdisciplinary tools – at the theoretical, conceptual, methodological, and practical level – to help us effectively capture, analyze, and respond to issues of global health.

Theme 2: There is a Need for Greater Innovation in National and Global Health Governance

As was suggested by Slim and others above, the governance structures related to international humanitarian operations are often poorly organized without clear delineations about who is in charge, what needs to be done, and what resources can be relied upon. As a result, a second overarching theme between the chapters of this volume relates to a general view that despite key political, financial, and technological innovations in global health, the current system of global health governance remains underdeveloped and lacking in resources, proper coordination, and meaningful cooperation. Where there has been some headway is in relation to reaching an agreement on setting MDG targets as well as renewed commitments for increasing cooperation by building strategic "partnerships" between key stakeholders at the global, national, and local levels (Global Fund (2012) Framework Document; OECD (2008) Paris Declaration; and UN (2012) MDG 8). As argued by Moran and Stevenson (Chapter 28), "the centrality of health to the MDGs shows that health is no longer a 'second order element' of 'low politics' and is recognized as a central pillar of foreign policy." Because of this, "the MDGs provide an important normative framework for those working in development and a means for measuring and tracking progress toward eight broad development goals – three of which are directly health-related."

Accompanying these uniform MDG targets were governance innovations connected to what Moran and Stevenson call the "partnership moment." This moment is when the MDGs were "buttressed by global health partnerships, which have led to increased resources for tackling diseases that disproportionately affect low and lower-middle income countries – particularly communicable diseases." By developing global partnerships for health, argues Jeremy Youde (Chapter 27), the aim was to coordinate a multitude of organizations that combine human and/or financial resources to work together on a health issue of cross-border concern. As mentioned before, these partnerships led to an unprecedented increase in coordinated financial assistance, which between 2002 and

2006 increased 25 percent annually, with health partnerships receiving a large share of the funds (Dodd and Lane 2010: 364). As Youde notes, "successful ... [partnerships] can leverage the competitive advantages of the partner organizations to produce health outcomes that exceed what each partner could do on its own." Using the Global Fund as an effective case study, Youde suggests that the "health partnership introduced significant opportunities for public and private entities to collaborate in a mutually beneficial manner to promote good health internationally." These benefits offered hope that it was possible for an international organization (with a multitude of interests) to pursue a clear mission as well as to develop new multisectoral governance mechanisms that promoted national ownership with higher levels of international accountability.

However, the success of global health partnerships is still to be determined and in the case of the Global Fund there are increasing doubts about its claimed successes as well as its ability to fund health initiatives in the future (Arie 2012). As Youde notes, not only have donors recently raised concerns about the Global Fund's ability to provide credible anticorruption oversight, but many donors have also used these concerns as a way to decrease development aid more generally, which has only been exasperated and further justified in the face of the global economic crisis. What this suggests is that health partnerships are only as successful as their partners will let them be and that successful "partnership" will not only require the political will of each stakeholder to make the partnership work, but also a collective commitment by all stakeholders to build sustainable national health systems with the resources made available to do so. As Youde outlines, the most successful partnerships display seven key elements: (1) concrete goals and comparative advantage; (2) key staff related to aims; (3) processes of continuous assessment; (4) giving a voice to stakeholders; (5) equal deliberative ability for all partners; (6) the opportunity for real national buy-in and agenda setting; and (7) an aim to constantly improve by examining results. Without a good dose of these elements, argue Moran and Stevenson, health partnerships will continue to struggle to meet the MDGs and any future targets, since there is "a clear need for greater coordination between GHPs [global health partnerships], public and private donors, and national health systems to improve the efficacy and effectiveness of health aid."

Whereas partnership has clearly become a master concept in health development (Barnes and Brown 2011), another policy development that has mobilized significant financial and political resources for global health is what Simon Rushton (Chapter 15) describes as the "securitization of health" (i.e., the way in which certain health issues have come to be understood as security threats). As Rushton suggests, "security language, concepts, practices and institutions have become increasingly evident in national and global health policy, the result of moves by both public health policy-makers and foreign and security policy communities towards treating health as a security issue." Although framing health as a security threat can raise disease awareness and mobilize political and financial support, Rushton suggests that there are worrying side effects of such framing and that securitization of health should be used with a high degree of caution. Politicizing health as a security priority will tend to fetishize communicable diseases at the expense of ignoring NCDs and in the process legitimate narrowly targeted resources that prioritize the abatement needs of developed countries over those of the LMICs.

In response, Stefan Elbe and Nadine Voelker (Chapter 16) claim that politicization based on protecting self-interest is simply part and parcel of securitization more generally and that many global health security policies now mirror the forms of brinksmanship usually associated with securitizing other national interests. As an example, Elbe and Voelker examine Indonesia's refusal to share H5N1 viral samples with the WHO for most of 2007 (Garrett and Fidler 2007), suggesting that this viral sovereignty claim represents a by-product of the language of securitizing national health. The authors argue that "presenting highly pathogenic avian flu as a pressing global security threat contributed to a re-politicisation of existing virus sharing mechanisms, and also enabled countries like Indonesia to use access to H5N1 virus samples as a diplomatic bargaining chip for fundamentally reforming the international virus sharing system." As a result, the securitization of H5N1 "rendered international health co-operation a matter of more narrow and calculated national interest, prompting Indonesia to assert its 'viral sovereignty' over the virus." The downside of this is that these moves significantly undermine genuine cooperation in global health governance, which can have lasting effects on how we tackle global health priorities.

Issues of health security are further complicated by the reality that states face clear external risks and a level of preparedness and security is required. In his chapter outlining current pandemic preparedness (Chapter 29), Adam Kamradt-Scott argues that the "nature of an influenza pandemic requires governments to develop comprehensive – or 'whole-of-government' – pandemic preparedness plans that minimize economic and social disruption while also protecting human health." To do so, would entail "bringing multiple interest groups such as government, civil society, business, and industry together" so as to critically "understand the various roles and responsibilities" needed "as well as identifying and addressing vulnerabilities." For Scott, the key to preparedness is having robust contingency plans that have the buy-in of all key sectors and that have thought through the important ethical issues about how to balance the rights of the individual with protecting societies as a whole.

Theme 3: Health Aid to Developing Countries Requires Re-engineering

The "halcyon days of global health financing," are over, say Marco Schäferhoff and colleagues (Chapter 19). Since 2010, in the wake of the global financial crisis and austerity programs in high-income countries, annual DAH has stagnated (IHME 2012). This flat-lining of aid for health has provoked a reassessment of the achievements and failings of the aid enterprise. *The Handbook of Global Health Policy* goes a long way in critically examining DAH and laying out potential pathways towards a more sustainably financed global health system. The halcyon days were characterized by the emergence of multiple global health financing partnerships that brought tremendous innovation in raising and channeling funds. Schäferhoff and colleagues describe creative mechanisms that have been used to mobilize DAH. UNITAID, for example, has used a tax on airline tickets (a "solidarity levy") to fund HIV, TB, and malaria interventions (Atun *et al.* 2012).

What lay behind this mushrooming of new global health entities? Ruairí Brugha and colleagues (Chapter 1) give three reasons: the energy arising from the MDGs; the "growing perception of poor past performance by UN agencies and the need to do things differently;" and the assumption that these new vehicles could attract funding to develop drugs for neglected infectious diseases of poor countries. These vehicles, they say, brought much-needed urgency to tackling infectious diseases through targeted, vertical programs.

Although Christopher J. Coyne and Claudia R. Williamson (Chapter 20) question the overall value of aid for systematically improving health outcomes, they acknowledge that "recent micro-level studies find some evidence of successful health aid interventions," such as scale-up of immunizations. Other scholars in this handbook view the evidence on health aid much more favorably. Sonia Bhalotra and Thomas Pogge (Chapter 11) argue that transfers of wealth from rich to poor countries to pay for infectious disease programs will have profound *long-term* pay-offs, including through "multiplier effects," such as boosting economic growth and childhood education outcomes. Targeted interventions, they say, "also tend to generate positive spillovers for richer countries," such as through reducing the externalities of infectious diseases.

Nevertheless, a recurring theme in this handbook is that the financing of global health is in crisis. The multiplicity of actors, say Schäferhoff and colleagues, has led to fragmentation and unclear role responsibilities. Support for vertical programming has created "fragile, isolated islands of sufficiency" (Ooms *et al.* 2009), with insufficient attention paid to building strong health systems. Rajaie Batniji and Francisco Songane (Chapter 3) argue that DAH has distorted national priorities: recipient governments understandably follow the money, prioritizing donor-supported, one-size-fits-all, "quick win" campaigns to control infectious diseases over longer-term health concerns.

Donors have largely ignored the core functions of global health, such as disease surveillance and knowledge generation and sharing – witness, for example, WHO's budgetary crisis, which threatens its very existence (Nebehay and Lewis 2011). WHO has been left to wither on the vine, an alarming situation given the crucial roles that the organization plays in providing technical and policy support to countries and in defining and articulating evidence-based global norms and standards. As one of us has previously argued, in a paper called "Why does the world still need WHO?," "if we, the international health community, want WHO to carry out the tasks for which it has the comparative advantage, we need to provide it with adequate resources for these vital activities" (Yamey 2002).

In a novel framing of the crisis, Harman (Chapter 2) distils the crisis of global health policy formation into "the four Rs": *reaction* (health agendas are reactionary to donors); *repetition* (repetitive policies are applied uniformly across different country contexts); *results-orientation* (policy orientation is determined by achieving the results that donors want); and *raising funds* (health agendas become shaped by the need to constantly raise money). Underlying the crisis, she says, is a "dominance of market-based strategies in developing policy" that contradicts the rights-based approach to global public health. Market orientation can be seen, she argues, in the growing role of private actors in global health, including in public–private partnerships (PPPs), and in the way in which PPPs borrow from private sector approaches to maximizing efficiency.

What is the way forward out of the crisis? In *The Handbook of Global Health Policy*, public health practitioners, clinicians, and scholars in political economy offer a diverse set of policy options. Harman says that "hierarchies of decision-making" must be inverted, such as through greater engagement of the public in LMICs. Julio Frenk and colleagues (Chapter 23) say that we must go beyond the tired dichotomies that have plagued global health, such as vertical versus horizontal strategies or tackling social determinants of health versus building health services. A "diagonal approach" they say, in which certain health interventions are prioritized as a way to strengthen the overall structure and functions of health systems, can bring important health dividends. In a paired chapter (Chapter 24), Gorik Ooms and colleagues show how Ethiopia successfully used the opportunities provided by the global AIDS response to strengthen and expand its health system.

Vanessa Kerry and colleagues (Chapter 26) propose an entirely new set of "rules of the road" for DAH, which they call *an accompaniment approach*, one that seeks to boost national capacity through long-term partnerships. This approach, which seems both pragmatic and yet potentially revolutionary, includes supporting institutions that the poor identify as representing their interests; prioritizing local job creation; buying and hiring locally; and co-investing with governments to build strong workforces.

Although these options differ in their underlying orientation, they share at least two common features. First, they all argue for *a new kind of funding relationship* between donors and recipient countries, in which national governments in LMICs shape their own domestic agendas. Second, *financing of strong national health systems everywhere* is at the heart of the suggested reforms, and will be particularly important for tackling the NCD crisis in LMICs. There seems little doubt, particularly for MICs, that such financing will require "co-investment," in which DAH plays a small but catalytic role, whereas long-term funding increasingly comes from domestic sources. Donors have shown no willingness at all to provide financial assistance for tackling NCDs in developing countries. Indeed, NCDs are encountering "the leading edge of a maturing aid reform movement willing to conceptualize a world 'beyond aid' " (Marrero *et al.* 2012).

Theme 4: Scientific Evidence must be Balanced with Political and Ethical Considerations

A fourth theme is that while global health policy-making must be underpinned by robust evidence on disease burden and effective responses, it cannot be a "pure" technical enterprise. Evidence-based global health policy-making has undoubtedly had a major impact on mortality and morbidity. "Significant health gains could be achieved by leveraging such evidence to its full potential," argue Gavin Yamey and Jimmy Volmink (Chapter 7). But sound policy-making also has ethical and political dimensions. As editors, we wanted to reflect the two sides of the coin by pairing "scientific" with "ethical" chapters.

Many authors in *The Handbook of Global Health Policy* argue that global health actors have neglected or marginalized scientific evidence, to the detriment of public health. Batniji and Songane (Chapter 3) document cases of scientific complacency at the WHO and World Bank. Kerry and colleagues (Chapter 26) give the frustrating example of donors neglecting evidence on the link between food security and mortality in HIV-infected patients treated with antiretroviral medications. Neglect of food support costs lives: mortality in patients starting antiretroviral therapy is much higher in malnourished patients (World Food Programme 2012).

Global health policy-making becomes weakened, and potentially dangerous, without scientific evidence. Policy decisions, say Nancy Fullman and colleagues (Chapter 5), are compromised if they draw from an evidence base that is "incomplete, incomprehensive, or incomparable over time and across geographies." Without evidence, it is difficult for policy-makers to know how to prioritize resources, which interventions to scale-up, and whether policies are benefiting the population. With the stagnation of aid for health, it has become even more important to make sure that funds are targeted to proven, high-impact interventions. Fullman and colleagues give several powerful examples of how the generation of evidence led to important policy shifts. Mexico's Ministry of Health, for example, did not realize that out-of-pocket health expenditures were causing widespread impoverishment among Mexican families until publication of *The World Health Report 2000* (WHO 2000), which ranked WHO Member States by "fairness of financial contribution" for health services (Mexico was ranked 144th). The ministry responded by rolling out universal health insurance coverage, called *Seguro Popular* (described in Chapter 23). Similarly, studies of the global burden of disease, showing a very rapid epidemiological transition from infectious diseases to NCDs, helped to push NCDs, including mental health conditions, up the global health agenda (Marrero *et al.* 2012).

Now that NCDs have caught the attention of the global development community – the UN General Assembly even held a high level meeting on NCDs in September

2011 – empirical evidence must surely be used to guide the global response. A major modifiable risk factor is poor dietary quality. Ashkan Afshin and colleagues (Chapter 9) examine systematic reviews of the evidence on how best to improve global dietary quality. They conclude that population-based approaches, such as regulations to reduce specific components of foods (e.g., trans-fats, salt), subsidizing healthy foods, and taxing unhealthy foods and sugary sodas, should be widely adopted.

Food policy is an excellent example of how systematic reviews of the best available evidence, using explicit, replicable methods, can empower governments to take on powerful, vested interests, such as food corporations. Such companies are now aggressively promoting heavily processed foods high in calories, trans-fats, salt, and sugar to people in LMICs (Stuckler and Nestle 2012). Protecting populations from conditions such as cardiovascular disease and diabetes requires "activist" governments who are willing to push strong evidence-based public policies that may cut into industry's profits, such as banning marketing of unhealthy foods to children.

Although driving evidence into practical policy-making is an important tool for accelerating progress towards the MDGs and for curbing NCDs, there are still many barriers to evidence uptake. For a start, many low-income countries have weak systems for local data collection and evidence generation. While research enterprises such as the Global Burden of Disease Study 2010 (Wang et al. 2012) have used modeling methods to try and fill in the gaps, these modeled estimates are less reliable than locally generated "bottom-up" data. Peter Byass (Chapter 6) argues that the global health community must develop better tools and procedures to improve the collection and availability of bottom-up data.

While several authors in this handbook call for global health policy to become more evidence-based, Amy Barnes and Justin Parkhurst (Chapter 8) believe that such calls "raise a number of political debates, dilemmas, and potential ethical issues." These issues include whether evidence generation is adequately taking social concerns into account, how to value the various outcomes established by the evidence, and whose values should be represented in these assessments. Even the process of research itself, including which health topics to examine, they say, cannot be divorced from politics.

And even if global health policy-making *could* be de-politicized, *should* it be? Divorcing policy from questions of politics and ethics is as dangerous as ignoring scientific evidence. Policy-makers must of course use evidence, say Barnes and Parkhurst, but they need to also consider human rights concerns, as well as questions of justice, fairness, autonomy, and the deeper social and economic determinants of health: "Unequal structures of wealth, dominance, and poverty (which are typically allied to capitalist visions of economic development) can shape global health problems and policy interventions." Traditional forms of global health research, they argue, tend to *conceal* the macro-structures that socially and politically shape health. For example, HIV risk in South African mining towns is embedded in migrant workers' living conditions (Campbell 2003). The spread of TB and measles in sub-Saharan Africa has been linked with capitalist expansion (Doyal 1979).

Even the question of "who is at risk?" cannot be reduced to a technical answer alone. It has ethical, moral, and political dimensions. In Chapter 10, Christine Straehle examines the moral problem of being at risk, which she says "derives from the fact that to be vulnerable means to be unable to effectively protect one's fundamental interests." The concept of *morally problematic vulnerability*, she argues, can help us assess global health policy scenarios and help to shape our normative responses to them. She applies this framework to the problem of rich countries actively recruiting nurses and other health professionals from poor countries, which "leads to a risk of vulnerability to harm" since patients in

poor countries are being deprived of health professionals. "It is a duty to change recruitment to avoid inflicting harm," she concludes. And in Chapter 17, which tackles policies
towards humanitarian crises, François Grünewald and Veronique de Geoffroy show that
vulnerability to natural disasters is intricately linked to broad questions of justice, power,
and social positioning. "Acute urban poverty," they say "increases the likelihood of poor
urban dwellers settling in 'areas at risk,' on flood-exposed river banks or landslide-prone
areas."

Theme 5: Promoting Global Health is Clearly an Ethical Issue, But the Scope and Scale of Our Normative Commitment Remain Undetermined

Several ethical dimensions related to global health policy have already been noted
throughout this introduction. As we have seen, many of the issues involved in global
health policy either connect to, or are informed by, longstanding ethical and legal considerations and debates. For example, Lisa Forman (Chapter 25) argues that one political
and legal tool available to help assure that health obligations are fulfilled is to assign a
legal "right to health," which can "offer a guiding framework for global health equity."
According to Forman, not only is there evidence to suggest that a right to health can help
to assure access to adequate healthcare in domestic systems (e.g., guaranteed antiretroviral (ARV) drug access in many sub-Saharan African countries), but that a rights approach
can also, through strengthening existing international covenants, become "a powerful
tool for achieving global health equity." Yet, as Brown and Paremoer highlight (Chapter 4), the use of a rights approach to health can be problematic, because rights often
"only mitigate the impact of institutions that ultimately consolidate or deepen socioeconomic inequalities." Although rights can be useful to "protect citizens against the worst
excesses of unjust institutions," it is not necessarily the case that they can also transform
or dismantle those institutions. For that to be possible, argue Brown, Paremoer, and to
some extent Forman, these rights must be embedded in better understandings of social
justice and how health rights can act as tools for broader long-term structural change.

Another powerful ethical consideration within debates about global health involves
having access to medicines and understanding the structural impediments that allow some
people to have access to good health while denying this access to others. For Valbona
Muzaka (Chapter 22) the "World Trade Organization's TRIPS [Trade-Related Aspects
of Intellectual Property Rights] agreement brought about significant changes to pharmaceutical IP protection rules, many of which restrict the availability of affordable medicines
worldwide" so as to favor powerful corporate interests. This uneven distribution of benefits and burdens, according to Muzaka, requires reassessment of the pharmaceutical
intellectual property (IP) regime – what she calls "freeze, roll-back, and reassess" – so
that social needs can be factored into IP alongside other legitimate concerns about maintaining research and development (R&D) incentives. One such recommendation for how
to do this comes from Bhalotra and Pogge (Chapter 11), who suggest that the TRIPS
regime could be "relaxed" by establishing a global "Health Impact Fund." Such a fund
would incentivize pharmaceutical R&D through a system of global payments based on
a company's overall health impact, in return for promised lowest cost production as well
as access for generic manufacturers. Although this fund could be a potentially transformative mechanism for stimulating R&D for neglected diseases of poverty, Manica Balasegaram and his colleagues at Médecins Sans Frontières (Chapter 13) argue that concerns about access go beyond medicines and relate more broadly to "essential health
commodities." For them, as for Muzaka, Bhalotra, and Pogge, "commercial imperatives

driving medical innovation mean that many urgently needed health commodities are left undeveloped and many existing commodities are often unsuitable for use in developing countries or are unaffordable."

As suggested by some authors in this book, voluntary industry-driven means to lower commodity prices have, with some exceptions, been largely unsuccessful and pharmaceutical companies have largely resisted reforms. Nevertheless, Mary Moran's in-depth survey (Chapter 12) of the opportunities available for developing new tools for diseases of poverty reminds us that there is a place for both "market-based" and "non-market-based" solutions. An example of a market-based intervention is a "milestone prize" to incentivize companies to develop new vaccines, diagnostics, and treatments for diseases of poverty – a company gets rewarded for taking commercial risks at key points along a product development pathway. An innovative example of a non-market-based approach is the Medicines Patent Pool (http://www.medicinespatentpool.org/, last accessed February 2014): pharmaceutical companies put their IP rights into a public pool, from which non-exclusive licenses can be given to as many generic firms as are interested.

What is common between the authors in *The Handbook on Global Health Policy* is a profound concern for entrenched structural inequalities that have perversely negative effects on global public health and that create a wide range of "neglected diseases" that remain somehow outside policy focus (Chapter 12). What is also common, and fitting with the other themes captured in this volume, is a normative appeal to locate alternative models of innovation that can effectively respond to the needs of developing countries and those whose health is most at risk.

Since the focus of this book is on global health, it is not surprising that many of the ethical discussions that take place in these chapters are also global in scope. In particular, there is consensus about a need to alter inequities in global health. In some cases the appeal from authors to restructure current systems is made from a practical or evidence-based position, suggesting that there is simply a more effective or efficient way to tackle global health priorities. Nevertheless, even these more empirically driven appeals to alter existing health structures rest on an implicit concern for the well-being of human beings and are premised on a moral belief that the health of human beings matters. In most cases, the arguments presented in the volume are explicitly normative and are clearly grounded in moral or ethical sentiments. What is most striking is that there is normative agreement that health is a key component for human beings to live minimally decent lives, that human beings matter morally, and that we have certain moral responsibilities and obligations to reform and design policies that can reasonably respond to human health needs. In Chapter 4, Brown and Paremoer take this argument to its logical extreme. They suggest that if we hold certain claims to be morally important about the worth of human beings and their health, and if existing economic, legal, and political structures are known to negatively affect human health at the global level, then there are "relational" reasons to argue that reforming these structures is the right thing to do. Such reform, they argue, is also a matter of justice, so we are obligated to act – both domestically as well as globally.

Conclusions

The Handbook of Global Health Policy is being published just as the MDGs era is coming to a close. We will soon be entering a new era of "sustainable development goals" or SDGs (Kenny 2013). At the time of writing this, there are strong indications from high-level discussions within the development community, particularly within the UN system, that health will continue to feature prominently in the SDGs (High-Level Panel

2013). Such prominence is entirely appropriate, as major global health challenges still loom large. These include high rates of avoidable infectious, reproductive, maternal, and child deaths in developing countries; a global pandemic of NCDs and injuries; health impacts of climate change and environmental degradation; and the impoverishing effects of medical expenditures in countries without universal health coverage.

The five cross-cutting themes in this book alert us not only to the weaknesses in current global health policy formulation but also to the tremendous opportunities for a new kind of policy-making fit for the SDGs era. Such policy-making must be pro-poor in its orientation, ensuring that those "on the periphery" are no longer forgotten and no longer bear the global burden of risks and diseases. *The Handbook of Global Health Policy* points to the potentially catalytic effects of new collaborations across sectors, including health, education, labor, and the environment; new forms of global health governance to better support national policy-making processes; and new "rules of the road" for DAH. Huge progress in health could be achieved through policy that puts evidence at its core, while also acknowledging the important moral, ethical, and political dimensions of decision-making. Throughout this book, there is a repeated call for international collective action to become more focused on a set of essential functions, such as knowledge generation and sharing, R&D for neglected diseases, and international disease surveillance, while also providing direct support to the most vulnerable countries through long-term, equitable partnerships ("accompaniment").

The MDGs era brought great achievements in global health. Today, five million fewer children are dying every year than in the year 2000, when the MDGs were established. A quarter of a million fewer women are dying every year during or shortly after pregnancy. We hope that the insights, debates, and policy guidance in *The Handbook of Global Health Policy* can play a role in accelerating these trends to achieve even more dramatic progress in human health over the coming generation.

References

Arie S. 2012. Global health. Make or break for the Global Fund? *BMJ* 345, e7561.

Atun R, Knaul FM, Akachi Y, Frenk J. 2012. Innovative financing for health: what is truly innovative? *Lancet* 380, 2044–9.

Barnes A, Brown GW. 2011. The idea of partnership within the Millennium Development Goals: context, instrumentality and the normative demands of partnership. *Third World Quarterly* 32(1).

Bhutta ZA, Chopra M, Axelson H *et al.* 2010. Countdown to 2015 decade report (2000–10): taking stock of maternal, newborn, and child survival. *Lancet* 375, 2032–44.

Brown GW. 2012. Distributing who gets what and why: four normative approaches to global health governance. *Global Policy* 3(3), 292–302.

Campbell C. 2003. *"Letting them Die": Why HIV/AIDS Prevention Programmes Fail.* Oxford: James Currey.

DFID (Department for International Aid). 2011. *The future of UK aid.* https://www.gov.uk/government/news/the-future-of-uk-aid (last accessed December 2013).

Di Cesare M, Khang Y-H, Asaria P *et al.* 2013. Inequalities in non-communicable diseases and effective responses. *Lancet* 381(9866), 585–97.

Dodd R, Lane C. 2010. Improving the long-term sustainability of health aid: are global health partnerships the way to go? *Health Policy and Planning* 25(5), 363–71.

Doyal L. 1979. *The Political Economy of Health.* London: Pluto Press.

Eisenberg JM. 2002. Globalize the evidence, localize the decision: evidence-based medicine and international diversity. *Health Affairs* 21, 166–8.

Elovainio R, Evans DB. 2013. *Raising and Spending Domestic Money for Health*. Chatham House Working Paper, May. http://www.chathamhouse.org/publications/papers/view/191335 (last accessed January 2014).

Garrett L, Fidler DP. 2007. Sharing H5N1 viruses to stop a global influenza pandemic. *PLOS Medicine* 4(11), e330.

Global Fund (Global Fund to Fight AIDs, Turberclosis and Malaria). 2012. *The Framework Document*. Geneva: Global Fund. www.theglobalfund.org/documents/ . . . /framework/Core_GlobalFund_Framework_en/ (last accessed December 2013).

High-Level Panel (High-Level Panel on the Post-2015 Development Agenda). 2013. *A New Global Partnership: Eradicate Poverty and Transform Economies through Sustainable Development*. http://www.post2015hlp.org/the-report/ (last accessed December 2013).

IHME (Institute for Health Metrics and Evaluation). 2012. *Financing Global Health 2012: The End of the Golden Age?*. Seattle, WA: IHME. http://www.healthmetricsandevaluation.org/publications/policy-report/financing-global-health-2012-end-golden-age (last accessed December 2013)

Kenny C. 2013. What should follow the millennium development goals? *BMJ* 346, f1193.

Legge D, Sanders D. 2013. New development goals must focus on social determinants of health. *BMJ* 346, 22

Lozano R, Naghavi M, Foreman K *et al.* 2012. Global and regional mortality from 235 causes of death for 20 age groups in 1990 and 2010: a systematic analysis for the Global Burden of Disease Study 2010. *Lancet* 380, 2095–128.

Marrero SL, Bloom DE, Adashi EY. 2012. Noncommunicable diseases. A global health crisis in a new world order. *JAMA* 307, 2037–8.

McMichael AJ. 2010. Globalization, climate change, and human health. *New England Journal of Medicine* 368, 1335–43.

McNeil D, Jr. 2010. At front lines, AIDS war is falling apart. *New York Times* May 9. www.nytimes.com/2010/05/10/world/africa/10aids.html (last accessed December 2013).

Morel CM, Acharya T, Broun D *et al.* 2005. Health innovation networks to help developing countries address neglected diseases. *Science* 309, 401–4.

Nebehay S, Lewis B. 2011. *WHO slashes budget, jobs in new era of austerity*. Reuters, May 19. http://www.reuters.com/article/2011/05/19/us-who-idUSTRE74I5I320110519 (last accessed December 2013).

Oberth G. 2012. Who governs public health? Donor retreat and the shifting spheres of influence in southern African HIV/AIDS policy making. *Sociology Study* 2(7), 551–68.

OECD (Organisation for Economic Co-operation and Development). 2008. *The Paris Declaration on Aid Effectiveness and the Accra Agenda for Action*. http://www.oecd.org/development/effectiveness/34428351.pdf (last accessed December 2013).

Ooms G, Van Damme W, Baker BK, Zeitz, Schrecker T. 2009. The "diagonal" approach to Global Fund financing: a cure for the broader malaise of health systems? *Globalization and Health* 4, 6.

Smith D. 2013. South Africa warns aid cut means change in relationship with UK. *Guardian* April 30, http://www.guardian.co.uk/global-development/2013/apr/30/south-africa-aid-cut-uk (last accessed December 2013).

Stuckler D, Nestle M. 2012. Big food, food systems, and global health. *PLOS Medicine* 9(6), e1001242.

UN (United Nations). 2012. *Millennium Development Goals Report 2012*. New York: UN.

UN (United Nations) Inter-agency Group for Child Mortality Estimation. 2013. *Levels and Trends in Child Mortality Report 2013*. New York: UNICEF.

UNAIDS. 2012. *Global Report: UNAIDS Report on the Global AIDS Epidemic 2012*. Geneva: UNAIDS. http://www.unaids.org/en/media/unaids/contentassets/documents/epidemiology/2012/gr2012/20121120_UNAIDS_Global_Report_2012_with_annexes_en.pdf (last accessed December 2013).

Walz J, Ramachandran V. 2011. *Brave New World: A Literature Review of Emerging Donors and the Changing Nature of Foreign Assistance*. Center for Global Development (CGD)

Working Paper No 273. Washington DC: CDG. http://www.cgdev.org/content/publications/detail/1425691 (last accessed December 2013).

Wang H, Dwyer-Lindgren L, Lofgren KT *et al.* 2012. Age-specific and sex-specific mortality in 187 countries, 1970–2010: a systematic analysis for the Global Burden of Disease Study 2010. *Lancet* 15(380), 2071–94.

WHO (World Health Organization). 2000. *The World Health Report 2000. Health Systems: Improving Performance*. Geneva: WHO. http://www.who.int/whr/2000/en/ (last accessed December 2013).

WHO (World Health Organization). 2011. *Global Status Report on Noncommunicable Diseases 2010*. Geneva: WHO. www.who.int/nmh/publications/ncd_report_full_en.pdf (last accessed December 2013).

WHO (World Health Organization). 2014. *Human infection caused by the avian influenza A (H7N9) virus – highlights, 6 February 2014*. Geneva: WHO. http://www.who.int/influenza/human_animal_interface/influenza_h7n9/en/index.htm (last accessed February 2014).

World Food Programme. 2012. *HIV, AIDS, TB and Nutrition Fact Sheet*. Rome: World Food Programme. http://www.wfp.org/content/hiv-aids-tb-and-nutrition (last accessed December 2013).

Yamey G. 2002. WHO in 2002: why does the world still need WHO? *BMJ* 325, 1294–8.

Part I Global Health Policy and Global Health Governance

Chapter 1

Understanding Global Health Policy

Ruairí Brugha, Carlos Bruen, and Viroj Tangcharoensathien

Abstract

Global health policy comprises the goals, rules, and actions that address or have an impact on the health challenges and priorities that transcend individual countries and regions. This introductory chapter outlines some of the major events, contexts, processes, and actors (the people and organizations) that have contributed to what is a fluid and fast changing global health policy environment. The chapter charts the transformation of global health policy over the twientieth century, including the changing role of the state and traditional multilateral institutions, along with the rise and increasing power of new global health actors. Drawing on the examples of the GAVI Alliance and the Global Fund to Fight AIDS, Tuberculosis and Malaria, the authors discuss how non-state actors and new forms of global partnerships have become increasingly important players alongside states and traditional multilateral agencies in global health policy processes.

Case studies are used to outline key concepts and foundational theories for understanding policy-making and policy implementation. The case study on nutrition and obesity illustrates a failure to tackle vested food industry interests, preventing a coherent and coordinated global health policy response. New global partnerships involving non-state actors, global efforts to strengthen health systems, and global agreement on an international code of practice on health worker recruitment illustrate diverse policy processes, solutions, and instruments. Common to most global health policy issues is the political nature of policy-making, where recognition of actors' interests, power, and ability to mobilize resources are central. The chapter concludes with pointers for policy practitioners, researchers, and students when conducting health policy analyses. Analysts may be actors in policy processes and need to consider how their own institutional positions, resources, and values may influence their analyses.

The Handbook of Global Health Policy, First Edition. Edited by Garrett W. Brown, Gavin Yamey, and Sarah Wamala.
© 2014 John Wiley & Sons, Ltd. Published 2014 by John Wiley & Sons, Ltd.

Key Points

- Global health policy refers to the statement of goals, objectives, and means that create the framework for global health activities.
- Actors – individuals, organizations and their networks – are central to how priorities are established and how health policies are made and implemented.
- Understanding global health policy requires an understanding of the political nature of policy-making, the role of actors' interests, and the centrality of power.
- Policy theory, developed to analyze national health policies, can be applied to understanding global health policy processes and the influence of old and new actors.
- New global health partnerships, incorporating non-state actors who can mobilize large levels of resources, have become powerful players in setting global health priorities, policy-making, and implementation.

Key Policy Implications

- Global health policy is an inherently political and complex arena, where the positions, interests, and objectives of nations, organizations, and networks of individuals often determine what policies are formulated and implemented.
- While there is often consensus on the need for evidence-based policy-making, its achievement can be undermined by a failure to understand and analyze how power and the interests of different groups often shape and can determine global health policies.
- The application of theories of policy processes can deepen the understanding of the global health policy terrain, highlighting the political obstacles and opportunities for getting population health issues on to the policy agenda.

Introduction

Global health refers to issues that directly or indirectly impact on the health of populations and that can transcend national boundaries (Koplan *et al.* 2009). Solutions to global health issues often require global cooperation and policy actions that are beyond the capacity of individual countries. Building on Kent Buse and colleagues' definition of health policy (Buse *et al.* 2005), we define *global health policy* as the statement of goals, objectives, and means that create the framework for global health activities. Global health policy incorporates both policy *content*, the substance of policy comprising rules and guidelines, and policy *processes*, the purposeful, deliberate actions, methods, and strategies that influence the shape and impact of policy development and implementation (Jenkins 1978).

Global health policy, and its implementation, is shaped by a complex and dynamic set of individuals, groups, and organizations that form global, interrelated networks of actors. These networks have an impact upon the health of populations. Understanding such policy processes is a prerequisite for achieving global population health goals, such as universal health coverage (Kruk 2013), and for tackling the social and economic determinants of health, where causes and actions go beyond country borders. This opening chapter introduces the field of global health policy and provides a brief history of the main actors and processes in global health policy-making over the last 25 years. It also identifies further readings on policy theories, which can help to provide an understanding of how global health policies are shaped.

Actors are considered central to the analysis of how policies are made and implemented. Global and country policy actors include individuals and institutions, such as civil society organizations, research institutions, private sector and philanthropic organizations, governments and program managers, health workers, and community-based organizations. Policy analysis in global health can help explain how power and the interests and values of different global actors play an important role in shaping policies. Power and politics, which are implicit in all fields of knowledge and activity, are made explicit and thereby more transparent through policy analysis (Walt and Gilson 1994). There is a compelling case to be made for grounding global health policies in evidence (see Chapter 7), and an analysis of actors' power and interests may explain whether or not evidence gets used during policy formulation (Buse *et al.* 2007; Hutchinson *et al.* 2011).

Health policy analysis is a growing field, occupied by policy practitioners, including policy-makers and technical analysts, and by academic researchers and students (Gilson 2012). Practitioners are primarily interested in using policy analysis *prospectively* to help shape future policies (analysis *for* policy), and in bringing evidence from the clinical sciences, epidemiology, and economics to inform the content of health policies. In contrast, health policy researchers mostly conduct retrospective analyses of past policy processes (analysis *of* policy), recognizing that factors other than scientific evidence – policy context, processes, and actors – play an important role in determining policy content and outcomes (see Chapter 8).

Several papers in a 2008 special issue of the journal *Health Policy and Planning* help to outline the field of health policy, drawing particularly on lessons and evidence from low- and middle-income countries (Buse 2008; Gilson and Raphaely 2008; Walt *et al.* 2008). The ethics of whether or not health policy researchers should be actively involved in shaping policy has been debated (Buse 2008; Surjadjaja and Mayhew 2011). The risks of doing so, argue Surjadjaja and Mayhew, include jeopardizing the role of academics as "impartial" and credible researchers. Buse, however, argues that policy researchers *should* help

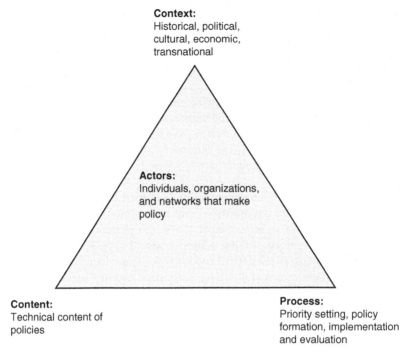

Context:
Historical, political,
cultural, economic,
transnational

Actors:
Individuals, organizations,
and networks that make
policy

Content:
Technical content of
policies

Process:
Priority setting, policy
formation, implementation
and evaluation

Figure 1.1   Health policy triangle (Walt and Gilson 1994).

to shape policy through prospective policy analysis if this helps to achieve international goals, such as the Millennium Development Goals or universal health coverage. Buse's view points to the importance of the relationship between researchers and policy-makers and the respective responsibilities of policy-makers and researchers to ensure evidence-based policies (see Chapter 7).

Walt and Gilson's (1994) health policy triangle provides a useful framework to identify key issues in health policy and how they impact on the health systems, policies, and health of populations (Figure 1.1). The framework can be used to move beyond a study of the *content* of policies to understand how political, historical, and cultural *contexts* influence the direction and feasibility of policy-making. The triangle emphasizes the importance of identifying the *actors* or stakeholders and the *processes* that lead to (or obstruct) health policy development and implementation. It is a flexible framework that can complement different policy theories to help explain which issues get on the policy agenda, and how these are formulated and implemented. There is now a large body of research on global health policy that has been conducted using this framework (e.g., see Schneider *et al.* 2006; Hanefeld 2010; Surjadjaja and Mayhew 2011). A particular value is that it can accommodate theories on rational and explanatory theories on how and why policies get made (as discussed later, in the section called "Contribution of Theory to Understanding Global Health Policy"). The health policy triangle can be used to illustrate some important contextual factors, actors, and processes influencing the content of global health policy, which are discussed in this chapter.

This chapter is aimed at readers who are interested in what *actually* happens in global health policy-making, and not just in what *should* happen, thereby assisting them to make strategic decisions about future policies and steer their implementation. We begin by outlining some of the major transformations in global health policy over the last few decades, linking these to global policy contexts, actors, and processes. We then identify important new global actors and policy instruments, and review how policy theories can be used to explain how global health policies are shaped. Throughout the chapter, we illustrate these concepts by providing "real world" case studies of policy responses (and non-responses) to recent major global health priorities. The chapter ends with a set of key conclusions on what can be learned from an analysis of global health policies.

Globalization and the Transformation of Global Health Policy

Global health policy should be situated within its historical context – in particular, processes of globalization have had a powerful influence upon policies and policy-making processes, a theme recurring throughout this *Handbook*. Following the establishment of the new institutions of the United Nations (UN), after the Second World War, international affairs were overseen by an ordered set of multilateral institutions with different models of national representation and decision-making. It may be more accurate to say that these institutions were *inter-national* (based on shared decision-making by nation states) rather than *global*. In the early decades, international health policy was mainly formulated through the World Health Organization (WHO), comprised of representatives from Member States. Newly independent countries were finding their place in the emerging international order throughout this period, with the WHO providing an important arena for them to influence international health policy-making (Brown *et al.* 2006).

From the late 1980s, however, the World Bank, and to a lesser extent the International Monetary Fund (IMF), stepped into a vacuum created by an increasingly ineffective and resource-limited WHO (Abbasi 1999; Yamey 2002; Brown *et al.* 2006). The World Bank and the IMF exerted influence on national policy-making by mobilizing and allocating financial resources to leverage policy change in the health and social sectors, as well as in economic policy, especially in low-income countries. This period was marked by a weakening in the role of the state in health policy and delivery. The multilateral financing agencies and other donors pressurized poorer countries to downsize the role of the state to providing basic services as a last resort, coupled with an increased role for the private sector in providing health services to rich and poor alike (Brugha and Zwi 2002). A notable feature of policy change at this time was the introduction of user charges for health services, previously provided free by many governments, as part of a wider set of market-based reforms (World Bank 1987).

A further transformation occurred towards the end of the twentieth century, which saw the globalization of, and changing context of cooperation for, international health (Buse *et al.* 2002). Several parallel developments help to explain this transformation, including: (i) a redefining of the traditional legitimacies of the nation state; (ii) escalation in the numbers of non-state actors in global health and the evolving configuration of relationships between new and traditional actors; and (iii) ongoing shifts in the distribution and location of power between stakeholders at global, regional, and national levels.

These global trends and processes, often viewed as aspects of *globalization* (Lee and Goodman 2002; see also Chapter 30), have had a direct impact on national health policy through increased interaction and interdependence between states. For example, shortages of health workers in low-income countries can be attributed to active and passive health worker recruitment by wealthier countries (Hagopian *et al.* 2005; see also Chapter 10 for an analysis of the ethics of such recruitment). Broader global inequities have also influenced the health of populations through the social determinants of health (see Chapters 14 and 21), where the conditions within which people live and work are increasingly determined by global commercial interests that affect opportunities to live healthy lives (Labonté and Schrecker 2007).

On a more positive note, the communications revolution has created possibilities for learning from the policy experiences of other countries and organizations and applying these ideas to different contexts, a process termed *policy transfer.* The scope and intensity of policy transfer activity across countries has been facilitated by dramatic improvements in digital communication, enabling policy ideas to spread, be reinterpreted in the transfer process, and adapted to fit new policy contexts (Evans 2004). Communication technology is connecting local actors with national and global ones, creating opportunities for new actors to enter the global health arena and to expand network relations (Walt *et al.* 2008). Civil society groups, for example, have used electronic communication and social media to operate outside the control of governments, particularly under repressive regimes. Such groups have also fought for (and have been given) global policy influence through the emergence of new forms of global health entities, such as the Global Fund to Fight AIDS, Tuberculosis and Malaria (the Global Fund) (Biesma *et al.* 2009). These new global initiatives have recognized the legitimacy that civil society groups have long claimed – sometimes resisted by aid recipient country governments and others – as advocates for health services that are more responsive to the poor and marginalized.

New Global Health Policy Actors

The transformation in the arena of global health policy has also come about through the unprecedented rise in development assistance for health (DAH), up from US$5.6 billion in 1990 to nearly $28 billion in 2010 (Figure 1.2). The steepest upward trajectory was in the decade from the turn of the new millennium. This decade saw the establishment in 2000 of a new, well-resourced global health partnership, the Global Alliance for Vaccines and Immunization (now called the GAVI Alliance or GAVI), formed largely due to the influence and contribution of the Bill & Melinda Gates Foundation (Box 1.1). This was followed shortly after by the establishment in 2002 of the Global Fund (Box 1.2). An important feature of the Global Fund is that a significant proportion of its funding is channeled through non-governmental organizations (NGOs), sometimes outside the control of recipient country governments. A recent analysis of the Principal Recipients (PRs) of Global Fund grants – i.e., those who implement services on the ground – found that from 2005 to 2010, civil society PRs performed better in implementing programs than governmental PRs (Global Fund 2011).

These two new organizations rapidly mobilized large amounts of disease-specific funding from donor governments, and from the Bill & Melinda Gates Foundation in the case of GAVI. For example, by the mid 2000s, annual donor funding for the control of HIV/AIDS in some African countries was estimated to exceed annual total government spending on health (Oomman *et al.* 2007). Nevertheless, since 2008, the banking and financial crisis has led to a stagnation or lowering of DAH. For example, while international assistance for malaria rose sharply from 2004 to 2009, it fell between 2009 and 2010 (WHO 2010).

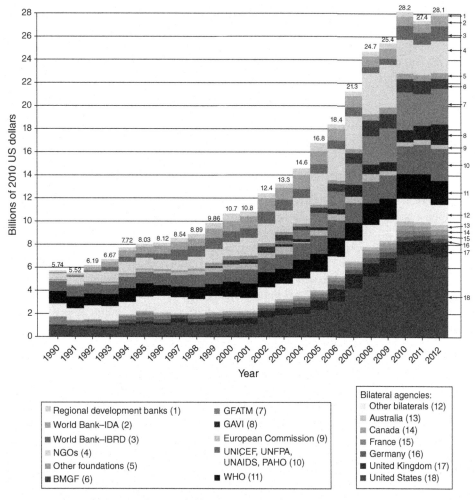

Figure 1.2 Development assistance for health by channel of assistance, 1990–2012. Source: Institute for Health Metrics and Evaluation (2012: 13).

Box 1.1   The GAVI Alliance

The GAVI Alliance (GAVI)[1] was launched in 2000, building on a start-up grant of $750 million from the Bill & Melinda Gates Foundation, with additional funds from donor governments (Norway, the Netherlands, and the United Kingdom). GAVI is a public–private partnership established to improve access to immunization services for children, expand the use of underused vaccines, accelerate the development of new vaccines and technology, and raise the priority of vaccines in global health policy. GAVI also seeks to strengthen the capacity of health systems to deliver immunization and related health services. It has developed new mechanisms for raising and distributing finances, including through the International Finance Facilitate for Immunization (IFFIm) and the pneumococcal advanced market commitment. The

Alliance is governed by a Secretariat based in Geneva and a Board comprised of representatives from both the public and private sectors. GAVI does not have a presence in countries and requires country-level Interagency Coordination Committees (ICCs) to coordinate its grants. Donor contributions are projected to reach over $14 billion by 2031.

[1] www.gavialliance.org (last accessed November 2013).

Box 1.2   The Global Fund to Fight AIDS, Tuberculosis and Malaria

The Global Fund to Fight AIDS, Tuberculosis and Malaria[1] was launched in 2002 as a public–private partnership dedicated to attracting, managing, and disbursing additional resources to control these three diseases. With most of its contributions coming from donor governments, the Global Fund had approved $22.6 billion worth of grants by the end of 2011. More than half of its resources have been distributed to disease control activities in sub-Saharan Africa, with some funds going to strengthening health systems. The Global Fund is managed by a Secretariat in Geneva and governed by a Board comprised of representatives from both public and private sectors. Uniquely, there are three civil society delegates with voting rights on its Board; they are from developed and developing country NGOs and from communities affected by the diseases. The Global Fund does not have a presence in countries, and awards grants directly to country Principal Recipients (PRs), who can be governments, NGOs, or multilateral agencies. The Fund engages at country level primarily through: (i) Country Coordinating Mechanisms (CCMs), which coordinate and submit proposals to the Global Fund; and (ii) Local Fund Agents (LFAs), who are employed by the Fund to provide financial oversight of grant disbursement. In 2014, the Global Fund replaced its "rounds-based" model, in which countries could only apply for financing during discrete time periods (rounds), with a more flexible funding model aimed at providing steadier and more predictable funding flows and increasing ongoing engagement between the Global Fund and potential finance recipients throughout the proposal development process.

[1] www.theglobalfund.org (last accessed November 2013).

GAVI and the Global Fund were established as alternatives to traditional bilateral and multilateral donor agencies, which were considered by many global health policy actors to be too slow in achieving global health goals. Both initiatives have prioritized disease-specific *vertical* interventions, as opposed to strengthening health systems, advancing comprehensive primary healthcare or other *horizontal* disease control strategies (WHO 2009). These organizations have a number of common innovative features, such as their emphasis on performance-based funding and their demand-driven approach (Feachem *et al.* 2010). However, they also work in somewhat different ways, and these differences are rooted in the influence of different stakeholders involved in their formation.

For example, the Bill & Melinda Gates Foundation was an important financial supporter and influencer of the governance structures and policy priorities of GAVI, advocating for greater private sector engagement and the use of private sector "know-how"

(Muraskin 2005). The Foundation leveraged its extensive ties with a small group of vaccine industry representatives and technical non-profit organizations, such as the Program for Appropriate Technology in Health (PATH). GAVI has since gone on to cultivate innovative financing mechanisms, including issuing of bonds on capital markets with the backing of long-term government pledges, where proceeds from bond sales function as cash resources for GAVI programs (Harmer and Bruen 2011).

In contrast, the establishment of the Global Fund involved a greater number of actors seeking to influence the structures, focus, and policy priorities of the new initiative, which was reflected in more participatory global governance structures when compared with existing organizations (Box 1.2). The Global Fund Board and committees have continued to provide a platform on which different interest groups are represented. These groups are formally distinguished by constituency, for example by developed or developing country NGO delegations, NGOs representing affected communities, private sector or private foundation representatives, multilateral organizations, as well as public representatives from donor or implementing government agencies. Relative to other global organizations, this platform has given unprecedented influence to NGOs and to a lesser extent private sector companies. However, the Global Fund's reliance on contributions from bilateral donors, such as the United States, the United Kingdom, and the Scandinavian donor countries, has ensured that these more traditional development actors continue to exert substantial influence over how the Global Fund operates (this issue is discussed further in the next section, including in Case Study 1.2).

In order to understand the birth and evolution of these initiatives from a global health policy perspective, it is important to identify the positions and actions of the different actors. For example, civil society advocates successfully mobilized around the scale-up of antiretroviral treatment (ART) needed for the large number of people affected by HIV/AIDS. Success was achieved by developing and mobilizing *transnational networks of influence* around a global response to treatment. These were networks of activists and NGOs with extended links to individuals from scientific communities, international organizations, donor agencies, and philanthropic foundations seeking to expand the response to HIV/AIDS. Civil society groups were successful in: (i) contributing to the increased political priority for HIV/AIDS treatment; (ii) shaping how the problem of HIV/AIDS was understood; and (iii) advocating for voting rights and influence in the Global Fund governance and decision-making processes as well as over policy implementation and service delivery activities (Smith and Siplon 2006).

The emergence of GAVI and the Global Fund occurred in the context of a massive increase in new global health partnerships and initiatives, creating a "mosh pit of global health governance" where new rules and ways of engagement were forged (Buse and Harmer 2009). From 1998 to 2002, there was a dramatic rise in the number of new global health partnerships, with around 12 new partnerships established annually (Brugha 2008). This explosion can be attributed to a number of factors, including: (i) the optimism and energy that emerged from the Millennium Development Goals (MDGs) summit in 2001; (ii) a growing perception of poor past performance by UN agencies and the need to do things differently; and (iii) a "copy-cat" assumption that new health products (drugs, diagnostics, and vaccines) and orphan diseases could best attract new funds through these new vehicles (Brugha 2008).

Taken together, new global health partnerships and initiatives have created new forms of governance at global and country levels. These partnerships have a major influence on how resources are mobilized and allocated, the procedures for decision-making, and the implementation of health policies at global and country levels. While these new initiatives certainly injected much-needed financing into the global health sphere and brought new stakeholders to the table, at the same time there has been increased fragmentation in national health policy implementation, conflicting with the harmonization and alignment agenda of the Paris Declaration on Aid Effectiveness (Box 1.3) (Biesma *et al.* 2009; WHO 2009).

Box 1.3 Paris Declaration on Aid Effectiveness

The 2005 Paris Declaration on Aid Effectiveness – with follow-up international meetings in Accra (2008) and Bhusan (2012) – was a landmark agreement between donor agencies, developing country governments, multilateral organizations, regional development banks, and international agencies. Its aim was to make aid more effective through adherence to five principles:

1. Country *ownership* of development policies and strategies.
2. Donor *alignment* with the priorities of developing countries, their institutions and procedures.
3. Donor *harmonization* and coordination at country level to avoid duplication.
4. All parties agree to *manage for results* and to develop tools and systems to measure impact.
5. To ensure transparency in the use of aid, *mutual accountability* between donors and developing countries is required, including to their citizens and parliaments.

GAVI, the Global Fund, the US President's Emergency Plan for AIDS Relief (PEPFAR), a multibillion dollar bilateral HIV initiative, and the US President's Malaria Initiative have helped to tackle complex infectious disease priorities more urgently and have spearheaded the political prioritization of children's vaccines, ART, and malaria control tools for poor countries. Recognizing that weak health systems were hindering the scale-up of these commodities, and in response to the concerns of European donors as well as implementing countries, these global health initiatives have expanded their portfolios to include health systems strengthening (HSS). For example, this shift towards HSS resulted in several of the major global health actors, new and old – the Global Fund, GAVI, and the World Bank – with technical support from the WHO, committing to establish a Health Systems Funding Platform in 2009 to coordinate and channel resources to support national health strategies. However, the platform has failed to galvanize the required support and commitment to meet its potential (Hill *et al.* 2011). In the wake of the Global Fund's 2011 political crisis, in which the organization was plagued by allegations of misappropriated funds (see Case Study 1.2), the Global Fund suspended its involvement in the platform, with other partners reviewing and gradually decreasing their engagement with the platform.

In addition to the new "players" in global health discussed above, middle-income countries have also emerged as influential global health actors. In particular, Brazil, Russia, India, China, and South Africa (the "BRICS") continue to increase their influence, due in part to shifting geographies of power and the economic and political motives of these emerging economies. Brazil and India, for example, have used flexibilities in intellectual property law to locally produce generic medicines that are up to 98% cheaper than branded medicines (UNDP 2012). China has also become an important actor in bilateral assistance for malaria control in high-burden countries in sub-Saharan Africa, investing $116 million from 2007 to 2012 (Jamison *et al.* 2013). While having a critical role in global health, such as through the production of health commodities, BRICS countries are only beginning to contribute to financing global health programs, from which they have traditionally been recipients. Brazil, for example, became a donor to GAVI in early 2011 after gaining legislative approval from the Brazilian Parliament, pledging US$20 million from 2012 to 2031 (GAVI Alliance 2012). This contribution is part of a larger trend whereby BRICS countries are increasing their foreign assistance budgets and exploring collaboration opportunities, such as the proposal by India to create a development bank funded by developing countries (GHSi 2012).

Global Health Policy Instruments and Levers

Despite the emergence of new entities in the global health policy field, a more complex mix of actors, and the growth in communication and networking there has been less change in the available forms of global policy instruments and levers. While informal policy levers like health diplomacy and elite buy-in can bring about policy change, it is the formal instruments that most often influence policy change in countries. As shown in Table 1.1, these instruments can be classified into *financial instruments* (e.g., principal-agent contracts between donors and implementing agents, incentivizing private markets to develop health technologies, or performance-based health financing) and *legal/regulatory instruments* (e.g., international health treaties).

The most pervasive policy influence continues to come from the hard power of financing. During the 1980s and 1990s, health reforms in low- and middle-income countries were initially driven by structural adjustment programs overseen by the World Bank and IMF, where reforms such as the introduction of user fees or limiting the role of the state in service provision were some of the conditions that needed to be met in order to gain access to loans and other forms of financial assistance. This had a profound impact on the availability of health goods and services, including a decline in the health status of poor populations (McInnes and Lee 2012). Other finance-driven approaches began to be introduced from the mid 1990s, the most common of which was the Sector Wide Approach (SWAp) favored by many European bilateral agencies, with policy input from the WHO and the World Bank. The SWAp model prioritized the pooling of donor funds, as a mechanism to reduce fragmentation and promote coordination of national health policy and implementation in several sub-Saharan African countries (Cassels and Janovsky 1998). These models were often bypassed, however, in response to changing global health priorities and channels for directing funding particularly as the new well-financed Global Health Initiatives (GHIs) began to have a greater impact and influence. Nevertheless, both structural adjustment programs (SAPs) and SWAps continue to exist as different strategies for influencing health policies (Peters *et al.* 2013).

While financial assistance can provide leverage over national policy in low- and middle-income countries, international funding agencies have not always been able to accurately monitor the impact of their finances in a complex implementation environment, particularly to the point of attribution (Victora *et al.* 2011). Performance-based funding models, such as those used by the Global Fund, have been proposed and implemented as a financial incentive for improving performance and for tracking results, as has been seen in Rwanda (Farmer *et al.* 2013). However, performance-based funding models have themselves shown mixed results (e.g., Montagu and Yamey 2011; Fan *et al.* 2013).

Table 1.1 Global financial and legal policy instruments.

Instrument	Description	Examples
Financial	Encompasses a range of tools to effect change or influence the behavior of different actors	• Conditionality models where access to finance is conditional on implementing specific policy reforms, e.g., (i) "hard-power models" such as the World Bank or IMF structural adjustment programs (SAPs), or (ii) "soft-power models" used by Global Health Initiatives, where access to finance is conditional on country policies aligning in some way with GHI objectives • Performance-based financing models, e.g., pay-for-performance or results-based financing used by the Global Fund • Push/pull mechanisms to incentivize research and development of life-saving medicines, e.g., pneumococcal Advance Market Commitment
Legal/regulatory	Often termed "command-and-control" instruments, where the command refers to standard setting and control refers to its monitoring and enforcement. The latter is not always in place	• International legally binding agreements and arbitration bodies, e.g., World Trade Organization TRIPS (Trade-Related Agreement on Intellectual Property Rights) Agreement and Dispute Settlement appellate body • International regulations, treaties, and guidelines, e.g., International Health Regulations; Framework Convention on Tobacco Control; International Health Partnership • Quality assurance and safety of medical products, e.g., Food and Agriculture Organization or WHO Department of Essential Medicines and Health Products

They have been implemented in a context of intense debate regarding the appropriateness, effectiveness, or best form from among a range of different performance-based financing models, including the model used by the Global Fund (e.g., Honda 2013; McCoy *et al.* 2013).

Regulations and legislation comprise a second set of policy instruments. For example, the International Health Regulations (IHR) provide a set of international legal instruments, binding on the Member States of the WHO, to prevent and respond to acute public health risks that have the potential to cross borders and threaten people worldwide (PLOS Medicine Editors 2007). These regulations remain one of the few global health policy responses that have elicited virtual unanimity across all countries, both on the need for and on the form of the response. In particular, the proposed revisions leading to the updated IHR in 2005 (IHR 2005), which requires Member States to notify WHO of "all events which may constitute a public health emergency of international concern" were hailed as "a great step forward for international public health practice" (Gostin 2004). Since being revised, the IHR 2005 nevertheless continues to face a number of hurdles – for example, many low-income countries lack sufficient financial resources to build the core surveillance and response capacity needed to comply with the updated regulations (PLOS Medicine Editors 2007).

Indeed, the feasibility of and capacity for enforcement of global health rules and regulations is often lacking in low-income countries. There may also be resistance to enforcement of such rules and regulations in high-income countries, for example where national or commercial interests are threatened. Globally, gaining collective agreement on legally binding and enforceable rules has proven to be a long process and not always a successful one. An example is the Framework Convention on Tobacco Control, developed from 1998 to 2003, where the interests of wealthy tobacco-producing countries led to the deletion of a robust implementation framework (Taylor and Dhillon 2011). Consequently, global efforts have tended instead to focus on gaining agreement on *non-binding* international agreements (so-called "soft laws"), such as the 2010 WHO Global Code of Practice on the International Recruitment of Health Personnel (for further discussion, see Case Study 1.4).

The area of global regulation and binding standards that has perhaps had the greatest impact on global public health has been trade and rules of engagement, e.g., through the Trade-Related Agreement on Intellectual Property Rights (TRIPs) (Box 1.4; see also Chapters 13, 22, and 25). These trade rules are "hard laws" governing state relations, through dispute settlement processes that have been formalized within the World Trade Organization (WTO) that allow for penalties and retaliatory measures, supported by changes of national laws to bring them into compliance with WTO standards. While focused on trade, there can be *policy spillover* to other sectors, sometimes converging and sometimes colliding, in that trade rules can impact on the capacity of governments to regulate the economic and social conditions that influence the health of their populations.

Box 1.4 Health and Trade: The TRIPs Agreement

Since 1995, binding commitments on trade liberalization have been overseen by the World Trade Organization (WTO) and adjudicated through its dispute settlement process, including the authorization of retaliatory measures. Obligations for the protection of intellectual property rights (IPRs) represent one pillar of the WTO, and are enshrined in the *Trade-Related Agreement on Intellectual Property Rights* (TRIPS). TRIPS sets out minimum standards of protection for intellectual property such as patents, copyright, trademarks, industrial design, and undisclosed or confidential information. It also sets out flexibilities for Member States. There are two flexibilities that are particularly important. The first is *compulsory licenses*. These allow an individual or company seeking to use a patent to do so without seeking the patent holder's consent, provided they pay the patent holder a set fee for the license. States are free to determine the grounds for granting compulsory licenses, and can exercise their right to pursue the local production of generic alternatives of individual inventions, such as a patented drug. The second is *parallel imports*. The TRIPs agreement states that the practice of parallel importation cannot be challenged within the WTO system, leaving it open to countries to determine their own policy around the importation and reselling of branded or patented products from another market, thus allowing them to take advantage of existing price differentials.

Policy processes and instruments are intertwined with the interests, influence, and actions of policy actors or stakeholders. For Buse and colleagues (2005: 20), policy-making is "a struggle between groups with competing interests, some in favor of change and others opposed to it, depending on their interests and ideas." Shiffman and Smith

(2007) expand on this notion of a struggle to outline the interplay between four key determinants generating political priority for different global health policies: (i) *actor power*; (ii) *ideas* (i.e., the way in which the health topic is framed); (iii) *political contexts*; and (iv) the characteristics of health issues (such as the burden of disease and the existence of simple, low cost treatments).

Actors and processes that can prevent or obstruct health-promoting policies are as important as policy enablers. Influential actors from some of the most important health policy spheres – tobacco, alcohol, and food – are often not at the policy table, and focus instead on lobbying policy-makers and on spinning, distorting, or suppressing the evidence. Large transnational corporations, like states, can strategically leverage the opposing interests of countries – and in some cases corporations can exploit countries' vulnerability to financial or other favors, cooption, and corruption. Through these strategies, companies have been able to promote global health policies that are favorable to commercial interests, but that sometimes run contrary to public health objectives (Case Study 1.1).

Case Study 1.1   Nutrition and Health – a Global Health Policy Failure?

Opposition to, and failures in, bringing about effective policy action are a feature of the global as well as the national policy terrain. Conducting policy analyses of these policy failures can yield important insights. For example, the health–food interface is a complex, political, and highly contested policy space distributed across sectors and levels of governance, with actors seeking to promote or limit food and drinks production, sales, and consumption.[1] Famines due to food shortages throughout human history have evolved in the late twentieth and twenty-first centuries into a double global burden of disease, characterized by both under- and over-consumption of food. The latter (discussed in Chapter 9), combined with reduced physical activity, has triggered pandemics in diet- and obesity-related ill health in low-, middle-, and high-income countries due to non-communicable diseases (NCDs) such as coronary heart disease, diabetes, and cancers (WHO/FAO 2003).

The 2004 WHO World Health Assembly agreed a Global Strategy on Diet, Physical Activity, and Disease that committed Member States to take steps towards improving population diet and activity, and to bring about changes to the food industry. However, a review of the commitments and practices of big food companies found that there was a low level of engagement by these companies (Lang *et al.* 2006). The 2006–2008 food commodity crisis shifted the focus to under-consumption and increasing access to food (Lang *et al.* 2009). Underlying all of these trends is the fact that current food systems favor maximizing profits over delivery of optimal human health. Actions to date have failed to tackle the vested interests that profit from the production and sale of unhealthy food (Stuckler and Nestle 2012). Factors that may help to explain the inadequate global policy response include (UNSCN 2011):

- Coalitions of economic and commercial interests at national, regional (especially North America and the European Union), and global levels benefit from over-production of products with higher price and cost surplus. These actors oppose mandatory regulations on food labeling, marketing, and distribution to children.
- Governance of global food policy is fragmented, in that several multilateral institutions and private sector actors form broad issue networks, but are also competing for authority over food-related policies. These multilateral actors include the

WHO, World Food Program (WFP), UNICEF, the Food and Agriculture Organization (FAO), and the WTO.

- Lack of trust or perceived conflicts of interest can present barriers to developing policy and strategic coherence on nutrition and effective frameworks to guide public sector engagement with the private sector.

There have been some country-level efforts and successes – for example, Mexico's 2010 Obesity Prevention Strategy, which removed sugar-sweetened products and high calorie, high saturated fat foods from government welfare and school programs. Activities such as these at the country level create opportunities for transfer of successful policies to other countries. This example from Mexico is part of a larger trend where innovative domestic health policies in middle-income countries are combining with shifts in power and influence to challenge the traditional global powers of the US and Europe in shaping global policy agendas (Lee *et al.* 2010; GHSi 2012).

[1] For more on the vested interests of the food industry, see the online *PLOS Medicine Series* on "Big Food" (multinational food and beverage companies) at www.ploscollections.org/bigfood (last accessed November 2013).

Contribution of Theory to Understanding Global Health Policy

The theoretical origins of policy analysis can be traced back to the years following the Second World War and the professionalization and institutionalization of policy or political science as a discipline in its own right (Dunn 1981). Policy analysis looks to the contributions of a range of academic disciplines in establishing an evidence base for policy, whether nationally or globally. Analysts also draw on a range of policy theories and models to explore and better understand policy processes. Theories provide alternative perspectives or frameworks that can be used to explore and analyze different types of policy questions and policy-making processes. These questions include how agendas are set, how issues are framed, and the roles of actors and networks in formulating or implementing policies. This section briefly outlines some of the foundational theories for understanding global health policy-making, using case studies to bring the issues alive.

The terms "framework," "theory," and "model" are often used interchangeably, whereas in fact they have different meanings. Schlager (2007) provides a very useful distinction between the three terms, one that we adopt in the rest of this chapter, based on the difference between classification (framework), explanation (theory), and prediction (model):

- *Frameworks* bound and organize an inquiry and lay out the critical features of the landscape being examined, but they do not provide explanations or predictions. The *policy triangle* discussed earlier in this chapter is an example of a framework.
- *Theories* assign values on some of the variables identified as important in a framework. They also suggest how the variables relate to each other. Theories explain the factors that influence an outcome and the mechanism of such influence. *Punctuated equilibrium theory* (see later) is an example of a theory.
- *Models* allow policy analysts to test theories. They are used primarily for prediction and they make precise assumptions about a limited range of variables. Examples of models include *functional rationality* and the *systems model* (see next section).

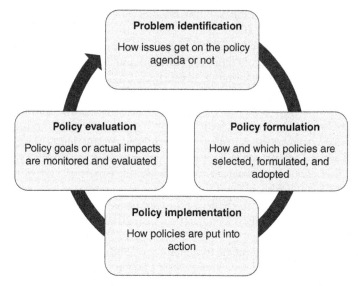

Figure 1.3   The policy cycle and its stages.

Functional Rationality: The Policy Process as a Set of Stages or a System

One of the earliest and most widely used models draws on the idea of the policy process as a rational and functional set of stages with inputs (problems) and outputs (policies) that, when taken together, form a *policy cycle* (Figure 1.3). This cycle is often termed the *stages heuristic* model. Early proponents used this model to make comprehensible the complexity of the policy process within political systems (see, for example, Easton 1965 and Lasswell 1956 in Parsons 1995). Each stage leads to and determines the next stage, with "feedback" from policy evaluation influencing future inputs into the system in a policy cycle. Feedback may or may not lead to a change in policy direction.

Figure 1.4 illustrates a related *systems model*, where change in one unit produces changes in another part of the system that may affect outputs and outcomes and may influence future policy inputs. Systems models (e.g., Jenkins 1978) can incorporate the

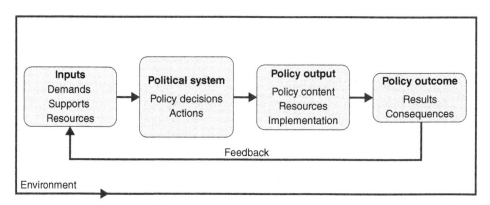

Figure 1.4   Systems model of the policy process.

wider environmental context, whether economic, political, or social. The value of these types of models lies in their ability to broadly conceptualize how different activities should occur at different times and how different components of complex systems are meant to function.

Cycle and systems models are preferred by scientists and decision-makers who assume that policy-making is normally evidence-based. These models have been criticized for being overly idealistic and prescriptive, for misrepresenting what *actually* happens, and for not being empirically grounded (Sabatier and Jenkins-Smith 1993). Despite the way in which the cycle or system is conceptualized, in reality the different stages or subsystems are not insulated from each other and the same actors may be involved at different times or in different subsystems. More importantly, actors may bring different interpretations of the evidence, different values and perspectives, and different interests to influencing the outcome of a policy process (see Chapter 8). Different and imperfect information, and complex interactions between the actors involved, mean that any simple, sequential, or functional model will always struggle to uncover the determinants and causal mechanisms in policy processes (John 2003).

Despite these limitations, stages and systems thinking and nomenclature continue to be widely used by policy practitioners as models for top-down planning and strategic decision-making. These approaches can help unpack and identify the complex stages in the policy process, including feedback loops that can incorporate new evidence and inputs leading to new developments during the policy life cycle. In the case of global health policy, stages and systems thinking has informed a range of useful analytic frameworks. These include frameworks for understanding health systems in their wider context (Atun and Menabde 2008), and more specific frameworks for assessing the effects of GHIs on countries' health systems (Bennett and Fairbank 2003; WHO 2009). An important recent advance relevant to global health policy-making is the synthesis of health systems and policy research, which seeks to understand what health systems are, how they operate, and what needs to be done to strengthen them. Gilson (2012), for example, has collected together a range of research and conceptual papers from low- and middle-income countries that address different aspects of this work and draws on a range of explanatory theories to support analysis.

Explanatory Theories of Policy Processes

Critical of the inability of stages or systems models to account for sudden changes in policy processes over time, Baumgartner and Jones (1993) were early proponents of the *punctuated equilibrium theory*. This theory proposes that patterns of abrupt change in policy occur during periods of instability, when new issues emerge and contribute to changes in institutional environments, relations between actors, and preferred policy ideas to resolve a given problem. The role of the media is vital, as it has the power to influence how institutions are perceived and the merit of different sets of ideas or *policy images*. Traditional authorities are weakened during periods of instability, opening up access to agenda-setting processes that had previously been monopolized by specific sets of actors in dominant institutions. Opportunities arise for new actors to promote new ideas that can compete for inclusion on the policy agenda, and – crucially – these new actors compete for influence in the new institutional arrangements that sometimes emerge. As these take shape, new rules and ways of working are agreed, following which a period of stability is established and the new policy ideas become mainstream. The punctuated equilibrium theory can usefully be applied to understand the evolution of the Global Fund (Case Study 1.2).

Case Study 1.2 Applying Punctuated Equilibrium Theory to Global Health Policy: The Global Fund

Key factors that led to the creation of the Global Fund in January 2002 included the recognition of HIV/AIDS as a health crisis; the perceived failure of existing institutions to effectively respond to this pandemic; and the formation of a transnational coalition of actors that promoted new policy images incorporating presumed private sector efficiencies. The launch of this new multilateral financing institution represented a turning point in the global response to HIV/AIDS and brought about significant changes in the institutional environment. The Global Fund quickly became a well-resourced and leading global initiative outside the UN system, and in the process shifted relations between actors in ways that opened up opportunities for new actors to influence policy priorities. For example, HIV/AIDS civil society groups played an important role in shaping the new policy images on how to respond to the crisis, such as through portraying HIV/AIDS as an exceptional disease requiring an exceptional response. As transnational networks of influence, these groups were a powerful lobbying force and contributed to media coverage of HIV/AIDS. Civil society highlighted the failure of existing institutions to respond to the epidemic, one that had previously been the restricted patch of governments and multilateral agencies. These longstanding actors were then forced to reposition themselves and relinquish some control over the global HIV/AIDS policy field (Smith and Siplon 2006).

Following a period of rapid innovation, from 2002 to 2005, new modalities for disbursing and overseeing aid became systematized and began to align with pre-existing aid mechanisms, introducing a period of stability (Biesma *et al.* 2009). In 2011, the Global Fund experienced a major crisis, triggered by: (i) evidence of financial misappropriation in recipient counties; (ii) representations of this issue in the media in the context of a global economic downturn and growing skepticism about development aid; (iii) a temporary withdrawal of financial support from some donors; and (iv) the discrediting of some senior officials in the Global Fund (McCoy *et al.* 2012). While this crisis did not lead to the demise of an existing institution, or the creation of a new one, it opened up opportunities for the introduction of new policy ideas as part of an institutional reform package. These reforms led to substantial changes in policy and institutional structures, in the appointment of senior staff with a different vision for the Global Fund that had the support of major donors, and a new funding model.

Kingdon's (1984) *policy streams model* has become popular in recent years among public health researchers. It comprises three streams that operate independently; a convergence of the three streams explains how issues rise to the top of policy agendas. The *problem stream* encompasses the many issues competing for the attention of policy-makers. As events occur that focus attention on specific issues, their importance is assessed and feedback provides information on whether or not these issues are being addressed.

The second stream is the *policy stream*, out of which comes the set of ideas and available solutions for addressing the problem. Crucial to the success of an idea are *policy communities* and *policy entrepreneurs*, who promote particular ideas through journals, conferences, and different forms of media. Ideas or solutions can be evaluated for their technical feasibility and compatibility with the dominant societal values; and lobbying and investment of resources can be used to promote particular ideas and shape the policy agenda.

The third and final stream is the *political stream*, typically consisting of politicians and decision-makers such as wealthy donors. Events such as elections, changes in public opinion, or pressure from organized political forces can combine to open up "political windows of opportunity." As Hafner and Shiffman (2013: 42) summarize, "issues are most likely to emerge on policy agendas when they have acquired status as problems, policy communities have generated consensus on workable solutions and political windows have opened, creating opportunities for policy entrepreneurs to link the three streams." Hafner and Shiffman (2013) applied the policy streams model to help understand why the global health community has begun to pay attention to HSS (Case Study 1.3).

Case Study 1.3 Applying the Policy Streams Model to Health Systems Strengthening (HSS)

Hafner and Shiffman (2013) use the policy streams model to explain the recent shift towards HSS in global health policy. They note that the *problem stream* has been dominated by concerns that disease-specific initiatives, such as the Global Fund, were unable to achieve their goals due to longstanding weaknesses in health systems. At the same time, HSS policy communities were building an evidence base to advance alternative ideas within the *policy stream*, drawing on: (i) the legacy of the 1978 Alma Ata Declaration on Primary Health Care (including the goal of "health for all by the year 2000"); and (ii) decades of debates on the relative merits of vertical disease-specific interventions versus horizontal HSS (e.g., Bradley 1998; Rifkin and Walt 1986). Policy solutions were proposed, such as "diagonalizing" vertical disease interventions in ways that would strengthen health systems (Sepúlveda *et al.* 2006; Ooms *et al.* 2008; see also Chapters 23 and 24).

Within the *political stream*, Hafner and Shiffman highlight how slow progress towards the health-related MDGs increased pressure on actors to find ways to achieve these goals. This pressure was heightened by the external influence of the Paris Declaration, which encouraged donors to align aid with the priorities and policies of national governments. Taken together, the authors suggest that the critical convergence of these three streams accounts for the increased level of attention towards HSS. However, the global financial crisis and a lack of technically feasible solutions to the strengthening of systems have raised questions about the sustainability of HSS as a set of policy ideas and actions to resolve current problems. Central to this question about the future of the HSS agenda is the fragmented nature of the HSS policy community, and a health systems research "image problem" that has not generated consensus on the evidence base (Hafner and Shiffman 2013).

Actors are central to most policy theories because they bring to the policy process negotiation skills, legitimacy, political connections, or financial backing. Actors engage in coalition building, network formation, or network leveraging (e.g., the way in which donors, multilaterals, or global health initiatives may leverage civil society networks for their own ends) in ways that can in turn maximize their impact and influence and bring about policy change. The *advocacy coalition framework* developed by Paul Sabatier and colleagues (e.g., Sabatier and Jenkins-Smith 1993) brings together a number of approaches and frameworks, including that of policy streams. Sabatier focuses on *policy subsystems* as the unit of analysis, where all public and private sector actors in a policy arena interact (Sabatier 1988). Within policy subsystems, actors sharing a set of core beliefs on a common problem may form an advocacy coalition, combine resources, generate technical and evidence-based information, and adopt strategies that will translate their beliefs into policy programs and institutional change. While the core beliefs of advocacy coalitions tend to be fixed, the secondary aspects of their belief systems, such as the best way to deliver a service, are open to change when new, convincing evidence or arguments are put forward. This change constitutes *policy learning*. While financial resources, expertise, or political connections can increase a coalition's chances of success, *policy brokers* play an important role in negotiating between competing strategies and coalitions. The advocacy coalition framework can be applied to understand the creation of the Global Code of Practice on the International Recruitment of Health Personnel (Case Study 1.4).

Case Study 1.4   Advocacy Coalitions in the Creation of the Global Code of Practice on the International Recruitment of Health Personnel

In 2010 the World Health Assembly (WHA) unanimously adopted the Global Code of Practice on the International Recruitment of Health Personnel. As a policy subsystem, the issue of health worker recruitment was highly contentious, with the debates driven by the needs and actions of different countries experiencing health worker shortages. Rather than rely on internal WHO committee processes, the WHO Department of Human Resources for Health entered into an alliance with an NGO, Realizing Rights, and the Global Health Workforce Alliance (GHWA), to form the Health Worker Migration Initiative (Taylor and Dhillon 2011). This advocacy coalition generated evidence, organized events and opportunities for policy learning, and secured high-level political support and engagement through a Global Policy Advisory Council. The Council's aim was to generate a workable policy solution that addressed three controversial issues impeding consensus: (i) financial compensation for countries losing health workers; (ii) the balance between the rights of health workers to travel and the health workforce needs in source countries; and (iii) the use of mandatory versus non-binding instruments.

At the May 2010 WHA in Geneva, national interests reappeared – notably on the part of the USA, EU, Canada and other health worker recipient countries – that threatened to water down the Code. An intensive negotiation process ensued from May 17 to the early hours of May 21 that required extensive brokering to bring opposing coalitions and interests together. On May 21, in the face of the efforts of wealthy countries who had up to that point dominated the discussions, "around 4.30 in the morning, the delegations from the African states ... established a united front in favor of maintaining the strong legal and institutional provisions in the final text against all efforts to modify and limit such provisions" (Taylor and Dhillon 2011: 11). The WHA formally adopted the Code later that day, a major achievement, and only the second Global Code to be unanimously adopted by the WHA in its history, the other being the International Code of Marketing of Breast-milk Substitutes in 1981.

Globalization processes have accentuated the role of networks and the development of *network theories* (Marsh 1998) in governance, policy-making, and analysis of interdependency relations. These theories have been applied in the context of global health policy-making, for instance, to account for the way in which global policy networks are formed, evolve, and change the way in which health policy is made, financed, and conceptualized (e.g. Lee and Goodman 2002). Theories on network forms of organization and governance are a contested domain, however, in that networks are not always a clearly separate form of socioeconomic coordination when compared with more traditional market or bureaucratic forms of organizational and institutional governance (Thompson 2003). For Ostrom *et al.* (2001) institutions play a fundamental role in the success or failure of efforts to address collective action problems that result in poverty, one of the biggest factors in poor health outcomes. Given the high stakes nature of decision-making and resource allocation or acquisition in global health governance and policy programs, differences in the motivating forces and financial resources of different actors can sometimes lead to narrow self-interest in the competition for resources. In turn this self-interest creates incentives and actions that can undermine global health goals. Consequently, the struggle to control or influence global health policy agendas, the institutions or organizations that shape them, and the incentives and behaviors they foster, remains a fiercely contested domain.

Conclusions and Pointers for the Health Policy Analyst

Health policy is inherently political, and global health policy and practice entail working in and understanding a highly complex and politically charged arena, where the positions, interests, and objectives of nations, organizations, and individuals are intertwined in complex ways. An understanding of the terrain enables the practitioner to become more aware of the political obstacles and opportunities to getting population health issues on to the policy agenda and implementing evidence-based policies to achieve health goals. This introductory chapter has mapped some of the key events, actors, and processes that have influenced a fast-changing and fluid global health policy environment. Later chapters will go into greater depth in reviewing these and other issues. This chapter also outlined a range of theoretical concepts and models that help to account for *what ought to happen* and for *what often happens* in policy-making, with references to useful readings on these theories. The utility of these theories and models for the student, practitioner, and researcher is that they help to organize and frame enquiry into a complex field.

The application of theory is quite different in health policy analysis than in epidemiology, where the principles and available methods are well established. The consideration of multiple policy theories is an accepted approach to some forms of policy analysis (Sabatier 2007), in the sense that different theories have different contributions to make in understanding the different stages of policy development and implementation processes. Where the policy arena is stable, the important actors and issues are clear, and when earlier policy analysis work has generated some clear propositions, a single policy theory may be more appropriate for guiding data collection and testing hypotheses. However, the arena of global health policy-making is quite fluid, and premature assumptions about who the important actors are may be dangerous, masking hidden issues or hidden participants in a policy process. This fluidity calls for a less prescriptive and more iterative application and consideration of different policy theories – before, during, and after data collection – where theory development may be one of the outcomes of policy analysis. Different policy theories may throw light on different dimensions of policy processes, though the analyst should comment on the utility or otherwise of the theories used in the analysis.

Researchers as well as practitioners can become actors in policy processes through participating in policy communities and issue networks, and through the process of researching the policy field. Students, researchers, and practitioners bring with them biases, perspectives, and preferences that have been influenced by geographic location, professional experience, gender, class, ethnicity, and a variety of other factors that shape experience and "position" them in relation to different policy issues. Researcher and practitioner positionality can influence the policy research agendas, the questions asked, or the analysis and interpretation of collected data (Walt *et al.* 2008). Since understanding global health policy-making requires the analysis of actor power, resources, and interests, researchers and practitioners also bear a responsibility for greater reflexivity in regard to how their own institutional positions, resources, and values influence their analyses.

Key Reading

Future Directions for Health Policy Analysis. Health Policy and Planning Special Edition 2008, 23(8).

Buse K, Mays N, Walt G. 2005. *Making Health Policy*. Buckingham: Open University Press, 2005

Gilson L (ed.) 2012. *Health Policy and Systems Research: A Methodology Reader*. Geneva: HPSR/WHO.

Merson MH, Black RE, Mills AJ. 2012. *Global Health: Diseases, Programs, Systems, and Policies*. Burlington, MA: Jones and Bartlett.

Sabatier P (ed.). 2007. *Theories of the Policy Process*, 2nd edn. Boulder, CO: Westview Press.

References

Abbasi K. 1999. The World Bank and world health: changing sides. *BMJ* 318, 865–9.

Atun RA, Menabde N. 2008. Health systems and systems thinking. In Coker R, Atun R, McKee M (eds) *Health Systems and the Challenge of Communicable Disease: Experiences from Europe and Latin America*, pp. 121–40. Maidenhead: McGraw Hill/Open University Press.

Baumgartner FB, Jones BD. 1933. *Agendas and Instabilty in American Politics*. Chigago: University of Chigago Press.

Bennett S, Fairbank A. 2003. *The System-Wide Effects of the Global Fund to Fight Aids, Tuberculosis and Malaria: A Conceptual Framework*. Bethesda, MD: Partners for Health Reformplus.

Biesma R, Brugha R, Harmer A, Walsh A, Spicer N, Walt G. 2009. The effects of global health initiatives on country health systems: a review of the evidence from HIV/AIDS control. *Health Policy Planning* 24(4), 239–52.

Bradley DJ. 1998. The particular and the general. issues of specificity and verticality in the history of malaria control. *Parassitologia* 40, 5–10.

Brown TM, Cueto M, Fee E. 2006. The World Health Organization and the transition from "international" to "global public health." *American Journal of Public Health* 96(1), 62–70.

Brugha R. 2008. Global health initiatives and public health policy. In Heggenhougen K, Quah S (eds) *International Encyclopedia of Public Health*, pp. 72–81. San Diego, CA: Academic Press.

Brugha R, Zwi A. 2002. Global approaches to private sector provision: where is the evidence? In Lee K, Buse K, Fustukian S (eds) *Health Policy in a Globalising World*, pp. 63–77. Cambridge: Cambridge University Press.

Buse K. 2008. Addressing the theoretical, practical and ethical challenges inherent in prospective health policy analysis. *Health Policy and Planning* 23(5), 351–60.

Buse K, Dickinson C, Gilson L, Murray SF. 2007. How can the analysis of power and process in policy-making improve health outcomes? *ODI Briefing Paper 25*. London: Overseas Development Institute.

Buse K, Drager N, Fustukian S, Lee K. 2002. Globalisation and health policy: trends and opportunities. In Lee K, Buse K, Fustukian S (eds) *Health Policy in a Globalising World*, pp. 251–81. Cambridge: Cambridge University Press.

Buse K, Harmer A. 2009. Global health partnerships: the mosh pit of global health governance. In Buse K, Hein W, Drager N (eds) *Making Sense of Global Health Governance: A Policy Perspective*, pp. 245–67. Basingstoke: Palgrave Macmillan.

Buse K, Mays N, Walt G. 2005. *Making Health Policy*. Maidenhead: Open University Press.

Cassels A, Janovsky K. 1998. Better health in developing countries: are sector-wide approaches the way of the future? *Lancet* 352(9142), 1777–9.

Dunn WN. 1981. *Public Policy Analysis: An Introduction*. Upper Saddle River, NJ: Prentice Hall.

Evans M (ed.). 2004. *Policy Transfer in Global Perspective*. Farnham: Ashgate.

Fan VY, Duran D *et al.* 2013. Performance-based financing at the Global Fund to Fight AIDS, Tuberculosis and Malaria: an analysis of grant ratings and funding, 2003–12. *Lancet Global Health* 1(3), e161–e168

Farmer PE, Nutt CT, Wagner VM *et al.* 2013. Reduced premature mortality in Rwanda: lessons from success. *BMJ* 346, f65.

Feachem R, Yamey G, Schrade G. 2010. A moment of truth for global health. *BMJ* 340, c2869.

GAVI Alliance. 2012. *Brazil: Proceeds to GAVI from Donor Contributions and Pledges (2011–2015) as of 30 June 2013*. http://www.gavialliance.org/funding/donor-profiles/brazil/ (last accessed November 2013).

GHSi (Global Health Strategies initiatives). 2012. *Shifting Paradigm: How the BRICS are Reshaping Global Health and Development*. New York: GHSi.

Gilson L (ed.). 2012. *Health Policy and Systems Research: A Methodology Reader*. Geneva: Alliance for Health Policy and Systems Research/WHO.

Gilson L, Raphaely N. 2008. The terrain of health policy analysis in low and middle income countries: a review of published literature 1994–2007. *Health Policy Plan* 23(5), 294–307.

Global Fund to Fight AIDS, Tuberculosis and Malaria. 2011. *PR Performance Analysis by Sector for all Grants from 2005 to 2010*. Geneva: Global Fund.

Gostin L. 2004. International Health Regulations – Comments from the Center for Law and the Public's Health. http://www.publichealthlaw.net/Reader/docs/IHR_comments.pdf (last accessed November 2013).

Hafner T, Shiffman J. 2013. The emergence of global attention to health systems strengthening. *Health Policy and Planning* 28(1), 41–50.

Hagopian A, Ofosu A, Fatusi A *et al.* 2005. The flight of physicians from West Africa: views of African physicians and implications for policy. *Social Science and Medicine* 61(8), 1750–60.

Hanefeld J. 2010. The impact of global health initiatives at national and sub-national level – a policy analysis of their role in implementation processes of antiretroviral treatment (ART) roll-out in Zambia and South Africa. *AIDS Care: Psychological and Socio-medical Aspects of AIDS /HIV* 22(S1), 93–102.

Harmer A, Bruen C. 2011. The Gavi Alliance. In Hale T, Held D (eds) *Handbook of Transnational Governance: New Institutions and Innovations*, pp. 384–94. London: Polity Press.

Hill PS, Vermeiren P, Miti K, Ooms G, Van Damme W. 2011. The health systems funding platform: is this where we thought we were going? *Global Health* 7, 16.

Honda A. 2013. 10 best resources on pay for performance in low- and middle-income countries. *Health Policy and Planning* 28(5), 454–7.

Hutchinson E, Parkhurst J, Phiri S *et al.* 2011. National policy development for cotrimoxazole prophylaxis in Malawi, Uganda and Zambia: the relationship between context, evidence and links. *Health Research Policy and Systems* 9(Suppl 1), S6.

IHME (Institute for Health Metrics and Evaluation). 2012. *Financing Global Health 2012: The End of the Golden Age?* Seattle, WA: IHME.

Jamison DT, Summers LH, Alleyne G *et al.* 2013. Global health 2035: a world converging within a generation. *Lancet* published online December 3.

Jenkins WI. 1978. *Policy Analysis: A Political and Organizational Perspective.* London: Martin Robertson.

John P. 2003. Is there life after policy streams, advocacy coalitions, and punctuations: using evolutionary theory to explain policy change? *Policy Studies Journal* 31(4): 481–98.

Kingdon J. 1984. *Agendas, Alternatives and Public Policies.* Boston: Little Brown.

Koplan JP, Bond TC, Merson MH *et al.* 2009. Towards a common definition of global health. *Lancet* 373(9679), 1993–5.

Kruk M. 2013. Universal health coverage: a policy whose time has come. *BMJ* 347, f6360.

Labonté R, Schrecker T. 2007. Globalization and social determinants of health: the role of the global marketplace (part 2 of 3). *Globalization and Health* 3(1), 6.

Lang TG, Barling D, Caraher M. 2009. *Food Policy: Integrating Health, Environment and Society.* Oxford: Oxford University Press.

Lang T, Rayner G, Kaelin E. 2006. *The Food Industry, Diet, Physical Activity and Health: A Review of Reported Commitments and Practice of 25 of the World's Largest Food Companies.* London: City University Centre for Food Policy.

Lee K, Chagas LC, Novotny TE. 2010. Brazil and the Framework Convention on Tobacco Control: global health diplomacy as soft power. *PLOS Medicine* 7(4), e1000232.

Lee K, Goodman H. 2002. Global policy networks: the propagation of health care financing reform since the 1980s. In Lee K, Buse K, Fustukian S (eds) *Health Policy in a Globalising World*, pp. 97–119. Cambridge: Cambridge University Press.

Marsh D (ed.). 1998. *Comparing Policy Networks.* Maidenhead: Open University Press.

McCoy D, Bruen C, Hill P, Kerouedan D. 2012. *A New Narrative for the Global Fund – Blowing the Ship Off Course?* Nairobi: Aidspan.

McCoy D, Jensen N, Kranzer K, Ferrand R, Korenromp E. 2013. Methodological and policy limitations of quantifying the saving of lives: a case study of the Global Fund's approach. *PLOS Medicine* 10(10), e1001522.

McInnes C, Lee K. 2012. *Global Health and International Relations.* Cambridge: Polity Press.

Montagu D, Yamey G. 2011. Pay-for-performance and the Millennium Development Goals. *Lancet* 377, 1383–5.

Muraskin, W. 2005. *Crusade to Immunize the World's Children.* Los Angeles, CA: USC Marshall Global BioBusiness Initiative.

Oomman N, Bernstein M, Rosenzweig S. 2007. *Following the Funding for HIV/AIDS: A Comparative Analysis of the Funding Practices of PEPFAR, the Global Fund and World Bank MAP in Mozambique, Uganda and Zambia.* Washington, DC: Center for Global Development.

Ooms, G, Van Damme W, Baker BK, Zeitz P, Schrecker T. 2008. The "diagonal" approach to global fund financing: a cure for the broader malaise of health systems? *Globalization and Health* 4(6).

Ostrom E, Gibson C, Shivakumar S, Andersson K. 2001. Aid, incentives, and sustainability: an institutional analysis of development cooperation. *Sida Studies in Evaluation 02/01:1.* Stockholm: Swedish International Development Cooperation Agency.

Parsons W. 1995. *Public Policy: An Introduction to the Theory and Practice of Policy Analysis.* Cheltenham: Edward Elgar.

Peters DH, Paina L *et al.* 2013. Sector-wide approaches (SWAps) in health: what have we learned? *Health Policy and Planning* 28(8), 884–90.

PLOS Medicine Editors. 2007. How is WHO responding to global public health threats? *PLOS Medicine* 4(5), e197.

Ravishankar N, Gubbins P, Cooley RJ *et al.* 2009. *Financing Global Health 2009: Tracking Development Assistance for Health.* Seattle, WA: Institute for Health Metrics and Evaluation, University of Washington.

Rifkin SB, Walt G. 1986. Why health improves: defining the issues concerning "comprehensive primary health care" and "selective primary health care." *Social Science and Medicine* 23(6), 559–66.

Sabatier P. 1988. An advocacy coalition framework of policy change and the role of policy orientated learning therein. *Policy Sciences* 21, 129–68.

Sabatier P (ed.) 2007. *Theories of the Policy Process*, 2nd edn. Boulder, CO: Westview Press.

Sabatier P, Jenkins-Smith HC. 1993. *Policy Change and Learning: An Advocacy Coalition Approach*. Boulder, CA: Westview Press.

Schlager E. 2007. A comparison of frameworks, theories, and models of policy processes. In Sabatier PA (ed.) *Theories of the Policy Process*, pp. 293–319. Boulder, CO: Westview Press.

Schneider H, Gilson L, Ogden J, Lush L, Walt G. 2006. Health systems and the implementation of disease programmes. *Global Public Health* 1(1), 49–64.

Sepúlveda J, Bustreo F, Tapia R et al. 2006. Improvement of child survival in Mexico: the diagonal approach. *Lancet* 368, 2017–27.

Shiffman J, Smith S. 2007. Generation of political priority for global health initiatives: a framework and case study of maternal mortality. *Lancet* 370, 1370–9.

Smith RA, Siplon PD. 2006. *Drugs into Bodies: Global AIDS Treatment Activism*. Westport, CT: Praeger Publishers.

Stuckler D, Nestle M. 2012. Big food, food systems, and global health. *PLOS Medicine* 9(6), e1001242.

Surjadjaja C, Mayhew SH. 2011. Can policy analysis theories predict and inform policy change? Reflections on the battle for legal abortion in Indonesia. *Health Policy and Planning* 26, 373–84.

Taylor AL, Dhillon IS. 2011. The Who Global Code of Practice on the International Recruitment of Health Personnel: the evolution of global health diplomacy. *Global Health Governance* 5(1).

Thompson GF. 2003. *Between Hierarchies and Markets: The Logic and Limits of Network Forms of Organization*. Oxford: Oxford University Press.

UNDP (United Nations Development Programme). 2012. *Risks, Rights and Health: Report of the Global Commission on HIV and the Law*. Geneva: UNDP.

UNSCN (United Nations Standing Committee on Nutrition) 2011. Nutrition and business: how to engage? *UNSCN News* 39.

Victora CG, Black R, Boerma J, Bryce J. 2011. Measuring impact in the Millennium Development Goal era and beyond: a new approach to large-scale effectiveness evaluations. *Lancet* 377, 85–95.

Walt G, Gilson L. 1994. Reforming the health sector in developing countries: the central role of policy analysis. *Health Policy Plan* 9(4), 353–70.

Walt G, Shiffman J, Schneider H, Murray SF, Brugha R, Gilson L. 2008. "Doing" health policy analysis: methodological and conceptual reflections and challenges. *Health Policy Plan* 23(5), 308–17.

WHO (World Health Organization), Positive Synergies Group. 2009. An assessment of interactions between global health initiatives and country health systems. *Lancet* 373(9681), 2137–69.

WHO (World Health Organization). 2010. *World Malaria Report 2010*. Geneva: WHO. http://www.who.int/malaria/world_malaria_report_2010/en/ (last accessed November 2013).

WHO/FAO (World Health Organization/Food and Agriculture Organization). 2003. *Diet, Nutrition and the Prevention of Chronic Diseases: Report of the WHO/FAO Expert Consultation*. WHO Technical Report Series. Geneva: WHO/FAO.

World Bank; Akin J, Birdsall N, de Ferranti D. 1987. *Financing Health Services in Developing Countries: An Agenda for Reform*. *World Bank Policy Study*. Washington, DC: World Bank.

Yamey G. 2002. WHO in 2002: have the latest reforms reversed WHO's decline? *BMJ* 325, 1107.

Chapter 2

Critical Reflections on Global Health Policy Formation: From Renaissance to Crisis

Sophie Harman

Abstract

Global health policy formation underwent a renaissance period from the late 1990s; however, in 2011, this renaissance underwent a period of crisis of purpose, leadership, and financing in which funding towards key diseases was cut, institutions such as the World Bank reduced their global health portfolio, and the World Health Organization was subject to continuous questions of reform and utility. This chapter explores the short- and long-term explanations for such a crisis of direction and financing and how they link to policy formation. In so doing it highlights issues of policy inertia and the paradox of success in policy formation, hierarchies within multisectoral decision-making, and the dominance of market-based strategies in developing policy. The chapter considers the role of intergovernmental organizations, aid donors, and emerging economies in policy formation while outlining three critical approaches to understanding health policy formation drawn from feminism, biopolitics, and historical materialism. The chapter concludes by offering several recommendations and key policy implications as a means of overcoming the reactionary, repetitive, results-orientated and raising-funds-based nature of global health policy formation.

The Handbook of Global Health Policy, First Edition. Edited by Garrett W. Brown, Gavin Yamey, and Sarah Wamala.
© 2014 John Wiley & Sons, Ltd. Published 2014 by John Wiley & Sons, Ltd.

Key Points

- Global health policy has gone from a renaissance to crisis over the last 20 years.
- Crisis in the short term can be explained by a lack of political will, changes in the global political economy, and the paradox of success.
- Crisis in the long term can be explained by problems with hierarchical forms of multisectoral decision-making, distorted partnerships, and the dominance of market-based principles to policy formation.
- Global health policy formation can be characterized by the four Rs: reaction, repetition, results, and raising funds.
- Critical approaches to global health highlight the utility of deconstructing the language of policy, looking at the power relations of context and who or what sets the agenda, and unraveling the influence of the market on global health issues.

Key Policy Implications

- Global health policy formation requires strong leadership that is able to separate policy from preoccupations with financing.
- The right to health, distributive justice, and equal access to primary healthcare must be at the cornerstone of health policy formation.
- Policy formation should be inverted so that local actors and their experiences have a direct impact on policy formation and implementation.

Introduction

The late 1990s saw the beginning of a renaissance period within global health. Key diseases such as HIV/AIDS were being placed at the heart of the political agenda of global agencies, new funding strategies and partnerships for promoting better health outcomes were being adopted in the United Nations (UN), and key individuals such as Jeffrey Sachs were teaming up with celebrities such as Bono to convene expert researchers and policy-makers to form strategic discussions, such as the Commission on Macroeconomics and Health of the World Health Organization (WHO). The result of these initiatives was large funding programs for key diseases, the formation of new finance mechanisms such as the Global Fund to Fight AIDS, Tuberculosis and Malaria (the Global Fund), and commitments from both the public and private sector to drive down the cost of treatment in developing countries. Combined, such activity suggested momentum within global health: it was finally occupying center stage in development debates, security agendas, and the personal agendas of wealthy philanthropists. This renaissance of global public health (now increasingly abbreviated to just global health to accommodate such private interests) suggests that policy-making and the global health agenda has worked. It has worked in getting the world to pay attention to issues of global health and it has worked in reversing the spread of diseases such as HIV/AIDS and polio. Yet emerging trends and unresolved tensions within global health policy-making suggest these slight gains will be relatively short-lived and that this period of renaissance has come to a point of crisis.

This chapter argues that problems in global health policy are not only emerging because of the ongoing financial crisis and turn to austerity by key health donors, but that they are symptomatic of issues regarding what actors inform policy and how. The chapter makes this argument by first outlining why the renaissance in global health is over and now entering into a period of crisis. It then explains how common problems of accountability and divisions between global agendas and national strategies have typically defined global health policy and in so doing have limited the effectiveness of global health and contributed to this crisis. Third, the chapter suggests that global health policy-making has come to rest on the four Rs – reaction, repetition, results, and raising funds – to the exclusion of politics and alternatives to the dominant liberal, market-based paradigm in which global health policy is made. Fourth, the chapter then outlines three critical lenses through which to understand health policy formation – biopolitics, historical materialism, and feminism – to highlight how such approaches unpack key assumptions about health and policy formation. Lastly, some recommendations are offered as to how to think differently about global health policy formation and overcome the causes of the crisis.

From Renaissance to Crisis

Global health governance underwent a renaissance from the late 1990s to 2010. This period saw a growth in investment for key health strategies (Harman 2012), the introduction of new actors, and the formation of new partnerships between the public and private sectors as a means of tackling old diseases such as malaria, and relatively new diseases, such as HIV/AIDS. Institutions like the World Bank developed billion dollar issue-specific health projects (World Bank 2007), bilateral donors such as USAID introduced multibillion dollar projects such as the President's Emergency Plan for AIDS Relief (PEPFAR) (PEPFAR 2012), and new philanthropic bodies such as the Bill and Melinda Gates Foundation have committed US$10 billion in vaccine development in an effort to eradicate polio and address common causes of child death in developing countries (BMGF 2012). In addition to the growth in financing, governments, the private sector, and civil society came together to form the Global Fund as a means to tackle what were then seen to be the biggest health concerns in developing countries and were committed to generate greater finance for global health from corporate forms of tax and social responsibility through initiatives such as UNITAID (UNITAID 2012). Ex-politicians such as Bill Clinton attempted to reduce the costs of some essential drugs and promote access to new products through the Clinton Global Health Access Initiative (CHAI) as part of his foundation (William J. Clinton Foundation 2012). Celebrities were keen to put their names to a range of health causes from infant mortality (footballer David Beckham as UNICEF Goodwill Ambassador) to malaria (actor David Arquette is an ambassador for Malaria No More!) to Stop TB (footballer Luis Figo) to maternal mortality (model Liya Kebede is WHO Goodwill Ambassador for maternal and child health). New actors in global health included both government and non-governmental actors on their boards and as recipients of aid money (Brown 2009; Harman 2010), and old actors such as the World Bank and WHO adopted operating principles of multisectoralism – the inclusion of state, non-state, local, national, regional, health-based, and non-health based actors in design and implementation of policy – in the delivery of flagship projects (Youde 2011; Harman 2012). This period was a renaissance in popular interest in global health not seen since the golden age of biomedical discovery in the late 1800s and the idealism of liberal institution building at the end of the Second World War.

Why this renaissance occurred can be understood by a number of different factors coming together at a similar time. First, the renaissance was a response to the stringent structural adjustment programs of the 1980s and early 1990s that reduced investment in global health spending and generated a range of criticism from practitioners (Farmer 2005), researchers (Cheru 2002; Thomas and Weber 2004), and organizations (WHO 2009) working in global health and development. Such widespread criticism suggested a need to rethink not only the type of policies developed for global health, but who is involved in policy-making and how inclusive it is. Second, policy focus on key diseases was in direct reaction to the accelerated spread of HIV/AIDS in sub-Saharan Africa, the continuing presence of malaria, and the resurgence of tuberculosis in the 1990s. Advocacy groups such as the Treatment Action Campaign (TAC) in South Africa responded to the growth of diseases such as HIV/AIDS by confronting stigma, highlighting the socioeconomic impact of the disease, and asserting the rights of people living with HIV to access treatment (Friedman and Mottiar 2005; TAC 2012). The third explanation is that intergovernmental bodies such as the World Bank and WHO had come to highlight the need to associate health concerns with development issues as part of their wider agenda. The World Bank made such a link through the positioning of health and diseases like HIV/AIDS at the forefront of its 1997 comprehensive development framework (CDF) agenda and by stressing the need to set up independent sectors within the Bank to address specific health issues alongside the Health, Nutrition, and Population Department (World Bank 1998). The basis of the Bank's commitment to health was established in the *World Development Report 1993: Investing in Health* that promoted the need for country-based growth, cost-effective spending on health, and the need for diversity in the financing and delivery of healthcare (World Bank 1993). The WHO had long recognized the relationship between socioeconomic development, rights, and access to health since its founding (Lee 2009) but reasserted this link through the 2001 report of the Commission on Macroeconomics and Health in its recognition of the relationship between health, economic development and global security, and the need for good governance (WHO

2001). The movement towards associating global health with development culminated in the inclusion of three stand-alone health objectives within the UN Millennium Development Goals (MDGs): goal 4, child health; goal 5, maternal health; and goal 6, combat HIV/AIDS and other diseases (see Chapter 28). The positioning of the three health goals within the MDGs was the most effective tool of global health policy of the late 1990s. Having clear goals that Member States of the UN were committed to achieving provided the impetus for the formation of actors such as the Global Fund and multilateral and bilateral aid commitments. The fourth explanation for such renaissance was the framing of a number of health issues – pandemic flu, HIV/AIDS – as threats to state security (see Chapter 15). The 2000 UN Security Council Resolution 1308 was the first time the Council discussed a health issue in the context of global peace and security. The presence of HIV/AIDS on the security agenda of the UN was heightened by the General Assembly Special Session (UNGASS) declaration on the disease. Arguably, for some, such inclusion was the precursor to HIV/AIDS exceptionalism and the distortion in money and attention attributed to AIDS at the expense of other health issues (McInnes and Rushton 2010). The fifth explanation is the growth of private philanthropy in the United States or what Bishop and Green (2010) call "philanthrocapitalism," which through initiatives such as the Bill and Melinda Gates Foundation's Global Health Program has earmarked health as a key site in need of financing and innovation. This has not only generated unprecedented funds towards global health initiatives, and impacted on how policy is delivered, but has helped to capture the public's attention towards global health.

The result of such a renaissance has been a year-on-year increase in total spending on global health between 2000 and 2010 (Harman 2012). The number of new HIV infections has declined by 21% since 1997 and 6.6 million people out of the 14.2 million people eligible are now taking antiretroviral treatment (UNAIDS 2011). By 2010, 18 million people received bed nets for malaria, an increase of 16.65 million people since 2006 (UN 2010). Multiple new community health centers and devolved health systems have been introduced to enable the poor in rural areas to access basic health services. According to the Bill and Melinda Gates Foundation (BMGF 2009) death from measles has reduced by 75% since 2000 and the number of polio cases has decreased by 99%. Such results suggest that the policy formation and ideas that underpin it have been a success. For some, global health policy formation may not be perfect, but is a good example of how public and private interests can work together, how economic resources and political will can be mobilized behind specific issues, and how some of the wealthiest people and lead researchers can combine to generate positive results (see Chapter 27). However, this only tells part of the story, particularly the happier part, as in effect the period of renaissance is coming to an end.

The continuing global financial events of the eurozone crisis, the uprisings in Egypt, Tunisia, and Libya, the conflict in Ivory Coast, and the death of Osama Bin Laden made 2011 a significant year in international relations. It was also a decisive year for global health. After a year of rumors and accusation, the Global Fund announced in November 2011 that it would suspend round 11 of funds (Global Fund 2011; see also Chapter 28). The WHO continued to face a decline in funding (Global Health Watch 2011) with cuts to budgetary support in areas such as essential medicines (Boseley 2012) as well as job losses. The World Bank no longer plans to fund stand-alone health projects – the current funding portfolio for the Africa region alone suggests the institution has refocused its attention to issues of infrastructure – and most of its large disease-specific programs have come to an end. Domestic health systems underwent increased scrutiny under the need to limit their costs in countries such as the United Kingdom and Spain. HIV prevalence in one of the countries hardest hit by the financial crisis, Greece, has risen by 52% since 2010 (Kentikelenis *et al.* 2011). Despite a large number of actors and different sources of funding, for some it would seem that the only show in the global health town is the Bill and Melinda Gates Foundation. This may be good for putting global health policy into practice, but less good for policy formation, as the Foundation has been subjected to increased criticism with regard to its funding portfolio, accountability structures, and focus on performance-based funding (McCoy *et al.* 2009). If 1997–2010 marked a period of renaissance, 2011 marked the turning point towards crisis – where funding was cut, leadership and strategic direction was lacking, and private wealth and personal interests dominated. This is not just down to changes in the global political economy, but can also be explained by a critical assessment of policy-making and the governance of global health during the previous period of apparent renaissance.

How can the Crisis in Global Health be Explained?

The basic explanation for the crisis in global health is that the money ran out and donors, politicians, and the public lost interest (see Chapters 14 and 21). The ongoing financial crisis of 2008 has led to fiscal austerity in overseas aid from Europe and North America. With tightened public spending and national budget cuts, international development aid seems like an obvious area for savings. Some countries such as the United Kingdom have ringfenced development spending as exempt from wider public budget cuts, but in so doing have also concentrated their priorities away from health to other areas and have been criticized for short-term interventions by key partners (Elliott 2010). Reduced bilateral aid can also impact on a reduction in states meeting target commitments to intergovernmental organizations and multilateral aid strategies. Multilateral funding bodies such as the World Bank have shifted their focus towards bigger, better projects that are less issue specific (see, for example, World Bank 2011). Beyond finance, uprisings in Africa and the Middle East, and the eurozone crisis, have pushed global health off the political agenda as politicians, agenda setters, and those in control of the global health budget have little space, time, or will to support these initiatives.

The problem of political will, however, goes beyond competing claims on politicians' time in the international arena. Part of the problem is the paradox of perceived success. A key way of securing political will and public support is by presenting specific issues as a crisis in need of attention or a threat to state security (see Chapter 15). Diseases such as HIV/AIDS are arguably seen as less of a global threat since trends in the epidemic began to reverse (UNAIDS 2011). With diminished threat comes diminished concern to control, prevent, or address specific health issues. There are multiple important issues that threaten the physical and mental being of people around the world, acutely in developing countries, yet slight changes to the availability of drugs, declining prevalence rates in diseases such as HIV, increased wealth in middle-income countries such as India and South Africa, has led to shifting perceptions of how acute these issues actually are and a reassessment of the role of external aid in financing interventions. The problem being that when donors, the general public, and political leaders perceive global health policy as a success, there is a paradox that less money and support is seen as being needed, whereas if anything more is needed. For example, the fights against both malaria and tuberculosis have seen boosts in efforts and progress when political will is forthcoming, only for them to be reversed once progress is made and the issues become sidelined (Harman 2012). Policy-makers have to strike the balance between the paradox of success and crisis fatigue among donors.

The paradox of success points to a wider problem with the influence of finance on policy formation and the current crossroads in health financing. The economic growth of China, India, and many African countries – such as South Africa, Botswana, and Namibia (Economist 2011) – challenges their position as aid recipients rather than aid givers. Traditional international aid donors in Western Europe and North America (Development Assistance Committee (DAC) members of the Organisation for Economic Co-operation and Development (OECD)) that have experienced negative or stalled growth may question why they continue to give aid to those countries that have greater, and in some cases accelerated, rates of economic growth. Many of these growing economies have started to develop their own international aid portfolios (Grimm 2011). Countries such as China have a history of medical interventions in countries in sub-Saharan Africa, specifically towards malaria programs (Anshan 2011), with such a presence likely to increase. However should DAC countries withdraw funding before alternative sources of aid and public spending are developed within these growing economies, systems of global health will collapse further. Moreover, the mechanisms of aid delivery developed under the aegis of South–South cooperation by such growing economies has faced increased questions with regard to transparency, disclosure, and aid effectiveness in regards to country-owned development strategies (Grimm 2011). Global health is not only at a crucial crossroads between sustaining support from more traditional donors and eliciting greater funding from emerging economies, but also has to ensure that policy on transparency, effectiveness, and country ownership is not compromised by new aid donors such as China.

The problem of who funds global health (and how) offers a different explanation as to why global health policy is in crisis. To explain these problems it is important to consider two phenomena within the global health renaissance period: the rise of multisectoralism and partnerships (see Chapter 27). As stated, the purpose of multisectoralism was to involve multiple actors in the policy formation and implementation of global health projects, with a specific emphasis on including participants from the non-health sector. Such multisectoral approaches to health policy were applied at the global, national, and local/regional levels of governance with the purpose of making global policy-making more responsive to, and reflective of, the local community, and in so doing more accountable to the people affected by global health policies. Despite rhetorical and financial commitment to such inclusion, multisectoralism generated a system of hierarchy between actors that favored the private sector and more established non-governmental organizations, blurred the lines of accountability, confused participants, and conflated issues (Harman 2010). At the institutional level, state interests continued to dominate the views of non-state partners and voting cleavages within organizations such as the Global Fund began to emerge (Brown 2009). As such, multisectoralism generated the dual problem of tokenistic inclusion of civil society organizations whilst absorbing criticism of the structures and processes of global health policy-making by including them within the system. In effect, full multisectoralism only exists at the implementation level with decision-making resting at the global level (Harman 2010): in other words civil society organizations implement projects on the ground and policy is decided by intergovernmental organizations and key private interests at the global level. The consequence of this for global health policy is the shrinking of space for alternatives and the reassertion of hierarchy in policy-making. Such hierarchy distorts the lines of who is accountable for what in global health, and instead of enhancing democracy in global health policy-making, restricts it.

The issue of public and private provision of healthcare is not new to global health and has been at the center of debate since market reform agendas permeated western and global health strategies from the late 1970s. The emergence of multisectoralism and public–private partnerships sought to resolve tensions in means of approach and purpose between these sectors by involving actors in institutional forms of policy formation, strategy, and co-financing (see Chapter 27). The risk being that embedding partnership can either promote solutions or embed tensions. In practice, partnerships did neither – instead they embedded a market-orientated approach to global health through principles of innovation, performance-based funding, and a shift away from social and public health policy to management strategies and business plans (Harman 2014). Whilst government agencies and principles of sovereignty remain central to the working operations and direction of the new partnerships, the approaches to governance they take and the solutions to the problems of health delivery remain linked to private sector commitments to efficiency, low cost delivery, and maximum profit (Harman 2014). Profit in this area is financial with regard to the money saved by lowering the cost of delivery and the maximum output or performance ratings for a specific initiative. However, performance-based indicators can overlook or sideline the causes of positive health outcomes that are tricky to measure, and ignore complex issues of social policy and the socioeconomic drivers of ill health that are difficult to address (Harman 2014). Moreover, such market-orientated principles are not the same as rights-based approaches to health, which is often the starting point for understanding global public health.

Market-orientated approaches and rights-based approaches are not necessarily diametrical, yet finding a compromise between the business sector and public health sector has been difficult (see Chapter 21). This has been a tricky compromise for the WHO to strike since its formation (Lee 2009) and is in part why the WHO is undergoing threats to its existence. The WHO needs to diversify funding sources to balance its budget and secure funds for neglected areas of global health but in so doing opens up policy-making to a variety of different actors with their own agendas. On the one hand this promotes a plurality of ideas, increases the pool of finance available for health, may refresh the WHO's approach, and offers new insights into old problems; on the other it may overlook any progress made by the WHO and assert a reform agenda that is contrary to the rights-based, accessible health mandate of the organization.

The WHO's mandate has been challenged by the growth of specialized health agencies such as UNAIDS, partnerships such as the Stop TB partnership, mission creep by the World Bank, the spending portfolio of the Global Fund, and the financial clout of the Bill and Melinda Gates Foundation. Whilst each of these agencies has close working relationships with the WHO, the organization has not been adept at exerting its own influence over these bodies. The main reason has been a lack of funding. A further reason has been leadership tensions within the WHO during the late 1990s which led to a degree of institutional statis and lack of direction at a crucial stage of the institution's development (Lee 2009; Lisk 2009). Margaret Chan has been seen as a relatively popular leader, both within and outside of the WHO, who is aware of the challenges facing the organization, yet in a bind as to how to address them without alienating core sources of financial aid to global health (Lee 2009).

The crisis of global health policy-making can thus be explained in the short term by problems within the global political economy and in the long term by ongoing tensions between the private and public sectors that have not been addressed through partnership. The net result for global health policy has been reduced to the four Rs: reactionary, repetitive, results-orientated and raising funds. Global hierarchy leads to repetition in the type of policy applied to country contexts. Dependence on finance makes health agendas reactionary to donors and changes in the global political economy and develops a preoccupation with raising funds rather than formulating policy. Performance-based funding and the need for efficiency create policy orientated on results set by donors.

Critical Understandings of Policy Formation

Health policy formation is commonly understood in a liberal, functionalist manner. As Chapter 1 suggests, policy-making is often seen to occur through a rational system of issue identification, response, and utility maximization where actors try to design policy to benefit the majority of a population as well as realizing their own objectives. This pragmatic, functionalist approach explains processes, but does not understand the politics of health formation and in many ways embeds the four Rs of health policy formation. Critical approaches to global health help us unpack the association between policy-making and health finance, the tensions between who makes policy, the global structural dynamics in which policy-making takes place, the language and assumptions of policy formation, and the politics of policy beyond consensus building and rational choice models of decision-making. Critical approaches can refer to a wide range of understandings and explanations of global health that are often quite divergent and based on fundamentally different epistemological and ontological positions. These approaches are often grouped together as critical because of their divergence from or critique of mainstream, liberal approaches to understanding policy formation, and/or for some, their lack of solution-orientated understanding or applicability to enhance policy change. This chapter acknowledges the fundamental differences between and within such approaches, but for the purposes of ease of exploration will apply historical materialist, biopolitical, and feminist lenses to global health policy formation and how we can critically understand the problems of reaction, repetition, results-orientation, and raising funds. What follows is not a comprehensive account of critical approaches but provides a general guide and introduction to understanding such approaches as a basis for further research.

Historical materialist approaches encapsulate a wide range of Marxist approaches that not only pinpoint how capitalism impacts on all aspects of life, including the provision, delivery, and consumption of healthcare, but seek to change such a capitalist system and to confront how capitalism is seen as the dominant ordering principle of social life. Applied to understanding global health policy formation, such approaches would argue that policy is made in the interests of capital and the embedding of capitalism within multiple aspects of state, society, and individual behavior. Hence policy is formed to manage the growth of capitalist expansion and embed market principles within such policy and practice. Global health policy ultimately acts in the interest of capital but also in that of the capitalist bourgeoisie who exploit the poor or the proletariat. Such an approach helps deconstruct the role of capitalism in shaping policy formation and the construction of a dominant market-based paradigm in which policy-making is made. In so doing, it challenges the assumption that market approaches and economic globalization are good for global health and questions the underpinnings of the private and public sectors' interests in health. This is particularly relevant to questions about the relationship between trade and health, pharmaceutical companies, notions of philanthrocapitalism, and the promotion of private sector principles through state partnerships with private companies. Historical materialism can also be used to challenge the idea of multisectoralism and civil society participation. For Marx, civil society represented the site of "crass materialism" in which individuals operate. This area of civic activity is increasingly defined by the interest of capital and thus the state (Bottomore *et al.* 1983). Hence multisectoralism would be an embedding of state or capitalist-defined activity. From a Gramscian perspective, multisectoralism suggests an embedding of the prevailing political order rather than a challenge to it, and hence any counterforce or counter-hegemony would occur outside such frameworks. Multisectoralism thus is a form of neutralizing discontent and absorbing resistance.

Marxist ideas of global health policy formation tend to underpin research into the relationship between neoliberalism and the reform of health policy from the mid 1980s onwards. Despite not being avowedly Marxist or drawn from historical materialist approaches, such research has been the cornerstone of much critical global public health theory that has sought to criticize and deconstruct the role of the market in global health (Labonté and Schrecker 2007; Labonté and Torgerson 2008; see also Chapter 21), structural adjustment reform, and evidence for the effectiveness of private sector provision (Brugha and Zwi 2002). In addition, historical materialism has a strong presence within medical sociology, particularly the work of Ivan Illich (1976). The application of historical materialist thought to understanding global health is thus quite common in research, yet critical engagement with such relationships remains at the sideline of the practice of policy formation.

The work of Michel Foucault has framed much critical discussion on global health projects and policies and offers a different critical take on policy formation to historical materialist approaches. The application of Foucault's biopolitics as the extension of political control to individual bodies suggests global health policy formation is about controlling, manipulating, and changing individuals' bodies and existence in a way that responds to changes in the broader population (Foucault 1976). Control is achieved through surveillance and the changing practice of behavior through the promotion of a specific discourse and specialized knowledge to define what is and what is not good behavior or practice. As such, global health policy formation seen through the lens of biopolitics produces and promotes specific rationalities of behavior based on a certain type of knowledge that then conditions the bodies of individuals within a population. Applied to contemporary policy formation, the critique relates to what knowledge is produced, how, and to which bodies and populations it controls. In addition, such a lens questions the use of surveillance practices and the assumptions that underpin their use and application, and problematizes the absorption of common "truths" and claims to knowledge within global health policy formation. Such approaches have been applied to understanding women's bodies, health institutions (Bashford 2006), population control, the global response to HIV/AIDS (Elbe 2005; Elbe 2008), and pandemic flu outbreaks in some detail. Taken together such studies suggest several common assertions to understanding global health policy. First is the need to deconstruct the claims to scientific truth and knowledge in global health policy formation to see what (or who) they represent, and who is being controlled. Second, the forms and justifications for surveillance strategies should be closely interrogated to see how they control specific bodies and populations. Third, what constitutes good or risky behavior, why, and how this is communicated needs to be considered. Fourth, functional approaches to global health policy formation should be deconstructed to explore the biopolitical dimensions of discourses and the production of truth, assumptions on risk, and the reproduction of certain rationalities.

Feminist approaches to understanding global health policy formation cut across historical materialist, biopolitical, and liberal understandings with feminist variants of these approaches. The common assertion for such an approach, however, is the need to see women and recognize gender in policy-making, implementation, and outcome (Murphy 2006). In current policy formation the issue of women is seen as having paramount importance for the realization of global health strategies (World Bank 2010). Yet in practice this has translated to leveraging money to support maternal and child health campaigns, including female quotas in decision-making processes, and measuring the rates of illness and burden among women (Harman 2012). Feminist scholars argue that global health policy needs to go beyond these efforts to also recognize the role of women in unpaid care roles, specifically at the community health level, the different experiences of women in accessing and receiving healthcare, women's bodies as a site of political contestation (Einstein and Shildrick 2009) and the socioeconomic factors that determine the context in which women experience healthcare and engage in social reproduction (Doyal 1995), and how economic crises impact on the health of women disproportionately to that of men (Mohindra *et al.* 2011). As such, health policy formation needs to not only build in strategies aimed at women, but to also consider the gendered dimension and impacts of policy and difference in women. Functionalist approaches to policy formation do not acknowledge difference or complexity in context. The problem of recognizing difference between people has been a key limitation to global health policy formation, which tends to be homogenous and repetitive in different countries and contexts.

Taken together, critical approaches to policy-making suggest a variety of ways to rethink policy formation and intent through: (i) the deconstruction of the language of policy; (ii) looking at power relations of who (dominant states or institutions) or what (norms, ideas, or capital) sets the agenda; and (iii) the environment in which policy-making takes place. In so doing such critical approaches allow us to unravel the influence of the market on global health issues and the framing of policy and specific outcomes and to who or what they benefit. Hence, when unraveling the shift from renaissance to crisis in the last 15 years of health policy, it is important to not only consider the functional operations of how policy was made, why, and with what impact, but to assess the power dimensions external and internal to these functions. Questioning the politics of health – how the balance between personal freedom and the promotion of health for all intersect with policy and distributive social justice; how justice and rights operate within market-based solutions to global health problems; and how inequality in access to healthcare and who is responsible for providing healthcare – helps us deconstruct problems of policy-making. Policy-making is less about functional amalgamations of actors and ideas in the process of *doing* global health policy, and more about the politics of global health: who decides what, when, how, and why and to who's benefit. Thinking about these questions will not solve all of the problems in global health but it will help pinpoint asymmetric power relations, opportunities for improvement, and space for reflection of meaning and purpose behind policy assertions.

Overcoming the Four Rs: Recommendations

Overcoming problems of reaction, repetition, results, and raising funds requires the following. The first is strong leadership to articulate a short- and medium-term vision, galvanizing support for such a vision both inside and outside an institution, and diversifying the funding base of that organization. Such diversification of funding cannot, however, contradict the strategic vision of the institution or the leadership. Strong leadership requires the building of coalitions within the broad and expansive global health community and relying less on donors to outline policy objectives. Hence those articulating global health policy must be separate to those who fund health policy. This is not easily achieved, as donors often want to know where their money is going and private philanthropists seek to invest in those causes they deem to be the most worthwhile. Actors should play to their strengths and assert their experience, expertise, and legitimacy. Global policy-making needs to be less driven by global finance for health. Money is intrinsic for the delivery of drugs, education campaigns, medical supplies, construction of health centers, health worker training, and a whole host of issues. However, the need to generate, maintain, and increase funds should exist separately to policy-making, otherwise policy-making is more reactionary and less visionary and strategic.

Second, key principles of public health – the right to health, distributive justice, questions of equality in access to healthcare, and how different people experience good or bad health – must be re-engaged with as a matter of policy practice (see Chapters 4, 10, 12, 25, and 28). Results-based frameworks and the need for a return on investment should not exclude such commitments and principles. One way of reintroducing these themes is to bring the public back into discussions on global health and making the private – including philanthropic organizations – subject to the same accountability and transparency structures as public bodies, whether governmental or intergovernmental. Whilst private actors may not be spending taxpayers' money, they have considerable influence on the health of the world's population. The plurality of actors and ideas is a unique and positive component of global health, yet such plurality needs to translate to decision- and policy-making and be held to account.

Third, global health policy must be designed in-country, by the government, as the elected government through public engagement and discussion sees fit. Global institutions such as the World Bank and the Global Fund should provide support through finance and as such can make recommendations, but such recommendations should not form the basis of conditional lending. Country-based agendas will make health strategies more context-specific, will reduce the burden on state-based health agencies that often have to juggle competing donor demands, and will avoid repetition in the formation of health policy. Focusing on country-based strategies will invert current structures of policy-making so that implementers of policy at the local level become the policy formulators and those who currently make policy at the global level concentrate on working with countries on effective implementation.

Conclusions

Global health policy underwent a period of renaissance from the late 1990s to 2010 that culminated in a crisis of funding, attention, and political will in 2011. This crisis in global health can be explained in the short term by a lack of attention or political will to address health concerns arising from more immediate crises in the economy and a lack of fear of health threats. Lack of political will has led to a decline in public spending on health and a crossroads in health financing where new actors are yet to come forward and the gap is filled by private finance. Efforts to generate political will remain dormant as the WHO continues to be subjected to questions of reform and other multilateral agencies retreat from health-specific interventions. Embedding such problems are the shortcomings in multisectoral participation, market-based strategies, and global centers of decision-making that lack accountability – typifying the last 10 years of global health policy-making. The result of which is that global health policy remains hierarchical, designed at the global level by those with the most money and flexibility in how it is spent. Policy is based on principles of maximum return and performance-based funding with only minimal feedback from local communities, patient groups, and those affected by the end result of global policy-making. Failure to separate policy-making from financing, invert hierarchies of decision-making, and exert leadership, will result in global health policy-making continuing to be characterized by the four Rs: reactionary, repetitive, results-orientated, and raising funds.

Key Reading

Elbe S. 2005. AIDS, security, biopolitics. *International Relations* 19(4), 403–19.

Global Health Watch. 2011. *Global Health Watch 3* (and other previous editions). London: Zed Books.

Green J, Labonté R (eds). 2008. *Critical Perspectives in Public Health*. London: Routledge.

Harman S. 2009. Fighting HIV and AIDS: reconfiguring the state? *Review of African Political Economy* 36(121), 353–67.

Illich I. 1976. *Medical Nemesis: The Expropriation of Health*. New York: Pantheon Books.

Kay A, Williams OD (eds). 2009. *Global Health Governance: Crisis, Institutions and Political Economy*. London: Palgrave MacMillan.

McCoy D, Chand S, Sridhar D. 2009. Global health funding: how much, where it comes from, and where it goes. *Health Policy and Planning* 24, 407–17.

References

Anshan L. 2011. *Chinese Medical Co-operation in Africa: with Special Emphasis on the Medical Teams and Anti-malaria Campaign. Nordiska Afrikainstitutet Discussion Paper 52.* Uppsala: Nordiska Afrikainstitutet.

Bashford A. 2006. Global biopolitics and the history of world health. *History of the Human Sciences* 19(1), 67–88.

Bishop M, Green M. 2010. *Philanthrocapitalism: How Giving can Save the World*. London: A & C Black Publishers.

BMGF (Bill and Melinda Gates Foundation). 2009. Progress Towards Immunization. http://www.gatesfoundation.org/livingproofproject/Documents/progress-towards-immunization.pdf (last accessed November 2013).

BMGF (Bill and Melinda Gates Foundation). 2012. *Decade of vaccines: why we're committing $10 billion*. http://www.gatesfoundation.org/Media-Center/Press-Releases/2010/01/Bill-and-Melinda-Gates-Pledge-$10-Billion-in-Call-for-Decade-of-Vaccines (last accessed December 2013).

Boseley S. 2012. WHO funding shortage risks harming essential medicines work. *Guardian* January 13. http://www.guardian.co.uk/society/sarah-boseley-global-health/2012/jan/13/pharmaceuticals-industry-world-health-organisation (last accessed November 2013).

Bottomore T, Harris L, Kiernan VG, Miliband R. 1983. *A Dictionary of Marxist Thought*. Oxford: Blackwell Publishers.

Brown GW. 2009. Multisectoralism, participation and stakeholder effectiveness: increasing the role of non-state actors in the Global Fund to Fight AIDS, Tuberculosis and Malaria. *Global Governance* 15(2), 169–77.

Brugha R, and Zwi A. 2002. Global approaches to private sector provision: where is the evidence? In Lee K, Buse K, Fustukian S (eds) *Health Policy in a Globalising World*, pp. 63–77. Cambridge: Cambridge University Press.

Cheru F. 2002. Debt, adjustment and the politics of effective response to HIV/AIDS in Africa. *Third World Quarterly* 23(2), 299–312.

Doyal L. 1995. *What Makes Women Sick: Gender and the Political Economy of Health*. Basingstoke: Macmillan.

Economist. 2011. Africa's hopeful economies: the sun shines bright. Economist December 3. http://www.economist.com/node/21541008 (last accessed November 2013).

Elbe S. 2005. AIDS, security, biopolitics. *International Relations* 19(4), 403–19.

Elbe S. 2008. Risking lives: AIDS, security and the three concepts of risk. *Security Dialogue* 29 (2–3).

Elliott L. 2010. Andrew Mitchell soothes charities' fears over planned DFID cuts. *Guardian* August 25. http://www.guardian.co.uk/business/2010/aug/25/andrew-mitchell-spending-cuts-aid-agencies (last accessed November 2013).

Einstein G, Shildrick M. 2009. The post conventional body: re-theorising women's health. *Social Science and Medicine* 69(2), 293–300.

Farmer P. 2005. *Pathologies of Power: Health, Human Rights and the New War in the Poor*. London: University of California Press.

Foucault M. 1976. *The History of Sexuality: Volume I: an Introduction*. London: Penguin.

Friedman S, Mottiar S. 2005. A rewarding engagement? The Treatment Action Campaign and the politics of HIV/AIDS. *Politics and Society* 33(4), 511–65.

Global Fund. 2011. Board decision: options for modification of the application, renewal and approval processes for new and existing investments. 25th Board Meeting, Accra, Ghana, November 21–25, 2011. Board Decision GF/B25/8.

Global Health Watch. 2011. *Global Health Watch 3*. London: Zed Books.

Grimm S. 2011. *Transparency of Chinese Aid: An Analysis of the Published Information on Chinese External Financial Flows*. University of Stellenbosch: Centre for Chinese Studies. http://www.ccs.org.za/wp-content/uploads/2011/09/Transparency-of-Chinese-Aid_final-for-print.pdf (last accessed November 2013).

Harman S. 2010. *The World Bank and HIV/AIDS: Setting a Global Agenda*. Abingdon: Routledge.

Harman S. 2012. *Global Health Governance*. Abingdon: Routledge.

Harman S. 2014. Innovation, multi-sectoral governance and the limits of rebranded privatisation in public health. In Payne A, Phillips N (eds) *The Handbook of the Political Economy of Governance*. Cheltenham: Edward Elgar Publishing.

Illich I. 1976. *Medical Nemesis: The Expropriation of Health*. New York: Pantheon Books.

Kentikelenis A, Karanikolos M, Papanicolos I, Basu S, McKee M, Stuckler D. 2011. Health effects of the financial crisis: omens of a Greek tragedy. *Lancet* 378(9801), 1457–8.

Labonté R, Schrecker T. 2007. Globalization and the social determinants of health: the role of the global marketplace. *Globalization and Health* 3(6), 1–17.

Labonté R, and Torgerson R. 2008. Interrogating globalisation, health and development. In Green J, Labonté R (eds) *Critical Perspectives in Public Health*, pp. 162–79. Abingdon: Routledge.

Lee K. 2009. *The World Health Organisation*. Abingdon: Routledge.

Lisk F. 2009. *Global Institutions and the HIV/AIDS Epidemic*. Abingdon: Routledge.

McCoy D, Kembhavi G, Patel J, Luintel A. 2009. The Bill and Melinda Gates Foundation's grant-making program for global health. *Lancet* 373, 1645–53.

McInnes C, Rushton S. 2010. HIV, AIDS, and security: where are we now? *International Affairs* 86, 225–45.

Mohindra K, Labonté R, Spitzer D. 2011. The global financial crisis: whither women's health? *Critical Public Health* 21(3), 273–87.

Murphy C. 1996. Seeing women, recognizing gender, recasting international relations. *International Organization* 50(3), 513–38.

PEPFAR (President's Emergency Plan for AIDS Relief). 2012. *About PEPFAR*. http://www.pepfar.gov/about/index.htm (last accessed November 2013).

TAC (Treatment Action Campaign). 2012. TAC's *campaigns*. http://www.tac.org.za/community/node/1983 (last accessed November 2013).

Thomas C, and Weber M. 2004. The politics of global health governance: whatever happened to "Health for all by the year 2007"? *Global Governance* 10(2), 187–205.

UN (United Nations). 2010. MDG *Monitor: combat HIV/AIDS, malaria and other diseases*. http://www.mdgmonitor.org/goal6.cfm (last accessed November 2013).

UNAIDS. 2011. *2011 World AIDS Day Report*. Geneva: UNAIDS.

UNITAID. 2012. *Innovative Financing to Shape Markets for HIV/AIDS*, Malaria and Tuberculosis. http://www.unitaid.eu/en/about/innovative-financing-mainmenu-105 (last accessed November 2013).

WHO (World Health Organization). 2001. *Macroeconomics and Health: Investing in Health for Economic Development*. Report of the WHO Commission on Macroeconomics and Health. Geneva: WHO.

WHO (World Health Organization), Maximizing Positive Synergies Collaborative Group. 2009. An assessment of interactions between global health initiatives and country health systems. *Lancet* 373, 2137–69.

William J. Clinton Foundation. 2012. *Access Initiative*. http://www.clintonfoundation.org/our-work/clinton-health-access-initiative (accessed December 2013).

World Bank. 1993. *World Development Report 1993: Investing in Health*. Washington, DC: World Bank.

World Bank. 1998. *Comprehensive Development Framework*. http://web.worldbank.org/WBSITE/EXTERNAL/PROJECTS/0,,contentMDK:20120725~menuPK:41393~pagePK:41367~piPK:51533~theSitePK:40941,00.html (last accessed November 2013).

World Bank. 2007. *The Africa Multi-Country AIDS Program: Results of the World Bank's Response to a Development Crisis*. Washington, DC: World Bank.

World Bank. 2010. *Better Health for Women and Families: The World Bank's Reproductive Health Action Plan 2010–2015*. Washington, DC: World Bank.

World Bank (Africa Region). 2011. *Africa's Future and the World Bank's Support to It*. Washington, DC: World Bank.

Youde J. 2011. The Clinton Foundation and global health governance. In Rushton S, Williams OD (eds) *Partnerships and Foundations in Global Health Governance*, pp. 164–83. London: Ashgate.

Chapter 3

Contemporary Global Health Governance: Origins, Functions, and Challenges

Rajaie Batniji and Francisco Songane

Abstract

"Global health governance" (GHG) is shorthand for the rules, norms, and formal institutions that mediate and facilitate international interactions related to health. These mediated interactions are more effective than direct state-to-state interactions at empowering scientists and weaker states. GHG makes international health financing, regulation, and cooperative research possible. Such activities, especially international financing, have grown rapidly since 2000. In recent years, several different frameworks have shaped the selection of global health priorities, from a "health for all" framework, to the global burden of disease and the Millennium Development Goals. These frameworks have shaped the aims and the priorities for GHG. In this chapter, we give an overview of recent developments in GHG. We also argue that the benefits to scientists and weak states that have distinguished GHG are under threat from efforts to dismantle equity in international institutions, the exclusion of poor countries from global health decision-making, and efforts to privatize global health.

The Handbook of Global Health Policy, First Edition. Edited by Garrett W. Brown, Gavin Yamey, and Sarah Wamala.
© 2014 John Wiley & Sons, Ltd. Published 2014 by John Wiley & Sons, Ltd.

Key Points

- "Global health governance" (GHG) is shorthand for the rules, norms, and formal institutions that mediate and facilitate international interactions related to health.
- These mediated interactions are more effective than direct state-to-state interactions in empowering scientists and weaker states.
- Functions of GHG include international health financing (now exceeding US$25 billion a year), regulation, and cooperative research, all of which have seen growth in recent years.
- The World Health Organization's (WHO) egalitarian one-country, one-vote system, where key policy decisions were to be made at the World Health Assembly (WHA), have historically allowed the priorities of developing nations to shape the global health agenda, even when these priorities were at odds with those of the richest nations.
- Recent trends in GHG – such as a reduced focus on equity, the marginalization of science, the prioritization of donor concerns, and the rise of privatization – threaten the benefits to scientists and weak states that have distinguished GHG.

Key Policy Implications

- In order to address unanticipated challenges and to establish lasting progress in global health, it is essential to revitalize the democratic decision-making processes that are crucial to empowering science and giving voice to poor countries.
- Increases in global health financing and new efforts at international regulation must be based on a process that prioritizes science and the views of poor countries.

What is Global Health Governance?

"Global health governance" (GHG) is shorthand for the rules, norms, and formal institutions that mediate and facilitate international interactions related to health. As the governance literature stems from political science, it is useful to further clarify our use of the term "institutions." While political economists often use "institutions" to refer to the full range of informal rules, norms, and formal institutions, we use the term here to refer only to formal international institutions, including international organizations and laws (North 1991).

While the phrase "global health governance" has recently caught on among academic researchers and, to a more limited extent, within the policy community, these interactions are not new. The renewed interest in GHG stems from the fact that these longstanding interactions have recently increased in intensity, frequency, and importance. The result is that some of the inequities and inefficiencies in GHG have become more obvious, in turn creating demands for reform.

In this chapter, we consider the functions of GHG and the challenges we face in optimizing international rules, norms, and formal institutions to create healthier societies. Our analysis is focused disproportionately on the impacts that GHG has on poor countries because their citizens have more at stake with international interactions relating to health.

What Purpose does Global Health Governance Serve?

An alternative to international interactions on health that are mediated by rules, norms, and international institutions are unmediated state-to-state interactions. Mediated interactions have two key advantages for persons whose primary concern is health. First, they can empower scientists and experts and facilitate discussion among them. Second, they can empower weaker states in a manner than unmediated interactions could not. While both of these benefits have been realized to some extent, they are presently under attack – as we discuss later in this chapter.

Institutions of GHG can empower scientists. Scientists and technical experts shape international public health norms and rules, and they compose much of the key staff at international health institutions. These technical experts have three key roles in policy-making: explaining the relationship between cause and effect; demonstrating interlinkages between different issues; and framing, proposing, and identifying regulations (Haas 1992). These experts are most effective when they have international presence and the clarity of scientific consensus.

International institutions often serve as a forum where experts interact and reshape interests (Haas 1993). Institutions give greater authority to science than it otherwise would have had. The earliest institutions on health, in the era between the World Wars, served as forums for sharing evidence on disease transmission, collecting information from around the world on epidemics, and, in turn, shaping trade and quarantine policies around scientific information and expertise. As they expanded, institutions broadened to include knowledge generation by sponsoring research and providing technical expertise to states as requested. International systems that have information-rich institutions are more disposed to cooperation when there is a new problem (e.g., HIV/AIDS, or other emerging infectious diseases), or when there is uncertainty associated with disease threats (e.g., pandemic influenza). Knowledge existing within an international institution is more likely to generate international action than knowledge that remains in national institutions or within the diffuse international scientific community.

Institutions of GHG can increase equity. While international institutions are often controlled by their most powerful members, moral principles have been embedded in their rules and charters perhaps contributing to the ability of institutions to lead cooperation on health that favors the poor. The constitution of the World Health Organization (WHO) declares as one of its principles "The enjoyment of the highest attainable standard of health is one of the fundamental rights of every human being without distinction of race, religion, political belief, economic or social condition" (WHO 1946). Keohane (1984) has pointed to the ability of institutional rules to reduce inequality: "most international regimes seem to be less constraining of the autonomy of weak states than politically feasible alternatives, which would presumably involve bilateral bargaining on the basis of power rather than of general rules" (Keohane 1984). International institutions allow weaker states to have a greater role in shaping international cooperation. For example, in voting on a budget allocation for smallpox within the WHO in 1966, the limited proposals supported by the 10 wealthiest nations was defeated by a more ambitious proposal supported by weaker and smaller states (Barrett 2007). Weaker actors were empowered again in creating the institutions for collective financing for HIV/AIDS. While the United States had initially proposed a Trust Fund for HIV/AIDS with a significant role for the pharmaceutical industry, the formalization of this process within an international institution ultimately gave the industry a more limited role (Poku 2002). A look at the WHO's constitution is a reminder that international institutions incorporate egalitarian principles that are missing from unmediated inter-state cooperation (WHO 1946).

The nature of institutions – including how the institutions themselves are governed – is important in determining the issues they take on and the participation they entice. Theorists of international relations have devoted much analysis to questions of institutional design. Here, we summarize a few of these key findings to guide thinking about how the design of institutions shapes global health action.

Abbott and Snidal (1998) suggest that organizations characterized by centralization and independence best facilitate cooperation. Centralization brings efficiency, and ability to pool resources and risks, thus making international cooperation on health more likely. Similarly, Keohane (1984) suggests that international institutions improve information-sharing and are able to raise the costs of violation of norms and rules. Independence brings neutrality and legitimacy for collective and individual actions and norms. Legitimacy of individual actions entices powerful states to participate, while neutrality demands that institutions be buffered from direct pressures of states, and allows international institutions to act as trustees, allocators, and arbiters, facilitating activities that might be otherwise unacceptable in interstate relations (Abbott and Snidal 1998). Levine (2004) has suggested that some key successes in cooperation on infectious diseases, such as the eradication of smallpox, can be attributed to a strong, centralized, and independent WHO that was able to make rules and execute programs with central authority.

Why Would a Powerful State Agree to Work through Global Institutions?

Poor and weak states are willing to give up autonomy to work through international norms, rules, and formal institutions because of the favorable redistributive benefits that accompany them. Small and rich states (e.g., Scandinavian countries) might be willing to give up their autonomy to work through international institutions because these institutions often offer these states authority and prestige that they would lack in unmediated international interactions. However, the most powerful states have less obvious incentives to work through international institutions and conform to international norms and rules. Given that powerful states do not always have the advancement of science-based international policy and equity as their top priorities, these states often have incentives to bypass or weaken international health institutions. Powerful states sometimes have the option to reject norms, rules, and international institutions, and "go it alone," or they might reshape these institutions to meet their own needs. They sometimes do, but not always.

The key question then becomes: under what conditions will powerful actors work through institutions of GHG? How can their behaviours and preferences be changed by these interactions? Building on work done on financial regulation, we can suggest that powerful actors are likely to work through international institutions when threats they face are diffuse or shifting (Simmons 2001). In contrast, when the threat is localized and distinct, or the benefit concentrated, these powerful actors will prefer to act unilaterally.

For example, with smallpox eradication, the potential sources for introducing the diseases were so wide that the United States did not seek to act unilaterally, despite the overwhelmingly favorable cost–benefit ratio. Similarly, with the threat of emerging infectious diseases, including pandemic influenza, where the threat is especially diffuse, the United States has championed working through and empowering the WHO. In contrast, in some cases, where threats were localized and distinct, the United States acted unilaterally. One example of such unilateral action was the eradication of yellow fever from the Panama Canal Zone to avoid the death of construction workers and to keep the passage safe from the disease (Harvard University Library 2012). Similarly, the United States preferred unilateral action in efforts to eradicate malaria from Latin America in the 1950s, in part because of the concentrated benefits of such "health diplomacy" efforts in relation to the Cold War (Siddiqi 1995). The United States also acted unilaterally in its early efforts to deliver antiretroviral drugs, through the US President's Emergency Plan for AIDS Relief (PEPFAR) (Dybul 2009) partly because of domestic pressures to achieve quick results, to favor US NGOs and corporations, and to build a coalition with the religious right opposed to abortion, needle exchanges, and sex education (Dietrich 2007).

Key Functions of Global Health Governance

In a seminal article on international collective action on health, Jamison *et al.* (1998) defined the core functions of international health organizations as the "promotion of international public goods (e.g., research and development), and surveillance and control of international externalities (e.g., environmental risks and spread of pathogens)." These functions are an important part of the work of international health organizations, often overlooked in debates about international health priorities that focus on international financing (WHO Maximizing Positive Synergies Collaborative Group *et al.* 2009). The authors suggest that WHO is the key provider of these core functions. For example, WHO creates formal rules in treaties and regulations, creates informal constraints through norms and codes of conduct, and serves as a facilitator of knowledge creation and consensus development (Yamey 2002).

However, a significant portion – if not the majority – of global health action is directed not to these core functions, but to "supportive functions" including financial and technical assistance to national health systems, and protecting the health of vulnerable groups (Jamison *et al.* 1998). For example, the massive investment in global HIV/AIDS programs in countries unable to provide care does not provide a global public good, but instead provides a (very valuable) local public good and sometimes a national public good. These efforts and the institutions that govern and mediate them are essential for local and national health in poor countries, even though they do not provide a global public good.

While several frameworks for thinking about international action on health have been proposed, here we consider three categories that allow us to consider a broad range of health efforts governed by international norms, rules, and institutions:

1. Jointly financed action in public health (e.g., the smallpox eradication program and the bilateral and multilateral efforts to provide HIV/AIDS treatment);
2. International regulation governing health policies (e.g., International Health Regulations and the Framework Convention on Tobacco Control); and
3. Health research and health surveillance (including the work of the WHO Secretariat in monitoring disease trends and research aimed at providing global public goods in health).

Internationally Financed Action

In 2010, development assistance for health approached US$27 billion (IHME 2010a). The rapid growth in development assistance for health, from about $5.8 billion in 1990 (Figure 3.1), may explain the focus on international health financing in discussions of GHG (IHME 2010a). To put current financing in context, during the intensified smallpox campaign, from 1967 to 1976, the average annual funding for smallpox was $40 million. In 1957, at the height of the malaria eradication program, $320 million went into the international financing of malaria eradication.

While international financing represents a minor component of overall health spending, accounting for 0.3% of total expenditures on health globally, and 14% of health

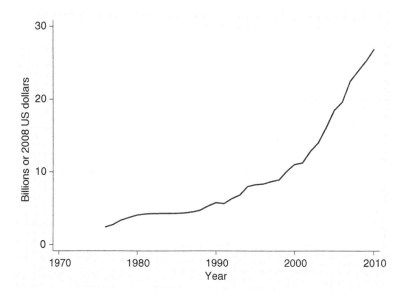

Figure 3.1 Development assistance for health, 1976–2010. Source: for 1976–1990 data, see Michaud and Murray (1994); for 1990–2010 data see IHME (2010b).

expenditures in WHO's Africa region (which excludes North Africa), international financing exerts a great influence on domestic programs and priorities in poor countries (WHO 2011). This influence exists because international financing supports most of the Ministry of Health budgets in many poor countries. Meanwhile, private spending, which is the bulk of health spending, is outside of any central direction (GEG 2008). Thus, seemingly minor variations in which diseases are targeted by international financing have big impacts on the arrangement of health services in poor countries.

International health financing has been criticized for promoting priorities at odds with disease burden and with country priorities, and for a lack of accountability and transparency from funding agencies (Sridhar and Batniji 2008). Further, critics have pointed out that the frequent changes in direction and priority for international financing have made it difficult for developing countries to set a health agenda (GEG 2008). These criticisms, and the efforts to address them, are discussed at the end of this chapter. At the same time, international health financing has succeeded in eradicating smallpox, reducing the mortality associated with HIV(Bendavid and Bhattacharya 2009), and reducing the burden of malaria (Murray *et al.* 2012).

International Regulation

International financing is not a requirement for cooperation on all health issues, some of which may be better addressed through international standards and regulation. For example, efforts to prevent the importation of plague from international trade were well addressed by international agreements in the nineteenth century that made international reporting requirements and established protocols for the prevention of disease (Cooper 1989). Similarly, cooperation on the control of tobacco, a shared cause of some of the most pervasive non-communicable diseases, has been pursued through international regulations that limit advertising and illicit trade of tobacco products (Roemer *et al.* 2005). International regulation governing health policies has been most robust in addressing the threats of emerging infectious diseases, such as avian influenza, with the 2006 International Health Regulations (Baker and Fidler 2006). These regulations give the WHO substantial power and authority, without requiring national ratification.

Research and Surveillance

One of the core, and earliest, functions of WHO and its predecessors has been disease surveillance and the facilitation of international research. Today, many organizations, most prominently the Bill & Melinda Gates Foundation, sponsor and facilitate the generation of knowledge to advance health around the world. The Gates Foundation disbursed nearly $9 billion in global health grants from 1998 to 2007, and now disburses over $1 billion annually, with about 40% of the funds directed to international organizations (McCoy *et al.* 2009). Just over one third of Gates Foundation grants were allocated to research and development, especially on vaccines and microbicides.

The WHO continues to have an essential role in disease surveillance. WHO's Global Outbreak Alert and Response Network (GOARN) is an international collaboration that identifies and coordinates response to disease outbreaks (WHO 2012). Operational since 2000, this network collects information from official and non-official sources and mobilizes resources to assist countries with disease outbreaks. However, this activity depends on continually raising funds from donors, as the network lacks any formal institutional funding.

Major Developments in International Health Institutions: New Players and New Priorities

Recent decades have seen the emergence of new norms and formal institutions for GHG. In the late 1970s, WHO stated a vision for health based on basic health services for all. This focus led WHO to (temporarily) abandon disease-focused campaigns by the early 1980s (Maciocco and Stefanini 2007). At the same time, the World Bank began disbursing loans and grants for health, based on recognition of the importance of health for development. In 1976, the World Bank funded its first health project ($19 million), and by 2005 the World Bank was disbursing nearly $4 billion for health annually (Michaud and Murray 1994). The World Bank quickly became a dominant financier of international cooperation on health (Abbasi 1999).

Historically, it appears that new institutions did not arise to fill a functional gap, but rather to establish a new set of priorities. The League of Nations Health Office was initially created to facilitate typhus control – left off the agenda by existing international health agencies. In response to the global HIV/AIDS epidemic, two major institutions were launched:

1. UNAIDS was launched in 1996 to coordinate the response of United Nations (UN) agencies to the epidemic and to reach beyond the health sector; and
2. The Global Fund to Fight AIDS, Tuberculosis and Malaria (GFATM) was created in 2002 to facilitate collective financing on the diseases.

By 2006, GFATM contributed two thirds of all donor resources for tuberculosis, half of resources for malaria, and one quarter for HIV/AIDS (Radelet and Siddiqi 2007).

In addition to new international institutions for cooperation on health, new institutional rules were adopted for selecting priority areas for cooperation. Three frameworks emerged that shaped the priorities for international cooperation on health. First, in 1977, WHO adopted a goal of "Health for All" based on a system of universal primary care. This was followed by the International Conference on Primary Health Care, in Alma Ata, Kazakhstan in 1978, where 134 countries and numerous non-governmental organizations (NGOs) adopted primary healthcare as the framework for achieving this goal. The Health for All agenda framed health as a development issue, firmly placed responsibility for health with governments, and linked health to issues of equity and universal access to care (Kickbusch 2000). The focus of the Health for All framework was on primary healthcare, nutrition, and sanitation, a focus that was reflected in international financing for health throughout the 1980s and 1990s.

The second framework shaping institutional priorities and rules for cooperation was based on the "Global Burden of Disease." This framework emerged from the World Bank in the late 1980s, partly in response to WHO's focus on universal primary healthcare. The Global Burden of Disease framework prioritized those diseases with the highest burden and most cost-effective interventions, creating a vision for "selective" (rather than universal) primary healthcare. The idea that the measurement of disease burden should guide the selection of institutional priorities was definitively stated by the World Bank in the 1993 World Development Report (World Bank 1993). By 1998, upon the election of Gro Harlem Brundtland as Director-General of WHO, this framework was also adopted by WHO. Brundtland imported the people and the ideas that had created the Bank's health strategy into a new WHO department, seeking to embed priority-setting processes based upon disease burden into WHO. The creation of a policy within WHO of directing funding towards those issues with the greatest global burden contributed to the prioritization of international tobacco control.

The third framework shaping institutional priorities and rules for cooperation was based on the Millennium Development Goals (MDGs). In 2000, 147 heads of state committed themselves to a series of development objectives, to be reached in the next 15 years. Known since 2001 as the Millennium Development Goals, six out of eight of the MDGs and eight of the 16 targets relate to health (Box 3.1). The three specific health MDGs (MDGs 4–6) seek to reduce child mortality, improve maternal health, and combat HIV/AIDs, malaria, and "other major diseases." The goals were initially formed from a review of the Organisation for Economic Co-operation and Development (OECD) development policy and evolved based on agreements among donor countries (Clemens *et al.* 2007). These objectives, and their associated targets, were explicitly used by the World Bank, WHO, and many bilateral agencies to establish priorities for international cooperation on health (Saraceno *et al.* 2007). Critically, donor agencies reshaped their programming to focus on the MDGs.

Box 3.1 Health-Related Millennium Development Goals (MDGs)

Nutrition (MDG 1): Reduce by half the proportion of people who suffer from hunger

Child Mortality (MDG 4): Reduce by two thirds the mortality rate among children under 5 years

Maternal Health (MDG 5): Reduce by three quarters the maternal mortality ratio

HIV/AIDS, malaria, and other diseases (MDG 6): Halt and begin to reverse the spread of HIV/AIDS and the incidence of malaria and other major diseases

Environment (MDG 7): Reduce by half the proportion of people without sustainable access to safe drinking water

Development (MDG 8): In cooperation with pharmaceutical companies, provide access to affordable essential drugs in developing countries

Source: adapted from http://www.who.int/mdg/goals/en/index.html and http://www.un.org/millenniumgoals/# (both last accessed December 2013).

The Current Crisis in Global Health Governance

In this chapter, we have argued that the core benefits of investing authority in international norms, rules, and formal institutions have been the advancement of science in policy and the empowerment of weaker members in the international arena. However, both of these benefits are under fire. Next we highlight some of the core challenges facing GHG today.

Dismantling Equity in International Institutions

WHO had been founded on an egalitarian one-country, one-vote system, where key policy decisions were to be made at the World Health Assembly (WHA). This system allowed smallpox eradication to become a priority for the organization, even though the intensified smallpox campaign was opposed by the 10 largest financial contributors to the organization. While still nominally in place, the WHA has diminishing impact on the priorities pursued by the agency, and a marginal impact on the allocation of WHO's budget. In fact, the WHO Secretariat only controls the distribution of about 25% of WHO's budget, as 75% of the budget comes through "extra-budgetary funds" from OECD and private donors that are tied to specific initiatives. Of note, in the early 1970s, this ratio of extra-budgetary to regular budget funds was inverted, with only 25% of funding outside of the agency's control. A recent study of the relationship between WHO's budgetary allocations and the global burden of disease showed that the WHO budget allocated by the Secretariat more closely matches disease burden than the (much larger) WHO budget earmarked by donor states, which favors infectious disease (Stuckler *et al.* 2008).

By largely abandoning its egalitarian principles, we would argue that WHO has compromised its ability to deliver health equity and to meet the demands of poor countries. As an African Health Minister commented, "The major international organizations are being distracted. They are looking for money because they are judged by the way they are mobilizing money. They are not guided by what has to be done" (GEG 2008).

While Member States work together to agree to resolutions and policy documents at the WHA, states then undermine these efforts by supporting specific disease initiatives based on sparse international consultation. Since 2000, there has been a rapid growth in global health initiatives, mostly targeting infectious disease, that have established their own decision-making bodies (WHO Maximizing Positive Synergies Collaborative Group *et al.* 2009). These initiatives are accountable to their own boards, rather than to the countries in which they operate, and they set their own policies, priorities, and conditions for engagement within countries. Despite frequent rhetoric, and some real efforts, there remains no proper synchronization of these initiatives with the activities, policies and priorities of WHO, thus leaving democratic decision-making in global health in a dismal state.

Furthermore, some of these initiatives increase their influence through the enforcement of conditions to access funds and resort to punitive sanctions when their policies and priorities are not adhered to, further limiting the autonomy of developing countries. A key problem with new global health initiatives is that each captures the limelight for a short period of time, shifting attention from one issue and approach to the next and making it difficult for developing countries to "stay the course" or build capacity (GEG 2008).

Marginalizing Science from the Policy Process

As discussed by Yamey and Volmink in Chapter 7, policy-making processes at international institutions have not kept up with the best of science. A 2007 study found that WHO's policy-making processes "usually rely heavily on experts in a particular specialty, rather than representatives of those who will have to live with the recommendations or on experts in particular methodological areas" (Oxman *et al.* 2007). A similar scientific complacency plagues the World Bank, which has been shown to replicate health programs, even in the face of evidence that the models are not delivering the desired outcomes (Sridhar 2008). International institutions, which are ideally positioned to advance science-based policy, have been falling short on their internal use of science and program evaluation.

Pursuing Donor Priorities

There is a double accountability problem in global health. In donor-dependent countries, governments are not accountable to their own populations, but rather to the donors that fund them. On the other hand, donors are not accountable to the populations to whom they are directing funds, but to their own constituents (i.e., their taxpayers and benefactors). The priorities and programs being pursued in global health today have been shaped in the context of this accountability problem. For example, in several countries PEPFAR operated outside of national health strategies. Reflecting on the refusal of PEPFAR to participate in the national approach agreed to by all other donors, one African health minister commented, "We have never put our foot down. We fear. We are cowards" (GEG 2008).

The increase in resources for global health has enabled countries and international institutions to face important health problems, and has saved lives through global health initiatives. However, these achievements may not be sustainable in the long run. While some research has shown improvements in overall mortality from disease-specific interventions (Bendavid and Bhattacharya 2009), much of the reported improvement has been based on indicators specific to diseases targeted by international financing, with little assessment of how countries have expanded their overall healthcare services. Donors have been framing their packages based on quick results (typically to be produced in 6–12 months), with funds often disbursed with strict conditions and the implementers only allowed to use the money in ways that will contribute to progress on selected indicators. Further, in the fight against HIV/AIDS in particular, key donors have largely directed funds to international NGOs rather than the government, limiting capacity-building in public services. In their pursuit of donor resources, aid-receiving countries have often had to set-aside their national strategies and priorities.

Privatizing Global Health

International institutions and donors have compromised their own accountability mechanisms through privatization and partnerships. These partnerships and the privatization of core functions have enabled global health efforts to expand rapidly, but they come at a cost. Some aid agencies, such as the US Agency for International Development (USAID), now contract much of their project implementation and evaluation out to consulting firms. USAID has seen its professional staff shrink from 4300 employees in 1975 to about 2500 employees by 2007 (Modernizing Foreign Assistance Network 2007). The agency now delegates responsibilities and programs largely to private contractors.

Similarly, WHO has entered into several partnerships with the private sector to address issues such as control of tuberculosis and malaria, polio eradication, and immunization (WHO Maximizing Positive Synergies Collaborative Group et al. 2009). These partnerships, like USAID's use of consultancies, have enabled a rapid growth in global health programs. Yet, these partnerships have been initiated by donor nations, are largely governed by "northern elites," and enable private companies (often not vetted for social responsibility) to have a greater role than they would have had the partnership not existed (Buse and Harmer 2004). Further, many global health actors have private-sector investments that are not compatible with their health-promoting interests (Stuckler et al. 2011). For example, the Gates Foundation has major holdings in the Coca-Cola corporation, even though rising consumption of Coca-Cola products, such as sugary drinks, has been linked with rising rates of non-communicable diseases in the developing world (Stuckler et al. 2011). While global health partnerships remain outside the scope of regulation, a lesson may be learned from the World Bank, which has in place guidelines for partnering with the private sector that allow staff to consider the true costs of a partnership (World Bank 2001).

Conclusions

The scale of global health efforts has grown rapidly, especially since 2000. The results from these efforts have had positive measurable impacts on the health of people in poor countries. However, recent trends in GHG – such as a reduced focus on equity, the marginalization of science, the prioritization of donor concerns, and the rise of privatization – should give those of us in the global health policy community cause for concern. In order to address unanticipated challenges and to establish lasting progress in global health, it is essential to revitalize the democratic decision-making processes that are crucial to empowering science and giving voice to poor countries.

Key Reading

Abbott KW, Snidal D. 1998. Why states act through formal international organizations. *Journal of Conflict Resolution* 42(1), 3–32.

Jamison DT, Frenk J, Knaul F. 1998. International collective action in health: objectives, functions, and rationale. *Lancet* 351(9101), 514–7.

Poku N. 2002. The Global AIDS Fund: context and opportunity. *Third World Quarterly* 23(2), 283–98.

Sridhar D, Batniji R. 2008. Misfinancing global health: a case for transparency in disbursements and decision making. *Lancet* 372(9644), 1185–91.

Stuckler D, King L, Robinson H, McKee M. 2008. WHO's budgetary allocations and burden of disease: a comparative analysis. *Lancet* 372(9649), 1563–9.

WHO (World Health Organization). 1946. Constitution of the World Health Organization. http://www.who.int/governance/eb/who constitution en.pdf (last accessed December 2013.)

WHO Maximizing Positive Synergies Collaborative Group; Samb B, Evans T, Dybul M *et al.* 2009. An assessment of interactions between global health initiatives and country health systems. *Lancet* 373(9681), 2137–69.

References

Abbasi K. 1999. The World Bank and world health: changing sides. *BMJ* 318, 865–9.

Abbott KW, Snidal D. 1998. Why states act through formal international organizations. *Journal of Conflict Resolution* 42(1), 3–32.

Baker MG, Fidler DP. 2006. Global public health surveillance under new international health regulations. *Emerging Infectious Diseases* 12(7), 1058–65.

Barrett S. 2007. The smallpox eradication game. *Public Choice* 130(1), 179–207.

Bendavid E, Bhattacharya J. 2009. The President's Emergency Plan for AIDS Relief in Africa: an evaluation of outcomes. *Annals of Internal Medicine* 150(10), 688–95.

Buse K, Harmer A. 2004. Power to the Partners?: The politics of public–private health partnerships. *Development* 47(2), 49–56.

Clemens MA, Kenny CJ, Moss TJ. 2007. The trouble with the MDGs: confronting expectations of aid and development success. *World Development* 35(5), 735–51.

Cooper RN. 1989. International cooperation in public health as a prologue to macroeconomic cooperation. In Cooper RN, Eichengreen B, Holtham G, Putnam RD, Henning CR. *Can Nations Agree? Issues in International Economic Cooperation*. Washington DC: Brookings Institution.

Dietrich JW. 2007. The politics of PEPFAR: the President's Emergency Plan for AIDS Relief. *Ethics and International Affairs* 21(3), 277–92.

Dybul M. 2009. Lessons learned from PEPFAR. *Journal of Acquired Immune Deficiency Syndromes* 52(Suppl 1), S12–S13.

Global Economic Governance (GEG). 2008. *Preliminary Report of a High-Level Working Group, 11–13 May 2008*. Oxford: Global Economic Governance Programme.

Haas PM. 1992. Introduction: Epistemic Communities and International Policy Coordination. *International Organization* 46(1), 1–35.

Haas PM. 1993. Epistemic Communities and the Dynamics of International Environmental Co-operation. In Rittberger V, Mayer P (eds) *Regime Theory and International Relations*, pp. 168–201. New York: Oxford University Press.

Harvard University Library. 2012. *Tropical Diseases and the Construction of the Panama Canal, 1904–1914*. http://ocp.hul.harvard.edu/contagion/panamacanal.html (last accessed November 2013).

IHME (Institute for Health Metrics and Evaluation). 2010a. *Development Assistance for Health Database 1990–2008*. http://www.healthmetricsandevaluation.org/record/development-assistance-health-database-1990–2008 (last accessed November 2013).

IHME (Institute for Health Metrics and Evaluation). 2010b. *Financing Global Health 2010:Development Assistance and Country Spending in Economic Uncertainty*. Seattle, Washington: IHME.

Jamison DT, Frenk J, Knaul F. 1998. International collective action in health: objectives, functions, and rationale. *Lancet* 351(9101), 514–7.

Keohane RO. 1984. *After Hegemony: Cooperation and Discord in the World Political Economy*. Princeton: Princeton University Press.

Kickbusch I. 2000. The development of international health policies: accountability intact? *Social Sciences and Medicine* 51(6), 979–89.

Levine R. 2004. *Millions Saved: Proven Successes in Global Health*. Washington, DC: Peterson Institute.

Maciocco G, Stefanini A. 2007. From Alma-Ata to the Global Fund: the history of international health policy. *Revista Brasileira de Saúde Materno Infantil (Recife)* 7(4), 479–86.

McCoy D, Kembhavi G, Patel J, Luintel A. 2009. The Bill and Melinda Gates Foundation's grant-making programme for global health. *Lancet* 373(9675), 1645–53.

Michaud C, Murray CJ. 1994. External assistance to the health sector in developing countries: a detailed analysis, 1972–90. *Bulletin of the World Health Organization* 72(4), 639–51.

Modernizing Foreign Assistance Network. 2007. USAID staffing. In *Obama-Biden Transition Project*: Obama-Biden Transition Project.

Murray CJ, Rosenfeld LC, Lim SS et al. 2012. Global malaria mortality between 1980 and 2010: a systematic analysis. *Lancet* 379(9814), 413–31.

North DC. 1991. Institutions. *Journal of Economic Perspectives* 5(1), 97–112.

Oxman A, Lavis JN, Fretheim A. 2007. Use of evidence in WHO recommendations. *Lancet* 369(9576): 1883–9.

Poku N. 2002. The global AIDS fund: context and opportunity. *Third World Quarterly* 23(2), 283–98.

Radelet S, Siddiqi B. 2007. Global Fund grant programmes: an analysis of evaluation scores. *Lancet* 369(9575), 1807–13.

Roemer R, Taylor A, Lariviere J. 2005. Origins of the WHO Framework Convention on Tobacco Control. *American Journal of Public Health* 95, 936–8.

Saraceno B, van Ommeren M, Batniji R et al. 2007. Barriers to improvement of mental health services in low-income and middle-income countries. *Lancet* 370(9593), 1164–74.

Siddiqi J. 1995. *World Health and World Politics: the World Health Organization and the UN system*. Columbia, SC: University of South Carolina Press.

Simmons B. 2001. The international politics of harmonization: the case of capital market regulation. *International Organization* 55(3), 589–620.

Sridhar D. 2008. *The Battle Against Hunger*. Oxford: Oxford University Press.

Sridhar D, Batniji R. 2008. Misfinancing global health: a case for transparency in disbursements and decision making. *Lancet* 372(9644), 1185–91.

Stuckler D, Basu S, McKee M. 2011. Global health philanthropy and institutional relationships: how should conflicts of interest be addressed? *PLOS Medicine* 8(4), e1001020.

Stuckler D, King L, Robinson H, McKee M. 2008. WHO's budgetary allocations and burden of disease: a comparative analysis. *Lancet* 372(9649), 1563–9.

WHO (World Health Organization). 1946. *Constitution of the World Health Organization.* Geneva: WHO.

WHO (World Health Organization). 2011. *World Health Organization, Global Health Observatory Data Respository 2011.* http://apps.who.int/ghodata/ (last accessed November 2013).

WHO (World Health Organization). 2012. *Global Outbreak Alert and Response Network 2012.* http://www.who.int/csr/outbreaknetwork/en/ (last accessed November 2013).

WHO Maximizing Positive Synergies Collaborative Group, Samb B, Evans T, Dybul M *et al.* 2009. An assessment of interactions between global health initiatives and country health systems. *Lancet* 373(9681), 2137–69.

World Bank. 1993. *World Development Report 1993: Investing in Health.* Washington, DC: World Bank.

World Bank. 2001. *Partnerships with the Private Sector: Assessment and Approval.* Washington, DC: World Bank.

Yamey G. 2002. WHO in 2002: why does the world still need WHO? *BMJ* 325(7375), 1294–8.

Chapter 4

Global Health Justice and the Right to Health

Garrett W. Brown and Lauren Paremoer

Abstract

There has been recent interest in the ethical considerations associated with global health. Underpinning many of these ethical concerns are claims that there exist duties of "health justice," which necessitate the establishment of corresponding rights and obligations to rectify existing global inequalities related to the poor delivery of health. When used in this way, "justice" refers to the idea that individuals ought to receive treatment that is fitting to them as dignified human beings as well as the assignment of corresponding rights and duties necessary to create an equitable distribution of benefits and burdens within a social order. The purpose of this chapter is to examine some key debates connected to arguments for global health justice and to explore their broad implications for global health policy. In doing so, this chapter outlines contemporary arguments for domestic health justice, reviews arguments for and against expanding the scope of justice to the global level, and explores the role that "a right to health" may have in furthering a more thoroughgoing condition of global health justice and the elimination of current global health inequalities. Through this examination we argue that if health is a key factor for living a minimally decent life, and if global health policy is correspondingly going to take human health seriously, then this requires the consideration of robust principles of global justice that transcend current state practices and which can reform existing inequalities of health.

The Handbook of Global Health Policy, First Edition. Edited by Garrett W. Brown, Gavin Yamey, and Sarah Wamala.
© 2014 John Wiley & Sons, Ltd. Published 2014 by John Wiley & Sons, Ltd.

Key Points

- There is widespread agreement that health is a key factor in living a minimally decent life and for the ability of people to be engaged citizens. As a result, most theorists agree that states have a moral duty of justice to promote citizen health via a fair distribution of resources and/or capabilities.
- If known global structures affect the health of those beyond borders, then based on the logic of domestic justice, principles of justice should also apply at the global level.
- Limiting the debate about the scope of justice to the domestic level produces a statist approach to global health policy that helps to enshrine a language of state securitization, the uneven distribution of health resources and capacities, and permits powerful states to feel a sense of reduced moral culpability.
- One way to distribute health fairly is through the use of justiciable rights, yet how these health rights are politicized can greatly affect broader health outcomes for better or worse and therefore require better understandings of their correspondence to social justice.
- If human health matters, and if global health policy is to take human health seriously, then a cosmopolitan approach to global health is best suited to prioritize the health rights of the individual as well as limiting the socioeconomic determinants of health that negatively affect the quality of that health.

Key Policy Implications

- Global health inequities cannot be significantly resolved without broader international commitments to distributive global justice.
- A rights-based approach is most viable if broader national and international commitments to social justice are structurally in place.
- Restructuring the institutional mechanisms that drive global health inequities will thus require radical new thinking away from traditional state-centric policies. These commitments will necessarily have to be grounded in new ethical and political commitments that will require greater international transfers of wealth, codified duties for fair economic relations, and a broader international recognition and response to the affects of globalization and their impacts on the social determinants of health.

Introduction

It is widely accepted that human beings require adequate health in order to maintain a minimally decent life. It is also widely accepted that states and their citizens have duties of justice to maintain health systems for the delivery of basic national health and the health needs of its population. Nevertheless, at the global level there is far less certainty about what moral duties exist in regard to the satisfaction of adequate health for those beyond borders. Although there is almost unified agreement that there are vast inequalities in global health and that more concerted efforts are needed to rectify these inequalities, there is also widespread disagreement about how to deliver these systems globally and the ethical principles that should underwrite such a system (Daniels 2008; Ooms and Hammonds 2010). As a result, there remains a general lack of consensus about what moral duties we have toward establishing more equitable global health initiatives and in regards to the values that should inform the "just" satisfaction of these moral duties in global health policy.

In order to provide some theoretical reflection about the role of justice in global health, the purpose of this chapter is to examine some key debates connected to arguments for health justice and to explore the broad implications these have on global health policy. In doing so, this chapter outlines several contemporary arguments for domestic health justice, reviews arguments for and against expanding the scope of justice to the global level, and explores the role that *a right to health* may have in furthering a more thoroughgoing condition of global health justice and the elimination of current global health inequalities. Through this examination we argue that human health is a matter of global justice and that the assignment of health rights and duties should be measured through the lens of cosmopolitan justice.

Debates about Health Justice at the Domestic Level

At the domestic level, debates about the relationship between health and justice are typically organized around two key questions. Do states have an obligation to promote the health of their citizens? Do states have an obligation to promote equity in access to healthcare and/or equity in health outcomes? If yes, what criteria should states use to fulfill this obligation in a just manner? Today, a broad consensus exists that states have an obligation to protect and promote the health of their citizens and, in some cases, the health of non-citizens within their borders. This consensus is codified in various international treaties – most prominently in Article 25 of the Universal Declaration of Human Rights, Article 12 of the International Covenant on Economic, Social and Cultural Rights, and General Comment 14 of the UN Economic and Social Council. These instruments compel states to promote the health and well-being of "everyone," not only citizens. Within states this normative consensus is typically reflected in laws and policies that promote citizens' access to preventative and curative healthcare services, and that prevent states and private corporations from actively undermining the health of citizens. This is true of both developed and developing countries, with 80% of developing states recognizing the right to health, healthcare, medical services, or health protection in their constitutions (Jung and Rosevear 2011).

Sociologists and historians have argued that modern capitalist democracies have come to recognize their "obligation" to promote citizens' health partly as a strategy for containing class conflict and encouraging political cooperation. One of the most prominent accounts in this tradition can be found in Marshall's 1964 essay on *Citizenship and Social*

Class. In this essay Marshall argued that social citizenship (i.e., the idea that citizens are entitled to a measure of substantive equality simply by virtue of their status as citizens) emerged in England towards the end of a centuries-long period of legal reforms designed to consolidate a conception of citizenship as a national-level status governed by a central state. During the course of this process, citizens were first granted civil rights and then political rights. However, in some respects these rights worked at odds with one another. Both civil and political rights promised citizens formal equality. Recognizing citizens' civil rights, including the rights of all citizens to sell their labor in the market, facilitated the emergence of the capitalist market system. In turn, this system generated material and status inequalities that undermined poorer citizens' practical ability to exercise their political rights. In the face of these inequalities, the formal promise of equal rights to political participation and voice were rendered meaningless. In order to resolve this contradiction, Marshall argues, a moral consensus emerged that the state should act as a guarantor of formal and substantive equality by implementing social policies that would eliminate or diminish material inequalities that undermined equal enjoyment of citizenship rights. This gave impetus to states recognizing the social rights of citizenship during the twentieth century. These rights were designed to ensure that citizenship status would guarantee that individuals would enjoy a basic measure of substantive equality simply by virtue of being citizens (Korpi 1983; Esping-Andersen 1990; Fraser and Gordon 1992; Skocpol 1992; Orloff 1993).

Social scientific scholarship has identified the material conditions and social relations that have historically contributed to the politicization of healthcare in capitalist democracies. However, this body of literature offers no systematic normative justification for the claim that states have an obligation to protect and promote the health of citizens, and/or to eliminate inequalities in health outcomes – regardless of the political pressure that is brought to bear upon it. For such an account we must turn to normative political philosophy.

Since its publication, Rawls' theory of justice as fairness has been hugely influential in shaping accounts of the liberal democratic state's obligations vis-à-vis its citizens. In *A Theory of Justice* (1971), Rawls argues that just societies should ensure that all citizens enjoy the same basic liberties. States should ensure that all citizens have fair equality of opportunity to serve in public institutions, and that social and economic inequalities are eliminated unless they improve the status of the worst-off members of the political community. This second principle of justice (known as the *difference principle*) requires that the state ensure that income, wealth, and public goods – notably education – are distributed in a manner that enables all citizens to participate in the life of the community, and to have equal prospects of succeeding in their goals, regardless of the circumstances in which they were born.

In developing his account of the just society, Rawls explicitly sets aside the reality that citizens experience ill health over the course of their lifetimes. Nonetheless, several prominent scholars have argued that Rawlsian principles offer important guidance to constitutional democracies that want to preside over a fair distribution of healthcare resources. These accounts generally frame health as a "good" which, like education, is a precondition for participating meaningfully in public life and for effectively pursuing one's private goals. However, amongst scholars working within the liberal tradition, who refuse to prioritize collective well-being or equality at the cost of individual freedom, serious disagreements exist about the desirability of promoting good health by focusing on the equitable allocation of resources, particularly in societies in which individuals experience multiple intersecting dimensions of marginalization. Daniels' (1985; 2008) application of Rawls' framework to the healthcare arena, and Amartya Sen's (2000) critique of the justice as fairness model are illustrative of this debate.

Both Daniels and Sen agree that formal and substantive opportunities for living a healthy life should be distributed in a fair and equitable manner. Daniels, like Sen, envisions a society in which health is defined as "normal functioning" (i.e., the absence of mental or physical pathologies) (Daniels 2006: 23). In a just polity, he argues, the state has an obligation to ensure that opportunities to access healthcare are distributed in accordance with the principle of justice as fairness (Daniels 2006: 23). In addition, the state has an obligation to ensure that social inequalities do not result in certain groups being systematically overexposed to conditions that are hazardous to their health. Under these conditions citizens should effectively enjoy equity with respect to their prospects of becoming ill and their opportunities to obtain effective treatment. Nonetheless, empirical research demonstrates that individuals from different socioeconomic backgrounds obtain differential benefits from seeking out universally accessible medical care (UCL 1967). It is thus likely that inequalities in health outcomes are likely to emerge, even if states ensure that healthcare resources and risks are distributed in a fair and equitable manner. In the face of this evidence, Daniels argues that differential health outcomes should be considered just, provided that they originate from the limited instances of inequality that are permissible within the framework of justice as fairness and the elimination of unfair inequalities in the social determinants of health (Daniels 2008).

Like Daniels and Rawls, Sen considers good health as important, and by extension the equitable distribution of risks and resources in healthcare, on the grounds that healthy individuals should be capable of performing autonomous and reasoned activities associated with citizens in liberal political theory. However, unlike Rawls and Daniels, Sen opposes the notion that a just society has the limited obligation of creating a basic structure that produces a fair distribution of health in the population. Instead, he regards good health as intrinsically valuable and argues that just societies have an obligation to eliminate inequalities in health outcomes (Ruger 2004: 1076). It follows that states that distribute opportunities for achieving good health equitably, but ultimately fail to address systematic inequalities in health outcomes, have fallen short of justice in healthcare. In Sen's view, this resistance to addressing inequalities in health outcomes arises from Rawls' (and by extension Daniels') unjustifiable focus on the distribution of resources per se, and not on the question of the ends individuals can achieve once they control these resources (Sen 1979; also see Cohen 1990). Sen argues that an equitable distribution of resources and opportunities in a society characterized by material and status inequalities cannot deliver on the promise of justice (i.e., on fair equality of opportunity) because such resource fetishism ignores the fact that individuals have unique social and personal characteristics that limit their capacity to convert resources into outcomes they value – such as health. As Sen suggests, "if the object is to concentrate on the individual's real opportunity to pursue her objectives (as Rawls explicitly recommends), then account would have to be taken not only of the primary goods the persons respectively hold, but also of the relevant personal characteristics that govern the *conversion* of primary goods into the person's ability to promote her ends" (Sen 2000: 74). What really matters, in Sen's view, is a social order that ensures equality of capabilities and not only fair equality of opportunity.

In this approach, equality requires that individuals be treated differently in order to ensure that individual capabilities are maximized in comparable ways. This formulation has a number of important implications. According to Sen, approaches to equality that prioritize equal allocation of resources risk reducing a normative ideal that affirms the equal worth of human beings to a technical procedure concerned with allocating individuals equality via quantities of goods and services. Sen also argues that giving analytical priority to the equal distribution of "things" amounts to a form of resource fetishism that neglects the question of how, in the context of societies characterized by relations of domination, specificities such as race, sex, or physical disability impinge on an individual's ability to use her allocation of goods and services as effectively as a more privileged compatriot. Thus, Sen's argument for the equality of capabilities approach compels political communities to constantly revisit the question of why equity is important and how it is constrained in specific contexts for particular types of people.

Sen's capabilities approach is open-ended in so far as he refuses to define the list of basic capabilities all individuals are entitled to. Instead, he argues that such a list should be generated through democratic deliberation within specific political communities, and not through an a priori claim (Sen 2000). In contrast, Daniels openly states that healthy functioning should be considered a basic precondition for equality of opportunity in all societies. However, he too acknowledges the importance of democratic deliberation in mediating political conflicts between reasonable individuals about the proper distribution of healthcare resources. Daniels argues that democratic deliberation characterized by publicity, relevance, and revisability gives citizens access to a fair procedure for deciding how healthcare resources should be rationed under conditions where, for example, there is reasonable disagreement about how inequality should be conceptualized, the grounds on which certain health needs should be given priority, and about the relative importance that should be assigned to individual needs versus aggregate outcomes (Daniels 2006: 23; Daniels and Sabin 2008).

Within the liberal tradition associated with Rawls, as well as the capabilities critique of this tradition, there is thus a consensus that health is a precondition for political participation and fair equality of opportunity, and that just societies are "good for health" because they eliminate unfair socioeconomic inequalities and facilitate access to healthcare services. In addition, just societies promote social solidarity by subjecting decisions about healthcare policy to reasoned deliberation rather than promoting a particularistic (and potentially politically contentious) principle for resolving all disputes about this matter. However, there is serious disagreement about the limit of states' obligations to eradicate or mitigate inequalities in health outcomes within their borders. In addition, critics of liberal theories of justice argue that these theories ignore the systemic constraints that states face in their efforts to promote a domestic order that is characterized by a commitment to equity. Because liberal theorists conceive of states as autonomous entities, they ignore the systemic global constraints that, in practice, limit a state's capacity to define the terms of the social contract pursued at the domestic level (see Chapter 21). It is with understanding how these constraints and global interconnections may require a broadened notion of global health justice that this chapter now turns.

Limiting the Scope of Health Justice to the State

There is general agreement within liberal thought regarding the role of good health in securing the possibility for individuals to lead minimally decent lives and for them to pursue interests associated with political citizenship. Nevertheless, there is considerable disagreement about what normative principles should ultimately underwrite the distribution of health and/or how external state relations should be considered when determining the demands of justice. In thinking about questions regarding the *scope of justice* there has been an active debate between liberal *statists* who argue that citizens should prioritize duties of justice to their local communities, versus more cosmopolitan minded scholars who suggest that everyone shares certain basic human rights to healthcare and that all states should have global responsibilities toward alleviating global health inequalities. In this regard, whereas most liberal statists consider reducing global health inequalities to be a less obligatory matter of humanitarian assistance, cosmopolitans argue that all human beings have an equal moral worth and that our decisions about the scope of justice must accord with universalized categories that prioritize basic human health regardless of where they happen to live.

Nevertheless, to be clear, statist arguments against broadening the scope of justice beyond the state does not exclude the possibility that we have some obligations to those abroad. What it stipulates is that these duties will not constitute the same level of "special obligation" that exists between family members, neighbors, co-nationals, and fellow citizens. In this way, determining the scope of justice is dependent on empirical conditions of mutual identity and social inclusion, in which normative determinations about the scope of justice must correspond to claims of existing solidarities and the intensity of obligations conditioned by the immediate proximity of co-patriots.

If we accept the empirical claim regarding communal belonging as the key to determining the scope of justice as correct, as many social justice theorists do, then it is possible to generate key normative arguments for why we should favor special obligations for justice between co-nationals as taking precedence over other individuals beyond our borders. As Miller argues, national and communal sentiments are important and necessary conditions in establishing the motivations for, and the reciprocal conditions of, social justice (Miller 1999). To ignore the meaningfulness of these special obligations upon our social lives would negate an important aspect of our human condition and the conditions upon which social justice rests. Although we should have some responsibilities to others beyond communal borders based on general humanitarian concerns, these responsibilities should remain a secondary "subduty" and that special duties of justice to co-nationals should take precedence over other international obligations (Miller 2007). In regards to how this may play out in relation to global health policy, Miller presents the following case:

> Suppose that a flu pandemic breaks out and the government only has sufficient vaccine to inoculate a limited number of vulnerable people against the disease. It does not seem wrong in this case to give priority to treating compatriots, that is to supply the vaccine to all those fellow-citizens identified by age or other relevant criteria as belonging to the vulnerable group, before sending any surplus abroad, even though it is reasonable to assume that some foreigners will be more vulnerable to the flu than some compatriots selected for vaccination. And this remains true even if we know that those more vulnerable foreigners will not receive the vaccine from their own health services. (Miller 2007: 45)

In making this determination Miller suggests that the context of "social justice" is different from normal appeals about just responsibilities, since "social justice is practiced among people who are citizens of the same political community" and "our thinking about justice should be conditioned by existing empirical realities" (Miller 2007: 16). As a result, "the idea of justice is contextually determined" and "we need to ask whether the institutions and modes of human association that we find within nation-states, and which form the context within which ideas of social justice are developed and applied, are also to be found at the international level, and if not, how we should understand human relationships across national borders" (Miller 2007: 14). In doing so, however, it is clear from Miller that proximity and relational duties are what matter in the formulation of just responsibilities and that when thinking about the scope of justice in regards to health we should not be afraid to appeal to our co-national "ethical intuitions" (Miller 2007: 45).

In line with Rawls and his understanding of distributing "public goods," Nagel suggests that "the nation state is the primary locus of political legitimacy and the pursuit of justice" because it constitutes "a form of organization that claims the political legitimacy and right to impose decisions by force" (Nagel 2011: 393). According to Nagel, since enforcement is a necessary requirement of justice, and this authoritative condition is missing at the global level, the idea of establishing duties of justice beyond borders remains an unintelligible "chimera" (Nagel 2011: 394). By reverting to a position that pegs the debate about justice to existing authority instruments, Nagel normatively demands that "egalitarian justice requires the internal political, economic, and social structure of nation-states and cannot be extrapolated to different contexts, which require different standards" (Nagel 2011: 394). In this regard, similar to the view held by Miller, when it comes to global health justice, although we do have some subduties to others beyond our borders, these duties cannot be obligatory duties of justice without the social and political mechanisms necessary to guarantee mutual identification and reciprocal obligation.

We can see this form of *relational justice* argument play out in contemporary ethical debates about health and the scope of justice as discussed in the last section. For example, in his recent exploration on justice and health, Daniels grounds his case for national health justice on a similar relational position as those espoused by Nagel and Miller, suggesting that we "should resist the pull of the cosmopolitan intuition" since this has the potential of weakening national health structures and the existing relational foundations of justice upon which they stand (Daniels 2008: 348). Although Daniels also rejects extreme statist versions of relational justice by suggesting that a middle position might be possible (Daniels 2008: 346), he does, ultimately, limit distributive priorities of health to the national level (Ooms and Hammonds 2010).

In unpacking these arguments it is important to highlight that a specific empirical understanding of globalization and its limited impact on the bounded properties of the state is being made. In essence, the argument is asserted that globalization and its transnational spaces do not represent a form of *relational* interdependency to a point where it resembles conditions of social cooperation and economic institutionalism as found within the state. In this regard, the current global order and its transnational structure does not (and possibly cannot) represent the basic institutional conditions analogous to the conditions under which Rawls argues justice should/can apply. In this case, the argument about the scope of justice rests on an empirical assessment about whether or not there is enough of an identification relationship between peoples at the global level or significant interactions to constitute relational interdependency. In other words, the debate about global justice involves evaluations about current solidarities regarding universal humanity, the "authenticity" of our economic and social interactions, our identification with these interdependent structures (if they exist), and whether these new transnational identities are strong enough to provide a *global horizon* for duties of global justice (Vertovec and Cohen 2002). As implied above, a common critique of the existence of a global horizon is that globalization and its transformational aspects have been "exaggerated" by more cosmopolitan minded scholars and that there are still justified arguments for national appeals when determining the boundaries of justice and political membership (Kymlicka 2011; Daniels 2008: 346).

The political manifestations of these sorts of arguments are evident within many current debates about global health policy. Perhaps most notably, this underwriting logic underpins what International Relations scholars call as a *statist* approach. As Davies suggests, "according to the statist perspective ... the health of individuals requires effective state structures ... [and] although this perspective recognizes the need for multilateral responses to some health crises, its central premise remains on securing the state" (Davies 2010: 21). From this, "the statist perspective holds that health issues must be addressed when they directly impact the economic, political and military security of the state" (Davies 2010: 14). Like above, the argument is not that we have no obligations to others at the global level, but that the prioritization of duties of justice relate specifically to the nation-state as the referent object and to the prioritized interests of that political community.

Since the referent object within this theory of justice is the bounded community (i.e., the state) and its security, it engenders particular normative conclusions in relation to global health responsibilities and policy. The basic premise is that because global health not only impacts upon the security of the state, but also because it can impact upon the stability of the state system as a whole, states should have responsibilities toward alleviating potential threats to the state (Price-Smith 2009). This is not only in regard to safeguarding the internal institutions required for domestic justice (Garrett 2001), but also in regard to pursuing international efforts to respond to key threats to national security (Fidler 1999). Nevertheless, to be clear, because of the overriding importance of state security, when determining duties of justice, the distribution should by necessity prioritize the security needs of the state first as well as frame all ethical considerations in relation to this prioritized demand.

Adherence to this position results in several idiosyncratic political formations and distributional models in relation to how capabilities and resources are distributed in existing global health policy. First, because national interests are often prioritized, there is a tendency for richer nations to engage in the *securitization* of global health and to think narrowly of international efforts as representing a form of *microbialpolitik* (Fidler 1999: 19). As a result, there is a propensity to give a prioritized focus to the securitization of transborder infectious diseases while ignoring other health-related emergencies or determinants. Although there are arguments to suggest that states are more willing to give increased resources when issues are framed in terms of security, it is also the case that security prioritization means that these resources remain narrowly targeted (McInnes and Lee 2006). One consequence of this is that normative appeals to security become most suitable for addressing an acute crisis, but often remain inadequate for addressing the underlying causes of infectious diseases, be they political, economic, social, or cultural (Youde 2005).

Second, addressing global health from a statist perspective can lead to what Wimmer and Glick Schiller have described as "methodological nationalism" and an uncritical acceptance "of existing national borders as the borders of society and as the necessary institutional nexus for citizenship" (Wimmer and Glick-Schiller 2002: 304). The problem being that by remaining anchored to existing political boundaries as delimiting the possible scope of health justice and effective collective action it can blindly overlook more appropriate and effective forms of political and social organization that could/should exist between states and beyond (Orbinski 2007). This problem is highlighted particularly well within the statist logic itself, which acknowledges a paradoxical situation where states represent the agents of prioritized interests while at the same time recognizing that many health threats are transborder phenomena or of a global socioeconomic nature, which cannot be addressed by a single state actor or a collection of states. This suggests that there is scope for more cosmopolitan inspired schemes of global justice, but because of narrow understandings of the scope of justice, these are often dismissed as only secondary components to the preferred position of state-based multilateralism.

Third, as Peterson (2006) and Rushton (2011) have suggested, if the normative argument about global health is framed solely in terms of security and "justice within borders," then most Western countries will not face the same threats as most of the world's population and they will therefore dedicate insufficient resources to those most in need (as Millers "ethical intuition" suggested). Since this distribution can be rationalized within the statist ideology, it will assist in "relieving Westerners of any moral obligation to respond to health crisis beyond their own national borders" (Peterson 2006: 46). This is because, if security is the overall specification of how to represent the objects within an overarching hierarchical relationship, then any normative command about justice must intonate and comply with the conditions of this overarching relationship. This will not only affect who we think we have duties of justice to, but also it will significantly limit the range of factors we think we have relational responsibility for.

Cosmopolitanism and Broadening the Scope of Health Justice

Whereas many liberals are committed to restricting the scope of justice to the state and to rely on weaker notions of humanitarian assistance to deal with global health, cosmopolitans argue that all human beings have an equal moral worth and that our ethical decisions about the scope of justice must accord with universalized demands for the satisfaction of adequate human health. The grounding for the cosmopolitan approach to global health is determined by three interrelated arguments.

First, cosmopolitans argue that any scheme of health justice based solely on state citizenship is morally arbitrary when comes to formulating its distributive principles. This is because it is simply a matter of happenstance whether a person is born in one place versus another. In other words, being born into one set of institutional relationships (i.e., a civilization or a state) is not a matter of moral choice by the individual who is born into that relationship. In fact, where a person is born is purely a matter of luck and, as many cosmopolitans argue, it is morally suspect to determine the level of health a person is entitled to solely on the good fortune of birth alone. As a result, many cosmopolitans have argued that the requirement of communal membership as an overriding precondition for determining the scope of justice is unconvincing and thus weakens the normative appeal of the statist position (Caney 2005). As an alternative, and as will be examined in the next section, most cosmopolitans adopt a rights-based approach to global health and argue that because all human beings are entitled to basic health satisfaction richer states (as well as the state in which a person resides) have corresponding duties of justice to advance the fulfillment of those rights.

When placed in comparison to the statist approach, the cosmopolitan argues that determining the scope of justice based on place of birth conflates luck with duty and as a result fails to appreciate the universal characteristics of human worth, vulnerability, and capabilities (see Chapter 10). As a contrasting theory, most cosmopolitans sustain that it is important to prioritize human moral worth (and thus the basic health of an individual) as a universally "protected public good" because this good captures what is distinctively human in our nature. For the cosmopolitan, it is imperative to consider ethical decisions in relation to whether the moral duty can also be conceived as universally valid. Otherwise, the idea of human morality no longer represents a self-imposed law onto oneself, but becomes a deterministic act of coercion outside the realm of moral agency. In this light, and like the arguments presented in Part I, the capability to self-legislate is the power to be an autonomous moral agent and represents the ultimate source of human dignity and existence (Rawls 1971; Sen 2000). Yet, unlike the statist position advocated by Rawls and others, cosmopolitans argue that there is no justifiable moral reason why the recognition of dignity must stop at state borders when it comes to basic duties of justice and the satisfaction of basic human interests.

In contemporary debates, this cosmopolitan morality has provided the inspirational ground for appeals to the protection of *universal human rights* (Pogge 2002) to the fulfillment of human *capabilities* in development strategies (Sen 2000; Nussbaum 2005; Venkatapuram 2011), to the notion of *human security* (Axeworthy 2001; Booth 2007), and to the establishment of mutually consistent maxims of universal public right (Benatar and Brock 2011). In relation to global health, and like the debates discussed in Part I, the ability to be an autonomous human being suggests that this would necessarily include a basic condition of individual health upon which one's human agency could have basic equality of opportunities to be a reasonably healthy human agent (WHO 2008a; Braveman *et al.* 2011).

Second, a cosmopolitan approach broadens the contextual conceptualization involved with relational theories of justice and by doing so seeks to undermine distributions that are strictly based on immediate communal membership. This logic suggests that if Rawls was right to claim that justice is the first principle of any scheme of social cooperation, and that globalization has "stretched" the need for cooperative relationships beyond the state, then the scope of justice should also extend beyond the borders of states. As several cosmopolitans have argued, international economic interdependency has come to resemble something like the conditions of social cooperation and "basic institutions" that originally motivated Rawls' domestic concern for distributive justice (Beitz 1992). As Beitz argues, under Rawls' own logic, "if evidence of global economic and political interdependence shows the existence of a global scheme of social cooperation, we should not view national boundaries as having fundamental moral significance" (Beitz 1979: 376). As Barry furthers, this form of impartial moral cosmopolitanism "shows itself to be distinctive in its denial that membership of a society is of deep moral significance when the claims that people can legitimately make on one another are addressed" (Barry 1998: 145). This is because cosmopolitanism morally demands that "human beings are in some fundamental sense equal" and that to satisfy this moral principle would require further principles of impartial justice that "others could not reasonably reject" (Barry 1998: 146).

A primary component of the statist position is the belief that globalization has not developed to a sufficient point of relational interdependence where debates about justice are held to apply. In relation to global health, theorists like Miller suggested that special duties to co-nationals should take precedence over other international obligations. In outlining his argument, Miller used an example of flu inoculations to illustrate how this prioritization to co-nations morally corresponds with our "ethical intuitions." A key aspect of Miller's justification is that whereas co-nationals are embroiled in a relational system of social justice, this relational element is not evident at the global level. As a result, when determining the scope of justice, "our thinking about justice should be conditioned by existing empirical realities" (Miller 2007: 16).

Nevertheless, given this very logic, there is increasing empirical evidence to suggest that, at a very minimum, there are causal components of interaction that exist at the global level that affect the health of those beyond borders (De Vogli 2011; also see Chapters 11, 14, 21, and 30). These interactions can be measured through locating key interdependent relationships produced by global markets, global economies, transnational spaces, and cultural cross-pollinations. In terms of global health, unlike Miller's assumption that each nation-state is largely self-contained and as result "self-responsible," there are several studies to suggest that the global economy and its existing political order have profound effects on the health and well-being of individuals across borders (Labonté et al. 2009; Brown and Labonté 2011). This has led some cosmopolitans, like Pogge, to suggest that our willing participation in the international market creates an "interactional context," and therefore implicates those benefiting from these global interactions with a set of mitigating responsibilities – such as responsibilities for global health (see Chapter 11). As Pogge proposes, there are injustices involved within the current interactional structure and this institutional architecture systematically violates the basic human rights of certain populations. Since the minimum demands of justice command that we do not violate the negative rights of others, and if one's involvement in the international structure systematically supports a violation of these rights, then there is "causal material involvement" and we are morally responsible to reform the system (Pogge 2004: 134–7).

Third, cosmopolitans often suggest that statist ideologies over-fetishize the status quo, which, although capturing some aspects of existing political solidarity, tends to lock-in existing political communities as static entities. Cosmopolitans counter this stance by suggesting that the state is simply a political construction that does not contain – in and of itself – an inherent moral worth (although they do suggest it has an instrumental worth). As some cosmopolitans argue, the state is the product of human invention and ingenuity and it is not a static entity that needs to be intrinsically protected from new forms of moral and political alteration. In this regard, the state is something that can be reconstructed, reformulated and, consequently, transformed into something else (Beck 2006). If this is true, then the state is merely a constructed institutional entity designed to coordinate the political relationships between people. If globalization has broadened the scope of those relationships beyond state borders, as even a statist position on global health admits, then the state loses its bounded saliency and relevance in favor of new political formulations that can better capture the interrelations that exist in a globalized world (Held and McGrew 2007). In terms of globalization and public health, if there are causal pathways between geopolitical and economic structures and they clearly impact on social determinants of health (Braveman et al. 2011), then there is significant ethical motivation to rethink current governance structures and the determinations(s) of justice that underwrite them (Friel and Marmot 2011).

From this there are three implications that follow from a cosmopolitan approach as it relates to global health policy and the determination of global health justice. First, given its focus on the deontological worth of human beings, cosmopolitanism demands a minimum moral subfloor in which to measure whether current global health policy satisfies the basic requirements of justice, as well as to provide a moral compass from which normative recommendations for reforming the current institutional structure should be generated. As Pogge argues, even if our duties of justice are only minimal, in that we are obligated to restrict systematic violations of negative rights, and if there is evidence of a systemic perpetuation of health inequalities that affect negative rights as a result of current global structures, then we have a moral obligation to reform these institutional structures in light of more equitable cosmopolitan concerns.

Second, unlike the statist approach, cosmopolitanism prioritizes the health of the individual as well as the socioeconomic aspects that affect the quality of that health. As a result, a cosmopolitan approach links nicely to debates about the social determinants of health and draws attention to correcting failures that continue to perpetuate key social inequalities and large disparities in individual health. In this regard, the cosmopolitan approach resonates with a growing body of literature that suggests that a greater focus on the social determinants of health (with a call for more radical deliberative and distributive reforms) is necessary in order to construct more equitable global health policies within state communities as well as between states (WHO 2008a; Putland *et al*. 2011).

Third, unlike the statist approach, cosmopolitanism recognizes that political participation beyond existing governance structures will be required for effective global health governance and that those at the periphery (who also have the greatest burden of health risk) will need to be better involved in policymaking if a more effective and successfully implemented system is to be possible (Commers 2002; Friel and Marmot 2011). Nevertheless, as most cosmopolitans argue, this will require a greater normative commitment to the idea of development "partnerships" as stated in the Millennium Development Goals as well as the distributive and deliberative commitments that are necessary to underwrite global health policies that will effectively tackle existing failures (Barnes and Brown 2011).

Fourth, most cosmopolitans, if not all, argue that one mechanism to safeguard participatory inclusion as well as the delivery of basic health needs is to present these interests as legally mandated human rights (both domestically and internationally). By doing so, a rights-based approach can be a valuable mechanism to reduce health inequalities both domestically and globally and the related suffering caused (Wolff 2012). Nevertheless, like most ethical prescriptions, a rights-based approach has attached benefits and burdens, and the next section examines a more detailed discussion of this approach as it relates to health justice.

Rights-Based Approaches to Health: Problematizing the Use of Rights Claims to Promote Social Justice at the Domestic and Global Level

Health activists, particularly those who view poor health outcomes as a function of political disenfranchisement, economic exploitation, and social marginalization, have frequently used the language of justice to advocate for policies aimed at eliminating health disparities (Alma-Ata Declaration 1978; Kim *et al*. 2000; Farmer 2005; Farmer *et al*. 2006). However, the language of justice and its emphasis on systemic reforms has found less resonance with intergovernmental organizations, transnational corporations, and the governments of developed states. Amongst these actors the language of rights is used more frequently than appeals to justice.

Depending on how rights claims are politicized, they can be rendered compatible with both resourcist and capabilities approaches to justice. In some states, for example, the right to healthcare is interpreted as imposing an obligation on the state to address the specialized needs of individuals or groups that would otherwise fail to attain capabilities comparable to those conferred on fellow citizens utilizing the same institutions. For example, the UK National Health Service (NHS) gives members of religious communities the right to consult doctors who share their religious commitments, access washing facilities, and wear hospital gowns that allow them to optimize their capacity to benefit from the resources provided at public health facilities. In Brazil, courts have recognized that the right to health places an obligation on the state to give specific HIV-positive individuals access to individualized treatment regimes in instances where standard treatment regimes have become ineffective or inaccessible (Biehl *et al*. 2009).

However, rights claims have also been interpreted as, at minimum, placing an obligation on states to provide everyone with an equitably distributed "minimum core" package of resources, so as to ensure they enjoy a decent quality of life. This interpretation of rights obligation does not necessarily impose an obligation on states to equalize individuals' capabilities. This resourcist interpretation is nonetheless influential. The United Nations Committee on Economic, Social and Cultural Rights, for example, has interpreted the International Covenant of Social and Economic Rights (ICESER) as imposing an obligation on states to realize citizens' and non-citizens' socioeconomic rights by providing them with the "minimum essential levels" of goods such as food, healthcare, housing, and education (Young 2008).

Many states – including those in the global South – now enshrine justiciable social rights, such as the right to health in their Constitutions (Gauri and Brinks 2008). In these polities. citizens (and in some cases, non-citizens) are legally entitled to request that courts evaluate the adequacy and fairness of the state's efforts to promote the rights to health and healthcare services. Recognizing the justiciability of these rights in unequal societies has several advantages. Justiciability places an explicit onus on the state to refrain from undermining extant infrastructure, policies, and laws that promote and protect better health outcomes for all – even when it has limited resources. It also compels the state to provide public reasons for undertaking practices that are perceived as being counter to its obligation to promote the right to health. In societies characterized by serious socioeconomic disparities, justiciability imposes a legally binding obligation on the state to expand citizens' access to the substantive resources that enable them to enjoy their formal status as free and equal citizens (Sachs 2000). Finally, justiciability allows courts to sanction practices that enjoy popular support and promote health, but nevertheless undermine a fair and equitable distribution of resources in society or that otherwise compromise the political community's commitment to principles such as equality, bodily integrity, and individual freedom (Scott and Macklem 1992; Wolff 2012).

Critics of social rights discourses acknowledge that legal entitlements to basic goods and services improve the material status of the most marginalized citizens. Nonetheless, they argue, these entitlements only mitigate the impact of institutions that ultimately consolidate or deepen socioeconomic inequalities. Rights claims do little to transform or dismantle unjust institutions; they only protect citizens against their worst excesses. As a result, critics suggest that there may be limits to using justiciable rights claims to bring about justice in the context of unequal societies. First, by their very nature, rights claims must be articulated using idioms of justice that are recognizable to the institutions adjudicating them (i.e., courts) and that are politically palatable to dominant classes in society. As a consequence, rights language risks reifying existing power structures while simultaneously mitigating their most extreme effects (Tushnet 1984, 1993; Crenshaw 1995). Ultimately, this implies that rights discourses may serve to legitimate unjust institutions rather than questioning them. Second, absent an analysis of the broader social injustices that characterize the polity, even states that show great generosity in recognizing citizens' rights may choose to honor these claims in a manner that further undermines the status of already marginal social groups (Orloff 1993). Third, some critics argue that governments faced with resource scarcity, competing commitments, and limited institutional capacity can only ever realize the right to health by providing citizens with a minimum core package of health services. This minimum core may be legally justifiable while falling short of citizens' expectations of what a right to health should entail, thereby invalidating the idea that a "right to health" can actually be achieved in practice. The risk, in all these cases, is that the law becomes complicit in bringing about incremental reforms that mitigate the most objectionable health effects of living in an unjust society. It does this by allowing the very social institutions that generate adverse health outcomes and unfair distributions of the social determinants of health to use the mechanisms of procedural justice (i.e., participation in reasoned deliberation adjudicated by courts) to promote incremental changes. The question of whether institutions that perpetuate injust inequalities should be dismantled is, however, deferred.

To what extent do discourses about universal rights help to clarify the transnational health obligations of political communities? Rights discourses emphasize the equal worth of all individuals and therefore require that certain goods (food), services (healthcare, education), and modes of recognition (e.g., dignity, life) be equitably and universally accessible to all people, regardless of their citizenship status or personal particularities. Whereas the domestic literature on health and justice focuses on the obligations we have towards members of our own political communities, rights discourses draw our attention towards another crucial question (i.e., what obligations do political communities have towards strangers; those who are not members of our political community?). At the same time, the language of rights claims offer outsiders a vocabulary for challenging democratic political communities that legitimate practices or laws that refuse to recognize outsiders' status as human beings with equal moral worth.

With respect to elucidating the obligations of states to promote non-citizens' access to healthcare, universal rights claims thus remind us that denying "strangers" access to healthcare services simply because they fall outside the boundaries of our political community is morally problematic if we claim to recognize the equal worth of all human beings. Moreover, rights discourses draw attention to the distinction between the state and the political community. In instances where the state is acting in a manner that ignores the wishes of the political community – for example, where citizens demand that the state do all it can to promote access to affordable medical care and medication both domestically and globally – rights discourses can function in a manner that expands non-citizens' access to medical care. For example, HIV/AIDS treatment activists in the United States have had some success in lobbying their government to promote antiretroviral access in the developing world, rather than being exclusively committed to defending US-based pharmaceutical companies' patent rights (Sell 2001).

Equally significant is the fact that this kind of transnational activism forges solidarity, and gives rise to concomitant moral and political obligations, which are not constrained by the geographic boundaries of the state. In other words, rights discourses enable forms of collective action that demonstrate that solidarity is not a "natural" function of national political communities, but a political sentiment that is produced through sustained political mobilization.

Finally, rights discourses offer individuals a framework for making demands on intergovernmental organizations, particularly those tasked with protecting, promoting, and recognizing human rights (e.g., the World Health Organization). By way of illustration: the language of human rights has enabled non-state actors to compel intergovernmental organizations to advocate for reforms that improve access to medical services and medication (e.g., creation of the Global Fund to Fight AIDS, Tuberculosis and Malaria at the UN General Assembly Special Assembly on HIV/AIDS of 2001), and which improve the social determinants of health at the global scale (e.g., the International Labour Organization's advocacy for legal reforms that protect workers' health and dignity).

It is nonetheless important to recognize that rights claims need not necessarily result in greater transnational solidarity or systemic reform. Conceptually, rights discourses emphasize individual entitlements and are concerned with limiting the extent to which the state or other powerful collectives can arbitrarily impose their will on individuals. The transformative potential of rights thus depends on the extent to which rights claims are situated within a theory of justice that prioritizes equity rather than individual freedom, and affirms a cosmopolitan vision of justice grounded in a commitment to preventing, or at the very least mitigating, the harm we inflict on others – at home and abroad – through our participation in unjust structures (Pogge 2004).

Conclusions

Most theorists believe that human health is a key factor in living a minimally decent life and a vital requirement for individuals to have opportunities to act as flourishing and engaged political participants. In addition, most theorists also argue that rectifying inequalities in health is a concern of justice because it acts as a foundational element in any social scheme of cooperation and social interdependency. In this chapter we argue that if human health is of moral concern, and if there are structures of international cooperation and interdependency that perpetuate unfair inequalities across borders, then the same logic for domestic justice should also apply at the global level. To think otherwise allows for extremely particularistic and statist distributions in health outcomes that greatly disfavor some while clearly benefiting others. Pursuing a statist approach to health based on a narrow definition of justice can create idiosyncratic global policies that encourage a state-based securitization approach, a reduction in moral responsibilities for unjust global economic structures, and the distributive prioritization of some groups over others based on nothing more than where someone was accidentally born. In contrast, we present arguments that favor a more cosmopolitan approach to global health policy as well as examine the use of a right to health as one particular mechanism to link cosmopolitan theory to practice. In doing so the underlying theme of this chapter is simple: if human health matters morally, and if global policy is to meaningfully reflect this moral concern, then considerations of global health justice will need to be more thoroughly incorporated into global policies if we wish to see better global health equity.

Key Reading

Benatar S, Brock G (eds). 2011. *Global Health and Global Health Ethics*. Cambridge: Cambridge University Press.
Lenard PT, Straehle C (eds). 2012. *Health Inequalities and Global Justice*. Edinburgh: Edinburgh University Press.
McInnes C, Lee K. 2012. *Global Health and International Relations*. Cambridge: Polity Press.
Venkatapuram S. 2011. *Health Justice*. Cambridge: Polity Press.
Wolff J. 2012. *The Human Right to Health*. London: Norton and Co.

References

Alma-Ata Declaration. 1978. (See sections II and V in particular.) April 15, 2013. http://www.who.int/publications/almaata_declaration_en.pdf (last accessed December 2013).
Axeworthy L. 2001. Human security and global governance: putting people first. *Global Governance* 7(1), 19–23.

Barnes A, Brown GW. 2011. The idea of partnership within the Millennium Development Goals: context, instrumentality and the normative demands of partnership. *Third World Quarterly* 32(1), 165–80.

Barry B. 1998. International society from a cosmopolitan perspective. In Maple D, Nardin T (eds) *International Society: Diverse Ethical Perspectives*, pp. 144–61. New Jersey: Princeton University Press.

Beck U. 2006. *Cosmopolitan Vision*. Cambridge: Polity Press.

Beitz C. 1979. Justice and International Relations. *Philosophy and Public Affairs* 4(4), 360–89.

Beitz C. 1992. International liberalism and distributive justice: a survey of recent thought. *World Politics* 52(1), 269–96.

Benatar S, Brock G (eds). 2011. *Global Health and Global Health Ethics*. Cambridge: Cambridge University Press.

Biehl J, Petryna A, Gertner AA, Amon JJ, Picon PD. 2009. Judicialisation and the right to health in Brazil. *Lancet* 373, 2182–4.

Booth K. 2007. *Theory of World Security*. Cambridge: Cambridge University Press.

Braveman P, Egerter S, Williams D. 2011. The social determinants of health: coming of age. *Annual Review of Public Health* 32, 381–98.

Brown GW, Labonté R. 2011. Globalization and its methodological discontents: contextualizing globalization through the study of HIV/AIDS. *Globalization and Health* 7(29), 1–12.

Caney S. 2005. *Justice Beyond Borders*. Oxford: Oxford University Press.

Cohen GA. 1990. Equality of what? On welfare goods and capabilities. *Louvain Economic Review* 56(3/4), 357–82.

Commers M. 2002. *Determinants of Health: Theory, Understanding, Portrayal and Policy*. Dordrecht: Kluwer Academic Publishing.

Crenshaw KW. 1995. Race, reform, and retrenchment: transformation and legitimation in anti-discriminatory law. In Crenshaw K, Gotanda N, Peller G, Thomas K (eds) *Critical Race Theory: The Key Writings that Formed the Movement*, pp. 103–22. New York: The New Press.

Daniels N. 1985. *Just Health Care: Studies in Philosophy and Health Policy*. Cambridge: Cambridge University Press.

Daniels N. 2006. Equity and population health: toward a broader bioethics agenda. *Hastings Center Report* 36(4), 22–35.

Daniels N. 2008. *Just Health: Meeting Health Needs Fairly*. Cambridge: Cambridge University Press.

Daniels N, Sabin J. 2008. *Setting Limits Fairly: Learning to Share Resources for Health*. Oxford: Oxford University Press.

Davies S. 2010. *Global Politics of Health*. Cambridge: Polity Press.

De Vogli R. 2011. Neoliberal globalization and health in a time of economic crisis. *Social Theory and Health* 9, 311–25.

Esping-Andersen G. 1990. *The Three Worlds of Welfare Capitalism*. Cambridge: Polity Press.

Farmer P. 2005. *Pathologies of Power: Health, Human Rights, and the New War on the Poor*. Berkeley, CA: University of California Press.

Farmer P, Niyeze B, Stulac S, Keshavjee S. 2006. Structural violence and clinical medicine. *PLOS Medicine* 3(10), 1686–91.

Fidler D. 1999. *International Law and Infectious Diseases*. Oxford: Clarendon Press.

Fraser N, Gordon L. 1992. Contract vs. charity: why is there no social citizenship in the United States. *Socialist Review* 22, 45–68.

Friel S, Marmot M. 2011. Action on the social determinants of health. *Annual Review of Public Health* 32, 225–36.

Garrett L. 2001. *Betrayal of Trust: The Collapse of Global Public Health*. Oxford: Oxford University Press.

Gauri V, Brinks DM. 2008. *Courting Social Justice: Judicial Enforcement of Social and Economic Rights in the Developing World*. Cambridge: Cambridge University Press.

Held D, McGrew A (eds). 2007. *Globalization Theory*. Cambridge: Polity Press.

Jung C, Rosevear E. 2011. *Economic and Social Rights in Developing Country Constitutions: Preliminary Report on the TIESR Dataset*, January 26, 2011. http://www.tiesr.org/TIESR%20Report%20v%203.1.pdf (last accessed December 2013).

Kim JY, Millen JV, Irwin A, Gershman J (eds). 2000. *Dying for Growth*. Monroe, ME: Common Courage Press.

Korpi W. 1983. *The Democratic Class Struggle*. London: Routledge.

Kymlicka W. 2011. Citizenship in and era of globalization. In Brown GW, Held D (eds) *The Cosmopolitanism Reader*, pp. 435–41. Cambridge: Cambridge University Press.

Labonté R, Schrecker T, Packer C, Runnels V (eds.). 2009. *Globalization and Health: Pathways, Evidence and Policy*. New York: Routledge.

Marshall TH. 1964. *Class, Citizenship and Social Development: Essays by T.H. Marshall*. New York: Doubleday and Company.

McInnes C, Lee K. 2006. Health, security and foreign policy. *Review of International Studies* 32(1), 5–23.

Miller D. 1999. *Principles of Social Justice*. Cambridge: Harvard University Press.

Miller D. 2007. *National Responsibility and Global Justice*. Oxford: Oxford University Press.

Nagel T. 2011. The problem of global justice. In Brown GW, Held D (eds) *The Cosmopolitanism Reader*, pp. 393–412. Cambridge: Polity Press.

Nussbuam M. 2005. Beyond the social contract: capabilities and global justice. In Brook G, Brighouse H (eds) *The Political Philosophy of Cosmopolitanism*, pp. 196–218. Cambridge: Cambridge University Press.

Ooms G, Hammonds R. 2010. Taking up Daniel's challenge: the case for global health justice. *Health and Human Rights* 12(1), 29–46.

Orbinski J. 2007. Global health, social movements, and governance. In Cooper A, Andrew F, Kirton J, Schrecker T (eds) *Governing Global Health: Challenge, Response, Innovation*, pp. 29–40. Aldershot: Ashgate.

Orloff AS. 1993. Gender and the social rights of citizenship. *American Sociological Review* 58(3), 303–28.

Peterson S. 2006. Epidemic diseases and national security. *Security Studies* 12(2), 43–81.

Pogge T. 2002. *World Poverty and Human Rights*. Cambridge: Polity Press.

Pogge T. 2004. Relational conceptions of justice: responsibilities for health outcomes. In Anand S, Peter F, Sen A (eds) *Public Health, Ethics, and Equity*, pp. 135–61. Oxford: Oxford University Press.

Price-Smith A. 2009. *Contagion and Chaos: Disease, Ecology, and National Security in the Era of Globalization*. Cambridge: MIT Press.

Putland C, Baum F, Ziersch A. 2011. From causes to solutions: insights from lay knowledge about health inequalities. *BMC Public Health* 11, 1–11.

Rawls J. 1971. *A Theory of Justice*. Cambridge, MA: Harvard University Press.

Ruger JP. 2004. Health and social justice. *Lancet* 364, 1076.

Rushton S. 2011. Global health security: security for whom? Security for what? *Political Studies* 54(4), 779–96.

Sachs A. 2000. Social and economic rights: can they be made justiciable? *SMU Law Review* 53, 1381–94.

Scott C, Macklem P. 1992. Constitutional ropes of sand or justiciable guarantees?: Social rights in the new South African constitution. *University of Pennsylvania Law Review* 141(1), 1–148.

Sell SK. 2001–2002. TRIPS and the Access to Medicines Campaign. *Wisconsin International Law Journal* 20, 481–522.

Sen A. 1979. *Equality of What?* The Tanner Lecture on Human Values. Delivered at Stanford University, May 22.

Sen A. 2000. *Development as Freedom*. New York: Anchor Books.

Skocpol T. 1992. *Protecting Soldiers and Mothers: The Political Origins of Social Policy in the United States*. Cambridge: Harvard University Press.

Tushnet M. 1984. An essay on rights. *Texas Law Review* 62(8), 1363–403.

Tushnet M. 1993. The critique of rights. *SMU Law Review* 47, 23–34.

UCL Research Department of Epidemiology and Public Health. 1967. *Whitehall II History.* http://www.ucl.ac.uk/whitehallII/history (last accessed December 2013).

Venkatapuram S. 2011. *Health Justice.* Cambridge: Polity Press.

Vertovec S, Cohen R. 2002. *Conceiving Cosmopolitanism: Theory, Context and Practice.* Oxford: Oxford University Press.

Wimmer A, Glick-Schiller N. 2002. Methodological nationalism and beyond: nation building, migration, and the social sciences. *Global Networks* 2(4), 301–34.

Wolff J. 2012. *The Human Right to Health.* London: Norton and Company.

WHO (World Health Organization). 2008a. *Closing the Gap in a Generation: Health Equity through Action on the Social Determinants of Health.* Geneva: WHO.

WHO (World Health Organization). 2008b. Chapter 19: Managing DR-TB through patient-centred care; and Annex 4: Legislation, human rights and patients' rights in tuberculosis prevention and control. In *Guidelines for the Programmatic Management of Drug-Resistant Tuberculosis: Emergency Update 2008.* Geneva: WHO. http://whqlibdoc.who.int/publications/2008/9789241547581_eng.pdf (last accessed December 2013).

Youde J. 2005. Enter the fourth houseman: health security and international relations theory. *Whitehead Journal of Diplomacy and International Relations* 6(1), 193–208.

Young KG. 2008. The minimum core of social and economic rights: a concept in search of content. *Yale Journal of International Law* 33, 113–75.

Part II Narrowing the Gap Between Knowledge and Action

Chapter 5

Measuring the World's Health: How Good are Our Estimates?

Nancy Fullman, Abraham Flaxman, Katherine Leach-Kemon, Julie Knoll Rajaratnam, and Rafael Lozano

Abstract

The increased attention and financial resources dedicated to global health over the last two decades demands heightened measurement of the world's health status. Our ability to quantify disease burdens over time and across geographies has substantially improved, but for much of the world's sickest and most impoverished populations, what we can currently measure still does not fully represent their health experiences and needs. In the absence of more complete health data collection throughout the world, a variety of population health metrics are used to estimate the world's health based on the data that are presently available. Not all data are equal, nor are the ways data are collected, analyzed, or interpreted. However, these distinctions are not always fully considered in global health policy-making as the data move from research and program domains into national and international agenda settings. Understanding the different dimensions of population health data – the sources, measurement types, estimation approaches, and resulting metrics – is critical to the development and execution of global health policies and programs based on the strongest available evidence.

The Handbook of Global Health Policy, First Edition. Edited by Garrett W. Brown, Gavin Yamey, and Sarah Wamala.
© 2014 John Wiley & Sons, Ltd. Published 2014 by John Wiley & Sons, Ltd.

Key Points

- Our estimates and analytic approaches for measuring the world's health have become more comprehensive, detailed, and rigorous in the last two decades.
- In spite of improving methods for measuring the world's health, many gaps remain and new challenges continue to emerge.
- There is no perfect metric or data collection system for measuring population health. Subsequently, the types of health indicators and estimation methods used must be carefully considered to best capture a specific population's health needs and to adequately correct for known biases.
- The most meaningful health metrics balance the need to capture the complexities of population health with the need to provide policy-makers an easily interpretable set of indicators.
- The pathways from the production of population health metrics to policy creation and implementation are influenced by several factors, including credibility of the source, timing, and comprehensibility.

Key Policy Implications

- Population health data and the metrics that capture them can determine which conditions warrant global attention and which do not. Thus, the production of health metrics and their dissemination can shape policy prioritization and decision-making, from local resource allocation to international target setting.
- Population health metrics are only as relevant as their alignment with the specific needs or objectives of a given population health stakeholder, the administrative level at which health services are delivered, and the time period during which a population experiences a particular health environment.
- Our current estimates of the world's health, however imperfect, support policy needs better than making decisions without any information; at the same time, it is necessary to continue improving upon the collection and assessment of global health data to best address the health challenges that the world faces.

What are Health Metrics, and Why do They Matter to Global Health Policy?

Imagine you are the recently appointed technical health advisor of a populous country with limited resources. You have been charged with understanding the landscape of health burdens for your country, deciding which conditions should receive the most attention, and developing a strategic set of policies that support the sustainable reduction of premature deaths and disease. What information would you need to do your job successfully?

At the very least, you would want to know which health problems exist and how their burdens compare. However, the mere presence of a disease is not very informative. Ideally, your health policy decisions would be informed by the country's historical and current experience with the disease, which populations have been affected and during what periods of time, and any trends associated with the fatal and non-fatal health outcomes of that disease. You would need to consider the quantifiable components of the disease (e.g., overall burden; the number of cases and/or deaths experienced each year; the availability, use, and effectiveness of interventions for the disease), as well as the less quantifiable (e.g., health priorities demanded by citizens; external funding offers for disease-specific programs; equity and ethical concerns). You would want this information for multiple health conditions, or else it may be challenging, if not impossible, to decide which diseases should receive more attention and resources than others.

Understanding what you need to know is a necessary step, but is far from sufficient. The information you need must also be collected in consistent, timely, and accurate ways. What should you do if some disease information was not collected for a period of time – or if no data were ever collected about a likely health problem facing your country? Or if certain populations at higher risk for a particular disease are not well represented by data collected at health centers because those populations have limited contact with service providers? Do you proceed with the information you have, recognizing that it provides an incomplete or skewed portrayal of your country's health outcomes? Or do you try to fill in the missing information or adjust for potential misrepresentation to the best of your ability? There are no easy answers, and these questions are very real ones faced today by poor and rich countries alike.

From the perspective of many population health researchers (Murray and Frenk 2008), health policy decision-making can be compromised or made more challenging if it draws from an evidence base that is incomplete, incomprehensive, or incomparable over time and across geographies. In South Africa, for example, the "true" magnitude of the HIV/AIDS epidemic was effectively masked for years because information about cause of death did not consistently accompany the documented large escalation in adult deaths (Groenewald *et al.* 2005; Setel *et al.* 2007). Even with its highly functioning health information system, Mexico's Ministry of Health was surprised to learn that out-of-pocket healthcare expenditures were bankrupting a substantial portion of its population (WHO 2000; Frenk 2006). Prior to the release of the World Health Organization (WHO)'s *World Health Report 2000*, it had been assumed that such economic catastrophes were less common because Mexico's health system was based on public funding (Frenk 2006).

Measuring population health and strengthening the science of its assessment can have a powerful influence on policy agendas and program orientations throughout the world. At the global level, mental illness was not viewed with significant concern, especially when considering the health loss due to infectious diseases in developing countries, until the Global Burden of Disease (GBD) 1990 study directly compared the high levels of disability associated with mental illness with those of malaria and tuberculosis (World Bank 1993). Because service delivery occurs at the district level in Zambia's decentralized health system, the provision of detailed maternal and child health intervention coverage trends from 1990 to 2010 by district, rather than national or even provincial estimates, enabled district health offices to better benchmark and adjust their programmatic approaches (IHME and UNZA, 2011). The latest iteration of the Global Burden of Disease study, GBD 2010, sought to further bolster the global health evidence base and corresponding policy generation by systematically quantifying the relative magnitude of health lost from diseases, injuries, and risk factors by age, sex, and geography for three specific points in time (Murray *et al.* 2012a). It produced 650 million estimates published in papers and appendices by *The Lancet* in December 2012. With the promise of annual updates, the GBD initiative has the potential to substantially inform policy-making processes worldwide through its emphasis on generating current, comparable, and comprehensive population health data and metrics.

The term "health metrics" describes both the science of measuring health and also the indicators, tools, and methodologies used to more fully understand the health status of individuals and populations (Murray and Frenk 2008). Health metrics for individuals are valuable for diagnosing and treating disease, as they permit healthcare providers to more precisely determine which ailments are affecting individuals, tailor interventions, and track longer term outcomes. Population health metrics, on the other hand, are useful when it comes to identifying health problems and designing health programs and policies that serve broader populations. In analogous terms, individual health metrics are to evidence-based *medicine* as population health metrics are to evidence-based *health policy* (Kohatsu *et al.* 2004): each set of metrics provides the information needed to tailor approaches to the corresponding recipient(s). As showcased by the GBD framework, population health metrics are critical for deciding which policies to implement, prioritizing how to allocate scarce resources, and evaluating whether interventions and programs are reaching – as well as benefiting – the populations who need them.

In this chapter, we introduce key health metrics, as well as data sources and the analytic methods used in their estimation. We also provide examples, at both the global and country level, that illustrate their use to shape policy.

Metrics for the World's Health

A taxonomy, or even comprehensive review, of the variety of health metrics in existence today would be too vast to summarize in just one chapter. Table 5.1 details a selection of commonly used and informative global health metrics that can feed into health policy and program decisions. This brief overview reflects the range of health domains that metrics cover and the types of data they represent, including measures that capture the number of people dying over a period of time (e.g., mortality rates); what they are dying from (e.g., cause-specific mortality rates); the number of people who are sick or hurt but do not die from their conditions (e.g., case counts; prevalence and incidence rates); and whether the people who need health interventions have access to or use them (e.g., coverage). Each of these metrics provides information that can be very helpful on its own and assist with tracking the progress toward specific targets for health achievement. At the same time, policy-makers often need condensed, yet comprehensive, information if they are to quickly understand whether health systems and policies properly align with a population's health outcomes and needs. Thus, it often can be useful to present policy-makers with summary or composite measures of health outcomes (e.g., combining information on premature loss of life and preventable ill health by disease cause) and health service delivery (e.g., combining data on health service use for multiple health interventions) through unified, simple but data-rich indicators.

Table 5.1 A selection of commonly used health metrics and definitions from a range of health domains.

	Types of health metrics	
Health domain	Metric	Definition
Mortality	Child mortality ($_5q_0$)	Probability that a child will survive for five years after he or she is born, assuming that age-specific mortality remains constant
	Adult mortality ($_{45}q_{15}$)	Probability that an adult will survive for 45 years (or to the age of 60 years), conditional upon living to age 15 and assuming that age-specific mortality remains constant
	Life expectancy at birth (E_0)	Average lifetime of an individual born at a given time, with the assumption that age-specific morality remains constant for the duration of his or her life and without adjusting for changes in environmental exposures or technology over his or her lifetime
Cause of death	Death count by cause	Tallies of the number of deaths per cause
	Cause-specific mortality rate (CSMR)	Ratio of deaths per cause to person-years of observation
Morbidity	Case count by cause	Tallies of the numbers of cases per cause
	Incidence rate	Ratio of new cases to person-years, or other specified time period, of observation
	Prevalence rate	Fraction of cases for a disease in an observed population at a particular point in time
Functional health status	Disability weight	Number on a scale from 0 to 1 that represents the severity of health loss associated with a health state
Health financing	Development assistance for health (DAH)	Financial and in-kind contributions from channels of assistance to improve health in low-income and middle-income countries
	Out-of-pocket expenditures	Any direct, private spending by households to health practitioners or suppliers of health services on health needs
Cost effectiveness	Dollars per DALY	Cost of preventing one year of disability-free life lost, in dollars, through exposure to a given intervention or set of interventions
Burden of disease/ comparative risk assessment	Disability-adjusted life-years (DALYs)	Number of years lost due to premature death and years lived with disability; serves as a single indicator for fatal and non-fatal conditions by combining individual measures of mortality and morbidity, cause-specific incidence and prevalence rates, and health weights that reflect the severity of health loss associated with non-fatal conditions
	Years of life lost (YLLs)	Years of life lost due to premature mortality
	Years lived with disability (YLDs)	Years of life lived with any short-term or long-term health loss
Health services/ health system performance assessment	Coverage	Percent of a population or other unit (e.g., households) that accesses or uses a health intervention, conditional on need for the intervention
	Effective coverage	Percent of a population or other unit (e.g., households) that accesses or uses a health intervention, conditional on need for the intervention and adjusted for the quality of the health intervention received or health gain actually provided by using the intervention

In this section, we focus on two health metrics: (i) *disability-adjusted life-years* (DALYs), which can give policy-makers a comprehensive view of overall population health; and (ii) *effective coverage*, which can provide insight into how well health systems are delivering services to the populations who need them.

Measuring Population Health Loss: DALYs

In the GBD 1990 study, researchers created a summary health measure, DALYs, which combined both fatal and non-fatal health outcomes into a single value that quantified the number of healthy years of life lost due to premature death and disability (World Bank 1993). With the standard that one DALY equals one year of healthy life lost, policy-makers and program managers could now tally DALY totals and make meaningful comparisons between very different health conditions. For example, DALY totals could compare the burden of prostate cancer to the burden of bipolar disorder. DALYs could thus provide a more comprehensive picture of the drivers of ill health and their consequences than only referring to cause-specific mortality rates or case counts alone.

Table 5.2, for example, shows the 20 leading causes of DALYs experienced by each region in the world for 2010 (Murray *et al.* 2012b). While some global trends clearly exist (e.g., non-communicable diseases rank as major drivers of DALYs), even at the regional level relative health burdens can vary substantially. Ischemic heart disease accounts for some of the highest percentage of DALYs in several regions, but despite its burden in absolute terms, there are 10 to 20 more pressing health problems in sub-Saharan Africa. Road

Table 5.2 Twenty leading causes of disability-adjusted life-years by GBD region in 2010. Lower numbers reflect a higher burden rank and higher numbers a lower burden rank.

Disease cause	Global	High-income Asia Pacific	Western Europe	Australasia	High-income North America	Central Europe	Southern Latin America	Eastern Europe	East Asia	Tropical Latin America	Central Latin America	Southeast Asia	Central Asia	Andean Latin America	North Africa and Middle East	Caribbean	South Asia	Oceania	Southern sub-Saharan Africa	Eastern sub-Saharan Africa	Central sub-Saharan Africa	Western sub-Saharan Africa
Ischemic heart disease	1	3	2	2	1	1	1	1	2	1	2	3	1	4	1	2	4	6	14	21	19	20
Lower respiratory infections	2	7	21	30	17	6	13	15	7	6	4	2	1	5	4	1	1	2	3	4	2	3
Cerebrovascular disease	3	1	3	5	7	2	3	2	1	4	11	1	3	11	4	3	12	11	7	16	14	16
Diarrheal diseases	4	46	52	53	48	77	44	49	49	26	14	8	18	8	11	8	3	3	3	4	2	3
HIV/AIDS	5	108	59	87	37	72	34	4	38	12	13	13	31	13	58	9	17	9	1	1	5	4
Low back pain	6	2	1	1	3	3	2	3	5	3	7	7	5	2	13	10	14	15	17	23	13	9
Malaria	7	163	162	157	155	163	166	163	169	145	154	22	162	142	66	56	44	5	20	2	1	1
Preterm birth complications	8	58	44	29	26	37	12	35	27	9	9	8	6	8	11	2	7	6	5	6	7	7
COPD*	9	18	7	3	2	7	7	10	3	10	16	9	11	18	13	22	5	18	9	20	20	22
Road injury	10	16	12	9	10	8	5	7	4	5	4	5	5	2	6	10	11	15	13	11	12	9
Major depressive disorders	11	12	4	4	5	5	4	5	8	6	5	6	6	3	3	7	14	12	10	13	17	19
Neonatal encephalopathy*	12	84	66	50	84	42	40	24	20	24	12	4	9	18	15	6	4	12	9	10	10	10
Tuberculosis	13	42	107	123	124	55	65	17	37	46	44	2	15	21	33	17	8	4	4	7	7	12
Diabetes mellitus	14	10	10	14	8	9	9	15	10	8	3	10	12	15	9	6	16	2	8	29	28	26
Iron-deficiency anemia	15	39	84	36	117	29	27	29	32	18	17	14	13	7	10	5	9	21	11	12	11	11
Sepsis	16	119	120	111	99	114	49	82	122	27	29	34	53	17	22	14	7	25	29	8	13	5
Congenital anomalies	17	41	35	27	30	32	13	25	16	11	10	16	10	7	16	15	17	17	18	8	18	18
Self-harm	18	5	15	18	14	11	14	6	13	29	25	29	14	32	38	33	13	26	27	32	37	69
Falls	19	11	6	7	15	6	17	14	11	23	21	20	28	19	21	20	7	25	29	43	33	21
Protein-energy malnutrition	20	114	119	117	116	122	80	123	99	59	34	49	68	35	37	32	19	20	36	6	3	6

Disease burden ranking legend: 1-10 | 11-20 | 21-30 | 31-50 | 51-90 | 91-176

*COPD = chronic obstructive pulmonary disease; neonatal encephalopathy = birth asphyxia and birth trauma.
Note: sepsis and other infectious conditions of the newborn.
Source: adapted from Murray *et al.* (2012b).

traffic injuries, a health burden that often receives relatively less international attention than conditions such as HIV/AIDs, tuberculosis, and malaria (Hazen and Ehiri 2006), rank as the second highest contributor of DALYs in Latin America. If you were a policy-maker in this region and only focused on infectious diseases, you may miss the opportunity to address a serious health challenge.

Calculating DALYs entails measuring the gap between the ideal of living a long life full of health and the reality of the health that populations experience (Murray *et al.* 2000). This computation requires two estimates: the years of life lost due to premature death (YLLs) and years lived with disability (YLDs). DALYs cannot be measured directly, and are derived by combining cause-specific mortality rates and prevalence rates. Disability weights, also known as health state weights, are applied to estimates of YLDs as a way to reflect the severity of health loss associated with each non-fatal outcome (Murray and Lopez 1997). These weights are based on individuals' perceptions, as measured by global surveys, of how much various conditions affect people's lives (Salomon *et al.* 2012).

DALYs are a useful summary health measure for understanding overall health burdens, as the metric combines fatal and non-fatal health outcomes into a single number that can be compared across geographies and different periods of time. At the same time, DALYs are limited by the availability and quality of the individual health metrics needed for their computation. These include indicators such as age-specific mortality rates, cause-specific mortality rates, and measures of disease prevalence. Combined, these metrics serve as the cornerstones for DALY estimation (Murray and Lopez 1997). Without supplementary information, though, such indicators can depict only partial pictures of overall health burdens. Child mortality, for instance, is a key health metric to track, as the metric provides a general benchmark against which countries can measure their progress in improving overall childhood survival over time (i.e., Millennium Development Goal (MDG) 4; Lozano *et al.* 2011). However, this measure does not provide information on the causes of child deaths, whether the composition of such causes is changing over time, or if children are suffering from non-fatal health impairments. Similarly, case counts of non-fatal health outcomes provide crucial information on the conditions that reduce the productivity and mobility of populations, but again, if case count data are used in isolation or without understanding their shortcomings, their usefulness for policy-making may be reduced. Case counts by cause can easily be skewed by changes in population size or age structure over time. Further, case data are often more challenging to measure than deaths as they are not captured by vital registration systems and thus rely on contact with the health system or self-report via health surveys.

As new analytic tools are developed and the science of global health measurement is advanced, it is incumbent upon those in the vanguard to increase the technical capacity of individuals and groups interested in better understanding the generation and use of these metrics. Such capacity can be increased through training workshops, increased collaboration, and clearly worded documentation of methods. In parallel, the international community should support further capacity-building in the production of in-depth national burden of disease studies. A host of organizations, including the Institute for Health Metrics and Evaluation (IHME), are developing new collaborations and approaches to assist with this goal (IHME 2013a).

Measuring Health System Performance: Effective Coverage

Quantifying whether, and how well, a health system is providing health services and interventions to its populations is one way to assess health system performance. Determining which components of health service delivery are working and which are not – as well as the degree to which delivery gaps persist – can provide the foundation for policy changes and incentives targeting performance improvement. There are many health metrics and approaches to assess health system performance, but here we will discuss the concept of coverage. Examples of coverage include the proportion of children using insecticide-treated nets against malaria or the fraction of mothers who give birth with the assistance of a skilled birth attendant.

While measuring coverage provides important information on whether health interventions or services are reaching target populations, it does not capture the quality of the received intervention or whether the interventions had their intended effects under routine conditions. Effective coverage unites intervention use, need, and quality by measuring the proportion of people who received or used a health intervention they needed and then adjusting that measurement for the quality of the intervention or the health gain actually provided by the intervention (Shengelia *et al.* 2005). To make the transition from measuring coverage to providing a measurement of effective coverage requires additional information, such as changes in a biological marker as related to the proper receipt or use of an intervention. This need for additional information makes effective coverage more challenging to assess than coverage alone.

To estimate the effective coverage of diabetes management, for example, information needs to be collected on the prevalence of diabetes (i.e., the population in need), the proportion of people with diabetes who receive treatment, and the effectiveness of their treatments. Data on effectiveness are infrequently collected, and, when they are, explicitly linking changes in health outcomes to intervention exposure may not be possible. However, when the requisite data are available for calculating effective coverage, informative analyses on treatment approaches and delivery options can be performed. In Iran, researchers measured the effective coverage of diabetes treatment across urban and rural areas (Farzadfar *et al.* 2012). They found that diabetes management through local health facilities in rural areas was associated with greater improvements in health outcomes (i.e., lower levels of fasting plasma glucose and systolic blood pressure) than diabetes management in urban areas.

Effective coverage can also provide helpful, as well as unique, insights into how well health systems are addressing health conditions. Since 2001, Mexico's Ministry of Health has used effective coverage estimates to assess its health system performance and incentivize further program improvements (Lozano *et al.* 2006). Before and during the roll-out of country-wide health reforms in 2004, the Ministry of Health took advantage of its extensive health information system to collect data on intervention need, utilization, and quality for several health conditions. The Ministry was able to pinpoint which states lagged behind in effectively delivering specific interventions. Figure 5.1 illustrates the range in both crude and effective coverage of hypertension treatment within and across states in Mexico during the implementation phase of health reform.

In terms of using effective coverage indicators to inform health policy decision-making, the Mexican health system performance assessment taught the global health field three main lessons (Murray 2009). First, Mexico showed that effective coverage could be used to develop a performance benchmarking system at the subnational level. Second, by using effective coverage indicators that not only included "more traditional" child and maternal health interventions but also interventions targeting non-communicable diseases, the Ministry of Health could identify the areas where the health system was performing better (e.g., poor children and mothers) than others (e.g., diabetes treatment). Last, and

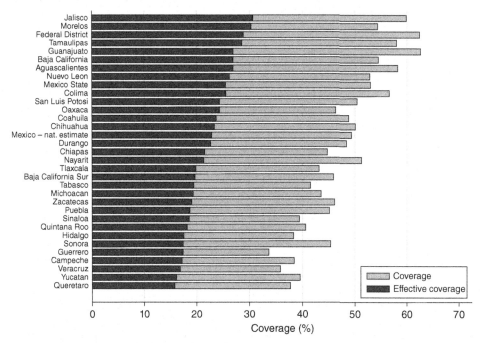

Figure 5.1 Crude coverage and effective coverage of hypertension treatment across Mexican states, 2005–2006. Source: adapted from Lozano *et al.* (2006).

perhaps most importantly, Mexico could point to a strong association between aggregated effective coverage indicators and total health system expenditures made by the government. This relationship was weaker between health outcomes and spending, which is not completely surprising given the number of potential confounding factors (e.g., the influences of education and poverty on health outcomes). However, finding that health system investments were associated with higher rates of effective coverage is an important piece of evidence in making the case for sustained, if not expanded, funding for health service provision (Murray 2009).

Data Sources for the World's Health Metrics

Health metrics, including DALYs and effective coverage, are estimated from several data sources. These sources can vary substantially in terms of the information they collect, the frequency with which data are collected and updated, and the populations they can accurately represent. Table 5.3 summarizes a range of data sources and how well a given data source can provide the information needed to estimate various health metrics. A thorough discussion of each data source is not possible within a single chapter, so in this section we focus on two types of key data sources that feed into the production of health metrics: vital registration (VR) systems and household surveys.

Vital registration systems continuously track civil events, which usually include births, deaths, and marriages, and thus can provide detailed information on fertility and mortality trends. VR data are currently the single best resource from which mortality trends can be disaggregated by causes of death (as designated by death certificates). However, these

Table 5.3 A selection of data sources frequently used in producing health metrics and how well their data support estimation.

Health domain	Health data source								
	Vital registration	Household surveys	Health examination surveys	Health service registries	Hospital discharges	Censuses	NHAs, budget and expenditure reports	Epidemiological studies	Health facility assessments
Mortality	Preferable	Possible				Possible		Possible	
Cause of death	Preferable	Possible			Possible			Possible	
Risk factors	Possible	Preferable	Possible	Possible		Possible		Possible	
Morbidity		Possible	Preferable	Possible	Possible	Possible		Possible	
Functional health status			Preferable					Possible	
Human resource inputs							Preferable		Possible
Health financing							Preferable		Preferable
Cost effectiveness	Preferable	Preferable	Preferable	Possible	Preferable				Preferable
Health services		Possible	Possible	Possible	Possible	Preferable		Possible	Preferable
Burden of disease/ comparative risk assessment				Summary health metrics – draws from multiple metrics above					
Health system performance assessment				Summary health metrics – draws from multiple metrics above					

NHA, National Health Accounts.
Source: adapted from Lozano and Mokdad (2009).

data are only as useful as the VR system's coverage (or inclusion) of a given population, the accurracy of cause of death designations, and the timeliness in which the data can be aggregated for population health needs. In 2003, only 64 of the 115 countries reporting deaths to the WHO had complete coverage of VR (Mathers *et al.* 2005). Among the annual deaths reported from 2000 to 2010 by VR systems in several countries in North Africa, the Middle East, and Southeast Asia (Figure 5.2), more than half of all deaths were assigned garbage codes (i.e., coded as a condition that cannot be an underlying cause) (Naghavi *et al.* 2010). The ramifications, ranging from political to financial, of accurately measuring only 50% of a country's deaths each year – and failing to understand which conditions account for the other half – could be substantial.

Household surveys aim to sample enough individuals and groups so that, through their answers and estimation procedures, they provide an accurate reflection of the larger population. Household surveys collect data on individual health through structured interviews and direct examination. There are several nationally representative household surveys conducted with some regularity that can inform the estimation of health metrics. These include the Demographic and Health Surveys (DHS), World Health Surveys (WHS), Malaria Indicator Surveys (MIS), Multiple Indicator Cluster Surveys (MICS), Reproductive Health Surveys (RHS), and Living Standards Measurement Surveys (LSMS). Surveys can provide many data advantages, such as purposely targeting individuals who live in rural areas, are less wealthy, or have other characteristics that make them less likely to be captured by administrative health data systems. As a result, survey data collected for these populations can be more representative, and surveys are often the only source of detailed information about these hard-to-reach populations.

In spite of their strengths, household surveys have three major weaknesses. First, surveys are expensive, with the DHS averaging about US$1 million per survey. Second, several survey types, including the DHS, MIS, and MICS, are meant to be representative at the national or provincial levels, yet many health services and corresponding policies are administered at lower administrative levels (i.e., district, city, village). Measuring coverage and effectiveness of health service delivery at these lower levels is of immense value to policy-makers, but doing so would require a much larger sample size, which can be prohibitively expensive. Third, surveys typically take place less often than routine data collection. Under ideal circumstances, such routine collection regularly updates health information and reports data up to health offices and ministries on a monthly basis (Lozano and Mokdad 2009). In contrast, DHS data collection generally occurs every five years in most countries, but in several places, such as Botswana, Paraguay, and Sudan, a DHS survey has not taken place in at least 20 years (Measure DHS 2013). It is likely that these countries use other data sources to inform their health system and policy needs, and are not significantly impaired by not having more frequent DHS. Nevertheless, infrequent DHS data collection may reduce the ability to compare or benchmark findings from other data sources (e.g., administrative health records) against those generated by household surveys (HIS Knowledge Hub and IHME 2009).

In many ways, health metrics can only be as informative as the data underlying them. It can therefore be helpful to researchers and policy-makers to have a better understanding of where population health data originated, as well as the benefits and challenges of using different data sources to estimate a given health metric. Through greater understanding of the underlying data, they can in turn better assess the degree to which they believe the health metrics they encounter and whether the information these metrics provide is useful to them.

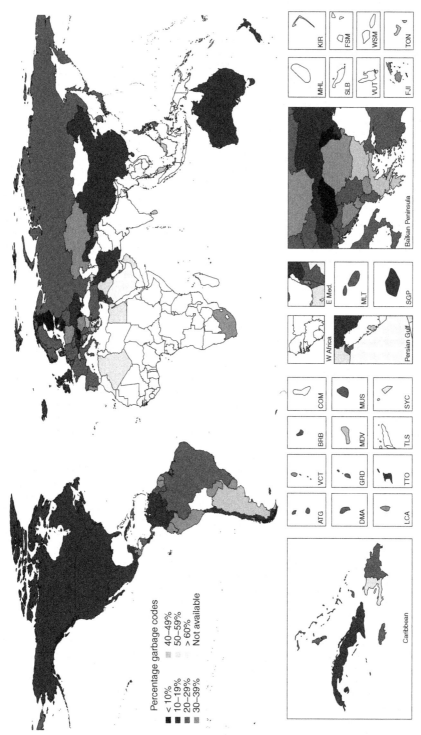

Figure 5.2 Fraction of deaths assigned as garbage codes from nationally representative vital registration systems, 2000–2010. Source: adapted from Lozano *et al.* (2012).

From Producing Health Metrics to Informing Policy: Are Our Estimates Good Enough?

Every day, population health data and health metrics are produced with the intention of informing global health programs and policy. We have identified some health metrics that, through their estimation, can provide very important information for policy-makers. We have listed a range of data sources, with a corresponding range of strengths and challenges, which serve as the basis for health metrics production. However, we have yet to consider what may be the most important question facing the field of health metrics and evaluation: is what we currently know about the world's health good enough? And, if not, how can we improve that knowledge?

Compared with our understanding of global health 20 years ago, we know a lot more, and in some respects, simply knowing more about the world's health is good enough. The progression from what we knew based on the original GBD 1990 study to what we know from the latest iteration highlights this increase in understanding the world's health. GBD 1990 resulted from a dearth of comprehensive, comparable, and timely information on a range of health outcomes and risk factors throughout the world (Murray and Lopez 1997). Many disease burdens experienced by populations remained hidden from policy-makers' awareness and were neglected by global agendas until GBD 1990 showcased their "true" impact on populations. At the same time, the scale of GBD 1990 was fairly limited. The collaborators worldwide involved in GBD 2010 recognized the value of adding more conditions and expanding the scope of the analysis. As a result, GBD 2010 helped to hone our understanding of the world's health by measuring the premature death and disability due to 291 diseases and injuries, 67 risk factors, and 1,160 non-fatal health states or sequelae in 21 regions, 187 countries, and 20 age groups for the years of 1990, 2000, and 2010 (Murray *et al.* 2012a). In addition, GBD 2010 researchers developed user-friendly data visualization tools in order to allow anyone to tailor the data produced from GBD 2010 to optimally align with their individual needs (to use GBD 2010 data visualizations, visit www.ihmeuw.org/GBDCountryViz, last accessed February 2014). IHME and its research collaborators are working to produce annual updates of the GBD estimates, beginning with a new publication in 2014, allowing decision-makers worldwide to see current trends in their countries and to benchmark their health performance in comparison to their peers.

On the other hand, the world's current estimates of health burdens and health system performance are far from capturing a complete picture of health for all populations, geographies, and periods of time. Although the information produced by GBD can fill knowledge gaps related to various diseases and health burdens, we still lack a fuller understanding of the complex dynamics underlying and driving health outcomes. We are good, or at least better than we used to be, at describing the world's health – as long as enough accurate data at a given geographic level has been collected to inform our estimates. But we are not nearly good enough at explaining *why* the world experiences the health it does and *how* these health burdens are best addressed.

The generation of health estimates needs to be timelier, more financially feasible, and more policy relevant. After all, the most sophisticated health metrics are not useful if the measurements are not available when decisions need to be made; or if the cost of generating measurements exceeds the cost of the programs or policies needed; or if the health metrics provided do not appropriately capture the disease burdens experienced by populations or health system priorities. On the other hand, friction often emerges when we try to balance the demand for simpler health statistics and estimation procedures with the challenge of developing nimble and robust modeling techniques that can accurately capture the complex nature of population health and be more accessible to broader audiences. Being able to understand the machinery underlying health estimation does not always lead to being able to produce the most accurate estimates of population health. Akin to weather forecasting, our world rightly calls for accurate models of health estimation, and the simplest models, while certainly preferred and sought whenever possible, cannot always deliver the accuracy we want (Foreman *et al.* 2012).

An additional factor that determines whether global health estimates are sufficient is the credibility of those estimates. The most accurate, precise, timely, and relevant health metrics will be rendered useless if they are not believed. Discrediting of health metrics can occur at the local level (e.g., confusion over differences in reported data to health ministries and estimates generated by international organizations) or globally (e.g., politically charged disagreements over optimal estimation methodologies and data use). There are many approaches that may demonstrate, solidify, or improve the credibility of health metrics and estimates, including but not limited to: rigorous peer review; friendly competition in the ideas marketplace; testing predictive validity of health metrics and estimates with out-of-sample populations; the promotion and application of reproducible computational research methods; the implementation of open-source software; and wider sharing of input data. Nevertheless, the efficacy of these approaches remains relatively undiscovered.

To understand further the need for advancement in timely and comprehensive health metrics, we consider two recent examples: MDG 5, aimed at reducing maternal deaths, and Mexico's *Seguro Popular* health insurance reform.

Measuring the Attainment of MDG 5: Reducing Maternal Deaths

Millennium Development Goal 5 resulted from an agreement among member states of the United Nations (UN) in 2000. The goal set a target for countries of reducing the maternal mortality ratio – the number of deaths of women during pregnancy, childbirth, or 42 days after delivery per 100,000 live births – by 75% between 1990 and 2015 (UN 2000). Working toward this target clearly would benefit mothers and overall population health, but in terms of program and policy prioritization, one major question emerged: were the data available to know if countries were making progress toward MDG 5?

Tracking maternal health outcomes has been widely viewed as necessary by the global health field, but how to produce consistent information on maternal mortality trends over time is less straightforward and far more challenging (Graham *et al.* 2008). Since maternal deaths are relatively rare and often occur away from health facilities, there is substantial risk that these deaths may not be counted toward maternal mortality ratios. Subsequently, maternal mortality data are often sparse, especially in lower-income settings, and both corrective and predictive statistics are needed in order to produce systematic, valid estimates for all countries and regions (Hogan *et al.* 2010). For example, Figure 5.3 highlights the overall lack of data for maternal mortality in Egypt and Saudi Arabia. The figure also shows how model estimates (the solid line) become more precise as more reported data are available (i.e., the dashed lines, or uncertainty intervals, move closer to the model estimate), particularly in the case of Egypt between 2000 and 2010.

For both Egypt and Saudi Arabia, these estimates show that at least some progress has been made in reducing maternal deaths. However, especially for Saudi Arabia, it is difficult to say *how* much progress the country has made, especially given the great amount of uncertainty associated with the estimates. Without a more precise understanding of the

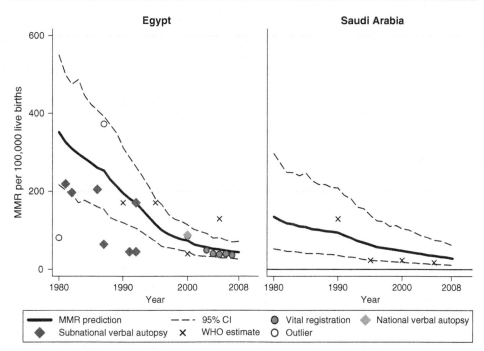

Figure 5.3   Maternal mortality ratio (MMR) estimates for Egypt and Saudi Arabia, 1980–2008. Source: adapted from Hogan *et al.* (2010).

ongoing risk for maternal mortality, program managers and policy-makers may struggle with appropriate program resource allocations and prioritization. On the other hand, even if the exact maternal mortality numbers could be produced, is it "good enough" to simply know what the health burdens are if we cannot understand what caused them, or if they are universally experienced within a given population? Luckily, this is a question that may be more easily answered in the future. For instance, the government of Saudi Arabia has invested in creating a real-time health surveillance system to strengthen the country's responsiveness to health burdens and policy needs for all citizens (IHME 2013b).

Measuring the Impact of Mexico's Health Reform: Seguro Popular

During its health system reform from 2004 to 2006, the Mexican government based its policy goals on data collected on the performance of the country's health system and on the levels and trends in population health prior to reform implementation (Lozano *et al.* 2006). The roll-out of *Seguro Popular* – the health insurance component of the system reform – took advantage of Mexico's high-quality surveillance systems to assess the impact of the reform. The implementation and subsequent evaluation of Mexico's *Seguro Popular* showed how health data could shape policy decisions and assess whether a national health policy had its intended effects (Frenk 2006).

The seeds of the health system reform date back to the assessment by the WHO *World Health Report 2000* of Mexico's health system performance (Frenk *et al.* 2006). Out of the 191 countries assessed, the Mexican health system was ranked 61st in terms of overall performance but 144th in "fairness of financial contribution[s]" for health services

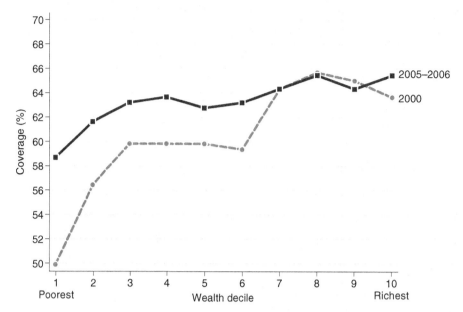

Figure 5.4   Changes in composite coverage by wealth decile between 2000 and 2005–2006 in Mexico. Source: adapted from Gakidou *et al.* (2006).

(WHO 2000). Prior to the report's release, Mexico's Ministry of Health did not know the degree to which out-of-pocket healthcare expenditures were affecting its citizens, especially the poor and uninsured (Frenk 2006). Mexican officials decided that one of the best ways to respond to the *World Health Report 2000* would be to extend health insurance coverage to all uninsured citizens. Before *Seguro Popular* was rolled out, though, Mexico's Ministry of Health made use of its extensive health data systems to capture the existing levels and trends for several health indicators by state. Then, during the quasi-randomized, phased implementation of *Seguro Popular* researchers were able to compare trends both pre- and post-reform and compare trends across states.

Between 2000 and 2006, the least wealthy populations in Mexico – *Seguro Popular's* targeted recipients – experienced significant increases in access to and use of health interventions (Gakidou *et al.* 2006). These increases effectively reduced health inequalities between the poorest and richest groups of people in Mexico (Figure 5.4). Although other factors may certainly have contributed to these improvements (e.g., implementation of other state-level health programs), the deliberate collection and analysis of health data linked to *Seguro Popular's* objectives and implementation provide evidence-based support for the program's success and overarching impact.

The ability to adequately evaluate the Mexican health reform relied on the availability of extensive health data sources and significant political will. The feasibility of conducting a similar assessment and evaluation in other countries is far less clear.

Moving Towards Better Health Estimates

In the last two decades, the metrics, data, and methods we use to measure the world's health have improved. We know much more about the health burdens experienced throughout the world, and in some cases, why these burdens have emerged and how to optimally address them. Nonetheless, the global health estimates we have today and the ways in which we ascertain them certainly have room for improvement. Decisions about how to further improve global health metrics and methodologies are not straightforward or easy. They involve determining which types of research and technical training to support, where and in what topical areas to strengthen data collection capacities, and how to better align the production of health data and estimates with health system demands.

Investing in the creation, expansion, and maintenance of health information systems serves as a foundational step for improving our knowledge of global health burdens and our abilities to address them. Without the ongoing collection of data on what ails individuals, what leads to their premature deaths, and which services the health system is providing them, important decisions about a population's health needs may be largely informed by modeling exercises, ideological views, or even guesses. In this type of information-sparse context, the path to achieving greater health for all becomes a steeper climb.

When population health data are available, their variable quality can remain as a substantial hurdle in moving toward better health estimates. Our metrics and measurement approaches, even the most sophisticated, can only do so much in the face of information that is incomplete, unrepresentative, or inaccurate, especially if we do not recognize the shortcomings of these data. Improving the quality of the health data collected and stored by monitoring systems, through actions like benchmarking exercises and routine system checks, can reduce the necessity of many modeling assumptions and estimation procedures, and thus tighten the divide between estimating population health and truly measuring a population's health.

From local health authorities to global agencies, these choices and debates on how to measure the world's health have substantial policy ramifications. After all, if a health need or condition is not measured, it is less likely to enter the discussions that inform health policy and programs. As a field, our ultimate goal is to improve population health. Deciding what to measure and how to do so shapes the way everyone, from researchers to policy-makers, views the progress, challenges, and prospects for global health. Continued work in health data collection, analysis, and interpretation is critical for ensuring that our estimates are strong enough to meet the health needs of all populations and ultimately improve the prospects for health achievement throughout the world.

Acknowledgments

We are most grateful for the assistance provided by several individuals at the Institute for Health Metrics and Evaluation (IHME), including William Heisel and Brian Childress for their editorial contributions, and Diego González-Medina and Charles Atkinson for GBD 2010 figure production.

Key Reading

AbouZahr C, Adjei S, Kanchanachitra C. 2007. From data to policy: good practices and cautionary tales. *Lancet* 369, 1039–46.

Boerma JT, Stansfield SK. 2007. Health statistics now: are we making the right investments? *Lancet* 369: 779–86.

Frenk J. 2006. Bridging the divide: global lessons from evidence-based health policy in Mexico. *Lancet* 368: 954–61.

IHME (Institute for Health Metrics and Evaluation). 2013. *The Global Burden of Disease: Generating Evidence, Guiding Policy.* Seattle, WA: IHME. www.ihmeuw.org/gbd (last accessed March 2014).

Mathers CD, Murray CJL, Ezzati M, Gakidou E, Salomon JA, Stein C. 2003. Population health metrics: crucial inputs to the development of evidence for health policy. *Population Health Metrics* 1(6).

Murray CJL, Frenk J. 2008. Health metrics and evaluation: strengthening the science. *Lancet* 371, 1191–9.

Walker N, Bryce J, Black RE. 2007. Interpreting health statistics for policymaking: the story behind the headlines. *Lancet* 369, 956–63.

References

Farzadfar F, Murray CJL, Gakidou E *et al.* 2012. Effectiveness of diabetes and hypertension management by rural primary health-care workers (Behvarz workers) in Iran: a nationally representative observational study. *Lancet* 379(9810), 47–54.

Foreman KJ, Lozano R, Lopez AD, Murray CJL. 2012. Modeling causes of death: an integrated approach using CODEm. *Population Health Metrics* 10(1).

Frenk J. 2006. Bridging the divide: global lessons from evidence-based health policy in Mexico. *Lancet* 368, 954–61.

Frenk J, González-Pier E, Gómez-Dantés O, Lezana MA, Knaul FM. 2006. Comprehensive reform to improve health system performance in Mexico. *Lancet* 368(9546), 1524–34.

Gakidou EE, Lozano R, Pier-González E *et al.* 2006. Assessing the effect of the 2001–06 Mexican health reform: an interim report card. *Lancet* 368, 1920–35.

Graham WJ, Foster LB, Davidson L, Hauke E, Campbell OMR. 2008. Measuring progress in reducing maternal mortality. *Best Practice and Research in Clinical Obstetrics and Gynaecology* 22(3), 425–45.

Groenewald P, Nannan N, Bourne D, Laubscher R, Bradshaw D. 2005. Identifying deaths from AIDS in South Africa. *AIDS* 19, 193–201.

Hazen A, Ehiri JE. 2006. Road traffic injuries: hidden epidemic in less developed countries. *Journal of the National Medical Association* 98(1), 73–82.

HIS Knowledge Hub (Health Information Systems Knowledge Hub) and IHME (Institute for Health Metrics and Evaluation). 2009. *Improving the Quality and Use of Health Information Systems: Essential Strategic Issues.* Health Information Systems Knowledge Hub Working Paper 5. http://www.uq.edu.au/hishub/wp5 (last accessed November 2013).

Hogan MC, Foreman KJ, Naghavi M *et al.* 2010. Maternal mortality for 181 countries, 1980–2008: a systematic analysis of progress towards Millennium Development Goal 5. *Lancet* 375(9726), 1609–23.

IHME (Institute for Health Metrics and Evaluation). 2013a. *The Global Burden of Disease: Generating Evidence, Guiding Policy.* Seattle, WA: IHME.

IHME (Institute for Health Metrics and Evaluation). 2013b. *Kingdom of Saudi Arabia Health Tracking Project.* http://www.healthmetricsandevaluation.org/research/project/kingdom-saudi-arabia-health-tracking (last accessed November 2013).

IHME (Institute for Health Metrics and Evaluation) and UNZA (University of Zambia). 2011. *Maternal and Child Health Intervention Coverage in Zambia: The Heterogeneous Picture.* Seattle, WA: IHME.

Kohatsu ND, Robinson JG, Torner JC. 2004. Evidence-based public health: an evolving concept. *American Journal of Preventative Medicine* 27(5), 417–21.

Lozano R, Mokdad A. 2009. *Role of Health Surveys in National Health Information Systems: Best-Use Scenarios.* Health Information Systems Knowledge Hub Working Paper 6. http://www.uq.edu.au/hishub/wp6 (last accessed November 2013).

Lozano R, Naghavi M, Foreman K *et al.* 2012. Global and regional mortality from 235 causes of death for 20 age groups in 1990 and 2010: a systematic analysis for the Global Burden of Disease Study 2010. *Lancet* 380(9859), 2085–128.

Lozano R, Soliz P, Gakidou E *et al.* 2006. Benchmarking of performance of Mexican states with effective coverage. *Lancet* 368(9548), 1729–41.

Lozano R, Wang H, Foreman KJ *et al.* 2011. Progress towards Millennium Development Goals 4 and 5 on maternal and child mortality: an updated systematic analysis. *Lancet* 378, 1139–65.

Mathers CD, Fat DM, Inoue ZM, Rao C, Lopez AD. 2005. Algorithms for enhancing public health utility of national causes-of-death data. *Bulletin of the World Health Organization* 83, 171–7.

Measure DHS (Demographic and Health Surveys). 2013. Survey search. www.measuredhs.com/What-We-Do/Survey-Search.cfm (last accessed November 2013).

Murray CJL. 2009. *Assessing Health Systems Performance using Information on Effective Coverage of Interventions.* Health Information Systems Knowledge Hub Working Paper 3. http://www.uq.edu.au/hishub/wp3 (last accessed November 2013).

Murray CJL, Ezzati M, Flaxman AD *et al.* 2012a. GBD 2010: design, definitions and metrics. *Lancet* 380(9859), 2063–6.

Murray CJL, Frenk J. 2008. Health metrics and evaluation: strengthening the science. *Lancet* 371, 1191–9.

Murray CJL, Lopez AD. 1997. Global mortality, disability, and the contributions of risk factors: the Global Burden of Disease Study. *Lancet* 349, 1436–42.

Murray CJL, Salomon JA, Mathers C. 2000. A critical examination of summary measures of population health. *Bulletin of the World Health Organization* 78(8), 981–94.

Murray CJL, Vos T, Lozano R *et al.* 2012b. Disability-adjusted life years (DALYs) for 291 diseases and injuries in 21 regions, 1990–2010: a systematic analysis for the Global Burden of Disease Study 2010. *Lancet* 380(9859), 2197–223.

Naghavi M, Makela S, Foreman K, O'Brien J, Pourmalek F, Lozano R. 2010. Algorithms for enhancing public health utility of national causes-of-death data. *Population Health Metrics* 8(9).

Salomon JA, Vos T, Hogan DR *et al.* 2012. Common values in assessing health outcomes from disease and injury: disability weights measurement study for the Global Burden of Disease Study 2010. *Lancet* 380(9859), 2129–43.

Setel PW, Macfarlane SB, Szreter S *et al.* 2007. A scandal of invisibility: making everyone count by counting everyone. *Lancet* 370, 1569–77.

Shengelia B, Tandon A, Adams OB, Murray CJL. 2005. Access, utilization, quality, and effective coverage: an integrated conceptual framework and measurement strategy. *Social Science and Medicine* 61(1), 97–109.

UN (United Nations) General Assembly. 2000. *United Nations Millennium Declaration.* A/RES/55/2. New York: UN.

World Bank. 1993. *World Development Report 1993. Investing in Health: World Development Indicators.* Oxford: Oxford University Press.

WHO (World Health Organization). 2000. *The World Health Report 2000 – Health Systems: Improving Performance.* Geneva: WHO.

Chapter 6

Achieving Better Global Health Policy, Even When Health Metrics Data are Scanty

Peter Byass

Abstract

There is often an unclear relationship between health metrics data and health policy-making, particularly in the global South, where adequate data are often simply unavailable. Evidence-based policy-making can only happen if at least some evidence of relevance to the policy-makers' settings is available in a suitably digested format. Health metrics data come from a variety of sources, including intensive local population surveillance, sample surveys, and health facilities, but synthesizing such data from different sources into coherent messages is not simple and may lead to complexities that do not facilitate understanding. Health facility users differ from non-users, and hence a population-based dimension is an essential component for the credibility of health evidence. Uncertainties in evidence, whether arising from inadequacies of quantity and quality, or from the technical basis of generalizing from sample-based data, add further difficulties to interpretation. Since all health data fundamentally derive from the lives of individuals, and sometimes from very private aspects of those lives, there are ethical imperatives in handling health data. Making health metrics data available in ways that do not compromise confidentiality presents further technical challenges. All of these considerations point towards the need for better evidence – and therefore better tools and procedures for gathering data – at grass-roots levels that correspond to policy-makers' domains. Overall improvements in global health evidence and policy depend critically on such bottom-up developments.

The Handbook of Global Health Policy, First Edition. Edited by Garrett W. Brown, Gavin Yamey, and Sarah Wamala.
© 2014 John Wiley & Sons, Ltd. Published 2014 by John Wiley & Sons, Ltd.

Key Points

- Evidence-based policy-making presupposes that the necessary health metrics data exist – but often they do not.
- Small-scale detailed data may be more useful than large amounts of largely uninterpretable data.
- Data need to be relevant to policy-makers' domains – at the national or subnational rather than global level.
- Strategies for obtaining better health metrics data must be affordable, manageable, and fit for purpose.
- Good global health policy needs to grow from the bottom up, in parallel with grass-roots evidence.

Key Policy Implications

- Countries and subnational areas need better tools for gathering and managing their own health metrics data, rather than being given external estimates of "their" parameters.
- Bottom-up approaches to information systems and policy-making need to be strengthened and closely integrated with each other.
- Evidence needs to be longitudinal and strongly population-based, including relating healthcare utilization data to surrounding populations.

What is Global Health Policy – and What Health Metrics Data are Needed?

Although some health policy concerns, such as the threat of new epidemics, are primarily considered at the "global" level (Dry 2008), in reality the decision-making processes for health usually go beyond the global level. Global health policy can be considered as a wide-ranging amalgam of national health policies, which are sometimes externally influenced by international agencies and donors, and which then filter down to subnational level. At that level, depending on within-country political and administrative structures, there may be further enhancement and interpretation of received policies. Processes coming from the *opposite direction*, for example from local politicians and civil leaders, as well as within lower levels of health systems, may well encounter top-down policies at the subnational level, and compromises may be needed to reconcile top-down concepts with bottom-up realities.

Although it is relatively easy to discuss these arrangements conceptually, it is hard to generalize about the precise mechanisms from country to country, because of the highly random nature of what nationhood entails (Byass 2009a) and the extent of regional autonomy within different countries. For reasons of politics, history, and geography, countries vary from mega-states such as China and India down to tiny island nations that might equate to single communities in other contexts. States or provinces within larger countries may operate with considerable autonomy and with health budgets that equate to national situations elsewhere.

This complexity presents a major challenge to making a coherent or systematic judgment about "global" health policy. Similarly, assessments of progress in global health are often confused by the need to measure issues at national level. For example, progress towards the Millennium Development Goals (UN 2011) is often popularly expressed in terms of the number of countries achieving (or likely to achieve) the targets – but this is a largely meaningless outcome measure if no consideration is given to the populations within those countries.

Some of the same considerations apply to health metrics data. Again, there is no single entity constituting "global health data" because information about health fundamentally originates from data on the lives of *individual people*. These data have to be aggregated up the various tiers of health and civil systems in order to make sense at different population levels. In turn, incompatibilities in systems and procedures mean that it can be difficult to achieve reliable aggregation, with the result that higher level evidence frequently undergoes some kind of modeling process as part of its interpretation. This process may have some advantages, but at the same time can result in evidence that seems somewhat detached from the original context of the constituent data.

In 2010, the open access global health journal *PLOS Medicine* published a series of essays giving different perspectives on the advantages and disadvantages of modeled estimates of global health (Boerma *et al.* 2010; Byass 2010; Graham and Adjei 2010; Murray and Lopez 2010; Sankoh 2010). Many health issues are currently receiving attention by means of modeled global estimates, though it is not entirely clear what the value of such estimates may be to policy-makers on a more local basis, for example at national or subnational levels.

Hence, to address the question of improving health policy on a global basis, without having all the desired data, one has to consider both data and policy on a more localized basis, as well as how aggregation from bottom-up processes to higher levels can be reliably achieved.

Scale of Health Metrics Data

The ideal strategy for health evidence at any population level would be to effectively gather and manage data on *every individual* residing at that population level, and report evidence on a non-sampled basis. The need for complex modeling and analysis would be minimized, and figures could largely speak for themselves. This is an approach to health evidence that was pioneered in Scandinavia in the eighteenth century (Sundin and Willner 2007) and which, at least in some settings, has settled down as the normative model. Most industrialized countries now adopt this approach. Known as universal registration, it presupposes a social infrastructure in which every individual is unambiguously identifiable, and it relies on a civil system in which the population trusts national and subnational authorities with their personal data, particularly concerning the confidentiality of sensitive issues (Ludvigsson *et al.* 2009). The costs of operating such a system tend to be subsumed and normalized within various branches of government – by no means exclusively within the health sector. It is actually very difficult to get an accurate handle on the costs of such a data system, because running the system is not a discrete activity in itself, but an integral part of the work of government.

However, due to infrastructural and economic constraints, most of the world's countries are still a long way from implementing and running a comprehensive data system that includes their complete population. The consequence is that we know a lot more about the populations of wealthier rather than poorer countries (Byass 2009b). Naturally this tends to introduce some bias into evidence at the global level, since we cannot simply suppose that the health status of poorer populations, which lack data, is the same, or even similar, to those of wealthier populations, about whom more is known.

To some extent the scale at which health evidence is needed depends on the purpose for which it is required. One example is the range of cause-of-death data that may be needed for different purposes and at different scales (Byass 2007). At one extreme, it may be very important to have clear medical evidence about the death of a particular individual, and medical and legal practitioners may invest considerable effort in a single case. At the other extreme, there is interest among international agencies in having reliable evidence about global patterns of causes of death, which is very far removed from the death of any particular individual. In between, and perhaps most importantly in terms of health policy, there are clear needs for health policy-makers to have reliable evidence that accurately relates to their particular level of responsibility. A district health manager mostly needs to know the cause-of-death patterns *within his or her own district*. It might be interesting for some purposes to make comparisons with adjacent districts or national levels, but in terms of deciding how to deploy health resources within the district, it is the health status of people within that area that counts. It is much less relevant to have evidence that only applies directly to a higher level, and which is not disaggregated.

The big question therefore is how to arrive at reliable health evidence that is clearly applicable to the levels at which it is needed, in settings where counting everyone is impractical. National cross-sectional sample surveys are often undertaken, but may be of limited use at the subnational level. The usefulness is limited since the surveys are normally designed with an emphasis on having a sufficient sample at national level, and even if data are broken down at subnational level, the numbers may be too small to be locally applicable.

One common example of this approach is the Demographic and Health Surveys (DHS) (Rutstein and Rojas 2006), as supported by the US government in many low-income countries. The DHS approach has a number of inherent strengths and weaknesses. A major advantage is that health data from the DHS are made available, on an open access basis, for countries that might lack any other such source. In any particular survey round, DHS achieve national coverage using a cluster sampling approach. Relatively closely standardized survey methodologies across all countries, apart from a small number of specifically local parameters, allow cross-country comparisons to be made (Garenne 2011; Hosseinpoor *et al.* 2011). However, it may be difficult to interpret differences in parameters between survey rounds because of the usual 5-year cycle between surveys, and because of the lack of any attempt to follow up individual participants from previous survey rounds. Recall bias effects, arising for example when asking women about their entire reproductive history, can also be difficult to interpret (Byass *et al.* 2007).

An alternative approach to a relatively thinly spread national sample is to take a more data-intense approach in one or more local areas. For discrete single areas, this approach is often known as the Health and Demographic Surveillance Sites (HDSS) (Evans and Abouzahr 2008; Bangha *et al.* 2010), although there are multiple approaches to designing such sites (Fottrell and Byass 2008). As with DHS, this approach also has its own strengths and weaknesses. Engaging with a defined population over an extended period of time means that individual lives can be followed longitudinally and aspects such as migration, partnership, and pregnancy can be ascertained without undue recall bias, through regular household update visits. An important, though sometimes overstated, potential weakness of single HDSS sites is a possible lack of representativeness or generalizability beyond the defined HDSS population.

If a number of such sites or areas are interlinked within a country, it is often referred to as sentinel area surveillance. China is a key example of a very large country where universal registration is likely to remain unrealistic for the foreseeable future, but which has a well-established network of sentinel surveillance areas known as the national Disease Surveillance Point (DSP) system (Yang *et al.* 2005). This DSP network combines the advantages of national representation (using 145 randomly selected locations) with detailed longitudinal follow-up of specific populations, but still amounts to a huge operation covering about 1% of the Chinese population, or 10 million people.

In both discrete HDSS and sentinel surveillance networks, the areas under enumeration are essentially microcosms of the universal registration approach, with detailed, longitudinal follow-up of individuals. In some ways this is a considerable advantage over the cross-sectional survey approach, particularly for monitoring changes over time without undue recall bias effects. However, there is also the frequently cited difficulty that there cannot be any hard data on how representative such enumerated areas might be of the surrounding non-enumerated ones. To some extent this issue can be addressed by comparing findings from surveillance areas with more widely distributed cross-sectional survey data, although the combined effects of different kinds of limitations applying to both kinds of data make such comparisons difficult (Bairagi *et al.* 1997; Hammer *et al.* 2006; Nhacolo *et al.* 2006; Fottrell *et al.* 2009; Garenne 2011).

It is also possible to analyze, within populations having universal registration, how a selected virtual local surveillance area might actually compare with its wider setting. This has been done using Swedish data from 1925, a time at which there were many similarities in population characteristics between Sweden and contemporary low- and middle-income countries (LMICs) (Byass *et al.* 2011). These analyzes suggest that localized population data may be more widely representative than is often supposed, even if that is hard to prove incontrovertibly. This in turn implies that policy-makers should possibly give more attention to evidence based on detailed, local data than on more superficial, wider data.

Population Basis of Health Metrics Data

Health evidence, as I have argued above, *must always be related* to the populations on which it is based. In any health system, it cannot be assumed that every individual has equal access to or take-up of the health services on offer, for reasons ranging from logistics and affordability to education and perceptions of health. This is just as true in industrialized countries as in developing countries (Notaro *et al.* 2011). Thus, while it is of course critically important for health facilities to keep accurate records concerning the use of their services, and feed these data into overall health information systems, it is just as important to get data on non-users of services in corresponding catchment areas.

Populations typically undergo several types of transition simultaneously when viewed longitudinally, and this can be seen both historically and in population projections. These transitions include changes in fertility, disease patterns, and mortality. As a result, the overall age–sex snapshot of a population, known as a population pyramid, changes shape over time, reflecting changes in the proportions of some population groups in relation to others. These structural changes in populations are of critical importance in the interpretation of health metrics data and for making policy decisions that will remain robust over a reasonable period of time. Any increase or decrease in morbidity or mortality from a particular cause can only be understood against the background of changes in susceptible segments of the population.

The global population is the ultimate example of this, as seen in Figure 6.1 (Byass 2008), reflecting overall reductions in fertility and increases in life expectancy over time, as well as changes in the proportions of people from countries at various stages of development. It is interesting to observe that the global population within any 5-year age group does not exceed 700 million either in 2010 or in 2050; yet the total projected population in 2050 (9.2 billion) is substantially greater than that for 2010 (6.9 billion), reflecting a substantial increase in life expectancy. The biggest single source of this difference will manifest as a rapidly increasing number of middle-aged to elderly people in less-developed countries, and this simple observation has major implications for health planning in those areas in the coming decades.

Any national or subnational population can be considered in a similar way. Data as basic as the pyramid for a local population tells a lot about likely health needs on a more local basis. Figure 6.2 gives several localized examples, all with the same horizontal scale

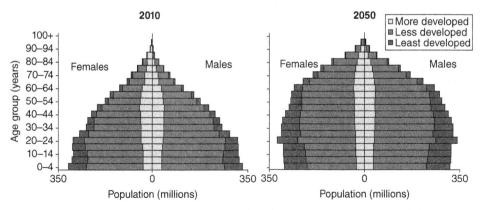

Figure 6.1 World population by age and sex groups in 2010 and 2050, for more-, less-, and least-developed countries. Source: Byass (2008), data from the UN Population Division.

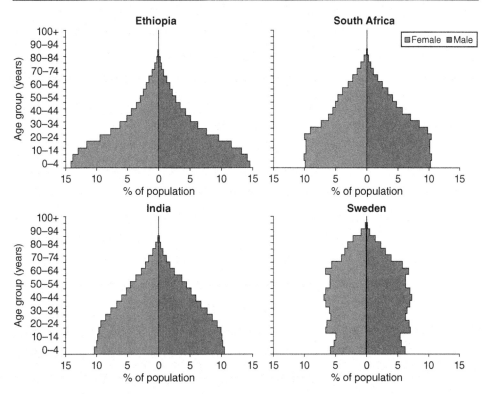

Figure 6.2 Age–sex population pyramids for four countries in 2010. Source: data from the UN Department of Economic and Social Affairs, Population Division (http://www.un.org/esa/population/unpop.htm; last accessed December 2013).

of percentage of total female or male population within each 5-year age band. Taking this example of four countries at different stages of demographic transition in 2010, it is very clear that there are huge policy implications deriving simply from the shape of these pyramids:

- In *Ethiopia* the population is still relatively young overall, and clearly child health services need to form a large part of service delivery.
- *South Africa* has a complex population structure deriving from the effects of the HIV/AIDS epidemic, with clear deficits in population among the younger adult groups. Not only does this illustrate the huge needs for HIV/AIDS services, but it also illustrates the problems of orphans and intergenerational households, with their particular health needs.
- *India* is undergoing rapid transition towards an older population, which has major implications for future health service needs.
- *Sweden* is at a late stage of transition, in which older people outnumber younger ones, which also has important implications for elderly care provision.

Changes in the shape of any particular population's pyramid over time mean that the size of population groups susceptible to particular health risks changes, and this has to be taken into account in formulating policies for various diseases and treatments.

Linking Health Service Encounters with the Everyday Lives of Citizens

A comprehensive understanding of population health can only be achieved by combining individual population data with health facility patient data. The full potential of health evidence is actually only realized when accurate linkages can be made at the individual level between health service encounters and the everyday lives of citizens. Ideally this synergy requires both universal registration, so that each and every citizen is unambiguously identified, and good health facility data that record every health service encounter by individual identifiers.

A more or less fully functional example of this at the universal registration level is evident in Sweden, where every individual is assigned a unique identity number at birth (or on in-migration to Sweden) which is then used as the identifier for every civil transaction, including at all levels of the health system (Norberg *et al.* 2010; Blomstedt *et al.* 2011). Other smaller scale examples exist where population surveillance and healthcare delivery activities are closely integrated (Serwaa-Bonsu *et al.* 2010), creating potential for much richer inputs to policy than is possible from either community-based or facility-based data alone.

Undertaking population-based surveillance, particularly on a selected rather than universal basis, also raises the possibility that the observed population may be influenced or changed in some way as a result of the surveillance, compared with the surrounding non-observed population. It cannot be assumed that counting people is a neutral activity – as with any other kind of scientific observation, there is the possibility of an associated Hawthorne effect (i.e., the population changes its behavior because it knows it is being studied) (Zwane *et al.* 2011). One can argue that counting populations is in itself an activity that might bring health benefits (Byass and Graham 2011).

Uncertainties in Measuring Health

It is undoubtedly true that for many scenarios adequate health metrics data are simply not available or are of poor quality. A different concern is the question of inherent uncertainties of measurement associated with *any* data. Any kind of data that are not based on successfully implemented universal registration inevitably have some kind of uncertainty associated with them as soon as any attempt is made to generalize findings beyond the population included in the measurement. These uncertainties are often expressed: (i) as 95% confidence intervals (meaning that there is a 95% chance that the true value for the generalized situation falls within the confidence interval around the measured value); or (ii) by using conceptually similar uncertainty bounds specified in some other way. In statistical terms, such uncertainty bounds may be a reasonably straightforward concept, but it is not something that is easy to understand in policy-making arenas. Evidence expressed as an interval, rather than a value, is much harder to interpret in terms of resource requirements, and apparent changes that actually occur within overlapping confidence intervals may be particularly confusing and difficult to interpret. Thus moving from confidence intervals to policy is often a particularly challenging process.

It is also the case that the complexity of calculating confidence intervals increases considerably when complex analytic approaches are used, as is the case in sophisticated global models (Byass *et al.* 2013). At the simplest level, such as a confidence interval around the value for a mean or a proportion, the interval will be equally distributed around the measured value, and its width will depend mainly on the size of the measured population. At the other extreme, such as in complex global estimates using multiple data

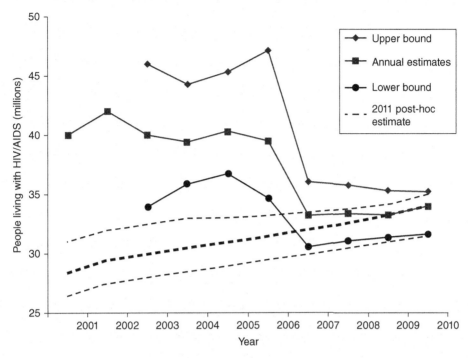

Figure 6.3 Global estimates of the number of people living with HIV/AIDS, made on an annual basis by UNAIDS, together with their 2011 post hoc estimates (and bounds). Sources: data from UNAIDS/WHO (2001–2005); UNAIDS (2007–20010); UNAIDS (2011).

sources, uncertainty intervals will not only be complex but also often asymmetric around the estimated value.

An interesting example illustrating these issues is the global estimate from UNAIDS for the number of people living with HIV. Figure 6.3 is actually a compilation of estimates from annual reports, which were not originally published together, plus post hoc estimates for the whole period published by UNAIDS in 2011 (UNAIDS/WHO 2001, 2002, 2003, 2004, 2005; UNAIDS 2007, 2008, 2009, 2010, 2011). Taken together, this is an example of evidence, issued on a regular basis, that might well lead to *increasing confusion as a basis for policy-making*. There are large year-on-year variations in the annual estimates, reflecting revisions to the estimation methods that were applied to compensate for the lack of reliable data on a worldwide basis (UNAIDS 2008). But as well as the changes in estimated values, the extent of the bounds around the estimated values also varies widely. These are not straightforward confidence intervals, but "plausibility bounds" that include some degree of interpretation as well as statistics, and for which methodologies were developed in parallel with the developing epidemic (Grassly *et al.* 2004). The reader, however, is left with questions as to whether the diminishing intervals over time reflect increasing data quality, or simply different methods of estimation. And how should the shift in the estimated values from the lower to upper regions of the intervals over time – which is manifest in the original annual estimates and in the post hoc series – be understood?

While a detailed consideration of the reality of HIV prevalence underlying these figures is beyond the scope of this chapter, these estimates do provide an interesting illustration of the difficulty of assembling reliable figures in the absence of adequate grass-roots data.

Ethical Issues in Health Metrics Data

Since health metrics data are fundamentally based on personal details, there are extremely important ethical considerations that have to be respected in any health information system. Standards and expectations of confidentiality and data integrity vary widely on a global basis. Industrialized countries commonly impose strict standards of data protection on any kind of computerized data, often including rights of access for citizens to any personal data relating to them, and the imposition of strict penalties for anyone failing to ensure the integrity and confidentiality of individual data. These considerations normally apply to any health-related data. However, similar standards of confidentiality and integrity may not apply to data in other settings, and this may become a major issue in terms of designing effective health information systems. If there is no widespread expectation or confidence that personal data will be held securely, there may be considerable doubts on the part of both individuals and health practitioners concerning committing personal data to computerized information systems.

Increasingly sophisticated medical technology also leads to new ethical challenges in terms of handling certain data. For example, if someone is diagnosed with a particular genetic defect or degenerative condition that may affect future health or life expectancy, that information has potential consequences beyond the purely medical context. Potentially, those data can therefore affect employment prospects, insurance premiums, and other important issues. The extent to which such information can safely be committed to computerized health information systems therefore becomes an important concern.

There is an increasing trend towards the view that data are essentially a public good, rather than a private commodity. This public good argument has important ethical implications for data that concern individuals, since such data have to be put into the public domain in ways that at the same time preserve confidentiality and individual rights (Van den Eynden *et al.* 2011).

In community-based surveillance, there are important reasons to anonymize data to ensure that anyone contributing responses to surveys cannot be individually identified or exploited as a result of their participation (Clark 2006). In recent years anonymization has become more complex if residential locations are identified and stored using global positioning system (GPS) technology. It has become very simple to accurately identify the location of anyone's household, simply by visiting it with GPS-equipped technology (and there are good reasons for doing so in terms of enabling spatial analyses). However, if such data are publicly released then effectively that household's confidentiality is compromised. One solution is to deliberately degrade the accuracy of any GPS data that are released into the public domain. Further concerns arise if cases of very rare health outcomes are identified, since they may be more readily identifiable if they are the only such case in a particular area.

Where health data are collected on a community basis, either as part of universal registration or in more localized surveillance operations, it can also be argued that undertaking such data collection carries ethical responsibilities when unexpected developments are discovered, such as particular epidemics (Fottrell and Byass 2009). This in turn implies that population data should be handled and processed as expeditiously as possible, so that important developments become obvious on a relevant timescale.

Moving from Health Metrics Data to Health Policy

It is often thought that researchers who generate evidence and policy-makers who wish to use evidence are fundamentally different beings, the so-called "two communities hypothesis" (Buse *et al.* 2005). The consequence is that much evidence does not find its way into the policy arena, and much policy-making is undertaken without adequate recourse to evidence. As discussed by Yamey and Volmink in Chapter 7, closing this gap is beginning to receive higher priority, at least in terms of higher expectations on researchers to provide evidence in policy-friendly formats. However, the processes for moving from evidence to policy are by no means clear or standardized and hence it is not necessarily the case in all settings that the possibly scant health evidence available is put to good use in policy terms.

Policy-makers are often caricatured as amazingly busy people with very limited quantitative understanding (even though many are in fact highly trained health professionals), while researchers and data providers are characterized as being obsessed with irrelevant detail and unable to see beyond their own noses. No matter how good and comprehensive health evidence may be, it is crucial to bridge this gap between evidence and policy in order to achieve effective evidence-based policy-making. In settings where evidence is fundamentally insufficient, however, it is much more difficult to achieve a high standard of evidence-based policy-making. There may even be perverse effects of insisting on evidence for policy-making in situations where evidence is available for some domains but not others. For example, if there is no evidence in a particular setting on mental health, and policy-making has to be evidence-based, then there will be no policy relating to mental health.

What is clear is that it is much easier for policy-makers to accept evidence if they are sure of its provenance – in other words, where it came from, how it was collected and interpreted, and its direct connection with their area of responsibility. This in turn means that coherent bottom-up data constitute a crucial part of any health service, being of much more certain provenance than externally generated or estimated values. The global health community has a major responsibility to facilitate this process by developing better tools and procedures to improve the collection and availability of bottom-up data.

The relationships between global health policy and global health metrics data currently remain somewhat serendipitous. In some instances, data exist but are not used effectively, while in other cases the necessary data are simply unavailable. There is a clear global imperative for better bottom-up data, in terms of quality and quantity, which is the only long-term basis on which to build better global health policy.

Key Reading

Byass P. 2009. The unequal world of health data. *PLOS Medicine* 6, e1000155.

Clark A. 2006. *Anonymising Research Data*. NCRM Working Paper Series 7/06. Leeds: ESRC National Centre for Research Methods. http://eprints.ncrm.ac.uk/480/1/0706_anonymising_research_data.pdf (last accessed December 2013).

Dry S. 2008. *Epidemics for All? Governing Health in a Global Age*. STEPS Working Paper 9. Brighton: STEPS Centre. http://www.episouth.org/doc/r_documents/Epidemics.pdf (last accessed December 2013).

Lindstrand A, Bergstrom S, Rosling H, Rubenson B, Stenson B, Tylleskar T. 2006. *Global Health, An Introductory Textbook*. Denmark: Studentlitteratur.

Sundin J, Willner S. 2007. *Social Change and Health in Sweden: 250 Years of Politics and Practice*. Stockholm: Swedish National Institute of Public Health. http://www.fhi.

se/PageFiles/4381/R200721_Social_change_and_health_in_Sweden0801.pdf (last accessed
December 2013).
Van den Eynden V, Corti L, Woollard M, Bishop L, Horton L. 2011. *Managing and
Sharing Data*. Colchester: UK Data Archive. http://www.data-archive.ac.uk/media/2894/
managingsharing.pdf (last accessed December 2013).

References

Bairagi R, Becker S, Kantner A, Allen KB, Datta A, Purvis K. 1997. An evaluation of the 1993–4 Bangladesh Demographic and Health Survey within the Matlab area. *Asia Pacific Population Research Abstracts* 11, 1–2.

Bangha M, Diagne A, Bawah A, Sankoh O. 2010. Monitoring the Millennium Development Goals: the potential role of the INDEPTH Network. *Global Health Action* 3, 5517.

Blomstedt Y, Emmelin M, Weinehall L. 2011. What about healthy participants? The improvement and deterioration of self-reported health at a 10-year follow-up of the Västerbotten Intervention Programme. *Global Health Action* 4, 5435.

Boerma T, Mathers C, Abouzahr C. 2010. WHO and global health monitoring: the way forward. *PLOS Medicine* 7, e373.

Buse K, Mays N, Walt G (eds). 2005. *Making Health Policy*. Maidenhead: Open University Press.

Byass P. 2010. The imperfect world of global health estimates. *PLOS Medicine* 7, e1006.

Byass P. 2007. Who needs cause-of-death data? *PLOS Medicine* 4, e333.

Byass P. 2008. Towards a global agenda on ageing. *Global Health Action* 1, 1908.

Byass P. 2009a. Epidemiology without borders: an anational view of global health. *Global Health Action* 2, 2052.

Byass P. 2009b. The unequal world of health data. *PLOS Medicine* 6, e1000155.

Byass P, de Courten M, Graham WJ *et al*. 2013. Reflections on the Global Burden of Disease 2010 estimates. *PLOS Medicine* 10, e1001477.

Byass P, Graham W. 2011. Grappling with uncertainties along the MDG trail. *Lancet* 378, 1119–20.

Byass P, Sankoh O, Tollman SM, Högberg U, Wall S. 2011. Lessons from history for designing and validating epidemiological surveillance in uncounted populations. *PLOS ONE* 6, e22897.

Byass P, Worku A, Emmelin A, Berhane Y. 2007. DSS and DHS: longitudinal and cross-sectional viewpoints on child and adolescent mortality in Ethiopia. *Population Health Metrics* 5, 12.

Clark A. 2006. *Anonymising Research Data*. NCRM Working Paper Series 7/06. Leeds: ESRC National Centre for Research Methods. http://eprints.ncrm.ac.uk/480/1/0706_anonymising_research_data.pdf (last accessed December 2013).

Dry S. 2008. *Epidemics for All? Governing Health in a Global Age*. STEPS Working Paper 9. Brighton: STEPS Centre. http://www.episouth.org/doc/r_documents/Epidemics.pdf (last accessed December 2013).

Evans T, Abouzahr C. 2008. INDEPTH @ 10: celebrate the past and illuminate the future. *Global Health Action* 1, 1899.

Fottrell E, Byass P. 2008. Population survey sampling methods in a rural African setting: measuring mortality. *Population Health Metrics* 6, 2.

Fottrell E, Byass P. 2009. Identifying humanitarian crises in population surveillance field sites: simple procedures and ethical imperatives. *Public Health* 123, 151–5.

Fottrell E, Enquselassie F, Byass P. 2009. The distribution and effects of child mortality risk factors in Ethiopia: a comparison of estimates from DSS and DHS. *Ethiopian Journal of Health Development* 23, 163–8.

Garenne M. 2011. Estimating obstetric mortality from pregnancy-related deaths recorded in demographic censuses and surveys. *Studies in Family Planning* 42, 237–46.

Graham W, Adjei S. 2010. A call for responsible estimation of global health. *PLOS Medicine* 7, 1003.

Grassly NC, Morgan M, Walker N *et al.* 2004. Uncertainty in estimates of HIV/AIDS: the estimation and application of plausibility bounds. *Sexually Transmitted Infections* 80(Suppl I), i31–i38.

Hammer GP, Kouyaté B, Ramroth H, Becher H. 2006. Risk factors for childhood mortality in sub-Saharan Africa: a comparison of data from a Demographic and Health Survey and from a Demographic Surveillance System. *Acta Tropica* 98, 212–18.

Hosseinpoor AR, Victora CG, Bergen N, Barros AJD, Boerma T. 2011. Towards universal health coverage: the role of within-country wealth-related inequality in 28 countries in sub-Saharan Africa. *Bulletin of the World Health Organization* 89, 881–90.

Ludvigsson JF, Otterblad-Olausson P, Pettersson BU, Ekbom A. 2009. The Swedish personal identity number: possibilities and pitfalls in healthcare and medical research. *European Journal of Epidemiology* 24, 659–667.

Murray C, Lopez A. 2010. Production and analysis of health indicators: the role of academia. *PLOS Medicine* 7, e1004.

Nhacolo AQ, Nhalungo DA, Sacoor CN, Aponte JJ, Thompson R, Alonso P. 2006. Levels and trends of demographic indices in southern rural Mozambique: evidence from demographic surveillance in Manhiça district. *BMC Public Health* 6, 291.

Norberg M, Wall S, Boman K, Weinehall L. 2010. The Västerbotten Intervention Programme: background, design and implications. *Global Health Action* 3, 4643.

Notaro SJ, Khan M, Bryan N *et al.* 2011. Analysis of the demographic characteristics and medical conditions of the uninsured utilizing a free clinic. *Journal of Community Health* DOI 10.1007/s10900-011-9470-7.

Rutstein SO, Rojas G. 2006. *Guide to DHS Statistics*. Claverton, MD: ORC Macro. http://pdf.usaid.gov/pdf_docs/PNACY778.pdf (last accessed December 2013).

Sankoh O. 2010. Global health estimates: stronger collaboration needed with low- and middle-income countries. *PLOS Medicine* 7, e1005.

Serwaa-Bonsu A, Herbst AJ, Reniers G *et al.* 2010. First experiences in the implementation of biometric technology to link data from Health and Demographic Surveillance Systems with health facility data. *Global Health Action* 3, 2120.

Sundin J, Willner S. 2007. *Social Change and Health in Sweden: 250 Years of Politics and Practice*. Stockholm: Swedish National Institute of Public Health. http://www.fhi.se/PageFiles/4381/R200721_Social_change_and_health_in_Sweden0801.pdf (last accessed December 2013).

UN (United Nations). 2011. *The Millennium Development Goals Report 2011*. New York: United Nations. http://www.beta.undp.org/content/dam/undp/library/MDG/english/MDG_Report_2011_EN.pdf (last accessed December 2013).

UNAIDS. 2007. *Annual Report 2006: Making the Money Work*. UNAIDS/07.19E. Geneva: UNAIDS.

UNAIDS. 2008. *Annual Report 2007: Know Your Epidemic*. UNAIDS/08.21E. Geneva: UNAIDS.

UNAIDS. 2009. *Annual Report 2008: Towards Universal Access*. UNAIDS/09.25E. Geneva: UNAIDS.

UNAIDS. 2010. *Annual Report 2009: Uniting the World Against AIDS*. UNAIDS/10.08E. Geneva: UNAIDS.

UNAIDS. 2011. *World AIDS Day Report 2011*. UNAIDS/JC2216. Geneva: UNAIDS.

UNAIDS/WHO (World Health Organization). 2001. *AIDS Epidemic Update 2001*. UNAIDS/01.74E. Geneva: UNAIDS.

UNAIDS/WHO (World Health Organization). 2002. *AIDS Epidemic Update 2002*. UNAIDS/02.58E. Geneva: UNAIDS.

UNAIDS/WHO (World Health Organization). 2003. *AIDS Epidemic Update 2003*. UNAIDS/03.39E. Geneva: UNAIDS.

UNAIDS/WHO (World Health Organization). 2004. *AIDS Epidemic Update 2004*. UNAIDS/04.45E. Geneva: UNAIDS.

UNAIDS/WHO (World Health Organization). 2005. *AIDS Epidemic Update 2005*. UNAIDS/ 05.19E. Geneva: UNAIDS.

Van den Eynden V, Corti L, Woollard M, Bishop L, Horton L. 2011. *Managing and Sharing Data*. Colchester: UK Data Archive. http://www.data-archive.ac.uk/media/2894/managingsharing.pdf (last accessed December 2013).

Yang G, Hu J, Rao KQ, Ma J, Rao C, Lopez AD. 2005. Mortality registration and surveillance in China: history, current situation and challenges. *Population Health Metrics* 3, 3.

Zwane AP, Zinman J, Van Dusen E *et al*. 2011. Being surveyed can change later behavior and related parameter estimates. *Proceedings of the National Academy of Sciences of the USA* 108(5), 1821–6. www.pnas.org/cgi/doi/10.1073/pnas.1000776108 (last accessed December 2013).

Chapter 7

An Argument for Evidence-Based Policy-Making in Global Health

Gavin Yamey and Jimmy Volmink

Abstract

From its early origins in the 1990s, evidence-based medicine has become a major driving force in healthcare improvement worldwide and has prompted other evidence-based "movements," including evidence-based policy-making (EBP) in global health. EBP approaches could help to narrow the "know–do gap," the gap between evidence (what is known) and policy implementation (what gets done), which is a major barrier to achieving the health-related Millennium Development Goals. Such approaches can also help to ensure that resources are not wasted on ineffective interventions, particularly in this time of global fiscal constraint. Proponents of EBP in global health acknowledge that policy-making is a messy non-linear process, in which evidence competes with other inputs, such as politics, sociocultural factors, and personal expertise. Nevertheless, scientific evidence should be a cornerstone of sound public health policies, and significant health gains could be achieved by leveraging such evidence to its full potential. Systematic reviews are a particularly valuable form of evidence for public policy-making, as they are less likely to produce misleading results. Such reviews are increasingly being used to address questions related to the governance, financing, architecture, and delivery of global health and to broader social, economic, and intersectoral issues. Important new approaches to synthesizing non-randomized studies, including observational, qualitative, and economic studies, and to integrating the synthesis of quantitative and qualitative studies, have been developed. These are paying large dividends in improving our understanding of how to tackle global health challenges. Nevertheless, there are still many barriers and challenges to adopting evidence-based approaches in global health policy-making. The global health community has made tremendous strides in tackling these difficulties, through a variety of initiatives aimed at improving the generation, synthesis, diffusion, and uptake of "evidence that matters" to policy-makers.

The Handbook of Global Health Policy, First Edition. Edited by Garrett W. Brown, Gavin Yamey, and Sarah Wamala.
© 2014 John Wiley & Sons, Ltd. Published 2014 by John Wiley & Sons, Ltd.

Key Points

- Evidence-based policy-making (EBP) in global health can be defined as the conscientious, explicit, and judicious use of evidence to guide and shape global health policies.
- EBP is becoming increasingly prominent, given its important role in accelerating progress towards the Millennium Development Goals (MDGs) and in helping to achieve "value for money" in global health programming.
- Evidence must compete with other factors that influence decision-making, such as power, politics, opinions, and vested interests.
- Policy actors may not prioritize research evidence in their policy-making decisions.
- An important challenge to EBP in global health is the relative lack of primary research and systematic reviews tackling problems of low- and middle-income countries (LMICs).
- Greater use of evidence in policy-making can be achieved by improving the generation and dissemination of "evidence that matters" to decision-makers in LMICs.

Key Policy Implications

- Scientific evidence remains a crucial foundation for improving global public health and significant health gains could be achieved by leveraging such evidence to its full potential.
- Systematic reviews can help global health decision-makers to answer crucial questions, such as the effectiveness, safety, and cost-effectiveness of an intervention, and they have had an important role in improving public health.
- Although there are many barriers to evidence-based policy-making in global health, including barriers to the local generation, synthesis, and dissemination of evidence, there has been a recent explosion in the number of initiatives aimed at increasing policy-makers' use of evidence.

Introduction

With philosophical roots extending back to nineteenth century France, evidence-based medicine emerged in the early 1990s as a new approach to patient care in which clinicians drew upon the most trustworthy, least biased research evidence as the basis for making clinical decisions (Sackett *et al.* 1996). Evidence-based medicine has been defined as "the conscientious, explicit, and judicious use of current best evidence in making decisions about the care of individual patients" (Sackett *et al.* 1996). McMaster University, Canada, has a leading role in promoting this approach to teaching and practicing medicine which has become a major driving force in healthcare improvement worldwide. The principles of evidence-based medicine are being adopted for guiding decisions across a wide range of healthcare disciplines, including public health, healthcare management, and policy-making.

The Cochrane Collaboration (www.cochrane.org; last accessed December 2013), an international network of over 28,000 people in more than 100 countries that prepares and disseminates high-quality information on the effectiveness of healthcare, including in low- and middle-income countries (LMICs), is pivotal to the practice of evidence-based decision-making. This initiative was inspired by the work of the British physician and epidemiologist, Archie Cochrane, who drew attention to our collective ignorance about the effects of healthcare, and pointed to the importance of developing an up-to-date repository of synthesized evidence from randomized controlled trials (RCTs) (Cochrane 1973). The Cochrane Collaboration gave rise to national agencies for promoting evidence-based health practice, such as the United Kingdom's National Institute for Health and Clinical Excellence and the New Zealand Health Technology Assessment. It also prompted the launch of many other evidence-based "movements," from evidence-based nursing, physiotherapy, and dentistry (Yamey and Feachem 2011) to evidence-based public health (Glasziou and Longbottom 1999; McMichael *et al.* 2005) and evidence-based social work (Roberts and Yeager 2006). "To this growing list," say Yamey and Feachem (2011), "we can now add evidence-based global health policy, a 'movement' that is gaining increasing prominence."

Evidence-based policy-making (EBP) in global health can be defined as the conscientious, explicit, and judicious use of evidence to guide and shape global health policies. There are two major forces driving its rise. The first is the growing recognition that a major barrier to achieving the health-related Millennium Development Goals (MDGs) is the "know–do gap" – the gap between evidence (what is known) and policy implementation (what gets done) (Pablos-Mendez and Shademani 2006; Yamey 2012). The second is the increasing need to ensure that limited global health resources are spent wisely. Although development assistance for health (DAH) has increased substantially over the last decade (Ravishankar *et al.* 2009), there are worrying signs that such assistance has flat-lined since the global economic crisis (Baker 2010; WHO 2010), making it even more crucial to ensure that these funds are spent only on interventions that work. As Garner *et al.* say, "wasting resources on ineffective interventions results in technical inefficiencies and substantial opportunity costs in countries least able to afford them" (Garner *et al.* 2004). The Global Fund to Fight AIDS, Tuberculosis and Malaria (the Global Fund), for example, faced widespread criticism in 2003 for purchasing large volumes of the malaria drug choloroquine, a drug that had become ineffective in much of sub-Saharan Africa as a result of parasite resistance (Yamey 2003; Attaran *et al.* 2004). As one prominent malaria researcher said at the time: "It is terrible to waste lives and money deploying a useless drug" (Yamey 2003).

These two forces are likely to intensify in the coming years, given that the 2015 MDGs' deadline is fast approaching and given the new "value for money agenda." Global health funding agencies and LMICs are trying to achieve better health outcomes despite constrained resources, sometimes referred to as "doing more for less" in global health. The growing chorus for achieving "value for money" in global health – in which funders and LMICs are trying to improve both the impact and efficiency of their investments – means that there is now a greater focus on investing in "the highest impact interventions among the most affected populations" (Center for Global Development 2012). Thus, we are likely to see an ever-increasing emphasis on using research evidence to define such interventions and populations.

Narrowing the Gap

As suggested by its title, this chapter argues that the global health community should work to close the gap between, on the one hand, the generation and synthesis of evidence relevant to global health, and, on the other hand, practical policy-making at national and global levels. We begin by discussing what we mean by policies that are "evidence-based" and what *kinds* of evidence are most valuable in global health policy-making. We discuss real world examples of how policies that are shaped by the best available evidence can have a profound impact on morbidity and mortality, and also of failures by global health actors to adopt evidence-informed approaches, failures that could have profound public health consequences. Finally, we explore the pathway from research to policy, laying out the barriers that prevent policy-makers from using evidence and the tremendous opportunities to improve the "evidence flow" from researcher to policy-maker.

The notion of EBP in public health is sometimes criticized for being overly simplistic and mechanistic (Greenhalgh and Russell 2009), and for implying that lives could be saved merely by giving policy-makers more evidence and just "urging" or "exhorting" them to use it. But proponents of evidence-based approaches, including us, do not adhere to a naïve view of the world in which global health policy-making is a simple linear process that links researchers to policy actors in a smooth uninterrupted flow. We fully acknowledge that policy-making cannot be divorced from its social and political context. We have previously argued, for example, that "policymaking is a messy, non-linear process, in which evidence is only one of many inputs" (Yamey and Feachem 2011) and that "health policymaking involves an uneasy balance of science, economics, and politics" (McMichael *et al.* 2005). Our practical experience in the world of global health policy-making has confirmed Black's assertion that, when shaping policy, "the other legitimate influences on policy (social, electoral, ethical, cultural, and economic) must be accommodated" (Black 2001). Sound policies must be shaped not only by rigorous evidence, but also by societal values, and such values do not need to be subject to clinical trials. Humphreys and Piot (2012), for example, say that "a rigorous study showing that people with an infectious disease could be cheaply and efficiently shipped off to colonies of isolation would be ignored in any humane society because respect for human dignity would rule out such a policy." Improving population health in LMICs will not happen from scientific improvements alone, but will require intersectoral cooperation, poverty alleviation efforts, and other social approaches (McMichael *et al.* 2005).

However, the focus of our chapter is *not* on the broader sociopolitical debates surrounding EBP, which are discussed in detail by Barnes and Parkhurst in an accompanying chapter (see Chapter 8). Instead, writing as two medical doctors, we take a somewhat more technical approach, examining some of the key opportunities for leveraging scientific evidence to help tackle the world's major global health challenges. A central argument of our chapter is that scientific evidence remains a crucial foundation for improving global public health and significant health gains could be achieved by leveraging such evidence to its full potential (Buekens *et al.* 2004). Or, as the UK Overseas Development Institute, puts it: "better utilization of evidence in policy and practice can help save lives, reduce poverty and improve development performance in developing countries" (Sutcliffe and Court 2005).

Why Should We Use Evidence? Which Evidence Should We Use?

Imagine for a moment that you are a health policy-maker in an LMIC. You are faced with a wide range of questions. For example, which childhood vaccinations should you prioritize? Your country has endemic malaria and you want to roll out a national prevention campaign, but which prevention tools should you choose? How best can you reduce your country's high maternal and newborn mortality rate? How can you tackle the high unmet need for family planning services? How will you plan preventive and therapeutic service provision for your burgeoning epidemic of obesity, diabetes, and cardiovascular diseases?

Whatever choice you make, you will be intervening in the lives of thousands or even millions of people. Given that health policies can have unintended effects, sometimes causing more harm than good, you surely have a duty to ensure that your interventions are informed by the best available evidence (Chalmers 2003); "good intentions and received wisdom are not enough" (Macintrye and Petticrew 2000). At its heart, evidence-based global health policy-making is about improving health outcomes by basing policies on the best available evidence, rather than on "opinion, whim, or political popularity" (Yamey and Feachem 2011). Proponents of EBP in global health envision that over time there will be "a shift away from opinion based policies being replaced by a more rigorous, rational approach that gathers, critically appraises and uses high quality research evidence to inform policymaking and professional practice" (Davies 2004) (Figure 7.1).

The World Health Organization (WHO) has repeatedly endorsed the necessity for policy-makers to use evidence to inform their decisions. In May 1998, the 51st World

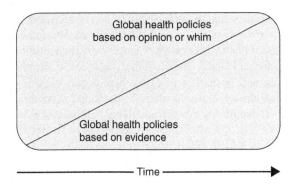

Figure 7.1 Dynamics of evidence-based policy-making in global health, showing a shift over time from policies based on opinion/whim to those based on evidence. Sources: Yamey and Feachem (2011); adapted from Sutcliffe and Court (2005).

Table 7.1 Example of a hierarchy of evidence; the highest
levels of evidence (levels 1 and 2) involve the most reliable
study designs – those least prone to bias.

Level of evidence	Study type
1	Systematic reviews, meta-analyses
2	Randomized controlled trials
3	Cohort studies
4	Case–control studies
5	Cross-sectional studies
6	Case series and case reports

Health Assembly urged all Member States to "adopt an evidence-based approach to health promotion policy and practice, using the full range of quantitative and qualitative methodologies" (World Health Assembly 1998), while the WHO's 2004 *World Report on Knowledge for Better Health* (WHO 2004a) called for greater use of research evidence in policy-making as a way to strengthen health systems. Using evidence helps policy-makers to prioritize between different health challenges, choose between policy solutions, and assess the impact and costs of different interventions (Shaxson 2005).

Adopting an evidence-based approach to policy decisions means that the relevant evidence is evaluated using a transparent and systematic process to identify as high a proportion as possible of existing reliable research (Chalmers 2003; Oxman *et al.* 2009). Not all evidence is created equal (Richards 2003); some types of evidence will be more valuable than others. One useful approach to help health policy-makers sift through the relevant research and assess its "evidential 'weight' and relevance" (Petticrew and Roberts 2002) is to use a "hierarchy" of evidence (Truman *et al.* 2000). Such hierarchies place greater weight on studies that are well designed and conducted and are therefore more convincing – the results are less likely to be explained merely by chance or bias. The most reliable types of study (systematic reviews and meta-analyses, followed by RCTs) are placed at the top of the hierarchy (Table 7.1).

For many crucial questions in global health (e.g., is this intervention effective, is it safe, is it worth the cost, is it better than the alternatives?), the greatest weight is given to systematic reviews and meta-analyses, such as those published by the Cochrane Collaboration. These use explicit, replicable, and systematic methods to find, select, appraise, and synthesize *all* research studies that addressed a specific question (Table 7.1). The likelihood that public policy-makers will be misled by research, say Lavis *et al.* (2004), is lower with systematic reviews than with individual studies. Systematic reviews are particularly valuable in global health because they place individual studies within the context of *the totality* of evidence. Placing single studies within the context of all other relevant research is in keeping with a mantra in global health that became prominent over the last decade: "globalize the evidence, localize the decision" (Eisenberg 2002). Localizing the decision means: (i) examining the best available "globalized evidence;" and (ii) considering local evidence (e.g., on availability of resources or the local expertise of policy-makers and clinicians) to inform judgments that shape health policy (Oxman *et al.* 2009) (Figure 7.2).

Systematic reviews of randomized or quasi-randomized controlled trials can help global health policy-makers to identify efficacious interventions. For example, Cochrane systematic reviews have shown the efficacy of condoms for preventing HIV transmission

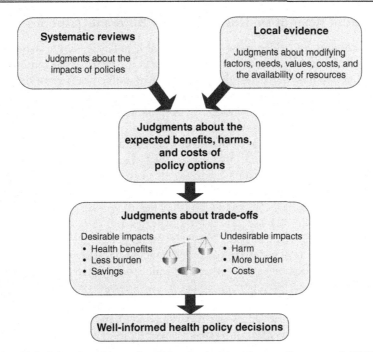

Figure 7.2   Globalizing the evidence, localizing the decision. Source: Oxman *et al.* (2009), figure 1.

(Weller and Davis-Beatty 2007), oral zinc supplementation for reducing the duration of childhood diarrhea (Lazzerini and Ronfani 2012), and mass administration of antibiotics for reducing the prevalence of active trachoma (Evans and Solomon 2011). In addition, given that global health policy is a field characterized by intense debates, disagreements, "turf" battles, conflicts of interest, and the championing of one preferred policy over another, systematic reviews have a crucial role in laying out what the best science shows about contested issues.

For example, the WHO argues that deworming drugs routinely given to all school-aged children will boost cognitive development so that these children can "earn their way out of poverty" (WHO 2005), yet a recent Cochrane systematic found that, for routine deworming drugs, the evidence in relation to cognition, school attendance, and school performance is "generally poor, with no obvious or consistent effect" (Taylor-Robinson *et al.* 2012). As Garner, one of authors of the review, said: "deworming schoolchildren to rid them of intestinal helminths seems a good idea in theory, but the evidence for it just doesn't stack up. We want policy makers to look at the evidence and the message and consider if deworming is as good as it is cracked up to be" (Garner 2012). Similarly, although many global health agencies promote directly observed therapy for tuberculosis (in which health workers, family members, or friends observe patients taking their medications), a Cochrane systematic review found no evidence that direct observation showed better cure rates than self-administered treatment (Volmink and Garner 2007). Implementing direct observation is expensive, and advocating its routine use makes little sense until we better understand the circumstances in which it may be beneficial (Volmink and Garner 2007).

Using Different Types of Evidence to Answer Different Questions

A common criticism of evidence-based global health policy is that systematic reviews focus narrowly on health intervention effectiveness at the expense of examining broader questions related to health systems, the architecture of global health, and social and economic factors in disease causation and treatment. However, while there is still much room for improvement, an important trend in recent years has been the growth of systematic reviews that examine broad "systemic" questions related to the financing, governance, and delivery of global health, many of which were conducted under the auspices of the Cochrane's Effective Practice and Organization of Care Group (Grimshaw *et al.* 2003; Lavis *et al.* 2004). For example, a review of the effects of using lay health workers (community members who receive basic training to promote health) on maternal and child health outcomes found that, compared with usual health services, using lay health workers probably leads to an increase in breastfeeding rates and rates of completion of child immunization schedules (Lewin *et al.* 2010). Increasing attention is also being given to the role of systematic reviews in improving understanding of the impact of policies on inequalities in health outcomes and on resource allocation and use, and guidelines have recently been developed for reporting equity-focused systematic reviews (Welch *et al.* 2012).

There have been other advances in promoting systematic reviews addressing wider social, systems, and intersectoral questions. For example, the Campbell Collaboration, launched in 2000, promotes EBP by supporting and disseminating systematic reviews in education, crime and justice, and social welfare (www.campbellcollaboration.org/about_us/index.php; last accessed December 2013). In 2011, the Australian Agency for International Development (AusAID), the UK Department for International Development (DFID), and the International Initiative for Impact Evaluation (3ie) launched an international call for proposals for systematic reviews of key intersectoral policy questions, including questions related to health, social protection, social inclusion, governance, fragile states, disasters, the environment, and aid effectiveness (International Initiative for Impact Evaluation 2011).

Critics of evidence-based approaches also argue that the "hierarchy of evidence" is flawed – "does the Emperor have no clothes?" they ask (Bigby 2001) – because of its slavish devotion to RCTs and its relative dismissal of other forms of scientific evidence. Again, this criticism is fast becoming out of date. First, a broad variety of study designs – including observational, qualitative, and economic studies – are increasingly being used to help shape global health policies. For example, observational, qualitative, and economic studies have found very low use of effective malaria drugs (artemisinin-based combination therapies (ACTs)) in sub-Saharan Africa and Southeast Asia, where 50–75% of malaria patients seek treatment in the private sector (WHO 2009), largely because of high drug costs. Data from these studies helped to inform the launch of the Affordable Medicines facility-malaria (Roll Back Malaria Partnership 2007), a highly innovative global drug subsidy that aims to lower the cost of ACTs (Yamey *et al.* 2012).

Second, important new approaches have been developed to synthesize non-randomized studies, including observational studies (Egger *et al.* 2008), qualitative studies (Britten *et al.* 2002), and economic studies (Shemilt *et al.* 2006), and to synthesize *both* quantitative and qualitative studies (Thomas *et al.* 2004; Harden *et al.* 2009). These are paying large dividends in improving our understanding of how to tackle global health challenges (Boxes 7.1 and 7.2).

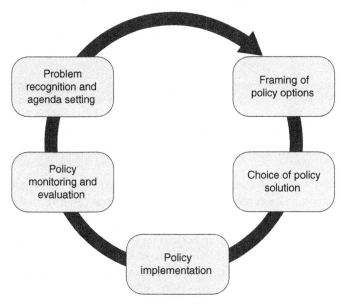

Figure 7.3   The policy cycle. Source: adapted from Young and Quinn (2002).

Third, far from being a "one size fits all approach," there is a growing realization that *different kinds* of research evidence are more or less applicable and valuable at *different stages* in the policy cycle, from agenda setting through to impact evaluation (Figure 7.3). For example, systematic reviews of prevalence studies showing the burden of disease are highly valuable at the agenda setting stage; systematic reviews of randomized or quasi-randomized trials can help guide policy-makers in choosing between different interventions or approaches); while operational and action research, including pilot or demonstration projects, can be valuable during policy implementation (Sutcliffe and Court 2005).

Box 7.1   Systematic Reviews of Qualitative Research that can Inform Global Health Policy

- *Understanding barriers to preventing and treating malaria.* Maslove *et al.* (2009) systematically reviewed qualitative studies (those involving focus groups and interviews) to examine the knowledge, attitudes, and practices of people living in malaria-endemic African countries. Barriers to malaria treatment included logistical obstacles (e.g., long distances from the nearest treatment facility), concerns about the safety and efficacy of conventional medicines, and use of traditional remedies. The authors conclude that "large-scale malaria prevention and treatment programs must account for the social and cultural contexts in which they are deployed."
- *Patient adherence to tuberculosis treatment.* In a systematic review of qualitative studies, Munro *et al.* (2007) found eight key factors associated with adherence to tuberculosis treatment, including health service factors (e.g., organization of treatment and care); social context (family, community, and household

influences); and the financial burden of treatment. "The findings of our review," conclude the authors, "could help inform the development of patient-centred interventions and of interventions to address structural barriers to treatment adherence."

- *End-of-life care in sub-Saharan Africa.* A systematic review of qualitative studies from 13 countries, by Gysels *et al.* (2011), challenged the notion that people prefer home-based care at the end of life and that the extended family care for the sick. The study found evidence of a preference for institutional care, which has important implications for service provision at the end of life.

Box 7.2 Systematic Reviews of Economic Research that can Inform Global Health Policy

- *Economic impacts of smoke-free policies on the hospitality industry.* A growing number of countries worldwide have instituted bans on smoking in bars and restaurants to help reduce the burden of disease and death caused by tobacco. Tobacco companies and the hospitality industry often argue that such bans reduce restaurant and bar sales and employment (Ritch and Begay 2001). However, a systematic review of the economic impacts of smoke-free policies found that "all of the best designed studies reported no impact or a positive impact of smoke-free restaurant and bar laws on sales or employment" (Scollo *et al.* 2003). This study, argue the authors, provides policy-makers with evidence to support legislation to protect workers and patrons from second-hand smoke without fears of adverse economic impacts.
- *Expenditure on primary prevention versus clinical care of cardiovascular disease.* Schwappach *et al.* (2007) systematically reviewed economic studies of cardiovascular preventive interventions, and found that far more public and private resources were directed at curative interventions than preventive strategies. For example, only 3.2% of government health expenditures went into the category "prevention and public health" in the 19 Organisation for Economic Co-operation and Development (OECD) countries for which recent data were available. These results, argue the authors, suggest that spending levels on prevention are suboptimal from a social welfare perspective.
- *One-to-one interventions to reduce sexually transmitted infections (STIs) and teenage pregnancies.* A systematic review of economic evaluations of one-to-one interventions (i.e., those delivered to one individual at a time) to reduce STIs and teenage conceptions found 55 studies that met the study inclusion criteria (Barham *et al.* 2007). Most interventions were found to be cost-effective, with the exception of HIV post-exposure prophylaxis, which must be targeted at high-risk individuals to fall within acceptable cost-effectiveness thresholds.

Evidence-Informed Policies Improve Public Health

The last decade has seen an extraordinary turnaround in global efforts to reduce the burden of malaria. This turnaround is a powerful example of how an evidence-based approach can help to shape effective national and global health policies that save lives.

The Roll Back Malaria campaign was launched in 1998, bringing together multilateral, bilateral, non-governmental, and private organizations to reduce the burden of malaria cases and deaths. It made a clear pledge: to halve malaria deaths by 2010 (Yamey 2000). However, the campaign got off to a very poor start and, by 2004, syntheses of observational data showed that the annual number of deaths worldwide from malaria was *higher* than it was in 1998 (Yamey 2004). The *Africa Malaria Report 2003*, published by the WHO and UNICEF, two of the most important actors in Roll Back Malaria, noted: "Roll Back Malaria is acting against a background of increasing malaria burden" (WHO and UNICEF 2003).

A reason for such poor progress was a huge mismatch between the amount of international funding dedicated to global malaria control and the amount needed for comprehensive control efforts. While the WHO was calling for US$1 billion annually in DAH for malaria (WHO 2004b), the international donor community was committing only 10% of that amount (Narasimhan and Attaran 2003).

The alarming data showing a rise in malaria deaths played an agenda-setting part in the policy cycle (Figure 7.3), helping to spur the donor community to action. Massive new funding was mobilized for malaria control, from just $300 million in 2003 to $1.94 billion in 2009 (Snow *et al.* 2010), mostly from three funders: the Global Fund; the US President's Malaria Initiative; and the World Bank. This funding was directed at supporting government-run campaigns to scale up two control tools that were backed by evidence from systematic reviews of multiple RCTs: insecticide-treated bed nets (ITNs) and ACTs.

A Cochrane systematic review, which included 14 cluster randomized and eight individually randomized controlled trials, found that ITN use can reduce child deaths by one fifth and malaria episodes by half (Lengeler 2004). In a dozen countries, aggressive scale-up of ITNs (together with scale-up of other tools, including ACTs and indoor residual spraying of households with insecticide) has been associated with a fall in reported malaria cases or deaths by over 50% since 2000 (WHO 2010).

Two recent studies on ITNs, led by the Institute for Health Metrics and Evaluation, have given a powerful demonstration of EBP "in action." The first study, which combined data from three different sources using Bayesian techniques, found that household ownership of ITNs across 44 malaria-endemic countries rose from an average of 2.2% in 1999 to 32.8% by 2008, and the proportion of children sleeping under a net rose from 1.5% to 26.6% over the same time period (Flaxman *et al.* 2010). Regression analysis found that this estimated increase in national ITN coverage was strongly related to the cumulative national DAH targeted for malaria over the same period. The second study, based on data from 29 surveys conducted in 22 sub-Saharan African countries, found that household ITN ownership was associated with a relative reduction in mortality of 23% in children aged 1 month to 5 years (Lim *et al.* 2011). Taken together, these studies suggest that DAH for malaria has been targeted effectively, based on sound evidence:

1. The rise in DAH for malaria has been associated with a rise in ITN coverage (each US$1 per capita of DAH for malaria was significantly associated with a 1.6% increase in childhood ITN use); and
2. This ITN rise in coverage has been accompanied by a significant fall in child mortality.

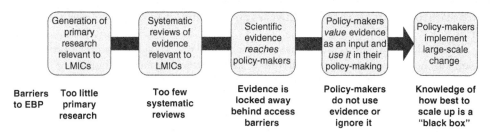

Figure 7.4 Idealized representation of "evidence flow" and barriers to evidence-based policy-making (EBP) in global health. LMICs, low- and middle-income countries.

"These findings," conclude Lim *et al.* (2011), the authors of the second study, "add to the body of evidence that ITNs are effective under usual program conditions and support the continued efforts to scale-up ITN coverage in sub-Saharan Africa."

Similarly, multiple systematic reviews have found evidence that ACTs are the most effective antimalarial for uncomplicated faciparum malaria (e.g., see the Cochrane review by Sinclair *et al.* 2009). Based on this evidence, and on the WHO's 2001 recommendation that ACTs should be first-line treatment (WHO 2001), there was a very rapid rise from 2001 to 2006 in the number of malaria-endemic countries adopting ACTs in their national treatment policies, from zero countries in 2001 to 67 countries by 2007 (Bosman and Mendis 2007). With support from external donors, some countries or regions, such as Zanzibar and KawaZulu-Natal, aggressively scaled up ACT availability in public health facilities, which was associated with a fall in the malaria burden (Barnes *et al.* 2005; Bhattarai *et al.* 2007).

What are the Barriers to EBP in Global Health?

We have argued that adopting EBP approaches can have profound public health benefits. However, in the "real world" of global health policy-making, which involves a complex interplay of multiple factors – such as power, politics, opinions, and conflicts of interest – policy actors may not prioritize research evidence in their policy-making decisions. Or, as Julius Court of the UK's Overseas Development Institute, put it: "The good news is that evidence can matter. The bad news is that it often does not" (quoted in Sutcliffe and Court 2011). So what gets in the way of the adoption of evidence into policy?

In this section, we briefly examine five major barriers (this is not an exhaustive list). Figure 7.4 gives a *highly idealized* representation of the way in which evidence would "ideally" flow from researcher to policy-maker to inform large-scale change in global health, showing where these five major barriers lie.

Mismatch Between Research Generation and Burden of Disease

Policy-makers look to locally generated evidence, because it has a crucial role in determining the preventive and therapeutic interventions that work best under local circumstances and in shaping local implementation strategies (Piot *et al.* 2008). But policy-makers in LMICs who wish to use locally generated research evidence may sometimes find that "the cupboard is bare" (Box 7.3). Most health research continues to be conducted in developed countries, even though developing countries bear the largest burden of disease

(Richards 2004) – known as the "10/90 gap" (less than 10% of global spending on research is spent on conditions accounting for 90% of the burden). Health research conducted in developed countries cannot simply be assumed to be transferable to LMIC settings, as it runs the risk of "exporting failure" (Miranda and Zaman 2010). There is also a well-described bias among medical journals against publishing research papers from developing countries (Horton 2003). "This cultural and geographical bias in the availability and relevance of published health literature," say McMichael *et al.* (2005), "is a significant problem."

Box 7.3   How Much Research on Tobacco Use and HIV is Generated in LMICs?

Tobacco consumption and HIV infection are ranked among the top five leading causes of death worldwide (Lopez *et al.* 2006). Ahmad *et al.* (2011) compared where research on these two global health priorities is conducted globally with where such research is needed. They identified 740 RCTs included in systematic reviews and 346 ongoing RCTs. For tobacco use, while LMICs accounted for 70% of mortality, only 4% of RCTs included in systematic reviews and 2% of ongoing trials were conducted in these countries. For HIV infection, 99% of the burden of mortality is in LMICs, but only 31% of RCTs included in systematic reviews and 33% of ongoing trials were performed in these countries. The results, conclude the authors, highlight "an important underrepresentation of LMICs in currently available evidence (RCTs included in systematic reviews) and awaiting evidence (registered ongoing RCTs) for reducing or stopping tobacco use and treating or preventing HIV infection."

Systematic Reviews Do Not Reflect the Health Priorities of LMICs

Similarly, a 2003 analysis of systematic reviews in two databases – the Cochrane Library and the Database of Abstracts of Reviews of Effects – found no correlation between the number of reviews about a disease and its global burden (Swingler *et al.* 2003). For many health risk factors that have a particularly high burden, such as maternal and child undernutrition and poor sanitation and hygiene, there are still too few reviews (Waters *et al.* 2006). This discrepancy is particularly alarming given the centrality of systematic reviews in informing public policy-making. One reason for the discrepancy is the underrepresentation of Cochrane reviewers based in developing countries (McMichael *et al.* 2005).

Policy-Makers in LMICs Cannot Access Research Evidence

Even though the United Nations has called for universal open access to the biomedical literature, in which all research papers would be universally free to read and free to reuse for legal purposes (UN Millennium Project 2005), nevertheless most of the world's health literature remains locked away behind access barriers. These barriers include exorbitant prices to read articles (a single research article in a medical journal typically costs $30–50 to access) as well as restrictive copyright licensing that makes it illegal to distribute articles, make copies, or translate them. The result of these barriers is that many policy-makers, researchers, clinicians, nongovernmental organizations, and others in LMICs simply cannot access research evidence.

Such restrictions also extend to Cochrane systematic reviews. While the publisher of the Cochrane Library, John Wiley and Sons, makes these reviews freely available or at low cost to selected low-income countries, this access policy excludes middle-income countries (MICs), such as Brazil, India, China, and Indonesia. Yet these MICs have large populations that continue to struggle with enormous health problems, and large populations living in poverty, and they have an acute and urgent need for health information (Yamey 2008) Indeed, most poor people now live in MICs rather than in low-income countries (Jamison *et al.* 2013).

Yamey (2008) has outlined the many ways in which such restricted access to the health literature impedes global public health, through preventing health workers from accessing information they need in their clinical practice; impeding health research capacity and sustainable development in LMICs; and hindering health systems strengthening. "Developing countries are poorer," argues the economist Stiglitz (2006), "not only because they have fewer resources, but because there is a gap in knowledge. That is why access to knowledge is so important."

Policy-Makers Do Not Use Evidence

Even when there is locally generated research and there are systematic reviews relevant to the challenges facing policy-makers, health policy actors may still not *make use* of such evidence. A recent systematic review of studies by Orton *et al.* (2011) that examined the use of evidence by health policy-makers identified several reasons why evidence may not be used (Orton *et al.* 2011). These reasons included: difficulties in understanding and interpreting the evidence, which is usually aimed at academic audiences (as Lavis [2009a] puts it, "policymakers hear noise instead of music"); a perceived gulf between research and policy that prevents evidence feeding into public policy; competing influences on decision-making, such as politics, time and resource constraints; and a preference for making decisions based on personal opinion. An earlier systematic review, by Innvaer *et al.* (2002), found that the most commonly reported barriers to the use of evidence by health policy-makers were the absence of personal contact with researchers, lack of timeliness and relevance of the research, mutual mistrust, and "power and budget struggles." Box 7.4 gives a case study by Volmink *et al.* (2001) of how politics trumped scientific evidence on preventing mother-to-child transmission of HIV (PMTCT). Evidence may even be ignored by policy-makers at the most influential multilateral health agencies, those that shape global health policy. For example, a study by Oxman *et al.* (2007) found that the WHO rarely uses systematic reviews in developing recommendations, often relying instead on expert opinion.

Box 7.4   Politics Trumps Evidence: A Case Study on PMTCT in South Africa

In the 1999, Manto Tshabalala-Msimang, South Africa's Minister of Health, commissioned the South African Cochrane Centre to conduct a literature review on the risks and benefits of interventions for PMTCT, with a particular focus on antiretroviral therapy (ART), especially zidovudine (AZT). The government was facing intense pressure from various stakeholders, including opposition parties and AIDS activists,

to roll out a national PMTCT policy that would offer ARVs to HIV-positive pregnant women, and wanted the literature review to be conducted urgently. At that
time, there was no political willingness or leadership to address the country's HIV
epidemic.

The Cochrane Centre researchers found strong evidence that both an intensive
AZT regimen (called the ACTG 076 protocol) and short course AZT reduced transmission, even among breast-fed populations. They also identified anemia as an
important side effect of the drug, particularly with the intensive regimen, but this
adverse effect resolved spontaneously once treatment ended. There was also limited
evidence that nevirapine, which was cheaper than AZT, was effective and safe.

The research team, led by Jimmy Volmink, sent a report of these findings to the
minister in December 1999. She declined to meet with the team to discuss the findings. The government did not act upon the evidence in the report – it refused to
adopt a national policy supporting ARVs for PMTCT, but gave no clear reasons
for its refusal. A 2001 policy analysis by Volmink *et al.*, examining the political and
epidemiological context of the government's inaction, concluded that "scientific evidence is not yet a powerful force in government decision-making in South Africa.
It appears to be eclipsed by political agendas and entrenched prior views that give
undue weight to unsubstantiated opinion" (Volmink *et al.* 2001).

The "Black" Box of Implementation

A fifth barrier to EBP in global health is that our knowledge of how best to scale up
evidence-based biological or behavioral interventions remains rudimentary. Evidence of
the effectiveness of an intervention is not sufficient to produce better health outcomes;
barriers and facilitators to its implementation must also be identified (Panisset *et al.*
2012). For example, an impact evaluation of UNICEF's Accelerated Child Survival and
Development Programme, which aimed to reduce childhood mortality by increasing coverage with three different evidence-based packages of interventions, found no difference
in survival between intervention and control districts (Bryce *et al.* 2010). It remains
unclear why the program had no survival benefit; the evaluation was unable, says Peterson (2010), to penetrate "the black box of implementation." Our lack of understanding of
this black box is impeding the large-scale implementation of evidence-based global health
tools (Yamey and Feachem 2011). Yet there has been little research attention towards, or
funding for, implementation research.

The New Landscape of Evidence Translation in Global Health

The good news is that in recent years there has been an explosion of initiatives aimed
specifically at overcoming these barriers and challenges to EBP in global health. These
initiatives fall under the umbrella of "knowledge translation," also known as "getting
research into policy and practice" (GRIPP). The Canadian Institute for Health Research
defines knowledge translation as "a dynamic and iterative process that includes synthesis,
dissemination, exchange and ethically-sound application of knowledge, through sustainable partnerships to improve the health of citizens, provide more effective health services
and products and strengthen the health care system" (Graham *et al.* 2006). Knowledge translation efforts in global health, discussed below, are designed to generate and

deliver evidence to decision-makers, particularly those in LMICs, packaged in a way that addresses their concerns and needs (Panisset *et al.* 2012).

Generation and Synthesis of Locally Relevant Evidence

An important recent trend has been the rise in the number of initiatives, networks, and partnerships aimed at strengthening primary research in LMICs and in producing more systematic reviews that are relevant to policy-makers in developing country settings. Examples of efforts to boost locally conducted research include INDEPTH (www .indepth-network.org), the International Network for the Demographic Evaluation of Populations and Their Health, whose members conduct longitudinal health and demographic evaluation of populations in LMICs; the Health Research Capacity Strengthening Initiative in sub-Saharan Africa, which serves as "a forum for African scientists to collate ideas on capacity building and to speak with a collective voice" (Whitworth *et al.* 2010); and the African Institutions Initiative, in which over 50 institutions from 18 African countries are partnered in seven international and pan-African consortia (Wellcome Trust 2009).

Such local research efforts have attracted increasing support from large foundations, such as the Bill & Melinda Gates Foundation, the Wellcome Trust, and the Rockefeller Foundation. Several Cochrane entities (e.g., the Cochrane Infectious Disease Group) are now prioritizing systematic reviews that address major contributors to the global burden of disease. The Cochrane Collaboration is also working more closely with the WHO, responding to specific needs for evidence by conducting full Cochrane reviews and rapid reviews and by preparing GRADE tables, which grade the quality of scientific evidence, for incorporation in guidelines. The Collaboration has been given official nongovernmental organization status in its relations with the WHO, which allows it to formalize projects the two organizations have been working on (such as the WHO Reproductive Library, at http://apps.who.int/rhl/en, and WHO Library of Evidence for Nutrition Actions, at http://www.who.int/elena/en/index.html; both last accessed December 2013) and to comment on WHO documents and proposed policies.

The Open Access Movement

The last decade has seen an extraordinary rise in international support for making *all* biomedical research papers open access (i.e., free to read, and free to reuse for all legal purposes with proper attribution). This support has come from a coalition or "movement" of funders, universities, governments, authors, journal editors, open access publishers (such as the Public Library of Science and Biomed Central), civil society organizations, patient advocacy groups, and the broader public. Angered by the rising cost of reading research articles, and empowered by the arrival of the internet, which offered a revolutionary mechanism for widespread dissemination of science at low cost, the open access movement has led to a growing proportion of the world's health literature being made open access (Yamey 2008). One obvious beneficiary is health policy-makers in LMICs.

New Initiatives and Tools for Packaging Evidence for Policy-Makers

Presenting research evidence in a clear accessible format – using language that a policy audience understands and addressing contextual factors that matter for policy-making – can increase the likelihood that health policies are informed by evidence (Lavis *et al.* 2005;

Orton *et al.* 2011). Global health policy-makers now have at their fingertips a wide array of short evidence "digests," including the following (Lavis 2009b):

- Short evidence-based policy briefs, such as those published by the SURE (Supporting the Use of Research Evidence) project, a collaboration between the Evidence-Informed Policy Network (EVIPNet) in Africa and the Region of East Africa Community Health (REACH) Policy Initiative (SURE 2012).
- Summaries of the key findings and policy implications of systematic reviews, such as those published by the SUPPORT (Supporting Policy Relevant Reviews and Trials) project (at the time of writing this chapter, 116 summaries are available in the SUPPORT database, at http://www.iecs.org.ar/support/iecs-visor-publicaciones.php; last accessed December 2013).
- Overviews of systematic reviews that lay out which policy questions have been addressed and which additional reviews are needed, such as those produced by IDEAHealth (International Dialogue on Evidence-Informed Action to Achieve Health Goals in Developing Countries) (Lavis *et al.* 2009).

Encouraging Linkage and Communication between Researchers and Policy-Makers

Systematic reviews (Lavis *et al.* 2005; Orton *et al.* 2011) have suggested that policy-makers are more likely to use evidence if there is two-way communication and interaction between researchers and policy-makers and if evidence can be presented to policy-makers at the right moment in time (particularly during "windows of opportunity," such as changes in the government). This evidence is the basis for a number of initiatives that see EBP in global health as a process that needs to be "actively managed," linking researchers and policy-makers in a continual two-way mutually valuable interaction. One prominent example is the Effective Health Care Research Consortium (http://www.evidence4health.org/; last accessed December 2013), which actively fosters linkages and exchange between researchers and policy-makers in LMICs. One potential approach to strengthening such linkages is "deliberative dialogues," participatory meetings in which researchers and policy-makers interact and share knowledge around a high priority policy issue (Lavis *et al.* 2009). National policy dialogues were used, for example, by EVIPNet in Burkina Faso and Cameroon to address low ACT coverage rates for malaria treatment (Lavis *et al.* 2009).

Conclusions

Adopting evidence-based approaches in public policy-making is a powerful tool for achieving global health goals, one that is likely to become increasingly more important as the MDGs' deadline gets nearer and as the international health community adapts to a new era of economic austerity. The tool can empower decision-makers in LMICs to prioritize interventions to achieve maximum impact and to help build stronger health systems (Moynihan *et al.* 2008). Although there are many barriers and challenges to EBP in global health, several of these are being overcome through a wide range of initiatives that seek to improve generation, synthesis, dissemination, and use of "evidence that matters." While there are many factors that will always influence global health policy-making, we believe that evidence should be a crucially important input – one that could profoundly improve global public health.

Key Reading

Chalmers I. 2003. Trying to do more good than harm in policy and practice: the role of rigorous, transparent, up-to-date evaluations. *Annals of the American Academy of Political and Social Science* 589, 22–40. Chalmers, one of the founders of the Cochrane Collaboration, which publishes systematic reviews on health interventions, makes a clear argument for using evidence in policy and practice.

Evidence-based policy-making in global health: the payoffs and pitfalls. An editorial, published in the journal *Evidence Based Medicine*, discussing both the public health benefits of evidence-based approaches to global health policy and also the challenges of adopting such approaches (see Yamey and Feachem 2011).

Evidence-Informed Policy Briefs, published by the SURE project (SURE: Supporting the Use of Research Evidence). http://www.who.int/evidence/sure/policybriefs/en/index .html (last accessed December 2013).

Guidance for Evidence-Informed Policies about Health Systems. A three-part series in *PLOS Medicine* that sets out how evidence should be translated into guidance to inform policies on health systems and improve the delivery of clinical and public health interventions (see Bosch-Capblanch *et al.* 2012; Lavis *et al.* 2012; Lewin *et al.* 2012).

Putting evidence into practice: how middle and low income countries "get it together." A team of researchers lays out key principles in evidence dissemination in developing countries (see Garner *et al.* 2004).

SUPPORT Summaries: Accessible summaries of policy-relevant trials and systematic reviews produced by the SUPPORT project (SUPPORT: Supporting Policy Relevant Reviews and Trials). The database of summaries can be found at http://www.iecs.org.ar/support/ iecs-visor-publicaciones.php (last accessed December 2013).

SUPPORT Tools for Evidence-Informed Health Policymaking. A collection of 19 articles, all open access, aimed at health policy decision-makers and those who support these decision-makers. http://www.health-policy-systems.com/supplements/7/s1 (last accessed December 2013).

References

Ahmad N, Boutron I, Dechartres A, Durieux P, Ravaud P. 2011. Geographical representativeness of published and ongoing randomized controlled trials: the example of tobacco consumption and HIV infection. *PLOS One* 6(2), e16878.

Attaran A, Barnes KI, Curtis C *et al.* 2004. WHO, the Global Fund, and medical malpractice in malaria treatment. *Lancet* 363, 237–40.

Baker B. 2010. *Flat Funding for AIDS: The Human Cost.* http://www.thebody.com/content/ 64488/flat-funding-for-aids-the-human-cost.html (last accessed December 2013).

Barham L, Lewis D, Latimer N. 2007. One to one interventions to reduce sexually transmitted infections and under the age of 18 conceptions: a systematic review of the economic evaluations. *Sexually Transmitted Infections* 83, 441–6.

Barnes KI, Durrheim DN, Little F *et al.* 2005. Effect of artemether-lumefantrine policy and improved vector control on malaria burden in KwaZulu–Natal, South Africa. *PLOS Medicine* 2(11), e330.

Bhattarai A, Ali AS, Kachur SP *et al.* 2007. Impact of artemisinin-based combination therapy and insecticide-treated nets on malaria burden in Zanzibar. *PLOS Medicine* 4(11), e309.

Bigby M. 2001. Challenges to the hierarchy of evidence: does the emperor have no clothes? *Archives of Dermatology* 137, 345–6.

Black N. 2001. Evidence based policy: proceed with care. *BMJ* 323, 275–9.

Bosch-Capblanch X, Lavis JN, Lewin S *et al.* 2012. Guidance for evidence-informed policies about health systems: rationale for and challenges of guidance development. *PLOS Medicine* 9(3), e1001185.

Bosman A, Mendis KN. 2007. A major transition in malaria treatment: the adoption and deployment of artemisinin-based combination therapies. *American Journal of Tropical Medicine and Hygiene* 77(Suppl 6), 193–7.

Britten N, Campbell R, Pope C *et al.* 2002. Using meta ethnography to synthesise qualitative research: a worked example. *Journal of Health Services Research and Policy* 7(4), 209–15.

Bryce J, Gilroy K, Jones G, Hazel E, Black RE, Victora CG. 2010. The Accelerated Child Survival and Development programme in West Africa: a retrospective evaluation. *Lancet* 375, 572–82.

Buekens P, Keusch G, Belizan J, Bhutta ZA. 2004. Evidence-based global health. *Journal of the American Medical Association* 291(21), 2639–41.

Center for Global Development. 2012. *Value for money: an agenda for global health funding agencies.* http://www.cgdev.org/section/topics/global_health/working_groups/value_for_money (last accessed December 2013).

Chalmers I. 2003. Trying to do more good than harm in policy and practice: the role of rigorous, transparent, up-to-date evaluations. *Annals of the American Academy of Political and Social Science* 589, 22–40.

Cochrane AL. 1973. *Effectiveness and Efficiency: Random Reflections on Health Services.* London: Nuffield Provincial Hospitals Trust.

Davies P. 2004. Is evidence-based government possible? Jerry Lee Lecture, presented at the 4th Annual Campbell Collaboration Colloquium, Washington, DC.

Egger M, Davey Smith G, Altman DG. 2008. Systematic reviews of observational studies. In Egger M, Davey Smith G, Schneider M (eds) *Systematic Review in Health Care: Meta-Analysis in Context*, 2nd edn, pp. 211–27. London: BMJ Publishing Group.

Eisenberg JM. 2002. Globalize the evidence, localize the decision: evidence-based medicine and international diversity. *Health Affairs* 21, 166–8.

Evans JR, Solomon AW. 2011. Antibiotics for trachoma. *Cochrane Database of Systematic Reviews* 3, CD001860.

Flaxman AD, Fullman N, Otten MW, Jr *et al.* 2010. Rapid scaling up of insecticide-treated bed net coverage in Africa and its relationship with development assistance for health: a systematic synthesis of supply, distribution, and household survey data. *PLOS Medicine* 7(8), e1000328.

Garner P. 2012. *Deworming: not all it's cracked up to be?* http://blogs.plos.org/speakingof medicine/2012/07/18/should-deworming-policies-in-the-developing-world-be-reconsidered/ (last accessed December 2013).

Garner P, Meremikwu M, Volmink J, Xu G, Smith H. 2004. Putting evidence into practice: how middle and low income countries "get it together." *BMJ* 329, 1036–9.

Glasziou P, Longbottom H. 1999. Evidence-based public health practice. *Australian and New Zealand Journal of Public Health* 23(4), 436–40.

Graham ID, Logan J, Harrison MB *et al.* 2006. Lost in knowledge translation: time for a map? *Journal of Continuing Education in the Health Professions* 26, 13–24.

Greenhalgh T, Russell J. 2009. Evidence-based policymaking: a critique. *Perspectives in Biology and Medicine* 52(2), 304–18.

Grimshaw J, McAuley LM, Bero LA *et al.* 2003. Systematic reviews of the effectiveness of quality improvement strategies and programmes. *Quality and Safety in Health Care* 12, 298–303.

Gysels M, Pell C, Straus L, Pool R. 2011. End of life care in sub-Saharan Africa: a systematic review of the qualitative literature. *BMC Palliative Care* 10, 6.

Harden A, Brunton G, Fletcher A, Oakley A. 2009. Teenage pregnancy and social disadvantage: systematic review integrating controlled trials and qualitative studies. *BMJ* 339, b4254.

Horton R. 2003. Medical journals: evidence of bias against the diseases of poverty. *Lancet* 361, 712.

Humphreys K, Piot P. 2012. Scientific evidence alone is not sufficient basis for health policy. *BMJ* 344, e1316.

Innvaer S, Gunn V, Trommald M, Oxman A. 2002. Health policy-makers' perceptions of their use of evidence: a systematic review. *Journal of Health Services Research and Policy* 7, 239–44.

International Initiative for Impact Evaluation. 2011. *AusAID-DFID-3ie Systematic Review Call*. http://www.3ieimpact.org/en/funding/systematic-reviews-grants/ausaid-dfid-3ie-systematic-review/ (last accessed December 2013).

Jamison DT, Summers LH, Alleyne G *et al.* 2013. Global health 2035: a world converging within a generation. *Lancet* 382, 1898–955.

Lavis J, Davies H, Oxman A *et al.* 2005. Towards systematic reviews that inform health care management and policy-making. *Journal of Health Services Research and Policy* 10(Suppl 1), 35–48.

Lavis JN. 2009a. Supporting evidence-informed policymaking. Presentation at the 8th Annual Symposium of the International Network Health Policy and Reform, Krakow, Poland. http://www.hpm.org/Downloads/Symposium_Krakau/Lavis_Supporting_evidenceinformed_policymaking.pdf (last accessed December 2013).

Lavis JN. 2009b. How can we support the use of systematic reviews in policymaking? *PLOS Medicine* 6(11), e1000141.

Lavis JN, Boyko JA, Oxman AD, Lewin S, Fretheim A. 2009. SUPPORT Tools for evidence-informed health Policymaking (STP) 14: Organising and using policy dialogues to support evidence-informed policymaking. *Health Research Policy and Systems* 7(Suppl 1), S14.

Lavis JN, Posada FB, Haines A, Osei E. 2004. Use of research to inform public policymaking. *Lancet* 364, 1615–21.

Lavis JN, Røttingen JA, Bosch-Capblanch X *et al.* 2012. Guidance for evidence-informed policies about health systems: linking guidance development to policy development. *PLOS Medicine* 9(3), e1001186.

Lazzerini M, Ronfani L. 2012. Oral zinc for treating diarrhoea in children. *Cochrane Database of Systematic Reviews* 6, CD005436.

Lengeler C. 2004. Insecticide-treated bed nets and curtains for preventing malaria. *Cochrane Database of Systematic Reviews* 2, CD000363.

Lewin S, Bosch-Capblanch X, Oliver S *et al.* 2012. Guidance for evidence-informed policies about health systems: assessing how much confidence to place in the research evidence. *PLOS Medicine* 9(3), e1001187.

Lewin S, Munabi-Babigumira S, Glenton C *et al.* 2010. Lay health workers in primary and community health care for maternal and child health and the management of infectious diseases. *Cochrane Database of Systematic Reviews* 3, CD004015.

Lim SS, Fullman N, Stokes A *et al.* 2011. Net benefits: a multicountry analysis of observational data examining associations between insecticide-treated mosquito nets and health outcomes. *PLOS Medicine* 8(9), e1001091.

Lopez AD, Mathers CD, Ezzati M, Jamison DT, Murray CJ. 2006. Global and regional burden of disease and risk factors, 2001: systematic analysis of population health data. *Lancet* 367, 1747–57.

Macintyre S, Petticrew M. 2000. Good intentions and received wisdom are not enough. *Journal of Epidemiology and Community Health* 54(11), 802–3.

Maslove DM, Mnyusiwalla A, Mills EJ *et al.* 2009. Barriers to the effective treatment and prevention of malaria in Africa: a systematic review of qualitative studies. *BMC International Health and Human Rights* 9, 26.

McMichael C, Waters E, Volmink J. 2005. Evidence-based public health: what does it offer developing countries? *Journal of Public Health* 27, 215–21.

Miranda JJ, Zaman MJ. 2010. Exporting 'failure': why research from rich countries may not benefit the developing world. *Revista de Saude Publica* 44(1), 185–9.

Moynihan R, Oxman A, Lavis JN, Paulsen E. 2008. *Evidence-Informed Health Policy: Using Research to Make Health Systems Healthier*. Rapport nr. 1-2008. Oslo: Nasjonalt Kunnskapssenter for Helsetjenesten.

Munro SA, Lewin SA, Smith HJ *et al.* 2007. Patient adherence to tuberculosis treatment: a systematic review of qualitative research. *PLOS Medicine* 4(7), e238.

Narasimhan V, Attaran A. 2003. Roll back malaria? The scarcity of international aid for malaria control. *Malaria Journal* 2, 8.

Orton L, Lloyd-Williams F, Taylor-Robinson D, O'Flaherty M, Capewell S. 2011. The use of research evidence in public health decision making processes: systematic review. *PLOS One* 6(7), e21704.

Oxman AD, Lavis JN, Fretheim A. 2007. Use of evidence in WHO recommendations. *Lancet* 369, 1883–9.

Oxman A, Lavis JN, Lewin S, Fretheim A. 2009. SUPPORT Tools for evidence-informed health Policymaking (STP) 1: What is evidence-informed policymaking? *Health Research Policy and Systems* 7(Suppl 1), S1.

Pablos-Mendez A, Shademani R. 2006. Knowledge translation in global health. *Journal of Continuing Education in the Health Professions* 26, 81–6.

Panisset U, Koehlmoos TP, Alkhatib AH *et al.* 2012. Implementation research evidence uptake and use for policy-making. *Health Research Policy and Systems* 10, 20.

Peterson S. 2010. Assessing the scale-up of child survival interventions. *Lancet* 375, 530–1.

Petticrew M, Roberts H. 2002. Evidence, hierarchies, and typologies: horses for courses. *Journal of Epidemiology and Community Health* 57, 527–9.

Piot P, Bartos M, Larson H, Zewdie D, Mane P. 2008. Coming to terms with complexity: a call to action for HIV prevention. *Lancet* 372, 845–59.

Ravishankar N, Gubbins P, Cooley RJ *et al.* 2009. Financing of global health: tracking development assistance for health from 1990 to 2007. *Lancet* 373, 2113–24.

Richards D. 2003. Not all evidence is created equal: so what is good evidence? *Evidence-Based Dentistry* 4, 17–8.

Richards T. 2004. Poor countries lack relevant health information, says Cochrane editor. *BMJ* 328, 310.

Ritch WA, Begay ME. 2001. Strange bedfellows: the history of collaboration between the Massachusetts Restaurant Association and the tobacco industry. *American Journal of Public Health* 91, 598–603.

Roberts AR, Yeager KR (eds). 2006. *Foundations of Evidence-Based Social Work Practice*. New York: Oxford University Press.

Roll Back Malaria Partnership. 2007. Affordable Medicines Facility – Malaria: Technical Design. Geneva: Roll Back Malaria Partnership. http://www.rbm.who.int/partnership/tf/globalsubsidy/AMFmTechProposal.pdf (last accessed December 2013).

Sackett DL, Rosenberg WMC, Gray JAM, Haynes RB, Richardson WS. 1996. Evidence based medicine: What it is and what it isn't. *BMJ* 312, 71–2.

Scollo M, Lal A, Hyland A, Glantz S. 2003. Review of the quality of studies on the economic effects of smoke-free policies on the hospitality industry. *Tobacco Control* 12, 13–20.

Schwappach DL, Boluarte TA, Suhrcke M. 2007. The economics of primary prevention of cardiovascular disease: a systematic review of economic evaluations. *Cost Effectiveness and Resource Allocation* 5, 5.

Shaxson, L. 2005. Is your evidence robust enough? Questions for policy makers and practitioners. *Evidence and Policy: A Journal of Research, Debate and Practice* 1(1), 101–11.

Shemilt I, Mugford M, Drummond M *et al.* 2006. Economics methods in Cochrane systematic reviews of health promotion and public health related interventions. *BMC Medical Research Methodology* 6, 55.

Sinclair D, Zani B, Donegan S, Olliaro P, Garner P. 2009. Artemisinin-based combination therapy for treating uncomplicated malaria. *Cochrane Database of Systematic Reviews* 3, CD007483.

Snow RW, Okiro EA, Gething PW, Atun R, Hay SI. 2010. Equity and adequacy of international donor assistance for global malaria control: an analysis of populations at risk and external funding commitments. *Lancet* 376, 1409–16.

Stiglitz JE. 2006. Innovation: a better way than patents. *New Scientist* 2569, 21.

SURE. 2012. *Evidence-Based Policy Briefs*. http://www.who.int/evidence/sure/policybriefs/en/index.html (last accessed December 2013).

Sutcliffe S, Court J. 2005. *Evidence-Based Policymaking: What Is It? How Does It Work? What Relevance for Developing Countries?* Overseas Development Institute. http://www.odi.org.uk/resources/download/2804.pdf (last accessed December 2013).

Swingler GH, Volmink J, Ioannidis J. 2003. Number of published systematic reviews and the global burden of disease: database analysis. *BMJ* 327, 1083–4.

Taylor-Robinson DC, Maayan N, Soares-Weiser K, Donegan S, Garner P. 2012. Deworming drugs for soil-transmitted intestinal worms in children: effects on nutritional indicators, haemoglobin and school performance. *Cochrane Database of Systematic Reviews* 7, CD000371.

Thomas J, Harden A, Oakley A *et al*. 2004. Integrating qualitative research with trials in systematic reviews. *BMJ* 328, 1010–12.

Truman BI, Smith-Akin CK, Hinman AR *et al*. 2000. Developing the Guide to Community Preventive Services: overview and rationale. The Task Force on Community Preventive Services. *American Journal of Preventative Medicine* 18(Suppl 1), 18–26.

UN (United Nations) Millennium Project, Task Force on Science, Technology and Innovation. 2005. *Applying Knowledge in Development*. London: Earthscan Publishing. http://www.unmillennium project.org/documents/Science-complete.pdf (last accessed December 2013).

Volmink J, Garner P. 2007. Directly observed therapy for treating tuberculosis. *Cochrane Database of Systematic Reviews* 4, CD003343.

Volmink J, Matchaba P, Zwarenstein M. 2011. Reducing mother-to-child transmission of HIV infection in South Africa. In: *Informing Judgment: Case Studies of Health Policy and Research in Six Countries*. Oxford: Cochrane Collaboration; New York: Milbank Memorial Fund.

Waters E, Doyle J, Jackson N *et al*. 2006. Evaluating the effectiveness of public health interventions: the role and activities of the Cochrane Collaboration. *Journal of Epidemiology and Community Health* 60(4), 285–9.

Welch V, Petticrew M, Tugwell P *et al*. 2012. PRISMA-equity 2012 extension: reporting guidelines for systematic reviews with a focus on health equity. *PLOS Medicine* 9(10), e1001333.

Wellcome Trust. 2009. *African institutions lead international consortia in 30 million initiative*. http://www.wellcome.ac.uk/News/Media-office/Press-releases/2009/WTX055742.htm (last accessed December 2013).

Weller SC, Davis-Beaty K. 2007. Condom effectiveness in reducing heterosexual HIV transmission. *Cochrane Database of Systematic Reviews* 4, CD003255.

Whitworth J, Sewankambo NK, Snewin VA. 2010. Improving implementation: building research capacity in maternal, neonatal, and child health in Africa. *PLOS Medicine* 7(7), e1000299.

World Health Assembly. 1998. *Resolution WHA 51.12 on Health Promotion*. Agenda Item 20, May 16, 1998. Geneva: WHO.

WHO (World Health Organization). 2001. *Antimalarial Drug Combination Therapy. Report of a WHO Technical Consultation*. Geneva: WHO.

WHO (World Health Organization). 2004a. *World Report on Knowledge for Better Health: Strengthening Health Systems*. Geneva: WHO. http://www.who.int/rpc/meetings/pub1/en/ (last accessed December 2013).

WHO (World Health Organization). 2004b. *More than 600 million people urgently need effective malaria treatment to prevent unacceptably high death rates*. http://www.who.int/mediacentre/news/releases/2004/pr29/en/ (last accessed December 2013).

WHO (World Health Organization). 2005. *The Millennium Development Goals. The evidence is in: deworming helps meet the Millennium Development Goals*. Geneva: WHO. http://whqlibdoc.who.int/hq/2005/WHO_CDS_CPE_PVC_2005.12.pdf (last accessed December 2013).

WHO (World Health Organization). 2009. *World Malaria Report 2009*. http://www.who.int/ malaria/world_malaria_report_2009/en/index.html (last accessed December 2013).

WHO (World Health Organization). 2010. *World Malaria Report 2010*. http://www.who.int/ malaria/world_malaria_report_2010/en/ (last accessed December 2013).

WHO (World Health Organization) and UNICEF. 2003. *Africa Malaria Report 1993*. http://www .rbm.who.int/amd2003/amr2003/amr_toc.htm (last accessed December 2013).

Yamey G. 2000. African heads of state promise action against malaria. *BMJ* 320, 1228.

Yamey G. 2003. Malaria researchers say Global Fund is buying "useless drug." *BMJ* 327, 1188.

Yamey G. 2004. Roll Back Malaria: a failing global health campaign. *BMJ* 328, 1086–7.

Yamey G. 2008. Excluding the poor from accessing biomedical literature: a rights violation that impedes global health. *Health and Human Rights* 10(1), 21–42.

Yamey G. 2012. What are the barriers to scaling up health interventions in low and middle income countries? A qualitative study of academic leaders in implementation science. *Globalization and Health* 8, 11.

Yamey G, Feachem R. 2011. Evidence-based policymaking in global health: the payoffs and pitfalls. *Evidence Based Medicine* 16(4), 97–9.

Yamey G, Schaeferhoff M, Montagu D. 2012. Piloting the Affordable Medicines facility-malaria (AMFm): what will "success" look like? *Bulletin of the World Health Organization* 90, 452–60.

Young E, Quinn L. 2002. *Writing Effective Public Policy Papers: A Guide To Policy Advisers in Central and Eastern Europe*. Budapest: LGI.

Chapter 8

Can Global Health Policy be Depoliticized? A Critique of Global Calls for Evidence-Based Policy

Amy Barnes and Justin Parkhurst

Abstract

Contemporary discourse about global health tends to dominantly frame policy-making as if it should be depoliticized: free from value-based choices or political judgments, and also from the corrupting influence of power, wealth, and material interests. This is exemplified in recent calls for evidence-based global health policy. This chapter considers these calls, and appraises whether policy-making can and should be depoliticized. It explores the following:

- Whether the generation of health sciences research evidence can itself be considered free from politics.
- Whether evidence from the health sciences alone can be used in an apolitical way to inform the global health policy agenda.
- Whether policies promoted under a banner of evidence-based global health policy can have problematic political effects.

The chapter argues that contemporary evidence-based discourse raises a number of political debates, dilemmas, and ethical issues – notably around which evidence should guide global health policy and whose values should be represented in fundamentally political decisions. The call for policy to only follow selected evidence bases tends not to fully recognize wider processes that are at work. This *obscures* the political nature of decision-making and risks limiting policy effectiveness and impact. Better ways to *govern* the use of evidence in health policy-making are needed to ensure that a range of evidence is debated and applied in valid and transparent ways, which are accountable to global publics, their values, and their multiple social interests.

The Handbook of Global Health Policy, First Edition. Edited by Garrett W. Brown, Gavin Yamey, and Sarah Wamala.
© 2014 John Wiley & Sons, Ltd. Published 2014 by John Wiley & Sons, Ltd.

Key Points

- Contemporary discourse about global health tends to dominantly frame policy-making as if it is, or should be, depoliticized; as exemplified in calls for evidence-based global health policy.
- The concept of evidence-based policy oversimplifies global health policy, obscuring the fundamentally political nature of, and value-based choices that are inherent to, decision-making.
- The production of evidence is political because research will be developed around issues with high political priority to begin with and because the "accepted" hierarchy of evidence, which promotes randomized controlled trials and systematic reviews, will skew decisions towards those interventions most easily explored via these research methods (e.g., those that are biomedical, clinical, and behavioral in nature).
- The selection and use of evidence in global health policy-making is also political because value-based choices must be made between different bodies of evidence; weighing evidence about health outcomes alongside evidence about other societal impacts.
- We need to govern global health policy in a way that allows engagement with the fundamentally political nature of decision-making, while also ensuring that there is space for the valid application of different bodies of knowledge.

Key Policy Implications

- Researchers, scientists, and experts should support (and advocate for) the use of multiple bodies of evidence to inform global health policy; preserving the importance of valid evidence use (accurately representing research findings), while acknowledging that evidence of different social outcomes may take different forms – for example, non-experimental evidence to explore complex and structural determinants of health, or qualitative research to understand societal beliefs about different social outcomes.
- Global health policy-makers must enhance their understanding of how different research methodologies produce relevant evidence to inform decision-making, while committing to transparent and open debate about how different bodies of evidence are valued in decision-making processes.
- Rather than calling for more evidence-based policy, the international research and policy community must work to establish best practice on, and institutional structures that support, the use of evidence in policy that follows principles of good governance.

Introduction

Contemporary discourse about global health tends to dominantly frame the health policy-making process as if it is, or should be, beyond politics (cf. Clarke 2004). It assumes that decision-making about global health issues and the implementation of programmatic interventions can and should be free from partisan values or political beliefs about the way world is or should be, and also free from the apparently corrupting influence of power, wealth, and material interests (Barnes and Brown 2011). In place of such politics is a call for a more technical framework for global health action, which is grounded in the logic of evidence-based policy. Here, the global health policy process is about finding out "what works" and then "getting it into policy and practice" research evidence is collated and expertly appraised, so as to identify particular global health problems and enable decision-making about efficient and cost-effective solutions (Lavis *et al.* 2004; Russell *et al.* 2008; Parkhurst *et al.* 2010). By combining what is apparently neutral and objective health sciences research evidence with reasoned scientific appraisal, politics is assumed to be excluded from the policy process. It is because of this that evidence-based policy comes across in contemporary discourse as an inherently good, legitimate, and, moreover, effective mode of global health action.

Yet is evidence-based policy-making as depoliticized as contemporary discourse dominantly seems to suggest? Moreover, what are the implications of this approach for global health-related action? The purpose of this chapter is to address these questions. It not only considers whether evidence-based global health policy-making *is* depoliticized (as it is currently practised); but also, and more fundamentally, whether it *can* and *should* be apolitical in the way that is suggested. While not wanting to dismiss the importance of valid and unbiased uses of evidence in global policy debates, this chapter seeks to question the assumption that policy-making cannot or should not be a political process.

We take as a starting point the understanding that decision-making about global health policy fundamentally involves making choices between, and allocating resources towards, competing alternatives, which have different values to society (Walt 1994; Hill 2009;). While valid evidence is needed to establish unbiased estimates of each possible outcome, we argue that the values placed on these competing outcomes cannot be removed from the policy-making process by appealing to evidence of health outcomes alone. Policy-makers are faced with "burdens of judgement" (cf. Rawls 1993), in that they have to consider and weigh up evidence about health outcomes alongside evidence about other societal outcomes – such as economic efficiency, human rights, social justice, or what might lead to a "good" society. As there are disagreements within society about the relative importance of these aspects, as well as more fundamentally about what a "good" society actually looks like (Tesh 1988; Stone 2002; Clark and Weale 2012), there is likely to be disagreement about which global health policy decisions will be acceptable to and appropriate for society.

Calls for health policy to be evidence-based – if stated with no qualifications – therefore raise a number of political debates, dilemmas, and potential ethical issues – notably around which social concerns to consider in gathering an evidence base of potential outcomes, how much to value the different outcomes established by the evidence, and whose values should be represented in these assessments. Furthermore, it is noted that bodies of evidence are typically created from political processes themselves: decisions about what to research, or on which health issues to develop an evidence base, will be made to the exclusion of other alternatives. Politically popular or publicly sensational health concerns, for instance, will no doubt have attracted more research attention and more funding to create an evidence base that can then justify action. Calling on policy-makers to only follow established evidence therefore implicitly skews policy attention to those issues that were initially politically popular. We argue that calling for global health policy to follow established evidence bases without recognition of these complexities obscures the inherently political nature of decision-making, allowing established power positions to remain unchallenged and potentially limiting policy effectiveness and impact.

The points that are outlined here are designed to provide a natural counterpoint to the arguments (and, indeed, the form of argumentation) put forward by Yamey and Volmink in Chapter 7. To be sure, the intention is not to dismiss the importance of increasing the use of rigorously gathered health sciences evidence, nor to deny the importance of valid use of those pieces of evidence considered (with validity defined by the methods and technical aspects of the research conducted). Rather, this chapter aims to promote a more critical (but more realistic) understanding about the political nature of global health policy-making and the potential "payoffs and pitfalls" (cf. Yamey and Feachem 2011) of depoliticized ways of thinking; that is to say, ways of thinking that deny or ignore important political dimensions.

The chapter starts by briefly revisiting the underlying logic of contemporary discourse about evidence-based global health policy. It then moves on to consider a number of critical political issues that are associated with both evidence generation and evidence utilization. In particular, the chapter explores:

1. Whether the generation of health sciences research evidence itself can be considered apolitical;
2. Whether technical evidence from the health sciences alone can be used to inform the global health policy agenda; and finally
3. Whether policies promoted under a banner of evidence-based global health policy can have problematic political effects.

Understanding Evidence-Based Global Health Policy

As suggested in Chapter 7, the idea of evidence-based global health policy evolved as an apparently natural extension of moves in the early 1990s from within the discipline of health sciences (including epidemiology, clinical medicine, and health economics) to promote "evidence-based medicine." The evidence-based medicine movement sought to ensure that clinical decision-making by doctors was based on the best available scientific research (Sackett *et al.* 1996). Abstracted upwards to global health policy, the broad idea is to ensure that decision-making by global actors, such as the G8/G20, World Health Organization (WHO), and World Bank, along with the programs and interventions that they fund, is based upon the best scientific research about what works for health; for this is assumed to be the most efficient and effective way to improve the health of the global population (Garner *et al.* 1998; van Kammen *et al.* 2006; Global Health Council 2010).

While Yamey and Volmink (see Chapter 7) provide more detail about the historical development and key characteristics of the evidence-based policy model, the vision is of a global policy-making process in which research evidence, typically implied to mean research from the health sciences – in contrast to political opinion, whim, or partisan judgement – is used to identify global health problems and select the right policy solutions (cf. Greenhalgh and Russell 2009; Yamey and Feachem 2011). This is to be achieved through the appropriate management of evidence throughout the policy cycle: from priority setting to programmatic implementation.

Importantly, within the health sciences, there is a commonly imposed hierarchy of evidence, within which experimental trials (specifically randomized controlled/clinical trials, RCTs) and systematic reviews (usually of multiple large-scale RCTs) are typically seen as the gold standard of research evidence (Sackett *et al.* 1996; Paxton *et al.* 2005; Padian *et al.* 2010). This hierarchy has migrated into contemporary policy discourse about evidence-based global health. As a result, experimental trials are commonly regarded as the "best" way to inform policy decisions about global health (Buekens *et al.* 2004; see also SUPPORT 2011). In a review of evidence for effective HIV prevention, Padian *et al.* (2010: 622) indicate, for example, that: "Randomized controlled trials (RCTs) are generally considered the gold standard to define the evidence base for HIV prevention programs and policies," using this to justify inclusion criteria for a systematic review that should inform policy-makers of HIV interventions that only considers RCT evidence. This is despite the fact that there are various issues associated with the limitations of RCTs in relation to several health and social policy goals (Victora *et al.* 2004; Cartwright 2011) and that most HIV prevention successes seen historically did not arise from the implementation of single interventions tested or evaluated in experimental trials (Auerbach *et al.* 2011).

We go on to consider some of the issues with RCTs later, but it is important to highlight here that the elevated hierarchical position of RCT evidence in calls for evidence-based global health policy is explained (at least in part) by certain assumptions about the way in which politics tends to get in the way of action for global health. In contemporary policy discourse, there is a tendency to see politics in a perjorative way (Siddiqi 1995; Barnes and Brown 2011); that is to say, as an obstacle to the unbiased use of health sciences research evidence and thus a barrier to effective policy-making for global health. As Gibson (2003: 302) explains, political judgment and the rational use of evidence tend to be portrayed as being "locked in a zero-sum game"; wherein the more policy is driven by values and interests, the less is the role played by evidence in decision-making, which limits policy impact. It is believed that the greater use of health sciences evidence, and especially the application of experimental trials, will move global health policy beyond politics (cf. Clarke 2004); resulting in decision-making and programmatic interventions that are more objective, efficient, and effective.

The Pejorative Influence of Politics in Global Health Policy

There are certainly well-documented cases in which policy-making has been biased to reflect the partisan agenda of particular (powerful) global actors. Examples range from the way in which major industrial countries of the West have dominated policy processes at the WHO (Walt 1993; Brown *et al.* 2006), to the way in which the United States, in particular, has shaped the global HIV/AIDS and reproductive health agendas, through the attachment of conditions to USAID and PEPFAR financing (Crane and Dusenberry 2002; Mayhew 2002; Barnett and Parkhurst 2005).

While these are valid and important observations, it is argued that there are actually deeper, more fundamental ways in which value-based political judgments shape global health policy, including in the production of research evidence itself. Although the particular type of partisan politics described above may well bias health policy towards the interests of powerful global actors, political dimensions are not always obstacles to good health policy. As the rest of this chapter shows, while research evidence from the health sciences can and should be generated by adhering to recognized quality standards, such evidence alone is never enough to guide global health policy decisions. These decisions are inherently political because they involve choices between competing outcomes, values, and interests. What is key is to make these choices and their associated valuations clear, so as to allow for more transparent, and therefore more democratic and representative, global policy-making (Schön and Rein 1994; Young 2000).

The next section considers the issues that arise when oversimplified calls for evidence-based policy fail to recognize the political nature of, and choices that are inherent to, policy-making. As we will see, it is for the reasons outlined below that global health policy simply cannot be depoliticized.

Producing Health Sciences Research: The Politics of Creating the Evidence Base

Contemporary discourse about global health suggests that research studies from the health sciences, and specifically from experimental trials like RCTs, are the gold standard to define the evidence base for health policies and programs. RCTs are particularly highly regarded because of their apparent methodological rigor. They aim to measure the effectiveness of health interventions accurately; giving the most valid possible assessment of a hypothesized cause–effect relationship that is assumed to exist between an intervention and a particular health outcome of interest, such as mortality or disease incidence (Victora *et al.* 2004). Here, the mechanism of action of the intervention is believed to operate in a relatively direct and universal way, and usually at the level of the individual – who is seen in isolation from their social context.

Although there are many supporters of RCTs, a number of issues have been raised with their superiority as a health sciences research methodology. While we are more concerned with the political implications of producing an evidence base for policy that is focused on RCTs, in order to explore this it is necessary to understand some of the criticisms that have been levelled at RCTs because, as we shall see, the two issues are interconnected.

A common criticism is that is that many successful health policy interventions have not been based on RCT evidence, which demonstrates that the field of health has not always been, and therefore does not now need to be, reliant on their use (Smith and Pell 2003; Sanson-Fisher *et al.* 2007; Worrall 2007). Another criticism comes from critical philosophers of science, who comment on the misleading way in which RCT studies attempt to "clinch" proof of effect of interventions through a deductive process, rather than build a broad evidence base that vouches for a feasible effect, as is typical in most other sciences (Cartwright 2007, 2011). A third criticism, and one that is of particular significance here, is that, for a wide range of non-clinical (non-biomedical) health phenomena, experimentation using a controlled trial is difficult and/or unethical, and, moreover, does not provide globally generalizable results because of the unrealistic assumptions that are made about how social context can be controlled for in implementing trialled interventions (also known as external validity problems) (Black 1996; Pawson and Tilley 1997; Victora *et al.* 2004; Kemm 2006; Sanson-Fisher *et al.* 2007; Worrall 2007).

While clinical or biomedical interventions (such as the provision of drugs or the use of a medical device) may have a relatively direct relationship between a causal agent and biological health outcome (irrespective of the wider social context), many social or structural interventions, which seek to change behavior, or to address the wider determinants of poor health (such as gender inequality, racial discrimination, social status, poverty) do not have such discrete and linear causal relationships with health outcomes (Victora *et al.* 2004; Raphael 2006; Marmot 2007; CSDH 2008). They tend to operate through more complex and non-linear webs of causation that may be context-specific, and will have health impacts over more prolonged periods of time (and potentially over the life course). As a result, they are difficult to define, measure, and assess as to whether they "work" in experimental research studies (Victora *et al.* 2004; Auerbach *et al.* 2011).

For many global health issues, researchers simply do not fully understand the complex ways in which different social or structural factors lead to poor health in different contextual settings, nor therefore how to design or implement interventions that will address them. We do not know, for example, what and how different types of social relationships or cultural norms shape the way in which health systems function in different country settings, and therefore whether and how particular health system interventions may work (Mills *et al.* 2008). Similarly, we may never fully know what definitively works to change sexual behavior in relation to HIV because of the complex social, economic, cultural, and political ways in which behavior may be influenced in different settings (Fisher and Fisher 1992, Carballo and Kenya 1994; Parkhurst 2008). What might work in one setting, and at one point in time, will likely be different in others (Mills *et al.* 2008; Brown and Labonté 2011). While researchers may have some plausible insights and generalizable ideas about these issues, and possible sociostructural interventions, health researchers will probably never have a comprehensive and universally applicable global evidence base about them, because they are fundamentally different from biomedical ones.

In consequence, if we prioritize experimental studies that explore cause–effect relationships on the global health research agenda, we may never fully explore and produce a substantial evidence base about what works to address the social and structural determinants of poor health, because it is simply not possible to investigate them with the requisite RCT level of precision and certainty (Sanson-Fisher *et al.* 2007).

This is significant point because it has political implications. Essentially, if the evidence base for global health is focused on a privileged set of experimental studies and we uncritically accept calls for more evidence-based policy, researchers will shape and, indeed, constrain the way global health policy is made. Decision-makers will be less likely to act upon those health issues that are not conducive to investigation through experimental trials in the first place, thus biasing their decisions towards those issues that time and resources have already been spent on building up a larger evidence base. In short, applying the hierarchy of research evidence (which was primarily developed for particular clinical and biomedical research validity), in order to guide valuation of evidence and policy attention, will skew global health policy towards addressing those issues and interventions where experimental trials have been most feasible – typically simple singular clinical or biomedical interventions like drug trials – to the exclusion of less well-understood and complex issues that require structural change – best exemplified by the social determinants of health (Marmot 2007; Navarro 2009). Calls for evidence-based policy may therefore end up favoring decisions and programmatic interventions that have a "[bio]medical rather than social focus, those that target individuals rather than communities or populations, and those that focus on the influence of proximal rather than distal determinants of health" (Rychetnik *et al.* 2002: 125).

Using Health Sciences Research: What to Value and How to Value Evidence in Decision-Making

A key political dimension to global health policy-making comes from the way in which available research evidence is selected and valued in decision-making processes. While experimental clinical or epidemiological trials can certainly provide valid evidence about certain global health issues, the idea (which has migrated from the evidence-based medicine movement) that this particular method provides the "best" evidence for policy-making is problematic because it conflates two rather different issues. The first is the validity of a particular research method (i.e., experimental trials) in generating evidence about, and assessing, a specific intervention and health outcome of interest, such as the effectiveness of a new vaccine or a new drug treatment reducing morbidity and mortality. The second is the importance of research evidence in decision-making when choosing what social outcomes to be concerned with, and how to value them when making choices about how society should act. It is a political decision to create global health priorities. The choice of whether to focus on malaria and HIV/AIDS, as opposed to, say, reproductive health, health systems strengthening, or any number of other possible global health concerns, will be made for a range of reasons beyond simply burden of disease and efficacy of treatments available (Shiffman 2006, 2007; England 2007; Patel *et al.* 2011).

There are also further social concerns that health policies touch upon, including cost implications, equity or equality issues, preservation of human rights, or promotion of socially desired behaviors (or alternatively promotion of the freedom to practice behaviors). There can be abundant evidence on what an intervention costs, whether it reproduces or reduces inequalities, whether it infringes on the rights of individuals, or whether it promotes a particular "healthy" or desirable set of behaviors. The balance of these, and judgment of which ones are important, are not answerable by epidemiological and biomedical means. They are only answerable through political debate where social values are presented to inform policy decisions (see Clark and Weale 2012).

There is a key difference then between valid measurement of outcomes (for which unbiased research evidence is needed), and choice and valuation of potential outcomes. This distinction tends to be obscured when advocates call for more evidence-based global health policy without qualification, or when it is implied that the ultimate policy decision can be made from the research evidence alone. The first is a methodological research issue. As indicated above, experimental trials are constructed to assess effectiveness, and to give the most valid possible assessment of an assumed cause–effect relationship between an intervention and a defined outcome of interest. The second, however, is a political concern, because it involves selecting and appraising evidence to prioritize and make choices about what we, as a global society, should focus on, intervene in, and evaluate.

There are a wide range of different threats to the health of the global population. Any number of health issues could potentially become the priority focus for global health policy. Decisions have to be made in order to "limit the realm" of action and inquiry (Schwartz and Carpenter 1999: 1175). This inevitably means that certain issues must be prioritized above others in global policy processes. To prioritize, global actors have to appraise multiple types of evidence. They will not only want to know the scale and distribution of various different health problems, and the efficacy of particular interventions (whether they "work" at individual or population levels in differing contexts), but they will also typically consider whether interventions are "worth" investing in (e.g., are they cost-effective). These tend to be the considerations most public health actors conceptualize when thinking about an evidence base for policy. Yet decision-makers will also base their decisions on whether policies work towards other social, political, or culturally acceptable goals.

Indeed, global health policy-makers will need to be mindful of whether particular priorities and interventions will be acceptable to global publics, and whether they are appropriate for different social groups. They will need to consider, for example, if particular interventions promote or hinder prevailing human rights concerns, or work to promote other societal goals, such as solidarity, justice, fairness, or autonomy (Clark and Weale 2012). Certain interventions, particularly those that are designed to address broader determinants of health, including economic opportunities, gender norms, and legal structures, are typically deeply contested. The nature of that contestation comes from competing values in society, and policy-makers have to take these different values into account when considering if global health policy will work.

No matter how rigorous the research method, clinical research alone cannot possibly provide evidence to address all of these policy considerations. Scientists can clearly contribute greatly here: supporting decision-making processes by deciding how best to undertake research inquiries, how to measure particular outcomes accurately, and generating evidence that could help inform policy-makers, but they cannot objectively tell policy-makers what the right or wrong policy choice is, or on which pieces of evidence the policy should be based (Brecht 1968). There are numerous bodies of evidence that need to be considered in order to make global health policy decisions: epidemiological evidence of health impact; economic evidence of cost and equity; legal evidence of human rights implications; survey evidence of behaviors and preferences; as well as more qualitative evidence of social values or meanings, and how interventions align with, or oppose, these locally held beliefs. Global health policy-makers will need to make judgments between the different sources of evidence, rather than basing policy on a single body of information.

The key point then is that the "right" global health policy approach cannot be reduced to technical issues of evidence alone. Evidence should clearly be utilized in the decision-making process, and utilized in valid ways, but when looking at the bodies of evidence available, policy-makers need to consider (to adapt a turn of phrase typically attributed to Albert Einstein) if what has been measured matters, and if what matters has been measured. When it is assumed that evidence-based policy has no politics, it not only obscures the fact that not all of the things that matter will necessarily have been measured to the same degree, but it misrepresents the nature of policy-making, where value judgments are part of any decision about what to focus on, where to intervene, and what to evaluate (Clark and Weale 2012).

These points can be illustrated by the example of the case of mandatory food fortification as a global health policy intervention. Although there is robust scientific evidence that this could reduce clinical symptoms of nutrient deficiencies, food is also a cultural, social, and commercial commodity. When faced with making choices about this issue, a key consideration for policy-makers might obviously be how much implementing a fortification policy would immediately cost for a particular state, but given that food is a commercial product, policy-makers would also want to appraise the likely impacts on the food industry. They might be concerned to understand how mandatory fortification would affect competiveness in global food markets; how different producers and suppliers would be impacted (would big companies and small-scale entrepreneurs have different opportunities and costs?); and also whether there is capacity to implement this approach in particular contexts. At the same time, policy-makers would need to balance this with evidence of public acceptability; not only taking into account whether there would be changes to food costs or the qualitative dimensions of food, but also whether this type of collective action would be culturally valued or seen instead as a impingement on individual rights (given that it may remove the right to choose not to eat fortified food) (Lawrence 2003, 2005). Similarly, policy-makers may also wish to consider alternative strategies to improve nutrition, such as upstream social and economic changes that might improve diet overall. A call for evidence-based policy alone may fail to highlight the multiple competing, yet relevant, considerations that policy-makers would want to make in this case.

Another example comes from the United Kingdom in relation to its illegal drugs policy. In a recent review of drug harms, a scientific advisory panel judged that the legal status of many drugs was not in line with their harmfulness to health – with illegal drugs, such as ecstasy (deemed class A – the most controlled), much less harmful than legal products like alcohol or tobacco (Nutt *et al.* 2007). The head of the panel went so far as to declare that use was less dangerous than horse riding (BBC 2009), to which government officials responded with denial and reprobation (and dismissal of the panel member involved) (Guardian 2009).

The failure of the UK government to change the drug classification system based on this health evidence is insightful because it illustrates the range of issues and concerns that policy-makers take into account when making decisions. While health professionals were asked to rank "harmfulness" (both individual and social), what was not considered were the other factors that may influence a policy-maker's decision on legality of different drugs. These include evidence of tax revenue; social acceptance; the roles that different drugs have in society; or pleasure or utility that users of drugs achieve – all of which could be affected by changes in the classification system (see Monaghan 2011). When considered in this light, there can be no single evidence-based drug policy, but only a political decision-making process that is based on a range of considerations.

In the UK drug case, the evidence of harm was made explicit, and the assessment of the advisory panel on harms was carried out in a transparent fashion allowing public and media scrutiny. One could argue that the other social values on which final decisions were made, however, could have been more clear or should have been explicitly laid out, to allow genuine democratic debate on the topic. Indeed, the original UK classification system was supposedly developed based on health harms, and the review of drugs shows it clearly is inconsistent on this ground alone. Assuming drug policy can be based on clinical evidence of harms alone obscures the real political issues that appear to be at stake in the decisions made about the control of different chemical substances.

These examples are provided to illustrate how societies have many values that they must equally consider alongside the pursuit of health outcomes. No matter what policy decision is made, there will inevitably be wider economic, social, and/or political implications. Inevitably, it is political choices that must be made about what multiple social values are deemed acceptable in pursuit of health. Medical ethics provides perhaps the most obvious example of this, whereby we have agreed not to sacrifice the rights of individuals in the name of a health-determined outcome (Gillon 1994). Ethical principles such as autonomy, beneficence (do good), and non-malfeasance (do no harm) explain, for example, why we as a global society typically tend to avoid forcibly quarantining individuals, or mandatory screening/testing programs for many conditions (despite potential medical efficacy). Other normative systems that are outside the basic remit of medical ethics are also commonly included in global health policy decisions, which may equally consider factors such as inequality, fairness, and social sensitivity (Kass 2001, 2004; Clark and Weale 2012; Parkhurst 2012).

Of course, this does not exclude the importance of the valid and fair use of those pieces of health science evidence deemed appropriate within the policy process. Study findings should not be doctored. Significance, study quality, and internal and external validity should also be equally understood and considered when looking at pieces of evidence. But we, as a global society, must understand potential impacts on health gains, alongside the other potential economic and social impacts. Difficult choices and judgments must be made between different bodies of evidence (Klein 2003). "What matters" in global health policy-making is not simply anything that reduces morbidity and mortality, but rather "what is *agreed* to be the overall desirable goal" (Greenhalgh and Russell 2009: 310, emphasis added; see also Sanderson 2003). As the UK drugs example illustrated, the process by which such agreement is reached is also crucial. Evidence can clearly be used in valid or non-valid ways. Evidence use can further be transparent and explicit, or unstated and implicit. Rather than making oversimplified calls for evidence-based policy, we must instead call for appropriate processes to be followed that ensure the transparent and appropriate use of evidence in decision-making. We revisit this concept in our conclusion, but first point to some other difficulties that can arise when taking an uncritical view of health evidence.

Wider Implications of a Depoliticized Approach to Evidence

A final key point to raise about a depoliticized approach to the use of health research evidence in shaping global policy is that uncritical acceptance of this approach has wider political implications because it obscures the broader macro-structural issues that shape global health and global health policy decision-making. As already mentioned above, in contemporary discourse, experimental studies are typically seen as the gold standard to define the evidence base for global health policy. While this type of research provides useful insight into the effectiveness of clinical or biomedical interventions, these studies tend to have very little to say about social factors or health inequalities and inequities (Asthana and Halliday 2006; Raphael 2006), and, moreover, often have little to say about the way in which macro-structural factors, or global political and economic processes, can shape decision-making and/or the implementation of health interventions. When social factors are included in health sciences research, they tend to be conceptualized in an individualized way; as individually owned measures of socioeconomic status (like income or education), and not, for example, as a function of wider structured power differentials, global trade or economic regimes, capitalist ideology, or issues of race, gender, or class hierarchy (Navarro 2009). Indeed, terms like economic globalization, liberal capitalism, trade flows, and class analysis are virtually absent from typical health science lexicons or research methodologies.

Interestingly, this is despite the fact that evidence from other disciplinary fields (including politics, development studies, anthropology, and sociology) has repeatedly illustrated how unequal structures of wealth, dominance, and poverty (which are typically allied to capitalist visions of economic development) can shape global health problems and policy interventions (Coburn 2000; Kay and Williams 2009; also see Chapter 21). For example, Doyal (1979) shows how the spread of communicable diseases (such as measles and tuberculosis), and also issues of malnutrition in Africa, are (at least in part) a product of capitalist expansion. Other examples bound. Navarro (2009) gives insight into the ways in which dominant social classes and elite alliances (re)produce conditions that lead to the underdevelopment of health; with maldistribution of land between dominant business classes and peasant/tenant farmers in countries like Bangladesh a case in point (Navarro 2009). Campbell (2003) has illustrated that HIV risk in South African mining towns is deeply engrained in the system of economic migrant workers' living environments. Other business practices associated with global capitalism, such as labour casualization (the shifting of workers to more flexible and "precarious" forms of employment), have also been seen to threaten health (Benach *et al.* 2007; see also Chapter 14). While more research is needed on this topic (Benach *et al.* 2010), Fraser and Lungu's (2007) work in Zambia, for example, has found that casualization in privatized mines is resulting in economic insecurity amongst communities in the country's Copperbelt, which may be influencing health outcomes in diverse ways: from the inability to afford adequate housing and nutrition, to increasing mental stress and the inability to purchase drugs when family members are sick.

Not only do health science professionals tend to see these political and economic issues as complex, unrelated, or removed from their area of focus (MacDonald and Horton 2009), but because these factors tend to operate through a web of direct and indirect channels, they are difficult to track and measure accurately using established methodologies (Smith *et al.* 2009). In consequence, these types of issues risk being routinely whisked "out of sight" (cf. Ferguson 1990: xv) in much health sciences research (see Chapter 21).

While clinical and traditional epidemiological research certainly provides insight into the ways in which more technical and individualistic factors shape and can be altered to affect health outcomes, it does not adequately deal with the issues raised here. As a consequence, uncritical calls for more evidence-based global health policy, which implicitly reduce policy decisions to assessment of epidemiological evidence, can actually conceal these macro-structures that socially and politically determine poor health. This is significant because it risks the perpetuation (albeit perhaps unintentionally) of a global system structured towards supporting the accrual of wealth and the more powerful social classes. It will ultimately result in the maintenance, rather than the confrontation, of global injustice, and a "band-aid" approach to dealing with the health problems it engenders.

Conclusions: A Way Forward?

There are clearly many issues associated with the way in which contemporary global health policy frames evidence-based processes in a technical and depoliticized way. We have argued that there are a number of reasons why global health policy cannot and should not be perceived as being beyond politics. While politics clearly can be a pejorative influence on decision-making, value-based choices and political judgments are actually inherent to the production and use of evidence in global health policy, not only shaping decisions about what goals and outcomes should be prioritized, but also the way in which evidence is created and appraised. Statements calling broadly and uncritically for evidence-based policy tend not to acknowledge fully the complex political and ethical dimensions of policy-making, which actually require a range of evidence be combined in normative judgments about appropriate courses of action (Sanderson 2006; see also Parkhurst 2012). This must be acknowledged by academics, aid donors, government officials, and health program managers if we are to find legitimate and sustainable solutions to global health problems. We need to find ways in which such politics can be embraced and converted into a powerful and creative force for the good of global health, alongside a more comprehensive and effective use of research evidence.

Indeed, we do not mean that research evidence is unimportant in global health policy. Rather, and to the contrary, it is argued that we need to find ways to broaden the scope for the inclusion of the diversity of evidence which is of importance to global health policies, while at the same time more effectively managing the competing values and political considerations that are inherent to decision processes. Managing competing values in policy processes does not mean ignoring or excluding them. Rather, it is fundamentally a question of governance; that is to say, about the way the policy process is managed, coordinated, and steered so that citizens' needs are met by those who legitimately represent them. Policy-making is a process, and that process will be shaped by the rules and institutional arrangements that are in place globally, and which we argue should encourage open reflection and balanced debate about the types of evidence on which to base health decisions (Cookson 2005; Fischer 2009). This conceptualization shifts the focus from one of using evidence as the basis for policy, to a focus on how health evidence can best be governed to inform policy-making. We argue that good governance of evidence and policy can only be achieved by setting up a democratic and deliberative approach, which is inclusive, explicit, transparent, and accountable to the needs of the people these decisions affect.

How can we start to move closer towards the "good governance of health evidence" in global health policy? What steps can be taken by academics, policy-makers, and health practitioners who are involved in global health? At the most basic level what is needed is a cultural shift on the part of researchers and decision-makers towards more "clarity through specificity" (cf. Cohen and Uphoff 1980); the making visible of the multiple values and frames of reference that shape global health policy, and how and why evidence has been generated and applied, and also the provision of clear and transparent explanations as to why particular decisions have been made.

More specifically, for scientists and experts, it involves commitment to support a "mixed economy" of research evidence (Petticrew *et al.* 2004), one that acknowledges the fundamental importance of RCTs and systematic reviews, but which is open to the use of other methodologies, including quantitative and qualitative social science methods to gather evidence on important considerations that are not easily reducible to experimental cause and effect testing. These are needed to explore the socioeconomic and political drivers of poor health, as well as the way in which values, norms, and power infuse research and policy processes. Within this, it is important that scientists and experts are more aware of the political dimensions of global health policy, so that they can find ways to support open reflection and debate about their evidence. Here also, it is important for researchers not to just "render advice," but to analyze and interpret findings in ways that are helpful to policy-makers and, equally importantly, to the publics that they represent (Fischer 2009: 5).

For global health policy-makers (including government officials, aid advisors, health managers, and civil society organizations), it is not only important to enhance understanding of the research methodologies that produce evidence to inform decision-making, but also to commit to transparently and openly engage in debate about such evidence in everyday contexts of practice. This requires policy-makers to become reflexive practitioners, who routinely question, and are open about, their own roles, relationships, and values, and how they include, exclude, or perhaps do not "hear" different bodies of evidence and engage with it in deliberative debate (Cunliffe 2009: 45). Embracing more explicit analytical models of decision-making, which encourage policy-makers to list all the possible outcomes they value, and transparently assign value weights to those outcomes (Sandersen and Gruen 2006), provides another concrete suggestion to ensure improved and better governance of evidence in decision-making.

Importantly, to achieve and subsequently sustain changes in decision-making processes typically requires those changes to be reified through establishment or alteration of institutional processes and structures. Emphasis needs to be placed on establishing structures that facilitate the use of valid and unbiased evidence, while allowing critical debate and appraisal of the reasoning and choices decision-makers make when using evidence. This could take the form of political institutions, including formal and participatory evidence review bodies, or regulatory norms (such as rules of independence of advisors, freedom of information, and transparency of decision-making). Best practice guidelines can further help to institutionalize a more sophisticated use of evidence – for example, guidance from health expert bodies to the media that explain that high quality questioning of policy-makers does not just ask if a policy is evidence-based but rather questions on which evidence it was based, why, and what value was placed on different bodies of evidence. Research evidence will not itself guide policy, but establishing good governance structures can help to ensure that evidence is used validly and transparently, and legitimately represents public values and interests. Establishing effective institutions may also increase the use of evidence by ensuring appropriate evidentiary reviews are conducted to inform policy debates. Overall, what is most important here is that we govern global health policy in a way that allows engagement with the fundamentally political nature of decision-making, while at the same time ensuring that there is space for the valid and reasonable application of different bodies of knowledge.

Key Reading

Lin V, Gibson B (eds). 2003. *Evidence-Based Health Policy*. Oxford: Oxford University Press.
Littlejohns P, Weale A, Chalkidou K, Teerwattananon Y, Faden R (eds). 2012. Special Issue: Social values and healthcare priority setting. *Journal of Health Organization and Management* 26(3) (see the paper by Clark S, Weale A. Social values in health priority setting: a conceptual framework, pp. 293–316.)
Stone D. 2002. *Policy Paradox: The Art of Political Decision-Making*. London: W.W. Norton and Company.
Worrall J. 2007. Evidence in medicine and evidence-based medicine. *Philosophy Compass* 2, 981–1022.

References

Asthana S, Halliday J. 2006. Developing an evidence base for policies and interventions to address health inequalities: the analysis of "public health regimes". *Milbank Quarterly* 84(3), 577–603.
Auerbach JD, Parkhurst JO, Cáceres CF. 2011. Addressing social drivers of HIV/AIDS for the long-term response: conceptual and methodological considerations. *Global Public Health* 6(Suppl 3), S293–30.
Barnes A, Brown GW. 2011. The Global Fund to Fight AIDS, Tuberculosis and Malaria: Expertise, Accountability and the Depoliticisation of Global Health Governance. In Williams O, Rushton S (eds) *Partnerships and Foundations in Global Health Governance*, pp. 53–75. Basingstoke: Palgrave Macmillan.
Barnett T, Parkhurst JO. 2005. HIV/AIDS: sex, abstinence, and behaviour change. *Lancet Infectious Diseases* 5, 590–3.
BBC. 2009. *Ecstasy 'not worse than riding'*. February 7, 2009. http://news.bbc.co.uk/1/hi/uk/7876425.stm (last accessed December 2013).
Benach J, Muntaner C, Santana V. 2007. *Employment Conditions and Health Inequalities. Final Report to the WHO Commission on Social Determinants of Health (CSDH)*. Employment Conditions Knowledge Network (EMCONET). http://www.who.int/social_determinants/resources/articles/emconet_who_report.pdf (last accessed December 2013).
Benach J, Muntaner C, Chung H *et al.* 2010. The importance of government policies in reducing employment related health inequalities. *BMJ* 340, c2154.
Black N. 1996. Why we need observational studies to evaluate the effectiveness of health care. *BMJ* 312, 1215–8.

Brecht A. 1968. *Political Theory: The Foundations of Twentieth-Century Political Thought*. Princeton, NJ: Princeton University Press.

Brown GW, Labonté R. 2011. Globalization and its methodological discontents: contextualizing globalization through the study of HIV/AIDS. *Globalization and Health* 7, 1–25.

Brown T, Cueto M, Fee E. 2006. The World Health Organization and the transition from international to global public health. *American Journal of Public Health* 96(1), 62–72.

Buekens P, Keusch G, Belizan J, Bhutta ZA. 2004. Evidence-based global health. *Journal of the American Medical Association* 291(21), 2639–41.

Campbell C. 2003. *"Letting Them Die": Why HIV/AIDS Prevention Programmes Fail*. Oxford: James Currey.

Carballo M, Kenya PI. 1994. Behavioral issues and AIDS. In Essex M, Mboup S, Kanki PJ, Kalengayi MR (eds) *AIDS in Africa*, pp. 497–512. New York: Raven Press.

Cartwright N. 2007. Are RCTs the gold standard? *Biosocieties* 2, 11–20.

Cartwright N. 2011. A philosopher's view of the long road from RCTs to effectiveness. *Lancet* 377, 1400–1.

Clark S, Weale A. 2012. Social values in health priority setting: a conceptual framework. *Journal of Health Organisation and Management* 26(3), 293–316.

Clarke J. 2004. Dissolving the public realm? The logics and limits of neo-liberalism. *Journal of Social Policy* 33(1), 27–48.

Coburn D. 2000. Income inequality, social cohesion and the health status of populations: the role of neo-liberalism. *Social Science and Medicine* 51(1), 35–46.

Cohen JM, Uphoff N. 1980. Participation's place in rural development: seeking clarity through specificity. *World Development* 8(3), 213–35.

Commission on the Social Determinants of Health (CSDH). 2008. *Closing the Gap in a Generation: Health Equity through Action on the Social Determinants of Health*. Geneva: World Health Organization. http://whqlibdoc.who.int/publications/2008/9789241563703_eng.pdf (last accessed December 2013).

Cookson R. 2005. Evidence-based policy making in health care: what it is and what it isn't. *Journal of Health Services Research and Policy* 10(2), 118–21.

Crane B, Dusenberry J. 2004. Power and politics in international funding for reproductive health: the US global gag rule. *Reproductive Health Matters* 2(24), 128–37.

Cunliffe AL. 2009. *A Very Short, Fairly Interesting and Reasonably Cheap Book about Management*. London: Sage Publications.

Doyal L. 1979. *The Political Economy of Health*. London: Pluto Press.

England R. 2007. Are we spending too much on HIV? *BMJ* 334, 344.

Ferguson J. 1990. *The Anti-Politics Machine*. Minneapolis, MN: University of Minnesota Press.

Fischer F. 2009. *Democracy and Expertise: Reorienting Policy Inquiry*. Oxford: Oxford University Press.

Fisher JD, Fisher WA. 1992. Changing AIDS risk behavior. *Psychological Bulletin* 111(3), 455–74.

Fraser A, Lungu J. 2007. *For Whom the Windfalls? Winners and Losers in the Privatisation of Zambia's Copper Mines*. Civil Society Trade Network of Zambia/Catholic Centre for Justice, Development and Peace.

Garner P, Kale R, Dickson R, Dans T, Salinas R. 1998. Getting research findings into practice: implementing research findings in developing countries. *BMJ* 317, 531–5.

Gibson B. 2003. Framing and taming "wicked" problems. In Lin V, Gibson B (eds) *Evidence-Based Health Policy: Problems and Possibilities*, pp. 298–310. Oxford: Oxford University Press.

Gillon R. 1994. Medical ethics: four principles plus attention to scope. *BMJ* 309, 184.

Greenhalgh T, Russell J. 2009. Evidence-based policymaking: a critique. *Perspectives in Biology and Medicine* 52(2), 304–18.

Guardian. 2009. Drugs policy: shooting up the messenger. *Guardian* October 31, 2009. http://www.guardian.co.uk/commentisfree/2009/oct/31/david-nutt-sacking-alan-johnson?INTCMP=ILCNE TTXT3487 (last accessed December 2013).

Hill M. 2009. *The Public Policy Process*. London: Longman.

Kass N. 2001. An ethics framework for public health. *American Journal of Public Health* 91(11), 1776–82.

Kass N. 2004. Public health ethics from foundations and frameworks to justice and global public health. *Journal of Law, Medicine and Ethics* 32, 232–42.

Kay A, Williams O. 2009. Introduction: The international political economy of global health governance. In Kay A, Williams O (eds) *Global Health Governance: Crisis, Institutions and Political Economy*, pp. 1–24. Basingstoke: Palgrave Macmillan.

Kemm J. 2006. The limitations of "evidence-based" public health. *Journal of Evaluation in Clinical Practice* 12(3), 319–32.

Klein R. 2003. Evidence and policy: interpreting the Delphic oracle. *Journal of the Royal Society of Medicine* 96, 429–31.

Lavis J, Posada FB, Haines A, Osei E. 2004. Use of research to inform public policymaking. *Lancet* 364(9445), 1615–21.

Lawrence M. 2003. Folate fortification: public health policy making in a food regulation setting. In Lin V, Gibson B (eds) *Evidence-based Health Policy: Problems and Possibilities*, pp. 110–26. Oxford: Oxford University Press.

Lawrence M. 2005. Challenges in translating scientific evidence into mandatory food fortification policy: an antipodean case study of the folate–neural tube defect relationship. *Public Health Nutrition* 8(8), 1235–41.

MacDonald R, Horton R. 2009. Trade and health: time for the health sector to get involved. *Lancet* 373(9660), 273–4.

Marmot M. 2007. Achieving health equity: from root causes to fair outcomes. *Lancet* 370(9593), 1153–63.

Mayhew SH. 2002. Donor dealings: the impact of international donor aid on sexual and reproductive health services. *International Family Planning Perspectives* 28(4), 220–4.

Mills A, Gilson L, Hanson K, Palmer N, Lagarde M. 2008. What do we mean by rigorous health-systems research? *Lancet* 372(9649), 1527–9.

Monaghan M. 2011. *Evidence Versus Politics: Exploiting Research in UK Drug Policy Making?* Bristol: Policy Press.

Navarro V. 2009. What we mean by social determinants of health. *International Journal of Health Services* 39(3), 423–41.

Nutt D, King LA, Saulsbury W, Blakemore C. 2007. Development of a rational scale to assess the harm of drugs of potential misuse. *Lancet* 369, 1047–53.

Padian NS, McCoy SI, Balkus JE, Wasserheit JN. 2010. Weighing the gold in the gold standard: challenges in HIV prevention research. *AIDS* 24, 621–35.

Parkhurst JO. 2008. "What worked?" the evidence challenges in determining the causes of HIV prevalence decline. *AIDS Education and Prevention* 20(3), 275–83.

Parkhurst JO. 2012. HIV prevention, structural change, and social values: the need for an explicit normative approach. *Journal of the International AIDS Society* 15(Suppl 1), 1–10.

Parkhurst JO, Weller I, Kemp J. 2010. Getting research into policy, or out of practice, in HIV? *Lancet* 375(9724), 1414–5.

Patel V, Boyce N, Collins PY, Saxena S, Horton R. 2011. A renewed agenda for global mental health. *Lancet* 378, 1441–2.

Pawson R, Tilley N. 1997. *Realistic Evaluation*. London: Sage.

Paxton A, Maine D, Freedman L, Fry D, Lobis S. 2005. The evidence for emergency obstetric care. *International Journal of Gynaecology and Obstetrics* 88, 181–93.

Petticrew M, Whitehead M, Macintyre SJ, Graham H, Egan M. 2004. Evidence based public health policy and practice: evidence for public health policy on inequalities. 1: The reality according to policymakers. *Journal of Epidemiology and Community Health* 58(10), 811–6.

Raphael D. 2006. Social determinants of health: present status, unanswered questions and future directions. *International Journal of Health Services* 36(4), 651–77.

Rawls J. 1993. *Political Liberalism*. New York: Columbia University Press.

Russell J, Greenhalgh T, Byrne E, McDonnell J. 2008. Recognising rhetoric in health care policy analysis. *Journal of Health Services Research and Policy* 13(1), 40–6.

Rychetnik L, Frommer M, Hawe P, Shiell A. 2002. Criteria for evaluating evidence on public health interventions. *Journal of Epidemiolgy Community and Health* 56(2), 119–27.

Sackett DL, Rosenberg WMC, Muir JA *et al.* 1996. Evidence based medicine: what it is and what it isn't. *BMJ* 312, 71–2.

Sanderson C, Gruen R. 2006. *Analytical Models for Decision Making*. Maidenhead: Open University Press.

Sanderson I. 2003. Is it "what works" that matters? Evaluation and evidence-based policy-making. *Research Papers in Education* 18(4), 331–45.

Sanderson I. 2006. Complexity, "practical rationality" and evidence-based policy making. *Policy and Politics* 34(1), 115–32.

Sanson-Fisher RW, Bonevski B, Green LW, D'Este C. 2007. Limitations of the randomized controlled trial in evaluating population-based health interventions. *American Journal of Preventive Medicine* 33(2), 155–61.

Schön DA, Rein M. 1994. *Frame Reflection: Toward the Resolution of Intractable Policy Controversies*. New York: Basic Books.

Schwartz S, Carpenter K. 1999. The right answer for the wrong question: consequences of type III error for public health research. *American Journal of Public Health* 89(8), 1175–180.

Shiffman J. 2006. Donor funding priorities for communicable disease control in the developing world. *Health Policy and Planning* 21, 411–20.

Shiffman J. 2007. Generating political priority for maternal mortality reduction in 5 developing countries. *American Journal of Public Health* 97, 796–803.

Siddiqi J. 1995. *World Health and World Politics: The World Health Organization and the UN System*. South Carolina: University of South Carolina Press.

Smith GCS, Pell JP. 2003. Parachute use to prevent death and major trauma related to gravitational challenge: systematic review of randomised controlled trials. *BMJ* 327, 1459–61.

Smith RD, Lee K, Drager N. 2009. Trade and health: an agenda for action. *Lancet* 373, 768–73.

Stone D. 2002. *Policy Paradox: The Art of Political Decision-Making*. London: W.W. Norton and Company.

SUPPORT. 2011. *SUPPORT – Supporting policy relevant trial and reviews*. http://www.support-collaboration.org/index.htm (last accessed December 2013).

Tesh SN. 1988. *Hidden Arguments: Political Ideology and Disease Prevention Policy*. New Brunswick, NJ: Rutgers University Press.

van Kammen J, de Savigny D, Sewankambo N. 2006. Using knowledge brokering to promote evidence-based policy-making: the need for support structures. *Bulletin of the World Health Organization* 84, 608–12.

Victora CG, Habicht JP, Bryce J. 2004. Evidence-based public health: moving beyond randomized trials. *American Journal of Public Health* 94(3), 400–5.

Walt G. 1993. WHO under stress: implications for health policy. *Health Policy* 24, 125–44.

Walt G. 1994. *Health Policy: An Introduction to Process and Power*. London: Zed Books.

Worrall J. 2007. Evidence in medicine and evidence-based medicine. *Philosophy Compass* 2, 981–1022.

Yamey G, Feachem R. 2011. Evidence-based policymaking in global health: the payoffs and pitfalls. *Evidence Based Medicine* 16(4), 97–9.

Young IM. 2000. *Inclusion and Democracy*. Oxford: Oxford University Press.

Part III   The Politics of Risk, Disease, and Neglect

Chapter 9

Dietary Policies to Reduce Non-Communicable Diseases

Ashkan Afshin, Renata Micha, Shahab Khatibzadeh, Laura A. Schmidt, and Dariush Mozaffarian

Abstract

Of the 53 million deaths worldwide in 2010, two thirds (35 million) were due to non-communicable diseases (NCDs). This global burden could be reduced through concerted policies that address modifiable NCD risk factors, such as smoking, insufficient physical activity, excessive alcohol consumption, and poor dietary habits. Approaches that target individuals (e.g., physician-provided counseling) have only a modest effect on behavior, whereas population-based strategies (e.g., regulation, economic incentives) can have broad and sustained impact. This chapter focuses on one specific risk factor, poor quality diet, as a major cause of NCD morbidity and mortality. Key dietary priorities for reducing the burden of NCDs include increasing consumption of fruits, vegetables, whole grains, nuts, and seafood, and reducing consumption of refined carbohydrates and starches, processed meat, industrial trans-fats, and sodium. Population-based approaches to improving diet that have a strong evidence base include multimodal media and education campaigns aimed at a specific food; food labeling as a way to influence industry behavior; economic incentives (e.g., subsidizing healthier foods and taxing less healthy foods); changes of local food environments; comprehensive school- and work-based interventions; restriction on advertising and marketing to children; and direct regulation (e.g., elimination of trans-fat).

Successful, sustainable implementation of these population-based interventions requires close collaboration among stakeholders occupying many different domains, including research, advocacy, policy development, policy implementation, capacity building, and monitoring and evaluation. Stakeholders must be engaged from a range of venues, including universities and research centers, advocacy groups, community-based organizations, schools and workplaces, agriculture and food industry, local and national governments, and international organizations. Governments and global economic and political institutions (particularly the World Health Organization, World Trade Organization, and World Bank) must take the lead to support, implement, and evaluate evidence-based population strategies to improve population dietary patterns.

The Handbook of Global Health Policy, First Edition. Edited by Garrett W. Brown, Gavin Yamey, and Sarah Wamala.
© 2014 John Wiley & Sons, Ltd. Published 2014 by John Wiley & Sons, Ltd.

Key Points

- Non-communicable diseases (NCDs) are now the dominant cause of death and disability worldwide, and a global action plan is needed to reduce this burden.
- Poor dietary quality is a key modifiable risk factor for NCDs, and improving global dietary quality is among the chief policy priorities of the twenty-first century
- The roots of poor dietary quality lie in suboptimal types and quality of foods consumed, including healthful foods missing from the diet.
- An array of factors influence food choices – these factors act at multiple levels: individual (e.g., nutritional knowledge), sociocultural (e.g., cultural norms), community (e.g., workplace food environment), agricultural industry (e.g., food marketing), government (e.g., food policies), and global (e.g. international trade agreements).
- The available evidence makes several specific dietary targets, and the effective population-based policies to address them, quite clear; it is now time for this evidence to be implemented in practice.

Key Policy Implications

- Given the roles of social and environmental factors in shaping dietary habits, population-based approaches should be a crucial component of efforts to improve diet; there is now a sound evidence base for several of these approaches.
- Effective strategies can be designed and implemented at the local level (e.g., schools, workplaces, community), as well as regionally, at the state level, and at national and supranational levels.
- An array of approaches are effective; including media and education campaigns, food labeling, economic incentives, changes of local food environment, comprehensive school- and work-based interventions, restriction on advertising and marketing, and direct regulation, providing flexibility to policy-makers and also allowing for synergistic multicomponent campaigns.
- Dietary policies for the twenty-first century aimed at reducing NCDs must engage stakeholders from a range of venues, including universities and research centers, advocacy groups, community-based organizations, schools and workplaces, agriculture and food industry, local and national governments, and international organizations.

Introduction

Non-communicable diseases (NCDs), the leading cause of mortality worldwide, principally include cardiovascular disease (CVD), cancers, diabetes, and chronic respiratory diseases. The Global Burden of Disease study found that in 2010, NCDs accounted for two thirds of all deaths worldwide, that is 34.5 million out of the 52.8 million (Lozano *et al.* 2013). The World Economic Forum and Harvard School of Public Health estimate that the overall economic burden associated with NCDs could reach US\$47 trillion by 2030 (Bloom *et al.* 2011).

In recent years, many national and international organizations have highlighted the critical need to reduce the health and economic burdens of NCDs (Bloom *et al.* 2011; UN 2011; WHO 2011). In September 2011, the United Nations (UN) General Assembly held a high-level meeting to address the need for global strategies to prevent and control NCDs worldwide (UN 2011). This was the second General Assembly meeting in the history of the UN to discuss a health issue, with the first, in 2001, on HIV. The 2011 UN meeting concluded with the adoption of a declaration laying out the burden of NCDs and calling for evidence-based interventions to reduce this burden. Unfortunately, the declaration stopped short of requiring data collection to track outcomes, specifying interventions that countries must adopt, or allocating funds toward prevention or treatment. Despite these limitations, a key achievement was increased awareness among policymakers of the global burden of NCDs – a critical first step towards addressing NCDs on a global scale.

The main modifiable lifestyle risk factors for NCDs include poor dietary habits, insufficient physical activity, excessive alcohol consumption, and tobacco use (WHO 2011). These "lifestyle risks" in turn can lead to obesity, high blood pressure, dyslipidemia (abnormalities of lipids in the blood), and high plasma glucose (Danaei *et al.* 2011a, 2011b). The term "metabolic syndrome," a precursor to NCDs, refers to clusters of such risk factors (Grundy *et al.* 2004). Over the past two decades (Lim *et al.* 2013; US Burden of Disease Collaborators 2013; Yang *et al.* 2013) scientists have quantified and monitored the national and global distributions of risk factors for NCDs. In 2010, lifestyle and metabolic risk factors accounted for 37% of global disease burden (measured in disability-adjusted life-years lost, or DALYs) (Lim *et al.* 2013). Suboptimal diet and insufficient physical activity alone were estimated to account for 10% of total DALYs (Lim *et al.* 2013).

With respect to virtually all of these risk factors, individual-based approaches such as physician-provided counseling have only modest impact on improving health behaviors and are often the most costly approaches (Artinian *et al.* 2010). Meanwhile, population-based interventions, such as regulatory strategies and altering economic incentives, can have broad and sustained impact (Mozaffarian *et al.* 2012). The World Health Organization (WHO) Global Strategy to Improve Diet and Physical Activity recommended that Member States actively engage all sectors to develop and implement such strategies at global, regional, national, and community levels (WHO 2004).

While a broad range of policies can improve lifestyle risk factors (Mozaffarian *et al.* 2012), a comprehensive review of all of these lifestyle risks for NCDs and their evidence-based interventions is beyond the scope of a single chapter. Here, we focus on diet as a key underlying cause of NCDs. We summarize the barriers to improving diet and review the evidence for effectiveness of a range of strategies to overcome these barriers. We also discuss the actions that should be taken in this field, the key actors and their roles, and several major gaps for future research. Although the focus of this chapter is on diet, many of the issues discussed here can be generalized to other lifestyle risk factors (Engelhard *et al.* 2009). Many of the individual studies and the meta-analyses providing evidence for this chapter have been previously summarized in detail in an American Heart Association Scientific Statement (Mozaffarian *et al.* 2012). Readers can find the individual citations, including detailed supplementary tables on their findings, in that report.

The Policy Problem

Policy approaches to reduce the global disease burden caused by suboptimal diet require an understanding of both the most relevant dietary priorities and the evidence-based interventions to change them. Global nutritional research has traditionally focused on caloric and selected nutrient deficiencies, broadly termed "undernutrition." However, poor dietary *quality* is a major cause of NCD mortality and morbidity (Mozaffarian and Capewell 2011; Lim *et al.* 2013). The term "overnutrition" (i.e., excess dietary quantity) is often used to describe such poor dietary quality. But "overnutrition" is a misnomer, because it obscures the roots of poor dietary quality that lay in suboptimal types and quality of foods consumed, including healthful foods missing from the diet (Lim *et al.* 2013; Mozaffarian 2008). Poor dietary quality, or true "mal"-nutrition, includes insufficient consumption of fruits, vegetables, nuts, whole grains, and seafood as well as excess consumption of refined grains, starches, sugars, processed meats, sodium, and trans-fats (Table 9.1). Individually, and in combination, the dietary risk factors shown in Table 9.1 substantially increase the risk for CVD, diabetes, obesity, and specific cancers (Lim *et al.* 2013; Mozaffarian *et al.* 2011b). Evidence on the key dietary priorities for reducing the risk of CVD, such as increasing the consumption of fruits, vegetables, and whole grains, are summarized in Table 9.2.

Determinants of Food Choices and Dietary Behaviors

As is illustrated by Figure 9.1, the influences on food choices are complex. At the individual level, taste preferences, personal and familial norms, education and income, nutritional and cooking knowledge and skills, and health status are all important determinants (Brug 2008). Related psychological factors also influence individuals' dietary behaviors: eating behaviors, attitudes toward food and health, incentives, motivation, and values (van't Riet *et al.* 2011). Additional lifestyle habits, such as sedentary behaviors (e.g., time spent watching television or looking at a computer, known as "screen time"; Hardy *et al.* 2010) and sleep duration, also influence patterns of food consumption (Robinson 1999, 2001; Patel and Hu 2008; Mozaffarian *et al.* 2011b)

Environmental influences affect food intake and choices, including accessibility (e.g., food availability, cost, and convenience), industry advertising and marketing, and the local (residential, school, workplace) food environment. Sociocultural determinants include cultural norms, social pressures to eat in normative ways, social class, social networks, and race/ethnicity (Brug *et al.* 2008). Each of these individual, environmental, and sociocultural determinants is shaped by, and in turn shapes, broader drivers of food choice: agricultural policy and production practices, food industry behaviors, and other market forces (Nugent 2011). Institutional, community, and governmental programs and policies further influence, and are influenced by, each of these factors.

Table 9.1 Dietary risk factors for non-communicable disesaes and their optimal consumption level.

	Optimal* consumption	Cardiometabolic outcomes	Cancer outcomes
Dietary risk factors			
Low intake of fruits	300 g/day	CHD, stroke	Mouth, pharynx, larynx, esophagus, lung
Low intake of vegetables	300 g/day	CHD, stroke	Mouth, pharynx, larynx
Low intake of whole grains[†]	2.5 (50 g) servings/day	CHD, diabetes	
Low intake of nuts	4 (1 oz) servings/week	CHD	
Low intake of milk	2 (8 oz) servings/day	Diabetes	Colorectal
High intake of unprocessed meat	1 (100 g) serving/week	Diabetes	Colorectal
High intake of processed meats	0	CHD, diabetes	Colorectal
High intake of starches, refined carbohydrates, and sugars	As low as possible[‡]	CHD, high BMI, diabetes	
High intake of SSBs	0	High BMI, diabetes	
Nutrients			
Low intake of PUFA replacing SFA	12%E	CHD	Colorectal
Low intake of seafood omega-3 fat	250 mg/day	CHD, stroke	
Low intake of dietary fiber	30 g/day	CHD	Colorectal
Low intake of dietary calcium	1200 mg/day		Colorectal, prostate
High intake of trans fatty acids	0.5%E	CHD	
High intake of dietary sodium	1000 mg/day	High blood pressure, stroke	Stomach

BMI, body mass index; CHD, coronary heart disease; PUFA, polyunsaturated fatty acids; SFA, saturated fatty acids; SSBs, sugar sweetened beverages.
*This represents the feasible level of intake associated with the lowest risk of disease. Higher (for protective foods) or lower (for harmful foods) levels of intake might be better but might not be feasible.
[†]In place of starches, refined carbohydrates, and sugars which should be reduced as much as possible.
[‡]Zero intake is likely not feasible. But many studies show that intake should be as low as possible. Feasible minimum intake needs to be determined in future research.
Source: adapted from Micha *et al.* (2012: 123), © 2011 Nature Publishing Group.

The Policy Solution

Given the key roles of social and environmental factors in shaping dietary habits, population-based approaches should be a crucial component of efforts to improve diet. Effective strategies can be designed and implemented at the local level (e.g., schools, workplaces, community), as well as regionally, at the state level, and at national and

Table 9.2   Selected dietary priorities to reduce cardiovascular mortality globally.*

Target changes and benefits	Reduction in RR of CVD mortality (%)	Estimated fewer global CVD deaths (range) in millions per year[†]
Reasonable target change		
Increase fruits by 1 serving/day	~8	1.6 (0.8–2.0)
Increase vegetables by 1 serving/day	~7	1.4 (0.7–1.8)
Increase whole grains by 1 serving/day[‡]	~10	2.0 (1.0–2.5)
Increase nuts by 2 servings/week	~11	2.2 (1.1–2.8)
Increase vegetable oils by 1.5 servings/day	~5	1.0 (0.5–1.3)
Increase seafood omega-3 fatty acids by 50 mg/day	~5	1.0 (0.5–1.3)
Reduce sodium by 0.8 g/day	~6	1.2 (0.6–1.5)
Reduce industrial trans-fats by 1% energy	~7	1.4 (0.7–1.8)

CVD, cardiovascular disease; RR, relative risk.
*This is a partial list of some key dietary priorities with strongest evidence. Examples of other priorities include reducing the intake of starches, refined carbohydrates, and sugars, in particular sugar sweetened beverages and reducing the consumption of processed meat.
[†]Range is based on the sensitivity assumptions of 50% less effectiveness and 25% more effectiveness.
[‡]In place of starches, refined carbohydrates, and sugars.
Source: adapted from Mozaffarian and Capewell (2011), © 2011 BMJ Publishing Group Ltd.

supranational levels. Several specific approaches have the strongest evidence base for effectiveness (Table 9.3). These include approaches that cut across several domains: media/education, labeling/consumer information, economic incentives, school/workplace approaches, local environment changes, and regulatory restrictions. Full details of the evidence, including individual studies, reviews, and meta-analyses, are described elsewhere (Mozaffarian *et al.* 2012).

1. *Media and education campaigns.* These can effectively improve diet when they are sustained, focused on specific foods, and multimodal (e.g., television, radio, print, mailing). Broader campaigns aimed at multiple dietary targets as well as other health-related behaviors simultaneously, or campaigns that use single modes of communication, have been shown to be less effective. Focused campaigns appear effective when continued, but have not yet shown sustained behavior changes after campaigns end. Evidence for the effectiveness of long-term campaigns (those lasting over three years) mainly comes from multicomponent interventions, leaving their independent effects difficult to quantify (Kelder *et al.* 1995; Sanigorski *et al.* 2008; de Silva-Sanigorski *et al.* 2010).

2. *Product or menu labeling.* Providing dietary information alone, through product or menu nutrition labeling, appears relatively ineffective for changing consumer behavior. In one experimental study in the United Kingdom, Sacks and colleagues tested the impact of front-of-pack "traffic light" labels, which used different colors to denote levels of saturated fat, sugar, and salt, on consumer food purchases (Sacks *et al.* 2009). The labeling had no effect on supermarket sales of the labeled products (Sacks *et al.* 2009). Similarly, mandatory menu calorie labeling on foods and beverages in New York City fast-food restaurants was not associated with lower calorie consumption in these restaurants, compared with either consumption prior to the introduction of labeling or with consumption in adjacent cities that had not introduced labeling (Elbel *et al.* 2009).

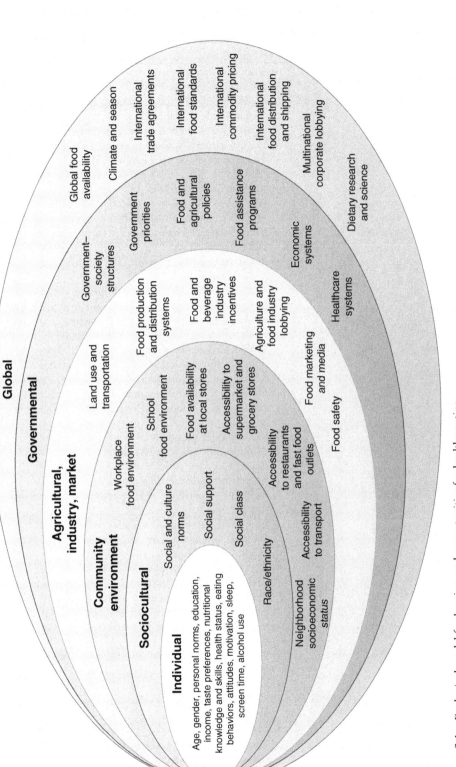

Figure 9.1 Ecological model for barriers and opportunities for healthy eating.

Table 9.3   Evidence-based population approaches to improve diet.[*]

Domain	Approaches
Media and education	• Sustained, focused media and education campaigns, utilizing multiple modes, for increasing consumption of specific healthful foods or reducing consumption of specific less healthful foods or beverages, either alone (IIa B) or as part of multicomponent strategies (I B)[†‡§] • On-site supermarket and grocery store educational programs to support the purchase of healthier foods (IIa B)[†]
Labeling and information	• Mandated nutrition facts panels or front-of-pack labels/icons as a means to influence industry behavior and product formulations (IIa B)[†**]
Economic incentives	• Subsidy strategies to lower prices of more healthful foods and beverages (I A)[†] • Tax strategies to increase prices of less healthful foods and beverages (IIa B)[†] • Changes in both agricultural subsidies as well as other related policies to create infrastructure that facilitates production, transportation, and marketing of healthier foods, sustained over several decades (IIa B)[†]
Schools	• Multicomponent interventions focused on improving both diet and physical activity, including specialized educational curricula, trained teachers, supportive school policies, a formal PE program, serving of healthier food and beverage options, and a parental/family component (I A)[†] • School garden programs including nutrition and gardening education and hands-on gardening experiences (IIa A)[†] • Fresh fruits and vegetables programs that provide free fruits and vegetables to students during the school day (IIa A)[†]
Workplaces	• Comprehensive worksite wellness programs with nutrition, physical activity, and tobacco cessation/prevention components (IIa A)[†] • Increased availability of healthier food/beverage options and/or strong nutrition standards for foods and beverages served, in combination with vending machine prompts, labels, or icons to select healthier choices (IIa B)[†]
Local environment	• Increased availability of supermarkets near homes (IIa B)[†¶]
Restrictions and mandates	• Restrictions on television advertisements for less healthful foods or beverages advertised to children (I B)[†] • Restrictions on advertising and marketing of less healthful foods or beverages near schools and public places frequented by youths (IIa B)[†] • General nutrition standards for foods and beverages marketed and advertised to children in any fashion, including on-package promotion (IIa B)[†] • Regulatory policies to reduce specific nutrients in foods (e.g., trans-fats, salt, certain fats) (I B)[†§]

Table 9.3   (*Continued*)

Agricultural	• Fiscal, trade, and regulatory instruments where feasible and proven effective to improve production, storage, and distribution of healthful foods (e.g., fruits, vegetables) • Developing mutual metrics that can be used to measure and evaluate the contributions of each relevant sector to improving diet

*The specific population interventions, listed here, are those that achieved either a class I or IIa recommendation together with an evidence grade of either A or B. The American Heart Association (AHA) evidence grading system is: *Class I*: evidence for and/or general agreement that the intervention is beneficial, useful, and effective; the intervention should be performed. *Class II*: conflicting evidence and/or a divergence of opinion about the usefulness/efficacy of the intervention. *Class IIa*: weight of evidence/opinion is in favor of usefulness/efficacy; it is reasonable to perform the intervention. *Class IIb*: usefulness/efficacy is less well established by evidence/opinion; the intervention may be considered. *Class III*: there is evidence and/or general agreement that the intervention is not useful/effective and in some cases may be harmful. The weight of evidence in support of the recommendation is classified as follows: *Level of evidence A*: data derived from multiple randomized clinical trials or, given the nature of population interventions, from well-designed quasi-experimental studies combined with supportive evidence from several other types of studies. *Level of evidence B*: data derived from a single randomized trial or non-randomized studies. *Level of evidence C*: only consensus opinion of experts, case studies, or standard-of-care. For brevity, we have not re-cited all of the 500+ individual studies reviewed in that AHA Scientific Statement. Readers can find the individual citations in that report.

†At least some evidence from studies conducted in high-income western regions and countries (e.g., North America, Europe, Australia, New Zealand).

‡At least some evidence from studies conducted in high-income non-western regions and countries (e.g., Japan, Hong Kong, South Korea, Singapore).

§At least some evidence from studies conducted in low- or middle-income regions and countries (e.g., Africa, China, Pakistan, India).

¶Based on cross-sectional studies only; only two longitudinal studies have been performed, with no significant relations seen.

**Such labeling strategies alone have limited effect if not complemented with environmental changes.

Source: adapted and revised from Mozaffarian *et al.* (2012), © 2012 American Heart Association, Inc.; Nugent (2011).

Yet some evidence suggests that front-of-pack icons and nutrient labels can influence industry behavior by encouraging more healthful products (Ratnayake *et al.* 2009; Vyth *et al.* 2010). While not necessarily changing consumer behavior, labeling may therefore still promote a more healthful food supply by altering industry behavior. Additional research is needed to confirm the types and extent of labeling influences on industry behavior.

3. *Economic policies*. Policies ranging from taxation to subsidization, price controls, and controls at the point of sales have been shown to be highly effective in altering diet (Mozaffarian *et al.* 2012). Both increases in prices of less healthful foods/beverages and decreases in prices of more healthful foods are effective. The magnitude of the dietary change correlates with the size of the price difference (Mozaffarian *et al.* 2012). Larger price changes, such as increases or decreases of 10–30%, appear most effective in changing consumer behavior (Powell *et al.* 2007; Andreyeva *et al.* 2009; Block *et al.* 2010; Duffey *et al.* 2010). Certain population subgroups, such as young people and those of lower socioeconomic status, are especially sensitive to economic incentives (Mozaffarian *et al.* 2012). In addition, taxation of less healthful foods can provide important revenue for use in prevention programs or for subsidizing the production of healthier foods.

4. *School- and work-based interventions*. Schools and workplaces are important venues for improving diet. Each weekday, up to two meals and several snacks are consumed at school or work. Based on randomized trials in schools, multicomponent interventions that simultaneously target both diet quality and physical activity are most effective (Mozaffarian *et al.* 2012). Successful programs typically involve educational curricula taught by trained teachers, supportive school policies, formal physical exercise programs, increased availability of healthier food and beverage options in school cafeterias and vending machines, and a parental or family component. School-based education alone, however, is ineffective. To work, education must be bundled with other policy components targeting the school, the food served, and the family. In a limited number of studies, other school-based strategies have increased fruit and vegetable consumption among children, including the use of school gardens for hands-on education and the provision of free fruits and vegetables during the school day. Such strategies have only been evaluated in high-income nations (Mozaffarian *et al.* 2012).

   Although often more costly, comprehensive worksite wellness programs may improve health behaviors, including diet, physical activity, smoking, and cardiometabolic risk factors. These interventions have greater impact if they target employees at higher risk, rather than all employees. The combination of worksite food labeling in cafeterias or vending machines with changes in the workplace food environment that alter the types and locations of foods and drinks served also effectively improves diet. This parallels the experience in schools where education and information alone, without environmental changes, has limited impact. (Mozaffarian *et al.* 2012).

5. *Changes in the local food environment*. In recent years, several studies that were mostly conducted in high-income western nations have observed associations between the community food environment and dietary habits or diet-related risk factors (Mozaffarian *et al.* 2012). These studies have found positive cross-sectional associations between neighborhood accessibility to supermarkets and consumption of more healthful foods, mainly fruits and vegetables, in both adults and children. Findings for grocery stores, convenience stores, and fast-food restaurants have been inconclusive. Nearly all studies of the community food environment have been cross-sectional, thereby greatly limiting the power to draw inferences about the causal nature of the associations. Overall, the hypotheses are compelling, but more prospective and quasi-experimental studies are needed to show that changes in the local food environment improve dietary behaviors.

6. *Regulatory strategies*. Strategies ranging from softer economic incentives to all-out bans have been repeatedly shown to improve diet at the population level. Restrictions on marketing and advertising to youth are effective strategies to reduce consumption of less healthy foods and beverages (Institute of Medicine 2009; Mozaffarian *et al.* 2012). Restricting the use of specific harmful nutrients, such as trans-fats or salt, also effectively reduces their consumption in the population. Following Denmark's lead, many regions and countries have regulated trans-fats in the food supply, either by banning or limiting amounts of trans-fats in fats and oils used for cooking or in the final food product.

7. *Agricultural policies*. Agriculture and food systems play major roles in population diets at local, national, and global levels (Nugent 2011). Evidence from US agricultural policy demonstrates that short-term economic strategies (e.g., subsidies) alone have a limited effect on food availability, price, or dietary habits at the population

level (Mozaffarian *et al.* 2012; Rickard *et al.* 2013). In contrast, sustained cross-sectoral efforts to create infrastructure that facilitates production, transportation, and marketing of healthier foods appear to have a greater long-term impact. Historically, global agricultural policies have often focused on increasing the availability of basic commodities – such as wheat, rice, corn, and soy – in efforts to augment available calories. Policies targeting the dietary concerns of the twenty-first century are likely to require a dramatic turnabout – one requiring more careful consideration of dietary quality rather than overall calories. Of course, agricultural policies are influenced by many considerations that go well beyond human health, including the need to economically protect farmers and food-producing industries. A range of agricultural development interventions can enhance capacity to produce healthier foods such as fruits, vegetables, vegetable oil crops, and nuts (Nugent 2011). Long-term policies should also focus on storage and transportation infrastructure to reduce postharvest losses of such foods.

In sum, many evidence-based population strategies can improve diet (Table 9.3). The literature provides clear guidance on the need to bundle policies to achieve greater effect, particularly by combining regulatory and educational strategies. Whichever interventions are used, the choice of the targeted dietary factors is also crucial. Interventions to reduce NCDs have historically focused on limited nutrient targets (e.g., total fat, saturated fat, dietary cholesterol). However, it is increasingly clear that a singular focus on these targets alone is unhelpful and, in some cases, could actually cause harm (Mozaffarian *et al.* 2011a). Any dietary policy may be prone to unintended consequences and those policies targeting specific dietary targets are especially vulnerable. For instance, policies that target sugars alone on the basis of their detriment to metabolic function could lead consumers to substitute other highly refined complex carbohydrates and starches that are equally harmful to health (Joint WHO/FAO Expert Consultation 2003). The key dietary targets with strongest evidence to reduce NCDs are summarized in Tables 9.1 and 9.2.

The Next Steps

Successful, sustainable implementation of population-based interventions requires close collaboration among stakeholders occupying many different domains, including research, advocacy, policy development, policy implementation, capacity building, and monitoring and evaluation (WHO 2004; Institute of Medicine 2010; Nugent 2011; Mozaffarian *et al.* 2012). Effective dietary policies for the twenty-first century must engage stakeholders from a range of venues, including universities and research centers, advocacy groups, community-based organizations, schools and workplaces, agriculture and food industry, local and national governments, and international organizations. While close collaboration of stakeholders in all steps of policy formulation, implementation, and evaluation is important, each group, based on its competencies and interest, should undertake specific actions (Table 9.4). Academic institutions should train investigators to conduct research on relevant dietary targets, on specific effective and cost-effective dietary policies, and on barriers to implementation. Advocacy groups should hold government and industry accountable on issues relating to diet and disseminate best practices to communities. Schools and workplace are also important settings for education, advocacy, and implementation of a range of diet-related policies.

Table 9.4 Policy recommendations for specific stakeholders to promote optimal dietary choices.

Stakeholder	Recommendations
Universities and research centers	• Train investigators to study diet-related chronic diseases • Conduct research on effectiveness and cost-effectiveness of policies • Advocate for research and policy on healthful diets • Investigate barriers to successful implementation of effective food policies • Evaluate impact and sustainability of implemented policies
Advocacy groups	• Advocate for policies to increase healthful diets and food supplies • Educate policy-makers about health risks and economic costs of poor-quality diets • Counter influence of industry lobbying and marketing • Establish and disseminate good practice in communities
Schools, workplaces, and community	• Educate students, teachers, parents, and employees on the components and benefits of a healthful diet • Create a supportive environment that increases the availability of healthful foods • Participate in local and national programs to promote healthy eating • Advocate for policy to increase healthful diets and food supplies
Agriculture	• Use trade and regulatory tools to improve production, storage, and distribution of healthful foods (e.g., fruits, vegetables) • Develop mutual metrics to measure the contributions of different sectors to improving diet • Advocate development of agricultural guidelines and policies to improve nutrition and health
Food industry (production, distribution, and retail)	• Develop and market products with greater health benefits and consistent with dietary guidelines, including corresponding education of consumers • Identify opportunities for mutually beneficial partnership with advocacy groups, governments, and agriculture to create commercial opportunities to shift sourcing from less to more healthy food ingredients • Fund research to characterize effects of diet and health and also monitor food supplies and composition • Adopt and develop technologies for creating more minimally processed foods • Support development of national and global policies and guidelines in agriculture and food sector that are designed to improve nutrition and health
Local government	• Implement fiscal policies and local ordinances to increase consumption of healthier foods and beverages and discourage consumption of less healthful foods and beverages • Ensure that publicly run entities such as after-school programs, recreation centers, and local government worksites implement comprehensive policies to promote healthier foods • Develop and advocate for nutritional guidelines related to health in federal, state, and local nutrition assistance programs • Promote media and social marketing campaigns on healthy eating • Increase community access to healthier foods through ordinances related to supermarkets, farmers' markets, and restaurants

Table 9.4   (*Continued*)

Stakeholder	Recommendations
National government	• Develop sustained agricultural priorities for farming, storage, and transport of healthier foods • Fund research on diets and health, on related policies, and on monitoring and evaluation • Institute surveillance of dietary habits, related risk factors and disease conditions, and related policies. • Promote participation of non-governmental organizations, civil society, communities, businesses, food industry, and the media in activities related to diet and health • Build incentives into healthcare and insurance to encourage patients, providers, and healthcare systems to promote healthier diets • Work to improve access to and availability of healthier foods • Regulate specific harmful additives (e.g., trans-fats, sodium) in foods • Restrict marketing of less healthful foods and beverages to children • Provide economic incentives to food industry and the consumer to select healthful foods and avoid less healthful foods • Align governmental policies across all sectors to support healthier diets and prevention of nutrition-related disease
International organizations	• Form cross-sectoral technical assistance teams to devise development plans, research translation, and policies for healthier diets in low- and middle-income countries • Prioritize research on connections between agriculture, dietary habits, and health and disease to better calibrate national-level policies • Set requirements and economic incentives for countries to promote healthier diets when making development loans • Align priorities across multiple sectors to emphasize healthier agriculture and foods • Use statutory powers to promote strategies that improve local, regional, and national food environments • Promote legal instruments and exemptions from trade restrictions that prevent nations from restricting distribution or marketing of globally produced less healthy food products

Source: adapted and revised from Nugent (2011: 54–8).

Agriculture and the food industry must also play key roles (Table 9.4). Agricultural policies including fiscal and regulatory tools should be used to increase production and improve storage and distribution of healthier foods. The food industry must use its technical expertise to formulate and market healthier products. Industry also has important roles to play in consumer education, product pricing, and marketing to promote dietary health. Agriculture and food industry should form mutually beneficial partnerships with advocacy groups and governments to replace less healthy foods with more healthful options.

Local and national governments must also prioritize healthier diets (Table 9.4). Based on development, economic, security, and health considerations, national governments should create a proactive environment to encourage and facilitate participation of other stakeholders in all steps of policy development, implantation, and evaluation. Government-led capacity building is crucial for the long-term sustainability of dietary policies, including in research, agriculture, and the food industry. For example, existing infrastructures and resources may be sufficient for certain policy interventions, but many others will require directed capacity building to ensure sustainability. An over-arching priority is to ensure sufficient agricultural capacity to supply healthier foods to the population, including facilities for storage, transportation, and distribution. Surveil-lance, monitoring, and evaluation of dietary habits and diet-related policies is crucial to design informed policies, determine whether implemented policies have the intended effects, evaluate heterogeneity among population subgroups, and assess unintended consequences.

Whereas national and subnational efforts are vital, global public health actions are also crucial to complement and strengthen the capacities of national and subnational gov-ernments. Organized global efforts are important in providing a countervailing political force with respect to highly organized, well-financed, multinational food industry lobby-ing. There is also a need to help policy-makers learn how to better navigate international trade laws and bilateral trade agreements that can make it difficult for governments to restrict access to less healthy food products. Key global economic and political institu-tions that must play more assertive roles in reducing the burden of NCDs include the World Health Organization, the World Trade Organization, and the World Bank. These organizations possess the technical expertise, statutory power, and access to key regional and national officials and should form technical assistance teams to formulate and imple-ment effective strategies in low- and middle-income countries. Development of the WHO Global Strategy on Diet, Physical Activity, and Health is an example of efforts undertaken by an international organization to improve diet globally (WHO 2004).

Conclusions

Poor dietary habits are a major cause of death and disability globally. Nearly every region in the world is undergoing an epidemiological transition in which diseases of undernutri-tion and infectious diseases are decreasing, while NCDs, driven to a great extent by poor diet quality, are escalating (Lim *et al.* 2013). These alarming trends produce tremendous burdens on both health and economic development (Institute of Medicine 2010) and improving global dietary quality is among the chief policy priorities of the twenty-first century.

Although there are still gaps in knowledge about certain dietary priorities or about the comparative effectiveness and cost-effectiveness of various dietary policies, advocacy and implementation of relevant policy strategies cannot await perfect evidence. The available evidence makes several specific dietary targets, and the effective policies to address them, quite clear. The relevant stakeholders must work together to formulate, implement, and evaluate policy measures to improve dietary quality. Governments and global economic and political institutions must take the lead and act by means of media and education campaigns, research and surveillance, agricultural policy, food pricing, and food and mar-keting regulation to improve population dietary patterns. This chapter has highlighted a specific set of evidence-based policy tools to improve diet. It is time for this evidence to be implemented in practice.

Key Reading

Ebrahim S, Pearce N, Smeeth L, Cases JP, Jaffar S, Piot P. 2013. Tackling non-communicable diseases in low- and middle-income countries: is the evidence from high-income countries all we needed? *PLOS Medicine* 10(1), e1001377.

Institute of Medicine (2010) *Promoting Cardiovascular Health in the Developing World: A Critical Challenge to Achieve Global Health*. Washington, DC: National Academies Press.

Mozaffarian D, Afshin A, Benowitz NL *et al.* (2012) Population approaches to improve diet, physical activity, and smoking habits: a Scientific Statement from the American Heart Association. *Circulation* 126(12), 1514–63.

Nugent R. 2011. *Bringing Agriculture to the Table: How Agriculture and Food Can Play a Role in Preventing Chronic Disease*. Chicago: Chicago Council on Global Affairs.

WHO (World Health Organization). 2004. *Global Strategy on Diet, Physical Activity and Health*. http://www.who.int/dietphysicalactivity/strategy/eb11344/strategy_english_web.pdf (last accessed December 2013).

References

Andreyeva T, Long MW, Brownell KD. 2009. The impact of food prices on consumption: a systematic review of research on the price elasticity of demand for food. *American Journal of Public Health* 100(2), 216–22.

Artinian NT, Fletcher GF, Mozaffarian D *et al.* 2010. Interventions to promote physical activity and dietary lifestyle changes for cardiovascular risk factor reduction in adults: a Scientific Statement from the American Heart Association. *Circulation* 122(4), 406–41.

Block JP, Chandra A, McManus KD, Willett WC. 2010. Point-of-purchase price and education intervention to reduce consumption of sugary soft drinks. *American Journal of Public Health* 100(8), 1427–33.

Bloom D, Cafiero E, Jané-Llopis E *et al.* 2011. *The Global Economic Burden of Noncommunicable Diseases*. Geneva: World Economic Forum.

Brug J. 2008. Determinants of healthy eating: motivation, abilities and environmental opportunities. *Family Practice* 25(Suppl 1), i50–i55.

Brug J, Kremers SP, Lenthe F, Ball K, Crawford D. 2008. Environmental determinants of healthy eating: in need of theory and evidence. *Proceedings of the Nutrition Society* 67(3), 307–16.

Danaei G, Finucane MM, Lin JK *et al.* 2011a. National, regional, and global trends in systolic blood pressure since 1980: systematic analysis of health examination surveys and epidemiological studies with 786 country-years and 5.4 million participants. *Lancet* 377(9765), 568–77.

Danaei G, Finucane MM, Lu Y *et al.* 2011b. National, regional, and global trends in fasting plasma glucose and diabetes prevalence since 1980: systematic analysis of health examination surveys and epidemiological studies with 370 country-years and 2.7 million participants. *Lancet* 378(9785), 31–40.

De Silva-Sanigorski AM, Bell AC, Kremer P *et al.* 2010. Reducing obesity in early childhood: results from Romp & Chomp, an Australian community-wide intervention program. *American Journal of Clinical Nutrition* 91(4), 831–40.

Duffey KJ, Gordon-Larsen P, Shikany JM, Guilkey D, Jacobs DR, Jr, Popkin BM. 2010. Food price and diet and health outcomes: 20 years of the CARDIA Study. *Archives of Internal Medicine* 170(5), 420–6.

Elbel B, Kersh R, Brescoll VL, Dixon LB. 2009. Calorie labeling and food choices: a first look at the effects on low-income people in New York City. *Health Affairs* 28(6), w1110–w1121.

Engelhard CL, Garson A, Jr, Dorn S. 2009. *Reducing Obesity: Policy Strategies from the Tobacco Wars*. Washington, DC: Urban Institute.

Grundy SM, Brewer HB, Jr, Cleeman JI, Smith SC, Jr, Lenfant C. 2004. Definition of metabolic syndrome: report of the National Heart, Lung, and Blood Institute/American Heart Association conference on scientific issues related to definition. *Circulation* 109, 433–8, doi 10.1161/01.CIR.0000111245.75752.C6.

Hardy L, Denney-Wilson E, Thrift AP, Okely AD, Baur LA. 2010. Screen time and metabolic risk factors among adolescents. *Archives of Pediatric and Adolescent Medicine* 164(7), 643–9, doi:10.1001/archpediatrics.2010.88.

Institute of Medicine. 2009. *Local Government Actions to Prevent Childhood Obesity*. Washington, DC: National Academies Press.

Institute of Medicine. 2010. *Promoting Cardiovascular Health in the Developing World: A Critical Challenge to Achieve Global Health*. Washington, DC: National Academies Press.

Joint WHO (World Health Organization)/FAO (Food and Agriculture Organization) Expert Consultation. 2003. *Diet,Nutrition and the Prevention of Chronic Diseases*. Geneva: WHO.

Kelder SH, Perry CL, Lytle, LA, Klepp KI. 1995. Community-wide youth nutrition education: long-term outcomes of the Minnesota Heart Health Program. *Health Education Research* 10(2), 119–31.

Lim SS, Vos T, Flaxman AD *et al.* 2013. A comparative risk assessment of burden of disease and injury attributable to 67 risk factors and risk factor clusters in 21 regions, 1990–2010: a systematic analysis for the Global Burden of Disease Study 2010. *Lancet* 380(9859), 2224–60.

Lozano R, Naghavi M, Foreman K *et al.* 2013. Global and regional mortality from 235 causes of death for 20 age groups in 1990 and 2010: a systematic analysis for the Global Burden of Disease Study 2010. *Lancet* 380, 2095–128.

Micha R, Kalantarian S, Wirojratana P *et al.* 2012. Estimating the global and regional burden of suboptimal nutrition on chronic disease: methods and inputs to the analysis. *European Journal of Clinical Nutrition* 66(1), 119–29.

Mozaffarian D. 2008. Promise of improving metabolic and lifestyle risk in practice. *Lancet* 371(9629), 1973–4.

Mozaffarian D, Afshin A, Benowitz NL *et al.* 2012. Population approaches to improve diet, physical activity, and smoking habits: a Scientific Statement from the American Heart Association. *Circulation* 126(12), 1514–63.

Mozaffarian D, Appel LJ, Van Horn L. 2011. Components of a cardioprotective diet: new insights. *Circulation* 123(24), 2870–91.

Mozaffarian D, Capewell S. 2011. United Nations' dietary policies to prevent cardiovascular disease. *BMJ* 343, d5747.

Mozaffarian D, Hao T, Rimm EB, Willett WC, Hu FB. 2011. Changes in diet and lifestyle and long-term weight gain in women and men. *New England Journal of Medicine* 364(25), 2392–404.

Nugent R. 2011. *Bringing Agriculture to the Table: How Agriculture and Food Can Play a Role in Preventing Chronic Disease*. Chicago: Chicago Council on Global Affairs.

Patel SR, Hu FB. 2008. Short sleep duration and weight gain: a systematic review. *Obesity (Silver Spring)* 16(3), 643–53.

Powell LM, Auld MC, Chaloupka FJ, O'Malley PM, Johnston LD. 2007. Access to fast food and food prices: relationship with fruit and vegetable consumption and overweight among adolescents. *Advances in Health Economics and Health Services Research* 17, 23–48.

Ratnayake WM, L'Abbe MR, Mozaffarian D. 2009. Nationwide product reformulations to reduce trans fatty acids in Canada: when trans fat goes out, what goes in? *European Journal of Clinical Nutrition* 63(6), 808–11.

Rickard BJ, Okrent AM, Alston JM. 2013. How have agricultural policies influenced caloric consumption in the United States? *Health Economics* 22(3), 316–39.

Robinson TN. 1999. Reducing children's television viewing to prevent obesity: a randomized controlled trial. *JAMA* 282(16), 1561–7.

Robinson TN. 2001. Television viewing and childhood obesity. *Pediatric Clinics of North America* 48(4), 1017–25.

Sacks G, Rayner M, Swinburn B. 2009. Impact of front-of-pack "traffic-light" nutrition labelling on consumer food purchases in the UK. *Health Promotion International* 24(4), 344–52.

Sanigorski AM, Bell AC, Kremer PJ, Cuttler R, Swinburn BA. 2008. Reducing unhealthy weight gain in children through community capacity-building: results of a quasi-experimental intervention program, Be Active Eat Well. *International Journal of Obesity (London)* 32(7), 1060–7.

UN (United Nations). 2011. *Political Declaration of the High-level Meeting of the General Assembly on the Prevention and Control of Non-communicable Diseases. September, 16, 2011.* http://www.un.org/ga/search/view_doc.asp?symbol=A/66/L.1 (last accessed December 2013).

US Burden of Disease Collaborators. 2013. The state of US health, 1990–2010: burden of diseases, injuries, and risk factors. *JAMA* 310(6), 591–608.

Van't Riet J, Sijtsema SJ, Dagevos H, De Bruijn GJ. 2011. The importance of habits in eating behaviour. An overview and recommendations for future research. *Appetite* 57(3), 585–96.

Vyth EL, Steenhuis IH, Roodenburg AJ, Brug J, Seidell JC. 2010. Front-of-pack nutrition label stimulates healthier product development: a quantitative analysis. *International Journal of Behavioral Nutrition and Physical Activity* 7, 65.

WHO (World Health Organization). 2011. *Global Status Report on Noncommunicable Diseases 2010.* Geneva: WHO.

WHO (World Health Organization). 2004. *Global Strategy on Diet, Physical Activity and Health.* Geneva: WHO. http://www.who.int/dietphysicalactivity/strategy/eb11344/strategy_english_web.pdf (last accessed December 2013).

Yang G, Wang Y, Zeng Y *et al.* 2013. Rapid health transition in China, 1990–2010: findings from the Global Burden of Disease Study 2010. *Lancet* 381(9882), 1987–2015.

Chapter 10

Ethical Reflections on Who is At Risk: Vulnerability and Global Public Health

Christine Straehle

Abstract

When thinking about who is at risk in a global public health context, a few preliminary concepts need to be defined. This chapter explores what it means to be at risk
and defines risk as being vulnerable to harm. Harm in turn is defined as not being
able to protect one's interest. This first part establishes vulnerability to harm as an
action-guiding principle in global public health. In the second part, I distinguish different types of vulnerability that point to different moral obligations. I then apply
this typology to contexts in global public health. I argue that we can understand
many public health measures as attempts to protect against risks – examples are
inoculation campaigns and preventative screening programs. Some vulnerabilities
are generated by constraints that define people's lives – like fees that are levied to
have access to vital tests, for example. This is morally problematic since we have a
duty to prevent harm from being inflicted. In the third part, I expand the analysis to
the global sphere. I show that individuals are made vulnerable to harm if developed
countries drain developing countries of healthcare workers. This is a neglect of the
duty to not inflict harm. It is also problematic for those who live in countries that
do not engage in active medical professional recruitment, because we all have an
obligation to prevent harm from happening.

The Handbook of Global Health Policy, First Edition. Edited by Garrett W. Brown, Gavin Yamey, and Sarah Wamala.
© 2014 John Wiley & Sons, Ltd. Published 2014 by John Wiley & Sons, Ltd.

Key Points

- To be at risk is to be vulnerable to harm.
- It is a moral duty to not inflict harm; while it is a moral obligation to prevent harm from happening.
- Vulnerability to harm in a global public health context can be construed as a lack of access to the means for a healthy life.
- Global public health needs to account for individual vulnerability.
- This implies a duty to not inflict harm, and an obligation to prevent harm from happening.

Key Policy Implications

- Health policy-makers need to account for individual vulnerability.
- Global public health concerns need to influence foreign policy – the benefits for one public cannot morally prevail over those of another; healthcare worker recruitment from countries under health stress cannot be justified.
- Justice demands global public health policy that regulates distribution of healthcare resources.

Introduction

How should we account for vulnerability in global public health? Who is at risk and what follows from this? Inequalities in health between those in health-rich countries compared with those living in health-deprived countries are well documented (see Chapters 9 and 12), whether these inequalities are defined as health outcomes, capabilities to health, or social determinants of health. So are the consequences of such inequalities. But what precisely we should conclude from these inequalities is less clear. One way of addressing the question is to think about the kinds of risks these inequalities bear.

To do so, some preliminary steps need to be taken. In particular, we need to know what it means to be at risk. Second, we need to know why it is ethically relevant that a person is at risk. Is it always morally problematic that somebody is at risk? Or is risk a factor of life that only gains moral relevance once it is unevenly distributed? Finally, linking risk with ethics in the context of this book raises the question of what the relevance of risk is, or should be, in our considerations of global public health. Should the goal of global public health be to reduce all kinds of unwanted risks? Is there a threshold at which risk becomes relevant for considerations of global public health?

In this chapter, I aim to do some of the preliminary definitional work that is necessary to make sense of the three components put before us – risk, ethics, and global public health. These components can be linked to several questions. What do we mean when we speak of risk? What does it mean for *a person* to be at risk? Why should we care? And why should we care, in particular, when thinking about global public health? Finally, what are our obligations towards those who are at risk? When we talk about ethics, this last question is the most important one, because it calls on us to define the kinds of obligations that flow from the fact that some are at a heightened risk, or so I will argue here.

Most theorists and practitioners of global public health usually put "risk" in terms of national or population health. A risk is a very specific category in public policy that needs to be hedged and contained. This stance is reflected in reports that shed light on the kinds of risks the world population faces in times of increased global sharing – of information, technology, but also diseases. Risk is then cast in terms of information that needs to be identified and assessed before countries can act together to address it (Brown and Harman 2011). Those who are at risk are most often sizable parts of, or entire populations; they are at risk of losing their standard of living, their health, or something similar that can be protected if nation-states act together in a decisive manner.

Here, instead, I want to propose that risk is first a category that characterizes individual lives. To be at risk in a global health ethics context means to be vulnerable to something. The moral problem arising from being at risk derives from the fact that to be vulnerable means to be unable to protect one's fundamental interests effectively. To make sense of this claim, I will provide a typology of vulnerability. I will accept that some conditions of vulnerability are not immediately morally problematic, even though they may become so if *vulnerability as a background condition of human life* is not accounted for in health policy-making. Second, I will construe *morally problematic vulnerability* as a specific kind of constraint on individual lives. Finally, I will explain how the concept of vulnerability can help us assess global health policy scenarios and help to shape our normative responses to them. Employing the idea of vulnerability, in other words, can help us assess the risks individuals find themselves in as well as help define the responsibilities we incur to address morally problematic risk.

What is a Risk?

So what is a risk? *The Oxford English Dictionary*, quite simply, defines a risk as the fact of being exposed to "the possibility of loss, injury, or other adverse or unwelcome circumstance; a chance or situation involving such a possibility." A risk is something we cannot fully know and which has unknown outcomes (Hansson 2003). A second distinction is important: between the unintended outcomes of our actions – we may know that we are running a risk when doing something, but we do not intend to put somebody at risk – and intentionally inflicting ill on somebody. Only the former can be called a risk in so far as it is unknown to us what the outcome of our actions will be. I will return to what this means when thinking about ethics later on; suffice to say, at this point, that moral philosophy is clear about prescribed conduct in the case of the latter – it is prohibited to inflict ill on somebody intentionally – while it is less clear what our moral obligations are in circumstances of risk and risk taking.

To run a risk may mean to come to harm or to be in danger to come to such harm. "Harm" is often used in a straightforward and literal sense – if I harm you, I inflict some kind of injury. A very standard definition of harm that I will adopt here is that to be harmed is to have one's fundamental interests negatively affected, where fundamental interests are interests that all persons share. To return to the original task of defining risk, we can then say, that to be at risk implies that some of our fundamental interests are not protected, but instead, that they are potentially exposed to being harmed. Put differently, we can say that they are *vulnerable* to harm. So when we think about who is at risk, we can say that those vulnerable to harm are at risk.

The connection between risk and harm to fundamental interests may explain why many theorists believe that most individuals are risk averse – if given the choice, most people would rather choose to be sheltered from risk than exposing themselves to it. Sometimes, however, risks are accepted; maybe because we expect a certain return or gain from taking the risk. This is to say that if not all else is equal, if individual gains are expected to outweigh the risk, we may think that we can "risk" it. As a result, we may choose endeavors that may potentially inflict harm, but that may also provide us with very high personal gains. Put differently, when thinking about morally problematic risk, we need to distinguish between the kinds of risks individuals may be willing to take – what we may call "tolerated or "accepted risks" – and the kinds of risks that individuals do not accept. Risks that are accepted do not prima facie pose a moral problem, whereas those we face without accepting or affirming them, do: if risk means to be vulnerable to harm, then such risk implies imposed vulnerability.

What does it Mean to be Vulnerable?

So assume that my interpretation is to be accepted, that to be at risk means to be vulnerable to having our interests harmed. Before assessing the content of the harm in global health policy, the idea of vulnerability warrants exploration. To be vulnerable may mean different things yet again. And not all forms of vulnerability are morally problematic in the way I want to argue here. Think about the kind of vulnerability that comes from being in a relationship with another person. Imagine two lovers who trust each other with their feelings and secrets – this makes each of them vulnerable to the other, potentially exploiting their sentiments for their own purposes. Yet, on the other hand, this also brings them very close to each other, because, in the good times at least, each can confide in the other. In fact, being vulnerable to the actions of another is to a large extent what it means to be in positive relationships with others (Frankfurt 1998). For most, the vulnerability that comes with relationships is something we accept; we risk getting into relationships, because the promise of our emotional gains outweighs the risk of having our interests harmed.

Another kind of vulnerability that I do not believe to be immediately morally problematic is vulnerability as a *background condition of human life* (Straehle 2010). To give quite an obvious example, the physical vulnerability of a newborn baby or a young child is a simple background condition of the life of a newborn baby or a child, even though we need not assume that most or even many children will be abused or neglected. The idea of human vulnerability then tries to account for human limitations and attempts to capture the "fragility of human life, action and achievement" (O'Neill 1998). What is important for my purposes here is that this kind of vulnerability is shared by all human beings – all newborn infants, we can say, are vulnerable in a very obvious, biological sense, and before any specific medical or social circumstance renders them more vulnerable than other newborn infants. To be sure, all newborn infants are *more* vulnerable to harm (through neglect, say) than all toddlers, and our responsibility towards all newborn infants are the same *qua newborn infants* as they are to all toddlers. The idea of human vulnerability in this sense simply underlines the moral responsibility towards those who are not able to protect themselves against their own fragility, like children, the ill, or the very old; but to experience vulnerability as a background condition as I construe it here does not designate a moral problem – something else has to happen for a moral problem to occur.

Note that this is not to say that we do not have obligations to *account* for this kind of vulnerability, especially in a health policy context. Namely, in order to *not* create a moral problem, governments are normally assumed to be under obligations to attend to the shared fragility of human life. I take it to be uncontroversial, for instance, that there is a moral responsibility for governments that have the necessary resources to inoculate against polio, which attacks mostly children and can cripple them for life. This obligation is simply due to the vulnerability of babies to be infected by the virus.

Obligations to account for background vulnerability are not limited to vulnerable babies or children, of course. I believe it fair to say that public health decisions like those for inoculation campaigns can best be understood as being motivated by the idea to shield individuals against risks that spring from such vulnerability. To illustrate, think of the outbreak of SARS in Canada in 2003. The onset and spread of the disease was remarkable for a developed country:

> As we write, over 3200 cases of severe acute respiratory syndrome (SARS) have been reported officially in 23 different countries. In Canada, 13 (12.4%) of 105 people with "probable" SARS have died. It is possible that milder cases are occurring without being reported, but it is too early to tell whether such cases might serve as a source of infection, further fuelling the epidemic. [...] There are reports of single people infecting up to 112 others. As health officials in Toronto continue to add cases to the SARS list, and quarantine hundreds of potential contacts, years of warnings about the implications of an easily travelled earth for infectious disease control have hit home. (Editorial 2003)

The fact that the disease spread as quickly and as seemingly uncontrolled as it did was promptly criticized: a report commissioned by the Canadian government in the aftermath of the outbreak castigated an environment of public health provision that was woefully unprepared to protect the members of the public from the disease. Put differently, it seemed as though "the years of warning" had only hit home after too many people had already been affected. The assessment by the commission is worth quoting at length, because it highlights to what extent the commissioners felt that public health provision had failed to account for the vulnerability of the population in a densely populated area such as Toronto:

> As a disease outbreak, SARS was relatively small. Nonetheless, the disease killed 44 Canadians, and caused illness in a few hundred more. The response to the outbreak paralyzed a major segment of Ontario's health care system for weeks, and saw more than 25,000 residents of the Greater Toronto Area placed in quarantine. Psychosocial effects of SARS on health care workers, patients, and families are still being assessed, but the economic shocks have already been felt. [...] As Canada recovers from this extraordinary set of events, the National Advisory Committee on SARS and Public Health has been weighing what lessons might be learned from the outbreak of SARS in Canada. The foregoing chapters indicate that there was much to learn – in large part because too many earlier lessons were ignored. (Public Health Agency of Canada 2012)

The underlying premise of this assessment of the outbreak is that Canada's government ought to have been prepared for such an outbreak, or at least that it should have been in a position to respond to it more promptly than it did (see Chapter 29). This is not to say that such epidemics happen regularly, or that governments can possibly be in a position to anticipate any such outbreak. Rather, it is to say that governments – if put in a position of being able to be prepared by warnings issued over time – are considered to *be* under a moral obligation to account for the vulnerability of individual citizens to be infected by highly infectious diseases, like SARS. And they are called upon to act accordingly. The idea, then, is to protect individuals against a vulnerability to harm that may indeed not materialize – but the extent of which is unknown and, if it were to materialize, the consequences of which would be too devastating for individuals and thus grievously harm their interests.

We can say, then, that even though vulnerability as a background condition of human life does not pose a moral problem in itself, a *lack of accounting for such vulnerability* will create a moral problem. Put differently, if we neglect this kind of vulnerability, then we may be putting individuals at risk. If public health policy neglects the eventuality of people becoming ill from highly infectious diseases, then it harms the interests of individuals to be protected against such infections. Thinking about vulnerability as a background condition of human life, then, provides us with an action-guiding principle in at least one way – it calls upon us to account for the fragility of human life.

An immediately more problematic case than that of vulnerability as a background condition of life is that of vulnerability *as a condition of constraint* or *circumstantial vulnerability*, both of which I use synonymously. This, it seems to me, is one type of vulnerability that many have in mind when thinking about moral obligations towards individuals. This kind of vulnerability describes the *specific* constraints an individual faces in her life, where these constraints make her life more open to the kind of harm that I described above, namely the harm to an individual's interest. In what follows, I will explore this kind of vulnerability in more detail. I will explain what precisely characterizes vulnerability as a condition of constraint, and show how it is related to the idea of unaccepted risk.

The kind of circumstances I have in mind are the specific conditions that frame decisions individuals can make about the protection of their fundamental interests. Some people live in circumstances that allow them to make decisions that promote and further their interests, and even though they may choose to act in ways that seem to outside observers to go against their interests, what is relevant for my purposes here is that the circumstances are such that they *could act* in ways that would promote their interests. An example that comes to mind is a well-endowed and talented person who chooses to use debilitating drugs. However, there are also circumstances that make it difficult if not impossible to promote and protect one's interests. If circumstances make individuals vulnerable to harm, I want to argue, they pose a moral problem and generate moral responsibilities. Such circumstances may be due to different things; for the purposes of this chapter, I will focus on circumstances that are due to health policy. Health policy as I understand it here is a set of rules that regulates the kind of access individuals have to the means of leading what they would consider healthy lives, among other things. To conceptualize this idea for the purposes of my investigation, I propose that the circumstances that determine an individual's vulnerability are circumstances that define to what extent a person can have access to reasonable means of healthcare provision in her country.

A first step on the way to determine whether or not we *need* access to healthcare provision are often preliminary tests that aim to determine potential health problems. Test programs are often in fact offered for sections of society simply as a precautionary measure, and based on the statistical evidence regarding what segments of society are most prone to the kinds of disease under investigation. Think of mammogram programs for women over 50, or prostate cancer screening for men of the same age. In most developed rich countries, these tests are offered free of charge even though there is no concern for the health of the greater public because cancer tests aim to determine non-communicable disease. In other words, even though danger of infection across populations is not given, governments assume the responsibility to provide for a section of society that is vulnerable to suffer from a disease. This is to say that circumstances defining access to healthcare are determined by the decisions of policy-makers in a given country about what kinds of tests to make available. Again, if governments have the resources to offer such tests, but would not do so, we can safely assume that their members would call upon them to fulfil their responsibilities and shield their members from the risk of having undetected cancers.

A similar rational as the one motivating cancer screening underlies prenatal HIV/AIDS tests for pregnant women to determine whether or not their fetuses are at risk of being infected with the virus – a risk that medication can reduce significantly (Cooper *et al.* 2002). One way of thinking about such tests is to postulate that they should be implemented based on our responsibility to protect the vulnerable fetus – thus falling into the earlier category of our moral responsibility to account for vulnerability as a background condition of human life. We can also hold, however, that these tests should be based on the interests individual women have to be responsible and provide well for their newborn children (see Chapter 11). Assume that this is a fundamental part of what pregnant women hold dear, that it is part of their interest as future mothers to have healthy babies. It would be obvious, then, that they would not accept the kind of risk that comes to them and their fetus if they forego such tests.[1]

Now, imagine that such tests were not available free of charge but that individual women could only obtain them for a fee. For most, this might not pose a hurdle and they could simply pay for such a test. For some, however, charging for the test may pose an insurmountable problem and they may have to forgo being tested. This kind of vulnerability is different from vulnerability as a background condition, because it is not a background condition of human life. Instead, it is the result of a *specific circumstance*, a constraint that is put into place by the requirement to pay for such a test. This is the first part of this kind of vulnerability that should give us moral pause. Some kinds of vulnerability, like those that are due to lack of access to funds for provision of healthcare, for example, are problematic because they *impose constraints* on individuals that may lead to harm.

The second aspect of this kind of vulnerability that raises moral concern is that this kind of vulnerability may be said to be *generated* by such constraints: without imposing a fee for such tests, we could speculate that there is no such vulnerability. To be sure, there may be vulnerability in the first instance due to the danger of HIV/AIDS infection; to my mind, however, this is a different category of vulnerability. We may say that being affected by a disease is a background condition of human life and illustrates the fragility of the human body. Recall that I accepted earlier that we have a moral obligation to account for this kind of vulnerability through health policies; in the case of HIV/AIDS infection, I side with those who argue for a global responsibility to combat HIV/AIDS (Kaida and Lenard 2012). Vulnerability due to a specific set of constraints, however, is in a different category of vulnerability because it is not vulnerability due to being human, but instead vulnerability *caused* by a specific constraint that some face and that constrain their ability to protect their interests. Such constraints can take different forms: in the example of HIV/AIDS, the constraint under discussion takes the form of a fee that would have to be paid to have access to a vital test. The point I wish to highlight here is simply that vulnerability as a condition of constraint is characterized by the fact that a person is made vulnerable to harm due to a constraint that is imposed. I will return later on to considerations of responsibility for such constraints, and to a treatment of how we should think about responsibility in specific cases, like that of circumstantial vulnerability due to a lack of access to medical professionals.

If we accept the premise I proposed earlier, which held that we have a moral obligation to protect the vulnerable from harm, then *creating* a constraint that *generates* vulnerability is particularly problematic, since it not only neglects our duty to protect those who are vulnerable but also neglects the duty *to not inflict harm*. Moral philosophers often argue about the relevance we should attribute to the distinction between letting something harmful happen to another person, and actively bringing about a harmful circumstance (Singer 1972). We are called upon to prevent harm from occurring; but we are positively prohibited from inflicting harm. I will distinguish here between a moral duty to not inflict harm and moral obligations to prevent harm from happening: both are binding, but the former is a stricter set of prescriptions than the latter. Or, to put this differently: "Although we are not always required to help, we are always required not to be indifferent" (Stohr 2011: 62).

I agree, therefore, with those who argue that there is a moral distinction between risk-taking and intentional ill-doing. Recall that I characterized risks as being unknown. Even though we are called upon to assess to what extent our actions carry risks, we are nevertheless not in a position to know for certain the outcome of our actions. Since risks are *precisely* defined by being unknown, we could say that we are on safe moral ground if we accept that we have thought in a reasonable way about certain risks, and that we have assessed the situation to the point that we think the risk acceptable, however "acceptable" is to be defined. We may imagine, for instance, that there is "only a slight risk" of a bad consequence to result from our actions. Or we may expect that the gain from choosing one course of action over another may far outweigh the risk we take. Assume that despite our best efforts at gauging the potential risk, our actions result in harm caused to another. Are we as blameworthy for taking the risk as if we had intentionally inflicted harm? Based on the distinction just drawn, we can say that we fulfilled our duty to not inflict harm, even though we may have failed our obligation to prevent harm from happening. If, instead, we intentionally inflict harm, we have violated our duty not to do so. There is, in other words, a morally relevant difference between harm that we knowingly inflict and harm that occurs despite our reasonable efforts to prevent it from happening. Put differently yet again, there is a difference between rendering people vulnerable and not preventing the circumstances that make them vulnerable to harm; however, we are called upon to avoid both.

Critics could object here that these are the kinds of distinctions that philosophers get excited about, but that they do not have much traction when thinking about moral action guiding principles. However, this criticism is not warranted, because such are the bases of principled arguments for some global health policies and the obligations that flow from them. To illustrate, think of a common example used to highlight risk and vulnerability in global public health, the case of brain drain of medical professionals. As is well known, many nurses and doctors from what we may call *health provision poor countries* choose to migrate to other countries to provide services and employ their skills there. This has led to a critical undersupply of doctors and nurses in their source countries, a situation defined by the World Health Organization (WHO) as less than 2.28 health workers per 1000 population, and less than 1.71 nurses per 1000 (WHO 2006: 15).

Earlier, I have proposed it to be uncontroversial that all individuals have a fundamental interest in having access to the means of leading healthy lives. To realize this interest, individuals need to have access to medical services if only to receive the kind of inoculation against polio or tests for HIV/AIDS infection discussed earlier. I also believe it uncontroversial to say that such an individual interest exists even though we may debate to what extent this interest can serve as the foundation for a human right to health (Weinstock 2011; Sreenivasan 2012; Wolff 2012; also see Chapter 25).

Now, if we accept my argument, we could say that a lack of healthcare professionals should be understood as a condition of constraint that inflicts a specific kind of vulnerability: without access to healthcare professionals able to provide basic healthcare services, individuals cannot protect their fundamental interest in leading lives free of easily preventable diseases; without inoculation against polio, to return to this example, children cannot protect their interest of not being crippled. Instead, they run the risk of being vulnerable to harm, in particular, the harm that comes with a lack of access to such means.

Vulnerability, Responsibility, and Moral Obligations

If the argument that some constraints imposed on individuals create vulnerability to harm is accepted, the next question in need of exploration is about the lessons to be drawn from this account. How can a vulnerability-based definition of risk help assess moral responsibilities and define action-guiding principles? I will develop an answer here again based on the example of brain drain.

One way of dealing with the question is to simply deny that it can be reasonably answered. We could hold that vulnerability that is created by outmigration of healthcare professionals is simply due to the fact that some countries cannot pay as much to their doctors and nurses as others can. The lure of greener shores is a fact of life just like the kind of basic human interconnection that is also responsible for epidemics and global health threats. According to this line of argument, we cannot attribute responsibility for the kinds of vulnerability that flow from a dearth of healthcare professionals. Instead, we would have to accept that it is part of the kind of background condition explained earlier. Note, though, that even in the cases of vulnerability as a background condition,

I argued, public policy has to account for such vulnerability in some way or other. Even if undersupply of health practitioners were simply a background condition of human life, a vulnerability-based account of risks would nevertheless demand that global health policy devise a way to account for the kind of vulnerability that individuals are faced with regarding health provision in poor countries.

Another way of answering the question about moral responsibilities in the case of medical brain drain is to accept that the emigration of health professionals is not simply a background condition, but a specific constraint that restricts the capacity of those staying behind in the countries of origin to protect themselves against harm. Recall here that I am interested in the kinds of circumstances that affect an individual's capacity to access reasonable means of healthcare provision. Earlier, I also stated that I construe such circumstances to be shaped by acts of health policy-makers in one's country, but also abroad as I will illustrate. To say, then, that constraints are imposed is simply to say that an individual would not have agreed to the kinds of circumstances she finds herself in. In this sense, the imposition could be either structural, due to the market in healthcare professionals described, or the lack of funds in one's country to retain healthcare professionals in the country. What concerns me here is that persons are prohibited from protecting their interests, thus becoming exposed to heightened risks. To address these risks, we need to be clear about their form and origin.

The constraint I have in mind is due to several factors that characterize provision of access to healthcare. First, the administration of healthcare is still mostly taken to be the responsibility of national governments. This includes the education and training of healthcare professionals, often at great expense to the country in question. This is of course particularly problematic for developing countries that have to spend scarce resources on the *training* of healthcare professionals in their countries rather than on *expanding* access to viable basic healthcare (Eyal and Hurst 2008). Second, and somewhat contrary to the principles of healthcare administration, we witness that competition for healthcare professionals is far from national; instead, national governments and health providers compete for talent *globally*. One consequence of such competition is the exorbitant advantage rich countries have compared to those countries who often educate and train health practitioners but which lose them to higher paying countries elsewhere (McAllester 2012). The effects on the countries of origins have been documented widely by now and go well beyond simply the loss of those trained in the developing country (Straehle 2012).[2] The constraint that results from brain drain is a lack of access to healthcare professionals. Individuals are vulnerable to not being able to protect their interests in leading a disease-free life if they lack access to healthcare professionals who can administer basic healthcare needs. This is the nature of the constraint. The origin of the constraint comes from the fact that healthcare practitioners are actively, and, as some say, aggressively recruited to move (Brock 2009).

I set out on this discussion in order to illustrate the moral distinction between taking a risk and inflicting harm. I argued that this distinction provides us with action-guiding principles: we are prohibited from actively inflicting harm, what I called a positive duty of justice, while we are called upon to prevent harm from happening, which is an imperfect obligation. If we accept that we have a duty to not inflict harm, and if my definition of risk as vulnerability to harm is plausible, then it seems to me that we also have a duty to not accept the kinds of risks that bear such vulnerability. The case of health professional recruitment illustrates, then, how vulnerability can help us assess moral responsibilities: if recruitment leads to a risk of vulnerability to harm, then it is a duty to change recruitment to avoid inflicting harm. Adopting an ethical perspective on global health policy, no government can justifiably engage in the kinds of recruitment practices that create the kinds of risks that leave people vulnerable to not be able to protect their fundamental interests in leading disease-free lives.

But what are the moral obligations for those who do not engage in such practices? Do they have any? The great advantage of a vulnerability-based analysis of risk is that it helps assess specific constraints that create specific vulnerabilities, as I explained earlier. However, much of the global health policy discussion is centred on problems, for which responsibility is not so easily assigned, as in the case of health worker recruitment. It is important, though, to remember the twofold character of our moral obligations (i.e., the distinction between duties and obligations to protect individuals from harm). The action-guiding principle described earlier is based on the duty not to inflict harm. However, we have also an obligation to prevent harm from happening. Even if our governments and healthcare administrators are not the ones aggressively recruiting in health provision poor countries, we are nevertheless under an obligation to prevent harm from being inflicted in these countries. Quite concretely, this implies that access to healthcare worldwide needs to be a concern for policy-makers in all countries. As the foreign ministers of the Oslo Declaration put it, health is a concern of foreign policy and the concern for health needs to be channeled into a resetting of foreign policy priorities nationally, and into collaborative measures across state borders in order to establish and promote global health security (Oslo Ministerial Declaration 2007; Labonté and Gagnon 2010).

Conclusions

Risk is often invoked as a moral consideration in debates about global health policy. Ideally, policy should aim to prevent risk or at least shield individuals from it as best as possible. I have argued that to be at risk is morally problematic because it means to be vulnerable to have one's fundamental interests harmed. I have then proposed a distinction between different types of vulnerability, the most immediately morally problematic is *vulnerability as a constraint*. A vulnerability-based analysis of risk explains and substantiates both duties to not actively inflict harm, and obligations to prevent harm from occurring. A vulnerability-based account of risk defines one important goal of global health policy: to protect individual fundamental interests in healthy lives.

Notes

1. Note here that I leave aside the question how individual women may have contracted the virus and whether or not their contracting the virus suggests that they have accepted the kind of risk they expose themselves and their fetus to (but see Stemplowska 2009 for a helpful discussion of attributing responsibilities in cases like these).

2. A look at actual figures may illustrate the problem best: in Kenya, for example, it is estimated that the cost to educate a doctor from primary school to university graduation amounts to $65,997 while educating a nurse costs $43,180 (Kirigia *et al.* 2006). Compare these figures with those published by the British Medical Association in January 2011, which put the training costs for British doctors between $436,000 and 620,500, depending on the level of specialization (BMA 2011). It is fair to say, then, that the current situation is a de facto subsidy that developing countries provide to their developed counterparts, by training what are to the latter inexpensive healthcare workers at a high cost to the former (Kapur and McHale 2006). Moreover, the pernicious consquences of skilled outmigration

go beyond losing valuable professionals: because public finances of sending countries dete-
riorate due to the loss in investment return, some countries then cannot actually employ
the health professionals that are in the country for lack of funds (WHO 2009).

Key Reading

Daniels N. 2008. *Just Health: Meeting Health Needs Fairly*. Cambridge: Cambridge University
    Press.
Goodin R. 1984. *Protecting the Vulnerable*. University of Chicago Press: Chicago.
Labonté R, Gagnon M. 2010. Framing health and foreign policy: lessons for global health
    diplomacy. *Globalization and Health* 6(1), 14.
Packer C, Labonté R, Spitzer D. Globalization and Health Worker Crisis. WHO Commis-
    sion on Social Determinants of Health. http://www.who.int/social_determinants/resources/
    gkn_packer_al.pdf (last accessed December 2013).
Vekatapuram S. 2011. *Health Justice*. Cambridge: Polity Press.
Wolff J. 2012. *The Human Right to Health*. W.W. Norton & Company.

References

British Medical Association. 2011. *How much does it cost to train a doctor in the United Kingdom?*
    http://www.bma.org.uk/press_centre/presstrainingcost.jsp (last accessed December 2013).
Brock G. 2009. Health in developing countries and our global responsibilities. In Dawson A (ed.)
    The Philosophy of Public Health, pp. 73–90. Aldershot: Ashgate.
Brown GW, Harman S (eds). 2011. Special Issue on Risk, Perceptions of Risk and Global Health
    Governance. *Political Studies* 54(4).
Cooper ER, Charurat M, Mofenson L *et al*. 2002. Combination antiretroviral strategies for the
    treatment of pregnant HIV-1-infected women and prevention of perinatal HIV-1 transmission.
    Journal of Acquired Immune Deficiency Syndromes 29(5), 484–94.
Editorial. 2003. Editorial: SARS: the struggle for containment. *Canadian Medical Association Jour-
    nal* 168(10), 1229, 1231. http://www.cmaj.ca/content/168/10/1229.full?ijkey=f05cc3575b7467
    cda21acf6373c5be5d56b7cbc8&keytype2=tf_ipsecsha (last accessed December 2013).
Eyal N, Hurst S. 2008. Physician brain drain: can nothing be done? *Public Health Ethics* 1(2),
    180–92.
Frankfurt H. 1998. Duty and love. *Philosophical Explorations* 1(1), 4–9.
Hansson SO. 2003. Ethical criteria of risk-acceptance. *Erkenntnis* 59, 291–309.
Kaida A, Lenard PT. 2012. Outlining the global duties of justice owed to women living with
    HIV/AIDS in sub-Saharan Africa. In Lenard PT, Straehle C. (eds) *Health Inequalities and Global
    Justice*, pp. 119–38. Edinburgh: Edinburgh University Press.
Kapur D, McHale J. 2006. Should a cosmopolitan worry about brain drain? *Ethics and Interna-
    tional Affairs* 20(3), 305–20.
Kirigia JM, Gbary AR, Muthuri LK, Nyoni J, Seddoh A. 2006. The cost of health professionals'
    brain drain in Kenya. *Biomed Central Health Services Research* 6, 89.
Labonté R, Gagnon M. 2010. Framing health and foreign policy: lessons for global health diplo-
    macy. *Globalization and Health* 6(1), 14.
McAllester M. 2012. Amercia is stealing the world's doctors. *New York Times*, March 7. http://www.
    nytimes.com/2012/03/11/magazine/america-is-stealing-foreign-doctors.html?pagewanted=all
    (last accessed December 2013).
O'Neill O. 1998. Vulnerability and finitude. *Routledge Routledge Encyclopedia of Philosophy*, Ver-
    sion 1.0, 467–99. London and New York: Routledge.

Oslo Ministerial Declaration. 2007. Oslo Ministerial Declaration – global health: a pressing foreign policy issue of our time. *Lancet* 369(9570), 1373–8.

Public Health Agency of Canada. 2012. *Learning from SARS: renewal of public health in Canada.* http://www.phac-aspc.gc.ca/publicat/sars-sras/naylor/12-eng.php (last accessed December 2013).

Singer P. 1972. Famine, affluence and morality. *Philosophy and Public Affairs* 1(2), 229–43.

Sreenivasan G. 2012. A human right to health? Some inconclusive scepticism. *Proceedings of the Aristotelian Society Supplementary Volume* 86(1), 200–16.

Stemplowska Z. 2009. Making justice sensitive to responsibility. *Political Studies* 57(2), 237–59.

Stohr K. 2011. Kantian beneficience and the problem of obligatory aid. *Journal of Moral Philosophy* 8, 45–67.

Straehle C. 2010. Cosmopolitan and national solidarity. *Contemporary Political Theory* 9(1), 110–20.

Straehle C. 2012. Healthcare migration, vulnerability and individual autonomy: the case of Malawi. In Lenard PT, Straehle C (eds) *Health Inequalities and Global Justice*, pp. 245–62. Edinburgh: Edinburgh University Press.

Weinstock DM. 2011. How should political philosophers think of health? *Journal of Medicine and Philosophy* 36(4), 424–35.

WHO (World Health Organization). 2006. *World Health Report 2006: Working Together for Health.* Geneva: WHO.

Wolff J. 2012. The demands of the human right to health. *Aristotelian Society Supplementary Volume* 86(1), 217–37.

Chapter 11

Ethical and Economic Perspectives on Global Health Interventions

Sonia Bhalotra and Thomas Pogge

Abstract

We suggest how contemporary global institutions shaping the development, pricing, and distribution of vaccines and drugs may be modified to deliver large improvements in health. To support a justice argument for such modification, we show how the current global economic order may contribute to perpetuating poverty and poor health in less-developed countries. To support an economic argument for such intervention, we adduce recent evidence which shows that improving early childhood health raises the future quality of life and, in addition, has multiplier effects, stimulating human capital investment and raising employment and earnings.

The Handbook of Global Health Policy, First Edition. Edited by Garrett W. Brown, Gavin Yamey, and Sarah Wamala.
© 2014 John Wiley & Sons, Ltd. Published 2014 by John Wiley & Sons, Ltd.

Key Points

- Disease in childhood causes poverty in adulthood and this, in turn, causes children of the next generation to start life in poor health. This causal chain runs across generations to create a poverty trap in which ill health is the primary mechanism. By their nature, poverty traps call for external intervention; there is no evident spontaneous mechanism by which they dissipate.
- Interventions that improve fetal or infant health tend to raise the productivity of subsequent investments in both health and education. In this way, health begets health, as well as education and earnings.
- Economists have documented the relevance of market, government, and political failures in contributing to incentive problems and other obstacles in the delivery of public health. We add that there is failure of the international political economy of global health marked by information constraints, commitment problems, poor representation of constituent preferences, and limited accountability.
- As disease is growing increasingly globalized, so is the management of disease. Contemporary global institutions shaping the development, pricing, and distribution of vaccines and drugs have raised the prices of new medicines in the developing world, making many treatments inaccessible to those who need them most. This is unnecessary, and modified arrangements can deliver large improvements in health.
- Richer countries have a moral responsibility to contribute to mitigating the disease burden in poor countries based on their contribution, through global institutional design, to the persistence of the poverty–disease cycle in the developing world.

Key Policy Implications

- Interventions targeted at early-childhood health may be among the best investments in poor countries – they are less easily appropriated than cash transfers, directly improve quality of life, generate education and income externalities, are likely to be cost-effective, and have built-in tendencies towards being self-sustaining.
- Since infectious diseases are most prevalent amongst the poor and children, their prevention and cure can lead to persistent reductions in health inequalities and thereby socioeconomic inequalities. However, the design of institutions and, in particular, equal opportunities for investing in schools and labor markets mediate this process.
- The TRIPS agreement can be relaxed in favor of an alternative feasible regime such as the Health Impact Fund, which would incentivize pharmaceutical R&D without aggravating health inequalities.

Introduction

Our approach is conditioned by three factors. First, the global burden of disease is largely borne by poor countries. Second, within poor countries, it is largely borne by children. Third, poverty heightens the risk of contracting disease and childhood exposure to disease causes poverty in later life and, plausibly, into the next generation.

The first factor may suggest that improving global health is essentially the duty of poor-country governments, but we present ethical and economic arguments against this view. The second and third factors suggest that health interventions may be self-financing and self-sustaining within the span of a generation and, overall, not only intrinsically desirable but also cost-effective. However, commitment problems arise in achieving international coordination of interventions, and these are enhanced by the fact that some costs of inaction flow in an intergenerational frame (familiar from debates about climate change). This motivates the consideration of global institutional reforms focused on alleviating disease burdens borne by children and especially by girls.

We suggest how contemporary global institutions shaping the development, pricing, and distribution of vaccines and drugs may be modified to deliver large improvements in health. We show how interventions that improve childhood health directly improve the quality of life and, in addition, have multiplier effects, producing long-term population and economic gains in poor countries. They also tend to generate positive spillovers for richer countries through reductions in population growth, migration, pollution, and the externalities of infectious disease. To support a justice argument for such modification, we show how the current global economic order may contribute to perpetuating poverty and poor health in developing countries. We argue that millions of poor people are caught in a poverty–disease "trap," the origins of which are typically in their early childhood and can be traced to their parents' childhoods. This suggests an explanatory role for past global institutions, in which slavery and colonial rule loom large.[1]

Recent estimates suggest that the gains in life expectancy in the United States over the twentieth century were worth more than US\$1.2 million per person to the current population (Murphy and Topel 2006). If we allow for the intrinsic value of life, for the longer horizon of life for children (as opposed to adults) saved from death, for next generation effects, and for socioeconomic gains from health, then the benefits for poor countries are possibly larger. Moreover, the costs of prevention and cure are likely to be lower in poor countries where studies suggest that substantial health gains can be achieved by interventions such as provision of clean water, micronutrients, oral rehydration therapy, insecticide-treated bed nets, vaccines, and generic antibiotics. In general, addressing infectious disease prevalence is much cheaper than addressing chronic diseases (e.g., cancer, diabetes), which are prevalent in richer countries and emerging rapidly in poorer countries. This is also pertinent to the case for interventions targeting infectious disease given that there is some evidence that preventing infectious disease in childhood lowers the risk of chronic disease in adulthood (Barker and Osmond 1986; Barker 1992).

The gap in life expectancy between rich and poor countries today is about 30 years, and the difference is due to child mortality. Someone born in Sierra Leone is about 87 times as likely to die in childhood as someone born in Sweden (Deaton 2007). Between 1850 and 1950, most high-income countries experienced historically unprecedented declines in child mortality from the control of infectious disease. This raised life expectancy at birth by nearly 30 years (Cutler *et al.* 2006). Today less than 1% of all deaths in richer countries are of children under the age of five, while child deaths still dominate mortality in poorer countries. Some 7.6 million children are dying each year before they turn five (UNICEF/WHO 2011) and avoidably so (Jones *et al.* 2003). The knowledge (e.g., concerning sanitation) and innovation (e.g., antibiotics) that were successful in richer countries are now available to poorer countries. Yet, in poorer countries only about 20% of children have access to safe water and only 20% of children who need antibiotics to treat pneumonia receive them (WHO 2010).

The costs of adequate nutrition and treatment are too small for poverty alone to explain the persistence of high levels of disease (Deaton 2007). But because poverty is a major contributor to morbidity and mortality, it is pertinent to note that the world poverty problem, which is so large in human terms, is small in economic terms. In 2005, the shortfall of the world's poor from an adequate standard of living amounted to about 2% of global household income or 1.2% of world income.[2] This global poverty gap could have been filled almost twice over, just from the *gain* in the share of the richest ventile during 1988–2005 (see the section "Health, Justice, and Global Institutions"). The widespread poverty we see today, like widespread ill health, is largely avoidable.

In this chapter we underline the role of a global political economy in generating significant barriers to improvements in both disease and poverty. The relevance of political factors at the national level is widely recognized. Foreign aid to the developing world is often characterized as being captured or dissipated by corrupt or failed governments (Temple 2010, section 7). The under-representation of women in government has been shown to result in the relative neglect of public health provision (Miller 2008; Bhalotra and Clots-Figueras 2014). What we underline here is the bearing of the broader international political economy upon this state of affairs and, further, on the shape of global institutional arrangements as they pertain to disease and poverty. Even where democratic governments have signed up to international agreements, they do not necessarily represent the preferences of their people. For these reasons, we suggest here a reconsideration of the current institutional order, focusing upon aspects that impinge upon health. The preservation of human rights provides an excellent starting point but we underline that this is a domain in which pursuit of this goal is compatible with widespread and lasting human capital and economic gains.

The chapter is structured as follows. The next section pulls together new evidence from epidemiology and economics that illustrates relevant causal pathways and demonstrates the costs of failing to intervene. This evidence demonstrates that health interventions in developing countries tend to directly produce improvements in early-life health and cognitive development and, by raising the productivity of investments, to stimulate subsequent human capital investments. This has been shown to translate into often very large impacts on labor market outcomes. We also underline the significance of investing in the nutrition and health of girls as this appears to be key to breaking the intergenerational persistence of ill health and poverty. We then argue that richer countries have not only the incentives to contribute to disease mitigation in poorer countries but also an active moral responsibility to do so.

Hidden and Long-Term Returns to Disease Mitigation

This section argues that mitigating infectious disease in poor countries and providing all children with a healthy start will bring about continued gains and convergence in health and socioeconomic status across the lifespan of the exposed generation and the next. Much of the literature on inequality of opportunity at birth focuses upon the influence of parental resources and attitudes on investments in children (Cunha and Heckman 2009). We highlight evidence from new work focusing on the importance of early-life health (Currie 2009; Almond and Currie 2011a).[3] The effect sizes in this literature are large enough to suggest that interventions against infectious disease (effectively targeting infant health) may be more effective at raising educational performance and income in poor countries than conventional interventions such as reducing class size (Miguel and Kremer 2004; Kremer and Holla 2009). Prioritizing the health of girls (who are widely disadvantaged today) can further enhance these long-term benefits because mothers are pivotal in the intergenerational transmission of health (Bhalotra and Rawlings 2010). We now develop these arguments in a natural sequence.

Infectious Disease: The Importance of Childhood

The primary proximate cause of death in poor countries is infectious disease. Pneumonia, HIV/AIDS, diarrhea, tuberculosis, and malaria exert the largest toll. Undernutrition lowers resistance to infectious disease, which in turn aggravates undernutrition.[4] Young children are especially vulnerable because their immune systems are immature and because the metabolic cost of nutritional deprivation is especially large in the peak years of human growth. Many children die. Others survive, assisted by adaptive physiological changes such as reduced body size or an altered kidney morphology. Recent research suggests that this short-term thrift may exert a penalty in the longer run, making survivors of childhood disease more likely to contract chronic diseases like cancer, cardiovascular problems, and diabetes later in life (Barker and Osmond 1986; Barker 1992; 1995; Almond and Currie 2011b). These adverse effects are thought to be larger when, as in many (growing) developing countries, the nutritional environment changes dramatically over the life course.

Chronic Disease

The "Barker hypothesis" suggests that the emergence of chronic diseases in poor countries may be aggravated by infectious disease exposure 50–60 years ago. This is when many of these countries were still under colonial rule or just emerging from it, and many were largely unexposed to the biomedical and technological innovations that reduced infectious disease in richer countries in the late nineteenth and early twentieth centuries. It also suggests that many less-developed countries today carry a double burden of disease: young children continue to suffer morbidity and mortality from infectious disease at an unnecessarily high rate while chronic disease is taking hold in the adult population.

Infectious Disease, Cognitive Development, and Poverty

Brain development consumes a very large share of metabolic resources in early life (85% compared with 25% in adults), and resource deprivation therefore endangers cognitive development (Eppig *et al.* 2010; Bharadwaj and Neilson 2011; Bhalotra and Venkataramani 2013; Venkataramani and Bhalotra 2013). Moreover, there is evidence suggesting: (i) the productivity of investments in an individual's health and education is lower when the endowments that they start out with are weaker; and (ii) investments in health and education are mutually reinforcing (Cunha and Heckman 2007; Glewwe and Miguel 2008). Related evidence shows that increases in life expectancy stimulate increased investments in education, consistent with the returns to education flowing over a longer horizon. This is nicely illustrated by Jayachandran and Lleras-Muney (2009), who show that a sharp drop in maternal mortality in Sri Lanka stimulated investment in the education of girls.

These dynamic complementarities imply that the damage incurred by poor fetal and infant health may grow larger rather than fade over time, and may scar not only future health but also adult cognitive attainment and, by these processes, adult earnings. In this way, early-life disease causes later-life poverty (Currie 2009; Bhalotra and Venkataramani 2012) which causes children of the next generation to start life in poor health. This causal chain runs across generations in an endogenous process that may be characterized as a poverty trap in which ill health is the primary mechanism (Currie and Moretti 2007; Bhalotra and Rawlings 2010, 2012). By their nature, poverty traps call for external intervention as there is no evident spontaneous mechanism by which they dissipate (Bonds *et al.* 2010).

There is widespread recognition that poverty leads to ill health (Gwatkin *et. al.* 2000; Friel and Marmot 2011). It is less widely known that ill health leads to poverty (or that health-promoting interventions produce educational and income gains).[5] One reason for this is that long-range longitudinal data are scarce and the causal impact of health on income or poverty takes time to emerge (the time from early childhood to employment or child rearing). Another reason is the difficulty of identifying causality when the relationship runs in both directions and is subject to confounders. Recent studies address this challenge. A 20-year follow-up of a randomized control trial involving de-worming in Kenyan schools estimated that treatment generated two to three additional years of schooling and a 21–29% increase in income (Baird *et al.* 2011). Other studies using cohort data on large-scale historical health interventions have arrived at remarkably similar estimates. Bleakley (2010) estimates that malaria eradication in the Americas increased wage income by 15–27%, and Bhalotra and Venkataramani (2012) estimate that the 30% drop in infant pneumonia mortality after the introduction of antibacterials was associated with a 19% income gain for survivors exposed to the disease in infancy.[6]

Health Inequalities and Institutional Design

Because infectious diseases are more prevalent amongst the poor, their prevention and cure reduce health and thereby socioeconomic inequalities. However, the design of institutions mediates this process. Here we present some compelling illustrations from recent US history, which are of generic relevance to our central thesis: that the full benefit of other changes (such as rising incomes in developing countries) may depend upon institutional change (or, the lifting of institutional barriers to access and opportunity).

Pneumonia was the leading cause of death in the early 1930s, twice as prevalent among (poorer) African-Americans as among whites. In both populations, infection rates were highest amongst infants. Upon the introduction in 1937 of sulfonamides, the first antibiotics, pneumonia fell sharply in both populations, but the absolute health gain for blacks was larger, in line with their higher pre-intervention exposure levels. Using econometric methods that isolate the impact of reduced pneumonia exposure in infancy on later-life outcomes, we find that the education and incomes of whites benefited enormously from being born just after 1937 as compared with just before, but there were, on average, no similar socioeconomic gains for African-Americans. We show that this can be traced to racial segregation in schools and labor markets (in the South in particular) that limited both the opportunities and incentives for blacks to make complementary human capital investments (Bhalotra and Venkataramani 2012). The results for whites illustrate how interventions that improve early-life health can produce large socioeconomic gains by encouraging reinforcing investments in health and education, while the results for blacks illustrate how this translation may be limited by "extractive" institutions that inhibit sections of the population from realizing potential returns.

Some 30 years later, Title VI of the 1964 Civil Rights Act, mandating desegregation among institutions receiving federal funds, provided a further positive shock to health endowments, this time, unique to African-Americans. The integration of hospitals led to a substantial narrowing of the racial gap in post-neonatal infant mortality (Almond and Chay 2007) and this has been shown to have been a key driver of the improved test performance of black teenagers in the 1980s (Chay *et al.* 2009).

Intergenerational Transmission of Health

The previous section outlines compelling evidence that childhood health interventions lead not only to immediate reductions in morbidity and mortality amongst children, but also to health and socioeconomic gains in adulthood. These, in turn, stand to raise the health and subsequent socioeconomic status of their children. In this way the benefits of a one-off intervention today persist into the future. There is some direct evidence of intergenerational impacts of early-life health interventions. For instance, girls exposed to the Great Chinese Famine grew up to have less healthy children (Fung and Ha 2010), and girls born into conditions of high infant mortality have children less likely to survive infancy (Bhalotra 2010). Immunization programs, as much as economic growth, have been shown to attenuate the intergenerational transmission of health at the low end of the maternal health distribution (Bhalotra and Rawlings 2012) – yet girls are routinely less likely to be immunized in many poor countries (Oster 2009; Bharadwaj and Nelson 2010). Since mother–child transmission of health tends to be stronger than father–child, these results imply that interventions that erase gender disparities in child health are supported by efficiency as well as equity considerations (see Bhalotra and Rawlings 2010 and references therein).

Health Interventions and Population Growth

Health interventions may influence population growth through their impacts on mortality, fertility (Galor and Weil 1996; Bhalotra and van Soest 2008; Galor 2012), and migration (Mesnard and Seabright 2009). Fertility may be expected to respond to the mother's health endowment and to changes in the health and survival prospects of potential offspring. Fertility declined just after the early-twentieth-century eradication of hookworm in the US South and, at the intensive margin, after the large-scale antibiotic treatment of pneumonia, consistent with parents substituting "quality" for "quantity" of children (Bleakley and Lange 2009; Bhalotra *et al.* 2012). The 1991 clean water reform in Mexico, which sharply reduced morbidity and mortality from diarrhea, also led to a decline in fertility (Bhalotra and Venkataramani 2013). The tendency for mothers to have fewer births once their (potential) offspring become more likely to thrive suggests a pathway from disease mitigation to lower population growth and more rapid economic growth (Galor and Weil 2000).

In sum, there is evidence of causal links flowing from improvements in early-life health to cognitive development, education, and earnings and some evidence that investments in the early-life health of women are particularly beneficial because they produce returns in the second generation. Drawing upon the evidence regarding fertility, we conclude that investments in child and especially girls' health promise lasting health and socioeconomic gains, alongside other (social and economic) changes that enable women to make productive contributions beyond childbearing.

Globalization of Disease

Human alteration of ecosystems in the processes underlying economic growth (e.g., urbanization, irrigation, deforestation) facilitates the emergence and spread of infectious diseases. Diseases evolve in unpredictable ways. The post-World War I global influenza epidemic of 1918–1920 killed an estimated 50–100 million people, including half a million in the United States alone. The current "swine flu" or H1N1 virus has evolved from an old form of ("Asian") flu which assimilated elements of avian and swine flu. Older diseases like malaria and tuberculosis are re-emerging on account of microbial resistance to existing drugs. Globalization, or the flow of information, goods, capital, and people across political and geographic boundaries, has helped spread some of the deadliest infectious diseases known to humans. In recent history, bubonic plague, influenza, SARS, and HIV/AIDS have spread from poor to richer countries. Disease crosses international borders more easily with increases in air travel (Lederberg 1997),[7] mass migrations due to wars or natural disasters (BBC 2004; Montalvo and Reynal-Querol 2007; Blattman and Miguel 2010), and trade in agricultural products. Globalization has increased not only the spread of infectious diseases from South to North, but also the risk of non-communicable diseases spreading by transmission of cultural behavior from North to South (Brown and Labonté 2011; see also Chapter 30).

Health, Justice, and Global Institutions

Building upon the empirical insights outlined so far, this section argues that richer countries have an active *moral responsibility* to contribute to mitigating the disease burden in poor countries, based on their ongoing contribution, through design and imposition of the current global institutional order, to the persistence of the poverty–disease cycle in the developing world.

Patents and Drug Prices

As disease is growing increasingly globalized, so is the management of disease. One central component of globalization has been the creation of an increasingly dense and influential supranational system of rules and actors that shape and regulate not only the ever-growing share of interactions that traverse national borders but also purely domestic interactions, profoundly shaping, for instance, trade, investment, innovation, working conditions, environmental protection, and the availability of weapons. In particular, the 1994 Trade-Related Agreement on Intellectual Property Rights (TRIPS) agreement, created with the World Trade Organization (WTO), has shifted important rules governing the development and sale of medicines from the national to the global level. The TRIPS agreement entitles pharmaceutical firms to protect their innovations with 20-year product patents, which enable them to suppress generic competition.[8] This has raised the prices of new medicines in the developing world to many times the marginal cost of production, thereby making many treatments inaccessible to those who need them most.[9]

A common defense of TRIPS is that the manufacture and sale of generic products are moral crimes ("theft," "counterfeiting," "piracy") that any just legal system ought to suppress (Nozick 1974: 182). But the defenders of this view have not managed to provide a convincing argument to show why the fact that one person has made a new product should give her a natural right to bar others from making a like product out of their own raw materials (Hollis and Pogge 2008, chapter 5). Patents fit poorly with libertarian views that celebrate property rights and freedom since they restrict the freedom to use one's property in novel ways.

Another defense states that poor countries signed the TRIPS agreement voluntarily. But many had little understanding of its implications at the time and they needed the improved access to rich-country markets that was then offered in return. The interests of the poor majority were often given little weight in the deliberations of those who held political power in less-developed countries (see Chapter 22).

In view of the difficulty of formulating convincing appeals to natural law or informed consent, most TRIPS defenders resort to pragmatic arguments stressing the need for economic incentives. The proposition is that potential innovators will develop new medicines only if this can earn them a decent return on their investment (WTO 2012); and such medicines, while immediately benefiting only the rich, will eventually go generic and then benefit poor patients as well. A weakness of this argument is that, by the time a medicine goes generic, its effectiveness may have been eroded by microbial adaptation or other changes. Another neglected drawback is the long-term cost of the delay arising from the intergenerational effects of poor childhood health, that is, children of a generation that experiences childhood in a pre-transition regime when drugs are inaccessible will carry a health penalty derived from their parent's health even if they grow up in a post-transition regime when drugs become more accessible.

Despite these problems, the status quo might be defensible if the development of important new medicines could be stimulated only through patent-protected mark-ups that exclude poor patients during the patent period. However, recent evidence suggests that the extension of strong patent protections into developing countries has not stimulated research and development (R&D) investment in the diseases prevalent there (Kyle and McGahan 2012). Plus, various plausible alternative mechanisms, designed to overcome existing access problems, have been proposed over the last decade.[10] Here we discuss one such mechanism, the Health Impact Fund (HIF), which would complement the existing system by offering innovators the option to register a new medicine or, under certain conditions, a traditional medicine or a new use of an existing medicine. By registering a product, the innovator would undertake to make it available globally, during its first 10 years on the market, at no more than the lowest feasible cost of production and distribution. The innovator would further commit to allowing, at no charge, generic production and distribution of the product after this decade has ended. In exchange, the registrant would during this decade receive annual reward payments based on its product's health impact.[11] Each reward payment would be part of a large, constant annual pay-out, with every registered product receiving a share equal to its share of the assessed health impact of all HIF-registered products in the relevant year.

The HIF is potentially beneficial on three fronts. First, it would foster development of important medicines for diseases concentrated among the poor. Pharmaceutical innovators are now neglecting such diseases because they have no realistic hope of recovering their R&D costs from sales to the poor (Moran *et al.* 2009). Second, the HIF would at any time support availability of a set of vital new medicines worldwide at very low prices. Third, the HIF would motivate registrants to ensure that their products are widely available, perhaps even below the price ceiling, and that they are competently prescribed and optimally used.[12] This is because, in the HIF scheme, registrants are rewarded not for merely selling their products, but for making them effective toward improving global health.

The HIF's annual reward pool might initially be set at $6 billion – about 0.03% of the gross national products of China plus the United States, or Brazil plus the European Union. If HIF-rewarded innovations were funded through taxes, affluent people would bear most of the cost and poor people would contribute little or nothing – just like under the current system. The key difference is that, instead of being excluded by large mark-ups, poor patients would gain access to HIF-rewarded medicines at prices that cover the cost of manufacture and distribution. By funding pharmaceutical innovation in this new way, affluent populations stand to benefit from lower drug prices (directly and through lower expenses for insurance, national health systems, and foreign aid), from better marketing of drugs for optimal health impact, from faster economic growth in poorer countries, and from reduced transmission of infectious diseases to richer countries.

By funding the HIF, affluent populations would also reduce their role in a grievous injustice. The HIF model shows clearly that the development of new medicines can be incentivized in a way that allows poor patients immediate access at the cost of manufacture and distribution. In view of this possibility, it is wrong for the affluent to choose to incentivize the development of important new medicines for themselves through the worldwide enforcement of temporary monopolies that prevent generic manufacturers from supplying cheap copies to poor patients.

Global Institutions and Social Justice

We first show that there are vast income inequalities across the world. We then illustrate how supranational institutional arrangements may be aggravating inequality and poverty worldwide (Pogge 2004). The final subsection sets out the tenets of a case for global health interventions from the standpoint of moral and political philosophy.

Poverty and inequality at birth   Some defenders of TRIPS contend that it is natural and not unfair that affluent people have all kinds of expensive things that poor people cannot afford to buy. This contention assumes an acceptable distribution of income and wealth. But are existing economic inequalities fair? They have accumulated over a history of colonial conquest, enslavement, exploitation, and genocide. Over 80% of income variability worldwide is explained by a person's country and socioeconomic class at birth (Milanovic 2009).

As Table 11.1 shows, the richest ventile (5%) of the global income distribution has gained substantially over the globalization period, while the poorest 90% have lost ground.[13] With the losses most severe in the poorest quarter, income has become more polarized: across 17 years, the ratio between the average income in the richest ventile and that in the poorest quarter has skyrocketed from 185 to 297. By 2005, the poorer two thirds of humanity had merely 6% of global household income and 3.34% of global private wealth (Keating *et al.* 2011: 14).

Table 11.1   The evolution of global income inequality.

Segment of world population	Share of global household income 1988	Share of global household income 2005	Absolute change in income share	Relative change in income share
Richest 5%	42.87%	46.36%	+3.49	+8.1%
Next 5%	21.80%	22.18%	+0.38	+1.7%
Next 15%	24.83%	21.80%	−3.03	−12.2%
Second quarter	6.97%	6.74%	−0.23	−3.3%
Third quarter	2.37%	2.14%	−0.23	−9.7%
Poorest quarter	1.16%	0.78%	−0.38	−32.8%

Global factors in the perpetuation of poverty and inequality   A familiar argument against foreign aid or other international interventions is that they do not reach the target population because of the corruption of developing country governments (e.g., Temple 2010). But corruption is often encouraged by the economic interests of richer nations. For instance, affluent countries and their banks may lend money to corrupt rulers and compel the country's people to repay it after the ruler is gone. Many poor populations are still repaying debts incurred, against their will, by kleptocrats such as Suharto in Indonesia, Mobutu in the Democratic Republic of the Congo, Abacha in Nigeria, and Mubarak in Egypt. Second, affluent countries facilitate the embezzlement of funds by public officials in less-developed countries by allowing their banks to accept such funds. This complicity could easily be avoided: banks are already under strict reporting requirements with regard to funds suspected of being related to terrorism or drug trafficking. Yet western banks still eagerly accept and manage embezzled funds, with governments ensuring that their banks remain attractive for such illicit deposits. Global Financial Integrity (GFI) estimates that less-developed countries have in this way lost $357–417 billion annually during the 2000–2008 period.[14] Third, affluent countries may facilitate tax evasion in less-developed countries through lax accounting standards for multinational corporations. Since they are not required to do country-by-country reporting, such corporations can easily manipulate transfer prices among their subsidiaries to concentrate their profits where these are taxed the least. As a result, they may report no profit in the countries in which they extract, manufacture, or sell goods or services, having their worldwide profits taxed instead in a tax haven where they only have a paper presence. GFI estimates that, during the 2000–2008 time period, trade mispricing deprived developing countries of $366–427 billion per annum.[15] Fourth, affluent countries and their firms often buy natural resources from the rulers of less-developed countries without regard for how such rulers came to exercise power. In many cases, this amounts to collaboration in the theft of these resources from their owners, the country's people. It also enriches their oppressors, thereby entrenching the oppression: tyrants sell their victims' natural resources and use the proceeds to buy the weapons they need to keep themselves in power (Pogge 2008; Wenar 2008).

Affluent countries also contribute to the problem by altering the environmental, political, and economic landscape. They account for a disproportionate share of global pollution. Their emissions are prime contributors to serious health hazards, extreme weather events, rising sea levels, food and water insecurity, and climate change, to which poor populations are especially vulnerable. A recent report by the Global Humanitarian Forum estimates that climate change is already seriously affecting 325 million people and annually causing $125 billion in economic losses plus 300,000 deaths, of which 99% are in less-developed countries (GHF 2009: 1, 60–1). Richer countries encouraged conflict within Africa during the Cold War (Dunning 2004). War has persistent impacts on health, human capital and hence long-term growth in poor countries (Blattman and Miguel 2010; Akresh *et al.* 2012). Richer countries have created a global trading regime that is cast as generating large collective gains through free and open markets. But the regime is rigged; it permits rich states to continue to protect their markets through tariffs and antidumping duties and to gain larger world market shares through export credits and subsidies (including some $227 billion annually in agriculture alone) which poor countries cannot afford to match.[16] Because production is much more labor-intensive in poor than in affluent countries, such protectionist measures tend to destroy many more jobs in poor countries than they create in more affluent countries.

The justice case   The core function of institutional arrangements – of the rules and practices structuring a national society or other social system – is to protect the freedom and well-being of the individuals whose lives are governed or profoundly affected by them. Physical and mental health is fundamental to both freedom and well-being. Institutional arrangements ought then to be designed and (if needed) reformed so as to enable those whose lives they profoundly affect to lead full and healthy lives.

This widely accepted thought is often connected with the value of solidarity (or risk-sharing). All human beings are vulnerable to various serious threats to their physical and mental health, and we can cope much better with these threats when we pool some of our resources. To be sure, participation in a scheme of organized solidarity will not be equally advantageous for all, even *ex ante*. Some will not be able to contribute a lot to the pool and some will foreseeably place greater burdens on it; such people are then likely to receive a share of the scheme's benefits that is larger than their share in the scheme's cost. But solidarity is a strong moral reason to include and to assist the more vulnerable among us.

While we endorse this call for solidarity, both within and beyond national borders, we also recognize that, on its own, it conveys an incomplete and potentially misleading picture. Institutional arrangements not merely address some of the health problems and vulnerabilities that individuals bring with them into society. They also shape these people and their environments, thereby profoundly affecting what health problems and vulnerabilities people face in the first place. Social institutions influence access to nutrients and patterns of environmental hazards, for example, and the resulting childhood exposure to malnutrition or lead pollution can have serious effects on people's health needs for the rest of their lives. Similarly consequential for health are a society's choices about public hygiene and sanitation, access to health knowledge, traffic rules, law enforcement, political competition, and protections against domestic and employer abuse. Persons whose health has been undermined by avoidable defects in any of these social factors can plead for solidarity, of course. But they can also invoke the more stringent value of justice.

One might say in response that, just like healthcare, the social determinants of health fall exclusively under the value of solidarity, which is lacking in a social order under which people are avoidably left to starve or must find their own way of protecting themselves from assault. We hold that such a social order is also unjust. Those upholding it are not merely insufficiently attentive to the needs of some of those on whom they impose it, but can also be said to be actively harming them. To be sure, one is not harming unemployed persons when one fails to provide them with the food they need to survive. But one is harming when one imposes institutional arrangements under which foreseeably some are avoidably unable to meet their basic needs.

Because human rights are constraints on government conduct, including that of upholding national and international institutional arrangements, governments may not be the most reliable judges of human rights. Their documents nonetheless deserve attention. The two most prominent references to health in these documents affirm that "Everyone has the right to a standard of living adequate for the health of himself and of his family, including food, clothing, housing and medical care and necessary social services" (Universal Declaration of Human Rights, Article 25.1) as well as "the right of everyone to the enjoyment of the highest attainable standard of physical and mental health" (International Covenant on Economic, Social and Cultural Rights, Article 12.1).

The latter formulation may need some explication. As the word "standard" indicates, it is not here postulated that each person has a claim to whatever resources may be needed to maintain her in, or restore her to, good health. The assertion is rather that each is entitled to enjoy whatever plausible overall standard can reasonably be achieved for all. Here three limiting considerations come into play. First, for some specific piece of health protection (a safe water supply, say, or some medical procedure) to count as "attainable," it must be achievable *for all* and not merely for some. Second, for a specific piece of health protection to count as achievable for all, it must be achievable not merely by itself, but as part of a plausible package of health protections that can be simultaneously achieved for all. This is why we speak of a *plausible overall standard*, one that covers a set of diverse health protections intelligently selected in light of a society's capacities and all relevant costs, opportunity costs, synergies, complementarities, etc. Third, there should be no requirement to assign absolute priority to health over everything else (such as culture, education, and leisure time). Even if a higher standard of health could be attained by eradicating all wild animals, for example, a society may judge this cost to be unreasonably high relative to the health gains attainable through it.

Some still claim supranational arrangements (such as TRIPS) as a morality-free zone in which the concept of justice has no application (Nagel 2005). But, on reflection, this claim is hard to justify.[17] If it is unjust for each of a group of governments to impose certain rules upon its own country's population, then it must also be unjust for this same group of governments to impose the same rules upon all their countries' populations pursuant to some international agreement.

The upholding of any institutional order involves a substantial element of coercion, which is morally justifiable only if the institutional order imposed meets certain requirements of social justice. What these requirements are is controversial, especially in the case of supranational institutional arrangements that govern people committed to a wide diversity of moral conceptions. But it is fairly uncontroversial that institutional arrangements must at least be human rights compliant, that is, must not foreseeably give rise to substantial and reasonably avoidable human rights deficits.[18]

Insisting on this minimal condition is especially important in regard to supranational rules that are not formulated through the kind of transparent, democratic procedures that characterize national law-making in those countries that have reached a basic level of domestic justice. Rather, supranational rules mostly emerge through intergovernmental negotiations that effectively exclude the general public and even the majority of weaker governments. Only a small number of "players" can exert real influence: powerful organizations, prominently including large multinational corporations and banks, very rich individuals, and ruling "elites" of the most powerful developing countries. They can reap huge gains from favorable supranational rules and can therefore afford to make large investments in acquiring the necessary expertise, forming alliances, and lobbying the stronger (G20) governments that dominate supranational rule-making. Ordinary citizens, by contrast, typically find it prohibitively expensive to acquire the necessary expertise and to form alliances that are large enough to rival corporate influence. In the absence of global democratic institutions, the shift toward global governance sidelines the vast majority of human beings, while greatly enhancing the rule-shaping powers of a tiny minority of those who are already the richest and most powerful. The latter's interests are diverse, and some elite players fail in their efforts to shape in their favor the rules that stand to impact them the most. Yet, the rules do get captured by some elite players and, as a group, they consequently grow their share of global wealth and expand their advantage over the rest of humankind. This, in turn, further increases their capacity to influence the design and application of the rules in their own favor and, unintentionally but no less inexorably, contributes to keeping the poorer section of humankind in poverty.

Conclusions

In poor countries infectious diseases cause high levels of morbidity and mortality that are avoidable at low cost. While recognizing more local barriers to progress on the demand and supply side, we have underlined the role of internationally imposed constraints on progress. We have indicated that interventions targeted at early-childhood health may be among the best investments in poor countries – they are less easily misappropriated than cash transfers, directly improve quality of life, generate positive education and income externalities, are likely to be cost-effective, and have built-in tendencies towards being self-sustaining. These factors strengthen the political case for intervening now. Against this backdrop, we have discussed ethical and pragmatic reasons for richer countries to undertake internationally coordinated commitments to tackle disease in poorer countries, focusing attention upon reforming the way pharmaceutical innovation is rewarded.

The present TRIPS system reflects the prejudice that innovation must be rewarded through large mark-ups, at the expense of access by the poor who, if they survive, gain access after patent expiration. We have made the following essential arguments against this regime. First, by an eclectic set of widely recognized ethical principles, including libertarian ones at one extreme, the current regime is unfair. Second, it is also unnecessary insofar as there is an alternative feasible regime that would incentivize pharmaceutical R&D without aggravating health (and thereby economic) inequalities. Third, we have highlighted evidence from epidemiology and economics suggesting that investment in disease mitigation among the poor today is economically wise and, with a lag, likely to pay for itself. Moreover, richer countries and richer people in poor countries have an incentive to contribute to making this investment because improving the health of the poor generates positive externalities for the rich.

A common depiction of the problems of ill health and poverty in poor countries is that they are complex and insurmountable. Furthermore, health problems are often shown to be demand-driven, for example, people may not have relevant information or sufficient education to process new information, leading to low uptake of publicly provided health goods (e.g., Banerjee *et al.* 2010). While this is valid, the existence of one sort of barrier does not justify imposing another barrier to progress. Economists have documented the relevance of market, government, and political failures in contributing to incentive problems and other obstacles in the delivery of public health. We add that there is also failure of the international political economy of global health marked by information constraints, commitment problems, poor representation of constituent preferences, and limited accountability.

Notes

1. Recent research in economics shows persistent impacts of slavery and colonial institutions on a range of contemporary outcomes including inequality, economic growth, and polygamy (Acemoglu *et al.* 2001; Sacerdote 2005; Fenske 2011).
2. This accords roughly with the World Bank's PPP-based tally which counted 3,085 million people as living in severe poverty in 2005 and estimated their collective shortfall – the global poverty gap – at 1.13% of world income (Pogge 2010: 69).
3. We provide relevant examples rather than a comprehensive survey of this literature.
4. There are two mechanisms for the latter. First, the immune response generated to fight infection is resource-intensive and taxes available nutritional resources (Crimmins and Finch 2004). Second, infectious disease tends to moderate appetite and to inhibit assimilation of nutrition (Scrimshaw *et al.* 1968).

5. As discussed earlier, this is relevant insofar as health interventions may eventually pay for themselves, but also insofar as it motivates the participation of richer countries that may stand to benefit from lower disease levels and higher levels of economic growth in developing countries.

6. These results, obtained on microdata, reflect partial equilibrium outcomes. Acemoglu and Johnson (2007) present an opposing view using cross-country data. They show that large-scale health interventions in the 1950s did raise gross domestic product (GDP) but as they also raised the population, there were no significant increases in per capita GDP. These results are contended in Bleakley (2006) and Bloom *et al.* (2009).

7. Air travel enables people to go to foreign lands, contract a disease and not have any symptoms of illness until after they get home, having exposed others along the way. The West Nile virus is believed to have reached New York City in 1999 via mosquitoes riding in airplane wheel wells.

8. The TRIPS agreement resulted from strong lobbying by the agribusinesses and pharmaceutical, entertainment, and software industries. Product patents allow patentees to veto the manufacture and sale of a patented molecule regardless of how it is produced. Before TRIPS, India granted only process patents, which allow patentees to veto merely a specific way of making a molecule. India is the leading supplier of medicines in the less-developed countries. See WHO (2010) and Chapter 22.

9. Parallel-import and reference-pricing problems notwithstanding, pharmaceutical firms often find it profitable to sell their patented products in poorer countries at lower prices. But even intranational inequalities are nowadays so large that in most less-developed countries an important medicine's domestically profit-maximizing sales price will place it out of reach of the majority of the country's population (Flynn *et al.* 2009).

10. Most of the more plausible proposals are described and discussed in the work of the WHO Consultative Expert Working Group on Research and Development (CEWG), available at www.who.int/phi/news/cewg_2011/en/index.html (last accessed December 2013).

11. Measured in quality-adjusted life-years saved. The QALY metric has been refined over the last 20 years and is already widely used, e.g., by public and private insurers deciding which new drugs to cover (Phillips 2009).

12. A registrant would want to offer its product below cost if and insofar as it expects its additional health impact rewards due to reaching additional patients to be larger than its loss on the sales price. A registrant would want to promote the wide and proper use of its product, especially by those who can benefit most from it, if and insofar as the additional health impact rewards due to such efforts exceed their costs.

13. The data used in this table were kindly supplied by Branko Milanovic, lead economist in the World Bank's Research Department, in a personal e-mail communication on April 25, 2010 (on file with authors). Milanovic is a leading authority on the measurement of socioeconomic inequality.

14. Kar and Curcio (2011: 3, 21, 37). This outflow is over four times larger than all official development assistance which, during this period, averaged $83.7 billion annually, of which only $8.1 billion was allocated to "basic social services" (United Nations, MDG Indicators, http://unstats.un.org/unsd/mdg/Search.aspx?q=bss%20oda, last accessed December 2013).

15. Ibid.: 37. This is the other 50.6% of illicit financial outflows.

16. OECD 2011: 18, also stating that in 2010 government subsidies accounted for 18% of gross farm receipts in OECD countries.

17. For further compelling critique of Nagel's view, see Cohen and Sabel (2006).

18. The word "reasonably" is meant to acknowledge not merely the limits of human foresight but also the possibility that the institutional reduction of human rights deficits may sometimes have high costs in terms of culture, say, or the natural environment. It is best to avoid the claim that human rights must never give way in such cases – certainly in

modern times, when human rights can be largely or fully realized through institutional reforms that would not entail such high costs.

Key Reading

Acemoglu D, Johnson S. 2007. Disease and development: the effect of life expectancy on economic growth. *Journal of Political Economy* 115, 925–85.

Almond D, Currie J. 2011. Killing me softly: the fetal origins hypothesis. *Journal of Economic Perspectives* 25, 153–72.

Bhalotra S, Venkataramani A. 2012. *Shadows of the Captain of the Men of Death: Early Life Health, Human Capital Investment and Institutions.* http://sites.google.com/site/soniaradhikabhalotra/ (last accessed December 2013).

Bhalotra S, Venkataramani A. 2013. Cognitive Development and Infectious Disease: Gender Differences in Investments and Outcomes. IZA Discussion Paper No. 7833. Bonn: IZA. http://www.iza.org/en/webcontent/personnel/photos/index_html?key=2905 (last accessed December 2013).

Cunha F, Heckman JJ. 2009. The economics and psychology of inequality and human development. *Journal of the European Economic Association* 7(2), 320–64.

Hollis A, Pogge T. 2008. *The Health Impact Fund: Making New Medicines Available for All.* Oslo and New Haven: Incentives for Global Health. www.healthimpactfund.org (last accessed December 2013).

Kyle MK, McGahan AM. 2012. Investments in pharmaceuticals before and after TRIPS. *Review of Economics and Statistics*, www.mitpressjournals.org/doi/abs/10.1162/REST_a_00214 (last accessed December 2013).

Pogge T. 2004. Relational Conceptions of Justice: Responsibilities for Health Outcomes. In Anand S, Peter F, Sen A (eds) *Public Health, Ethics, and Equity*, pp. 135–161. Oxford: Clarendon Press.

References

Acemoglu D, Johnson S. 2007. Disease and development: the effect of life expectancy on economic growth. *Journal of Political Economy* 115, 925–85.

Acemoglu D, Johnson S, Robinson J. 2001. The colonial origins of comparative development: an empirical investigation. *American Economic Review* 91(5), 1369–401.

Akresh R., Bhalotra S, Leone M, Osili U. 2012. War and stature: growing up during the Nigerian civil war." *American Economic Review Papers and Proceedings* 102(3), 273–7.

Almond D, Chay K. 2007. *The Long-Run and Intergenerational Impact of Poor Infant Health: Evidence from Cohorts Born during the Civil Rights Era.* New York: Columbia University.

Almond D, Currie J. 2011a. Human capital development before age five. In Ashenfelter O, Card D (eds) *Handbook of Labor Economics*, Vol. 4b, pp. 1315–486. Amsterdam: Elsevier.

Almond D, Currie J. 2011b. Killing me softly: the fetal origins hypothesis. *Journal of Economic Perspectives* 25(3), 153–72.

Baird S, Hicks JH, Kremer M, Miguel E. 2011. *Worms and Work: Long-Run Impacts of Child Health Gains.* Berkely, CA: University of California.

Banerjee AV, Duflo E, Glennerster R., Kothari D. 2010. Improving immunization coverage in rural India: a clustered randomized controlled evaluation of immunization campaigns with and without incentives. *British Medical Journal* 340, c2220, doi 10.1136/bmj.c2220.

Barker D. 1992. *Fetal and Infant Origins of Adult Disease.* London: British Medical Journal Publishing Group.

Barker D. 1995. Fetal origins of coronary heart disease. *BMJ* 311(6998), 171–4.

Barker D, Osmond C. 1986. Infant mortality, childhood nutrition, and ischaemic heart disease in England and Wales. *Lancet* 1(8489), 1077–81.

BBC (British Broadcasting Corporation). 2004. *Natural disasters "on the rise."* BBC News September 17. http://news.bbc.co.uk/2/hi/3666474.stm (last accessed December 2013).

Bhalotra S. 2010. *The Intergenerational Spillover of Early Life Conditions.* Colchester: University of Essex.

Bhalotra S, Clots-Figueras I. 2014. Health and the political agency of women. *American Economic Journal: Economic Policy* (in press).

Bhalotra S, Hollywood D, Venkataramani A. 2012. *Fertility Health Endowments and Returns to Human Capital: Quasi-Experimental Evidence from Twentieth Century America.* Colchester: University of Essex.

Bhalotra S, Rawlings S. 2010. Intergenenerational persistence in health in developing countries: the penalty of gender inequality? *Journal of Public Economics* 95(3–4), 286–99.

Bhalotra S, Rawlings S. 2012. Gradients of the intergenenerational transmission of health in developing countries. *Review of Economics and Statistics* (online print version available, journal version forthcoming).

Bhalotra S, van Soest A. 2008. Birth-spacing, fertility and neonatal mortality in India: dynamics, frailty and fecundity. *Journal of Econometrics* 143(2), 274–90.

Bhalotra S, Venkataramani A. 2012. *Shadows of the Captain of the Men of Death: Early Life Health, Human Capital Investment and Institutions.* http://sites.google.com/site/soniaradhikabhalotra/ (last accessed December 2013).

Bhalotra S, Venkataramani A. 2013. Cognitive Development and Infectious Disease: Gender Differences in Investments and Outcomes. IZA Discussion Paper No. 7833. Bonn: IZA. http://www.iza.org/en/webcontent/personnel/photos/index_html?key=2905 (last accessed December 2013).

Bharadwaj P, Neilson C. 2011. *The Role of Early Childhood Health Interventions on Mortality and Academic Achievement.* La Jolla, CA: University of California San Diego.

Bharadwaj P, Nelson L. 2010. *Discrimination Begins in the Womb: Evidence of Sex Selective Prenatal Care.* La Jolla, CA: University of California San Diego.

Blattman C, Miguel E. 2010. Civil war. *Journal of Economic Literature* 48(1), 3–57, doi 10.1257/jel.48.1.3.

Bleakley H. 2006. *Disease and Development: Comments on Acemoglu and Johnson.* Chicago: University of Chicago. http://home.uchicago.edu/~bleakley/ (last accessed December 2013).

Bleakley H. 2010. Malaria eradication in the Americas: a retrospective analysis of childhood exposure. *American Economic Journal: Applied Economics* 2, 1–45.

Bleakley H, Lange F. 2009. Chronic disease burden and the interaction of education, fertility, and growth. *Review of Economics and Statistics* 91(1), 52–65.

Bloom D, Canning D, Fink G. 2009. *Disease and Development Revisited.* NBER Working Paper 15137. Cambridge, MA: National Bureau of Economic Research.

Bonds MH, Keenan DC, Rohani P, Sachs JD. 2010. Poverty trap formed by the ecology of infectious diseases. *Proceedings of the Royal Society of London Series B* 277, 1185–92, doi 10.1098/rspb.2009.1778.

Brown GW, Labonté R. 2011. Globalization and its methodological discontents: contextualizing globalization through the study of HIV/AIDS. *Globalization and Health* 7(29), 1–12.

Chay K, Guryan J, Mazumder B. 2009. *Birth Cohort and the Black–White Achievement Gap: The Role of Access and Health Soon After Birth.* Federal Reserve Bank of Chicago Working Paper 2008-20. Chicago: Federal Researve Bank of Chicago.

Cohen J, Sabel C. 2006. Extra rempublicam nulla justitia? *Philosophy and Public Affairs* 34, 147–75.

Crimmins EM, Finch CE. 2004. Inflammatory exposure and historical in human life-spans. *Science* 305(5691), 1736–9.

Cunha F, Heckman J. 2007. The technology of skill formation. *American Economic Review* 97(2), 31–47.

Cunha F, Heckman JJ. 2009. The economics and psychology of inequality and human development. *Journal of the European Economic Association* 7(2), 320–64.

Currie J. 2009. Healthy, wealthy, and wise: socioeconomic status, poor health in childhood, and human capital development. *Journal of Economic Literature* 47, 87–122.

Currie J, Moretti E. 2007. Biology as destiny? short- and long-run determinants of intergenerational transmission of birth weight. *Journal of Labor Economics* 25(2), 231–64.

Cutler D, Deaton A, Lleras-Muney A. 2006. The determinants of mortality. *Journal of Economic Perspectives* 20(3), 97–120.

Deaton A. 2007. Global patterns of income and health: facts, interpretations, and policies. WIDER Annual Lecture, Helsinki, September.

Dunning T. 2004. Conditioning the effects of aid: Cold War politics, donor credibility and democracy in Africa. *International Organization* 58, 409–23.

Eppig C, Fincher CL, Thornhill R. 2010. Parasite prevalence and the worldwide distribution of cognitive ability. *Proceedings of the Royal Society, Series B* 277(1701), 3801–8.

Fenske, J. 2011. *African Polygamy: Past and Present.* Oxford: University of Oxford.

Flynn S, Hollis A, Palmedo M. 2009. An economic justification for open access to essential medicine patents in developing countries. *Journal of Law, Medicine and Ethics* 37(2), 184–208.

Friel S, Marmot MG. 2011. Action on the social determinants of health and health inequities goes global. *Annual Review of Public Health* 32, 225–236, doi 10.1146/annurev-publhealth-031210-101220.

Fung W, Ha W. 2010. Intergenerational effects of the 1959–61 China famine. In Fuentes-Nieva R, Seck PA (eds) *Risks, Shocks, and Human Development: On the Brink*, pp. 222–254. London: Palgrave Macmillan.

Galor O. 2012. The demographic transition: causes and consequences. *Cliometrica* 6(1), 1–28.

Galor O, Weil D. 1996. The gender gap, fertility, and growth. *American Economic Review* 86(3), 374–87.

Galor O, Weil D. 2000. Population, technology, and growth: from Malthusian stagnation to the demographic transition and beyond. *American Economic Review* 90(4), 806–28.

GHF (Global Humanitarian Forum). 2009. *The Anatomy of a Silent Crisis.* Geneva: Global Humanitarian Forum.

Glewwe P, Miguel E. 2008. The impact of child health and nutrition on education in less developed countries. In Strauss J, Schultz T (eds) *Handbook of Development Economics*, Vol. 4(5), pp. 3561–606. Amsterdam: Elsevier.

Gwatkin DR, Johnson K, Pande RP, Rutstein S, Wagstaff A. 2000. *India: Socioeconomic Differences in Health, Nutrition, and Population.* Working Paper No. 30544. Washington, DC: The World Bank.

Hollis A, Pogge T. 2008. *The Health Impact Fund: Making New Medicines Available for All.* Oslo and New Haven: Incentives for Global Health. www.healthimpactfund.org (last accessed December 2013).

Jayachandran S, Lleras-Muney A. 2009. Life expectancy and human capital investments: evidence from maternal mortality declines. *Quarterly Journal of Economics* 124(1), 349–97.

Jones G, Steketee RW, Black RE, Bhutta ZA, Morris SS and the Bellagio Child Survival Study Group. 2003. How many child deaths can we prevent this year? *Lancet* 362(5), 65–71.

Kar D, Curcio K. 2011. *Illicit Financial Flows from Developing Countries: 2000–2009.* Washington: Global Financial Integrity.

Keating G, O'Sullivan M, Shorrocks A, Davies JB, Lluberas R, Koutsoukis A. 2011. *Global Wealth Report 2011.* Zurich: Credit Suisse Research Institute.

Kremer M, Holla A. 2009. Pricing and access: lessons from randomized evaluations in education and health. In Easterly W, Cohen J (eds) *What Works in Development: Thinking Big and Thinking Small.* Washington, DC: Brookings Institution Press.

Kyle MK, McGahan AM. 2012. Investments in pharmaceuticals before and after TRIPS. *Review of Economics and Statistics*, www.mitpressjournals.org/doi/abs/10.1162/REST_a_00214 (last accessed December 2013).

Lederberg J. 1997. The future of infectious disease. Lecture at the College of Physicians of Philadelphia, April 1. http://articles.philly.com/1997-04-07/living/25529940_1_infectious-diseases-single-celled-organisms-genetic-information (last accessed December 2013).

Mesnard A, Seabright P. 2009. Escaping infectious diseases through migration? Qarantine measures under asymmetric information about infection risk. *Journal of Public Economics* 93, 931–8.

Miguel E, Kremer M. 2004. Worms: identifying impacts on education and health in the presence of treatment externalities. *Econometrica* 72(1), 159–217.

Milanovic B. 2009. *Global Inequality of Opportunity: How Much of our Income is Determined at Birth?* Cornell University Poverty, Inequality and Development Papers. Ithaca, NY: Cornell University. www.arts.cornell.edu/poverty/kanbur/InequalityPapers/Milanovic.pdf (last accessed December 2013).

Miller G. 2008. Women's suffrage, political responsiveness, and child survival in American history. *Quarterly Journal of Economics* 123(3), 1287–327.

Montalvo JG, Reynal-Querol M. 2007. Fighting against malaria: prevent wars while waiting for the miraculous vaccines. *Review of Economics and Statistics* 89(1), 165–77.

Moran M, Guzman J, Ropars A-L et al. 2009. Neglected disease research and development: how much are we really spending? *PLOS Medicine* 6(2), 137–46. www.plosmedicine.org/article/info:doi/10.1371/journal.pmed.1000030 (last accessed December 2013).

Murphy KM, Topel RH. 2006. The value of health and longevity. *Journal of Political Economy* 114(4), 871–904.

Nagel T. 2005. The problem of global justice. *Philosophy and Public Affairs* 33, 113–47.

Nozick R. 1974. *Anarchy, State, and Utopia*. New York: Basic Books.

OECD (Organisation for Economic Co-operation and Development). 2011. *Agricultural Policy Monitoring and Evaluation 2011: OECD Countries and Emerging Economies*. Paris: OECD.

Oster E. 2009. Does increased access increase equality? gender and child health investments in India. *Journal of Development Economics* 89(1), 62–76.

Phillips C. 2009. *What is a QALY?* www.medicine.ox.ac.uk/bandolier/painres/download/whatis/QALY.pdf (last accessed December 2013).

Pogge T. 2004. Relational conceptions of justice: responsibilities for health outcomes. In Anand S, Peter F, Sen A (eds) *Public Health, Ethics, and Equity*, pp. 135–161. Oxford: Clarendon Press.

Pogge T. 2008. *World Poverty and Human Rights: Cosmopolitian Responsibilities and Reforms*, 2nd edn. Cambridge: Polity Press.

Pogge T. 2010. *Politics as Usual*. Cambridge: Polity Press.

Sacerdote B. 2005. Slavery and the Intergenerational Transmission of Human Capital. *Review of Economics and Statistics* 87(2), 217–34.

Scrimshaw N, Taylor C, Gordon J. 1968. *Interactions of Nutrition and Infection*. OMS Monograph Series No 57. Geneva: WHO. http://whqlibdoc.who.int/monograph/WHO_MONO_57_%28part1%29.pdf (last accessed December 2013).

Temple J. 2010. Aid and conditionality. In Rodrik D, Rosenzweig MR (eds) *Handbook of Development Economics*, vol. 5, pp. 4415–523. Amsterdam: Elsevier.

Venkataraman A, Bhalotra SR. 2013. *Quasi-Experimental Evidence of the Consequences of Early Childhood Diarrhea for Education and Health Capital of Men and Women*. Mimeograph, University of Essex.

Wenar L. 2008. Property rights and the resource curse. *Philosophy and Public Affairs* 36, 2–32.

World Health Organization (WHO). 2010. *Pneumonia*. Factsheet No. 331. Geneva: WHO. http://www.who.int/mediacentre/factsheets/fs331/en/index.html (last accessed December 2013).

World Health Organization (WHO). 2011. *WTO and the TRIPS Agreement*. Geneva: WHO. www.who.int/medicines/areas/policy/wto_trips/en/index.html (last accessed December 2013).

World Trade Organization (WTO). 2012. *Intellectual Property: Protection and Enforcement*. www.wto.org/english/thewto_e/whatis_e/tif_e/agrm7_e.htm (last accessed December 2013).

Chapter 12

Global Health Policy Responses to the World's Neglected Diseases

Mary Moran

Abstract

Today many different pharmaceuticals are available to diagnose, prevent, and treat illnesses that are common in the West. But pharmaceutical products may not exist for diseases that disproportionately affect poor patients of the developing world, also known as neglected diseases. Governments usually entrust pharmaceutical research and development (R&D) to the market, which is motivated by profit and prioritizes R&D for medicines of high market value. Under this model, market-driven R&D for neglected diseases has been extremely limited. Fortunately, since 2000 there has been a remarkable resurgence of interest and activity in R&D for neglected diseases by the not-for-profit community, industry, and major philanthropists. But this renewed interest has not been matched by a similar policy commitment, with views divided on how to best fund and incentivize neglected disease R&D between market-based and non-market-based solutions. Market-based solutions, such as procurement funds, innovation prizes, and advance market commitments, use profits to "pull" or "push" the pharmaceutical industry to innovate, and have private intellectual property rights (IPRs) at their center. Non-market-based solutions, such as product development partnerships and patent pools, delink R&D from profits and allow the public and philanthropic sectors to directly pay for and control innovation. The tension between market-based and non-market-based solutions has become evident through a long and divisive debate on funding and incentive options for neglected disease R&D hosted by the World Health Organization. This tension has held up progress on neglected disease R&D funding policy for over a decade, with the debate increasingly taken hostage by discussions on public or private "ownership" of IPRs and pharmaceutical development for the developing world. To improve neglected disease R&D policy and to continue delivering new medicines to patients in the developing world, we must delink debates on R&D from debates on access to IP-protected commercial medicines.

The Handbook of Global Health Policy, First Edition. Edited by Garrett W. Brown, Gavin Yamey, and Sarah Wamala.
© 2014 John Wiley & Sons, Ltd. Published 2014 by John Wiley & Sons, Ltd.

Key Points

- Neglected diseases are diseases that occur predominantly in the developing world for which there is insufficient research and development (R&D) of suitable drugs, vaccines, diagnostics, and other pharmaceutical tools.
- Since 2000 there has been a resurgence of interest and activity in R&D for neglected diseases but this has not been matched by an effective policy commitment.
- Progress on neglected disease R&D funding policy has been held up by divisions between supporters of market-based solutions and supporters of publicly driven non-market solutions.
- Policy clarity has been obscured by conflation of neglected disease R&D issues (there is no market) with intellectual property rights and access issues (a market exists but does not include developing country patients).
- Improving neglected disease R&D policy is not about delinking R&D from profits but about delinking debates on R&D from debates on access to intellectual property (IP) protected commercial medicines.

Key Policy Implications

- Policy progress will continue to flounder without acceptance that there are workable solutions that support both market and non-market approaches to making new neglected disease medicines.
- The debate on funding and incentive policies for neglected disease R&D needs to be revitalized and clarified by separating it from debates on access to IP-protected commercial medicines.

What is a Neglected Disease?

Today, many different pharmaceuticals are available to diagnose, prevent, and treat serious illnesses such as cervical cancer, asthma, or heart disease as well as less life-threatening conditions such as hay fever or insomnia. However, for millions of patients in the developing world who have diseases such as sleeping sickness, Chagas' disease, or malaria – which are rarely found in the West – the situation is very different: diagnostic tests, drug treatment, or suitable vaccines may not exist, even for the most life-threatening diseases. Such diseases of the South that lack control tools are called the "neglected diseases." The Commission on Macroeconomics and Health (2001) classifies diseases into three types, of which types II and III are considered to be neglected (Box 12.1).

Box 12.1   The Commission on Macroeconomics and Health's Classification of Diseases

- **Type I:** Diseases that occur in both the North and South, such as diabetes, hypertension, and pneumonia. Given the potential for pharmaceutical companies to make large profits from sales in the North, there is substantial market-driven R&D related to type I diseases.
- **Type II:** Diseases that occur predominantly but not exclusively in the South, such as tuberculosis and malaria, with some market-driven R&D but not enough or not suitable to the South.
- **Type III:** Diseases that are virtually all in the South, such as the classic "tropical diseases of poverty" (Hotez 2011), including sleeping sickness, leprosy, and worm infestations, with no market-driven R&D.

In this chapter, I begin by exploring why such diseases are neglected and how the outlook for neglected diseases has begun to change over the last decade. I then examine potential policy solutions, including market-based solutions, such as "pull" and "push" incentives, procurement funds, innovation prizes, and advance market commitments, as well as non-market solutions, such as patent pools and non-profit drug development companies. The chapter ends by looking at some of the key debates and controversies surrounding these various policy approaches. Throughout the chapter, the term "medicines" is used as shorthand for all pharmaceutical products including drugs, vaccines, diagnostics, microbicides, and vector control products.

Why are They Neglected?

Governments have placed the responsibility for research and development (R&D) of new drugs, vaccines, and diagnostics in the hands of the market, in particular pharmaceutical companies. Companies make R&D choices, fund the research, do the work, and take the risks – and then charge sufficiently high prices to governments and patients to recover their investments and losses and maximize profits. Under this model, innovation – the creation of new medicines – is stimulated by the promise of profits, which are in turn created and protected by intellectual property rights (IPRs) such as patents. As discussed in greater detail in Chapter 22, patent owners can reap profits because the patents grant them a monopoly right to the market for their product: a patent is thus only as valuable as the market it represents.

Governments on the whole have a low appetite for risk, short-term horizons, and a mixed record of picking winners, and they are highly sensitive to accusations of failure. Most therefore see major benefits in leaving the risky project of pharmaceutical development to the private sector. However, doing so has two key drawbacks. First, it leads to high prices for those medicines that are successfully developed, because prices must not only cover costs but also deliver profits to shareholders who have risked their funds. These high prices in turn reduce access for poor patients. Second, it means that diseases of low market value are neglected, since R&D priorities are selected by companies based on potential profits rather than on public health criteria. Such selection based on profit potential explains the lack of commercial activity for both orphan diseases in the West, defined as rare diseases that affect only a very small percentage of the population, and neglected diseases of the developing world.

Although these two problems – lack of access and lack of R&D – have very different causes, mechanisms, and solutions, they are frequently conflated. This conflation has resulted in significant confusion in the policy debate on neglected diseases, impeding the ability of policy-makers to agree the way forward.

The Decade of Change

Prior to 2000, there was very little R&D for neglected diseases. The medicine pipelines were empty, investment was limited, and there were few incentives to develop new commodities (and none of these were tailored specifically to developing world diseases). Of the 1393 new products marketed between 1975 and 1999, only 16 were for neglected diseases (Trouiller *et al.* 2002). The lack of medicines for these diseases was not on the radar of the international health community, whose attention was focused elsewhere, including on the complex issues of patents and access to medicines that had been spotlighted by the impact of HIV/AIDS on the developing world (see Chapters 13 and 25).

However, since 2000 there has been a remarkable resurgence of interest and activity in R&D for neglected diseases. The not-for-profit community began to highlight lack of R&D as well as lack of access in its campaigns; major philanthropists such as the Bill & Melinda Gates Foundation began putting up the funds needed in this high-risk entrepreneurial area; and industry – surprised and confronted by the reaction to its antiretroviral medicines patent policies – saw the need to address other areas of corporate social responsibility, including neglected disease R&D.

The inception of Product Development Partnerships (PDPs) for neglected disease R&D was also a key factor. For the first time, these provided a route for academics, industry, and public institutions to contribute to making neglected disease products without having to take on the entire risk and cost alone, since the PDP brought in other collaborators and funders. PDPs were energetic advocates for neglected disease R&D, raising not only attention but also billions of dollars in grants from governments and R&D contributions from companies who had previously been unaware, uninterested, or unable to see a safe controlled way to contribute to the multimillion dollar task of making not-for-profit medicines. Between 2007 and 2010, PDPs raised over US$2 billion for neglected disease R&D (Moran *et al.* 2011).

The public sector has been both less agile and less committed in the field of neglected disease R&D, with a handful of honorable exceptions, including the United States, United Kingdom, and several smaller countries that are relatively large contributors of R&D funding, such as Ireland, the Netherlands, Norway, and Sweden. However, most G20 governments – and some G8 governments – provide less than $10 million per year to

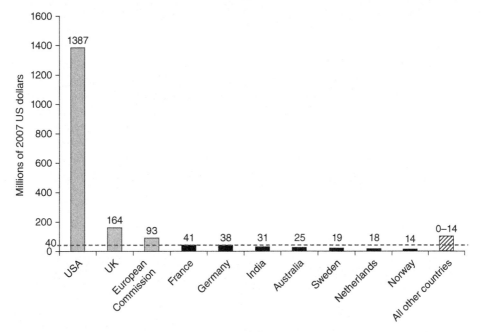

Figure 12.1   Government funding of neglected disease research and development, 2010. Source: Moran *et al.* (2011: 71).

neglected disease R&D (Moran *et al.* 2011), a paltry sum for these multibillion dollar economies (Figure 12.1).

Policy Responses to Neglected Disease R&D

This renewed vigor and commitment in the R&D arena has not been matched by a similar policy commitment. The World Health Organization (WHO) has hosted a long and divisive debate on which funding and incentive options might work best; while policymakers, working in parallel, have suggested or tried a range of funding and incentive options themselves. However, as of 2012, views still diverge on how best to fund and incentivize neglected disease R&D.

The key to understanding this fraught area is to realize that, underneath the multiplicity of complex and sometimes technical proposals, there is a simple but strongly held ideological divide between proponents of health R&D proposals based on market approaches and private IPRs, and those based on public approaches and public health goods. This divide explains both the diversity of proposals and the difficulty of reaching consensus. Similar debates have been seen in other areas that involve provision of essential services to populations, including water, electricity, telecommunications, health insurance, and education, with some firmly believing these are public responsibilities and others equally firmly believing the market mechanism is more efficient.

Market-Based Solutions

Market-based solutions to create medicines for neglected diseases are based on the profit principle: these solutions use profits to incentivize the pharmaceutical industry to innovate, and have private IPRs at their center.

Market supporters believe theirs is the most efficient system. They distrust government intervention (and sometimes judgment), are averse to creating public systems in parallel to the private market, and strongly support private IPRs as a key tool in profits, markets, and innovation. Some supporters also believe that only the private pharmaceutical industry has the necessary skills to create, develop, and manufacture new products for neglected diseases. Market-based solutions are often supported by originator pharmaceutical companies and western governments who host these. For instance, the United States has led the way on several of the market-based solutions outlined below, including orphan incentives and Priority Review Vouchers (PRVs), and is now discussing market-based prizes.

There are two types of market-based solutions: those that increase neglected disease profits from private markets (consumer sales), and those that use public funds to create neglected disease markets where no private market exists.

Increasing neglected disease profits from private markets (consumer sales)

These approaches aim to make neglected disease R&D more commercially attractive by increasing profits, though increasing financial returns ("pull" incentives), decreasing R&D costs ("push" incentives), or both (Box 12.2).

Box 12.2   Pull and Push Incentives for Neglected Disease R&D

Pull incentives (consumer-funded)

- Orphan legislation gives 10 years of market exclusivity on sales of a neglected disease product registered in the United States or Europe. However, it has a very low incentive value as there are so few consumers (patients with neglected diseases) in these regions.
- In the United States, PRVs reward companies who register a new drug for neglected diseases with rapid regulatory review of an unrelated commercial drug, which can then get to market sales more quickly. The estimated value of a PRV ranges from $50 million to $300 million (Ridley *et al.* 2006).
- Transferable IPR (TIPR) is a proposal to give several years of additional patent life on an unrelated commercial product as a reward for making a neglected disease product. Its estimated value is in the tens of billions if the extension were on a "blockbuster" product.

Push incentives (government funded)

- R&D grant programs – such as the US Small Business Innovation Research Program and the UK Small Business Research Initiative – give research grants to small businesses to support their neglected disease programs.
- Some governments give companies a tax credit for a fixed proportion (e.g., 50%) of their neglected disease R&D expenses.
- Orphan legislation normally also includes some push funding in the form of grants, faster regulatory review, or tax credits.

How does industry deal with low-profit neglected disease markets? When faced with low-profit markets, companies often reduce their R&D investment to match the size of

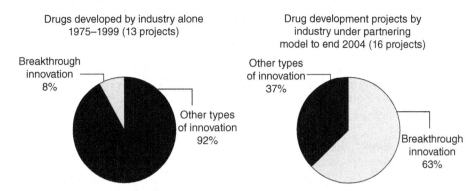

Figure 12.2 Level of innovation in company neglected disease programs. Source: Moran *et al.* (2005: 51).

the reward. Between 1975 and 1999, only 8% of neglected disease drugs developed by industry were breakthrough innovation (Trouiller *et al.* 2002), with companies squeezing a profit out of these areas by focusing on lower cost label extensions, reformulations, and re-registrations. Industry activity and innovation levels increased significantly after 2000 when companies could work in partnerships that provided grant support to company programs (Figure 12.2).

Creating public markets   Unlike private market approaches, public market incentives do not attempt to make developing country markets more commercial. Instead, they use public and philanthropic funds to create a neglected disease "market" that will act as a "pull" incentive to stimulate industry innovation.

Two common public market approaches are procurement funds and market-based prizes (prizes can also be constructed outside the market, as discussed later), while the recent Advance Market Commitment (AMC) is a combination of both.

Multilateral procurement funds   Procurement funds have, over many years, successfully created a multibillion pharmaceutical market using public and philanthropic cash. Three multilateral financing agencies alone – UNITAID, the Global Fund to Fight AIDS, Tuberculosis and Malaria (the Global Fund), and the GAVI Alliance (GAVI) – received over $4 billion from public, private, and philanthropic donors in 2011 (GAVI Alliance 2012; Global Fund 2012; UNITAID 2012). Although chiefly designed to buy products that already exist, some of these billion-dollar procurement funds have also recently begun to have a role in stimulating R&D.

In the past, procurement funds focused on stretching their dollars by competitively driving prices down to manufacturing-cost levels that excluded R&D cost, and therefore primarily created a market for generic versions of existing products rather than stimulating costly R&D of novel products. This focus has recently begun to change. Some funds have begun publishing specifications for desired new product combinations or formulations that do not yet exist, thus generating (admittedly low) innovation from generic companies. GAVI is increasingly looking at its potential influence or role in upstream R&D and also hosts the AMC, discussed later. In the R&D field, these funds have the added advantage that they use a model that industry understands and responds to. Companies develop the products on their own, retain full IPRs to them, and negotiate commercial contracts with the funds at prices that deliver them a profit.

Market-based prizes Market-based prizes are the opposite of procurement funds in the sense that they use public and philanthropic funds to pay for R&D (the innovation) but not for purchase of the final products. Prize proposals may therefore need to be twinned with purchase agreements to complete the circle.

In market-based prizes, the winner receives a one-off payment (the prize) for successfully creating the stipulated product, and retains the IPRs and market rights to that product. Examples include:

- *The "Innocentive" prizes.* Inventors compete to solve a problem and can then sell their successful solution to a pharmaceutical firm or convert it into equity in that firm. Innocentive prizes are mainly for early research and in the commercial area, although the Rockefeller Foundation has put up a similar prize in the neglected disease area.
- *Milestone prizes.* Rather than a single end-prize, these propose a series of prizes sized to match commercial risk and profit profiles at key points along a product development pathway. One proposal, the BIO Ventures for Global Health (BVGH) milestone prize for a developing country fever diagnostic, includes a proposed attached purchase agreement of $2–5 per test (funded by public and philanthropic donors) to make up for the lack of a commercial market.

Advance market commitment Under the AMC, GAVI has offered companies a $1.3 billion advance procurement agreement, funded through public and philanthropic dollars, as an incentive to adapt commercial pneumonia vaccines to include developing country strains. The AMC is essentially a cross between a prize and a procurement fund: a prize in the sense that a payment was offered for creating a product that did not yet exist, and a procurement fund because the payment was in the form of a guaranteed purchase of hundreds of millions of doses at a profitable average price. The AMC was a world first in that it generated higher innovation products by deliberately offering a higher per unit vaccine price that covered company R&D costs and included a modest profit margin.

Do market-based incentives work for neglected disease R&D? Market-based incentives can undoubtedly generate innovation, but they are generally undersized as public funders are rarely willing to put up the large amounts needed to create a true market. Such incentives also have a high risk of creating products that are unaffordable for patients in the developing world without additional or complementary public subsidy or purchase funds. They therefore work best in lower cost, lower innovation areas. In higher cost, higher innovation areas they tend to primarily act as top-ups to existing neglected disease R&D programs rather than standalone incentives (Figure 12.3).

Governments often like market incentives as they leave the risks, choices, and management of neglected disease R&D to industry: the government "only pays for success." However, these incentives are not a natural fit with neglected diseases – it is politically difficult and often prohibitively expensive to turn a non-market into a market. Billions of dollars would normally be required to incentivize companies to devote their R&D programs, staff, infrastructure, and shareholder funding to development of a drug for neglected diseases rather than a commercial antihypertensive, and these billions would need to be provided over many years to draw in and retain sufficient companies to create a sustainable neglected disease industry and product pipeline. Even one-off market incentives to create a single neglected disease product are expensive, since "one-off" does not

	PRIVATE MARKET {CONSUMERS}		PUBLIC MARKET	
MARKET PULL	• PRV and TIPR (western consumers)	•Orphan (western ND patients)	•Procurement funds / AMC	• Prizes (market based)
PUBLIC PUSH FUNDING	• R&D grants and tax credits			

Figure 12.3 Market-based incentives. AMC, Advance Market Commitment; ND, neglected disease; PRV, priority review voucher; R&D, research and development; TIPR, transferable intellectual property rights.

really exist in the world of research, where years of investment and long pipelines may be needed to create one successful product.

Thus, while governments like the notion of hands-off management and low risk that market incentives imply, they tend to underestimate (or shy away from) the scale of profits needed to create a successful neglected disease market incentive. Incentives that are large enough to motivate companies, such as the proposed billion dollar TIPR, often also meet resistance from taxpayers ("Why should we give billions to already-rich companies to make products for Africa?").

On the other hand, more modestly sized private market incentives (e.g., orphan incentives and the PRV) are generally too small to generate more than low-cost, low-innovation R&D. The only "new" neglected disease drug to claim a PRV was the antimalarial artemether-lumefantrine (Coartem), which had been used in developing countries for over a decade prior to being registered in the United States to trigger the PRV "payout." Similarly, a 2005 review showed that 70% of neglected disease orphan products registered in the United States were low or no innovation (Moran *et al.* unpublished data). However, groups with existing neglected disease R&D programs can find these incentives a useful source of "top up" funding for their programs. For example, PDPs applied for orphan benefits for the antimalarial dihydroartemisinin-piperaquine (Eurartesim), the tuberculosis drug candidate PA-824, and paromomycin to treat visceral leishmaniasis.

Public market incentives share the same "sizing" difficulty as their private market brethren. Procurement funds are rarely, if ever, large enough to cover the costs of innovation, and are intrinsically less reliable than private market incentives driven by largely stable consumer demand. Governments struggling with economic downturns can cut or cancel their contributions, as happened with the Global Fund in 2011, and funds can change their purchasing policies mid-stream, when companies have already made substantial R&D investments (e.g., changing antiretroviral (ARV) protocols).

While market-based prizes avoid these uncertainties – once a prize is in place it is very unlikely to be revoked – they share the general problem of undersizing seen with virtually all publicly funded incentives. No firm would invest $0.5 billion into malaria vaccine

R&D merely to secure a breakeven $0.5 billion prize. To be successful, prizes therefore either need to be large enough to compete with other commercial markets (hundreds of millions of dollars in addition to R&D cost coverage, except for very low cost areas such as simple diagnostics) or they need to be attached to a procurement agreement that guarantees a volume of profitable sales, such as the BVGH prize proposal.

At first sight, GAVI's pneumococcal vaccine AMC seems the exception to the mismatch problem between commercial expectations and funder willingness. The AMC raised $1.3 billion in public and philanthropic funds, and successfully stimulated GlaxoSmithKline (GSK) and Pfizer to develop pneumonia vaccines adapted for developing countries. However, on closer inspection, this was not because the public market pull was big enough to create a new developing world vaccine (it was not), but because the R&D costs could be heavily cross-subsidized from companies' commercial pneumonia vaccine programs (commercial sales of Pfizer's 13-valent pneumococcal conjugate vaccine (Prevnar 13) exceed $3 billion per year (VisionGain 2012)). Even so, the subsidized $1.3 billion price tag left many public funders baulking at the thought of another AMC.

Public push funding, on the other hand, makes no pretence of being anything other than a welcome top-up, aimed at tipping the return on investment equation for those with existing R&D programs. In this, such funding has been successful: 70% of companies involved in registering new neglected disease products since 2000 received public funding support (Policy Cures 2012).

Access and equity   For patients in the developing world, private market-based approaches can present a fundamental problem. Private market incentives are designed to cover R&D costs and include profit margins, but developing countries often cannot afford these higher prices without negotiation of charitable pricing programs or development of additional public subsidy or procurement programs. For instance, the AMC includes a public subsidy for GAVI countries, who pay $0.20 per vaccine instead of the $7 per vaccine price negotiated under the AMC. The price of artemether-lumefantrine (Coartem) fell from $2.40 per treatment in 1999 (WHO 2002) to an average of $0.76 per treatment a decade later (Medicines for Malaria Venture 2009). Most of this price drop was achieved through an agreement with the WHO to aim for $1 per dose (WHO 2012), and to economies of scale in manufacturing and a drop in the price of raw artemisinin (the main ingredient). Private market incentives that do not include, or are not affiliated with, a public subsidy program can mean greatly reduced – or even no – access for patients in the developing world. For instance, many neglected disease products developed in response to US orphan incentives, but without accompanying procurement agreements, were essentially unavailable to developing countries, such as amphotericin B (AmBisome) for visceral leishmaniasis at $350 per treatment and 4-aminosalicylic acid (PAS) for tuberculosis at $2700 per treatment (Moran *et al.* 2005).

Whether affordable or not, all private market approaches necessarily reduce access to the final product for patients in developing countries, since the number of patients that can be treated at any for-profit price point is logically lower than the number that could be treated at a not-for-profit price point. Supporters of market-based incentives argue that this is a reasonable price to pay if the R&D would otherwise not be done, or would be done more slowly. Others note that additional public funding can be used to subsidize developing world prices, but this is a circular argument since these public funds could still have been used to buy more lower priced product for more patients. The debate continues.

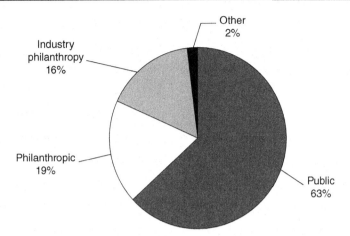

Figure 12.4   Neglected disease research and development funders. Source: Moran *et al.* (2011: 69).

Non-Market-Based Solutions

In contrast to market approaches, non-market solutions accept that neglected diseases are an area of market failure, and therefore a public rather than an industry responsibility.

Under these approaches, innovation is not stimulated by profits generated through price mark-ups to paying patients, nor is it funded through these profits (by definition these are non-existent for neglected diseases). R&D is therefore said to be "delinked" from price. This delinkage removes both the incentive for R&D (profit) and the funding source for R&D (shareholder funds), therefore the public and philanthropic sectors must now pay for and control innovation directly.

Non-market approaches have two hallmarks. The first is that R&D is directly funded by the public and philanthropic sectors, including industry philanthropy (Figure 12.4). Since the costs of R&D are covered, the resulting products can be manufactured at close to manufacturing cost-price by the intellectual property (IP) holder (usually a company) or through non-exclusive licenses to generic firms.

The second hallmark of non-market approaches is that, in the absence of profits, IPRs are largely valueless; they therefore no longer have a central or incentivizing role, instead being chiefly used for functional management of ownership and contracts. Because IPRs have little or no value they tend to be shared more freely through patent pools; licenses tend to be non-exclusive; and product development is often collaborative between the IPR holder and others.

There are many examples of non-market approaches:

- The most common are PDPs such as the Meningitis Vaccine Project (MVP), Medicines for Malaria Venture (MMV), TB Alliance, and International AIDS Vaccine Initiative (IAVI). These are not-for-profit organizations that bring together academics, originator companies, generic companies, and contract research organizations to discover and develop new neglected disease products, with public and philanthropic investors providing the funding. PDPs generally manage a portfolio of products, using industry principles and management styles to do so, but they select R&D based on health returns rather than returns on investment and the final products are produced at low or non-profit prices.

- Company not-for-profit neglected disease ventures. Most large companies now partner with PDPs (e.g., GSK through its Tres Cantos Medicines Development Campus in Spain, and Novartis through the Novartis Institute for Tropical Diseases in Singapore), while some also have standalone neglected disease operations (e.g., the Sanofi-aventis malaria program).

An important variant   There is an important variant of the non-market approach. Supporters of the non-market approach believe there is little or no place in health R&D for the market, profits, or the private IPRs that are the engine of these profits. The market, they believe, leaves R&D choices at the mercy of industry profit-seeking and bars poor patients from access to high-priced patented drugs controlled by companies. Instead, supporters of non-market approaches seek a new system of pharmaceutical development, controlled and funded by the public sector, which is focused "on patients not profits." Intrinsic to this stance is a belief that there should be no private ownership of intellectual property in the health field (and sometimes in other fields also): "no private ownership of the right to life." Thus, even if a company produces neglected disease medicines as a philanthropic activity or at non-profit prices this is still not enough. Or rather, it is not as good as the company handing over control of their IP through non-exclusive licensing to generics or, even better, putting the IP in the public domain for anyone to use.

These approaches prioritize proposals that minimize the role of IPRs and IP holders in favor of development of inventions as non-exclusive generics or as public goods, including the following:

- *Patent pools.* Companies put their IPRs into a public pool, from which non-exclusive licenses can be given to as many generic firms as are interested. An example is the Medicines Patent Pool, established by UNITAID in December 2009 and now an independent legal entity (Evidence to Policy initiative 2011), under which IP holders donate patents to their HIV drugs for use by generic firms.
- *Open source.* Open source is an IP-free approach, similar to Linux in software. Multiple collaborators are encouraged to work on a problem and to share their ideas and findings publically, with IP being in the public domain.
- *Non-market prizes.* These differ from market prizes in that the inventor hands over their IPRs to the prize-giver in return for the reward (i.e., inventors do not hold the IPRs or marketing rights to the product they have developed). This allows the IPRs to move into the public domain and to be reproduced cheaply by generic firms for health needs.

The binding convention on R&D to meet the health needs of developing countries
The Binding Convention was proposed by the WHO Consultative Expert Working Group on R&D (CEWG), who included it as a recommendation in its report to the 2012 World Health Assembly (WHA) (Consultative Expert Working Group on Research and Development 2012). The Convention proposes a new way to fund health R&D, especially product development, for the developing world. It is based on the R&D Treaty initially proposed by the Consumer Project on Technology (CPTech) and Tim Hubbard from the Sanger Institute together with a range of civil society organizations (CPTech 2005). A form of treaty or convention have been discussed in the WHA since 2003 and Member States agreed at the 2012 WHA to consider the proposed Binding Convention in the run-up to the next World Health Assembly in 2013.

The Binding Convention would mandate signatory countries to invest 0.01% of their gross domestic product into publicly funded and managed global health R&D for developing countries. Governments would preferentially use non-IPR-based approaches such as patent pools, open source, and non-market prizes and the resulting research and products would ideally be put in the public domain, free of IP ownership. Up to 20–50% of this funding would be channeled to a central organization (managed by the WHO or a similar multilateral organization) with the remainder under the control of governments themselves. The Convention would cover R&D for neglected diseases, as well as research to address specific developing world needs for type I diseases (e.g., R&D of a heat-stable insulin).

Those with more stringent views on IP ownership believe the Convention should also fund public R&D of essential medicines for type I diseases such as cancer, high blood pressure, and heart disease. They argue that this investment is needed to improve access to life-saving essential medicines for developing countries, and is a necessary step in removing pharmaceutical industry control over development of essential health products.

Do non-market approaches work for neglected disease R&D? Non-market approaches work: they have generated 80% of new neglected disease drugs and vaccines registered since 2000 (Policy Cures 2012). However, they require substantial ongoing public funding, and high levels of government intervention, decision-making, and risk.

Non-market approaches dominate neglected disease R&D: there are currently over 350 product candidates for type II and III diseases in development and over 40 new neglected disease products were registered between 2000 and 2011 (Policy Cures 2012), supported by over $3 billion per year in public and charitable funds (Moran *et al.* 2011).

These approaches have a number of advantages. They give governments full control over R&D choices and are usually substantially cheaper than industry R&D: for example, $250 million to create a novel drug (Policy Cures 2011) compared with the industry estimate of $1.3 billion (Tufts Center for the Study of Drug Development 2011). However, perhaps the greatest advantage of non-market approaches is for patients in the developing world. Products developed under these approaches are generally highly suitable for patients in developing countries (from the start, R&D is targeted at these countries, and not at commercial use) and are nearly always provided at low or non-profit prices. For instance, PDPs have developed a meningitis A vaccine for $0.50 per dose, and the Shanchol cholera vaccine for $1.85 per dose (Maskery *et al.* 2011). Prices are kept low because companies working in these non-market areas agree to use the "no profit, no loss" approach, and access pricing is a standard condition in PDP contracts.

But there are drawbacks. As with all publicly funded initiatives (including public "markets"), non-market approaches rely on consistent long-term government and philanthropic funding – which is at the mercy of politics, domestic financing, and global economic crises. And they are very hard work for governments. Since industry is not in control, the public sector has to take on the risks, costs, scientific choices, and repeated failures of pharmaceutical development itself. Some governments manage this by funding through PDPs, who conduct these tasks on their behalf. Indeed, small funders can find that PDPs are the only feasible way to provide neglected disease R&D funding in these complex areas. For example, aid agencies in the Netherlands, Ireland, Norway, Spain, and Belgium provide 100% of their neglected disease R&D funding through PDPs (Moran *et al.* 2011). However, many other governments simply drop the ball, providing little or no neglected disease R&D funding through PDPs or otherwise.

There are also specific difficulties associated with variants that focus primarily on IPRs, as these can sometimes leave aside or deprioritize R&D aspects. For instance, the most stringent advocates against private IP ownership not only decry private market solutions for neglected disease R&D but also many non-market approaches – even when these promise to create, or have created, effective new non-profit medicines for developing countries. For instance, these advocates have been highly critical of PDPs and of the HIV Medicines Alliance, which is a proposed collaboration between multilateral agencies, governments, donors, pharmaceutical companies, and generic manufacturers to create optimized low-cost ARVs for the developing world, seeing these public–private collaborations as "smokescreens" that continue to underwrite private company ownership of IP (Don't Trade Our Lives Away 2012).

Debates and Controversies

The tension between these two very different sets of policies and proposals – between those who believe health R&D should be left to the market and those who believe it is the responsibility of the public sector – has held up progress on neglected disease R&D funding policy for over a decade.

R&D for neglected diseases has increasingly been taken hostage by IP "warriors" on both sides of the fence. On one side are pharmaceutical companies, who come to this issue from a background of protecting their IP, the lifeblood of their business. On the other side are developing countries and non-governmental organizations, who come to this issue through the terrible inequity of access to patented AIDS and cancer drugs.

The terrible irony is that IP issues are largely irrelevant in the neglected disease area where markets, by definition, do not exist; where IPRs are valueless and widely shared; and where health-focused R&D, cost-pricing, and public funding and control of R&D are the norm. R&D for neglected diseases is already delinked from profits (there are none to be had) and the public and philanthropic sectors (including industry philanthropy) have been addressing their responsibilities in this area for over a decade to remarkable effect.

The current landscape of R&D for neglected diseases is not perfect. More could be done. Nevertheless, it is largely working. While IP debates have been raging, funders and developers have been quietly getting on with creating and registering dozens of new neglected disease products, and dozens more are in the pipeline. Such funders and developers have made the first pediatric antimalarial medicine, a meningitis vaccine that has transformed the African meningitis belt, and the first visceral leishmaniasis treatment that is affordable for developing countries.

Yet the debate continues as heatedly as if the last decade had never happened. Partly this reflects the nature and interests of the protagonists, but there has also been a disturbing tendency in policy debates to link or conflate neglected disease R&D with IPRs and access issues. This linkage is sometimes due to a genuine misunderstanding of their differences, but it has also been used deliberately in an attempt to use widespread global support for increased neglected disease R&D to shoehorn in the less widely supported notion of a more open global IPR regime for pharmaceuticals. This policy conflation between R&D and access has featured prominently in the WHO processes, from the Commission on Intellectual Property Rights, Innovation and Public Health (2003) through the Intergovernmental Working Group on Public Health, Innovation and Intellectual Property (2006–2008), Expert Working Group on Research and Development Financing (2008–2010) and CEWG (2010–2012).

In practice, this linkage has proved very unhelpful, slowing down progress on neglected disease R&D without adding to the debate on access to medicines. Improving neglected disease R&D policy is not about delinking R&D from profits (such profits are already delinked when it comes to neglected diseases). Rather it is about delinking debates on R&D from debates on access to IP-protected commercial medicines. These two important problems have different causes and mechanisms, and will need different solutions if we are to deliver new medicines to patients in the developing world – patients who continue to die while patiently waiting for the global health community to settle its differences.

Key Reading

Center for Global Health R&D Policy Assessment. 2012. *Policy Innovations. 2012.* http://healthresearchpolicy.org/innovation (last accessed December 2013).

CEWG (Consultative Expert Working Group on Research and Development: Financing and Coordination). 2012. *Research and Development to Meet Health Needs in Developing Countries: Strengthening Global Financing and Coordination.* http://www.who.int/phi/CEWG_Report_5_April_2012.pdf (last accessed December 2013).

De Ferranti D, Griffin C, Escobar ML, Glassman A, Lagomarsino G. 2008. *Innovative Financing for Global Health: Tools for Analyzing the Options.* Global Health Financing Initiative, Working Paper No. 2. Washington, DC: Brookings Institution.

Hecht R, Wilson P, Palriwala A. 2009. Improving health R&D financing for developing countries: a menu of innovative policy options. *Health Affairs* 28(4), 974–85.

Moran M, Guzman J, Abela-Oversteegen L *et al.* 2011. *Neglected Disease Research and Development: Is Innovation Under Threat?* Sydney: Policy Cures.

Toreele E, Usdin M, Chirac P. 2004. *A needs-based pharmaceutical R&D agenda for neglected diseases.* Geneva: World Health Organization. http://www.who.int/intellectualproperty/topics/research/Needs%20based%20R&D%20for%20neglected%20diseases%20Els%20Pierre%20Martine.pdf (last accessed December 2013).

Trouiller P, Olliaro P, Toreele E, Orbinski J, Laing R, Ford N. 2002. Drug development for neglected diseases: a deficient market and a public-health policy failure. *Lancet* 359(9324), 2188–94.

References

CEWG (Consultative Expert Working Group on Research and Development: Financing and Coordination). 2012. *Research and Development to Meet Health Needs in Developing Countries: Strengthening Global Financing and Coordination.* http://www.who.int/phi/CEWG_Report_5_April_2012.pdf (last accessed December 2013).

Commission on Macroeconomics and Health. 2001. *Macroeconomics and Health: Investing in Health for Economic Development.* http://whqlibdoc.who.int/publications/2001/924154550x.pdf (last accessed December 2013).

CPTech. 2005. *Letter to ask World Health Organization to evaluate new treaty framework for medical research and development.* http://www.cptech.org/workingdrafts/rndsignonletter.html (last accessed December 2013).

Don't Trade Our Lives Away. 2012. *Brook Baker: Proposed HIV Medicines Alliance – promise or peril.* http://donttradeourlivesaway.wordpress.com/2012/07/10/brook-baker-proposed-hiv-medicines-alliance-promise-or-peril (last accessed December 2013).

GAVI Alliance. 2012. *Key figures: donor contributions and pledges.* http://www.gavialliance.org/funding/donor-contributions-pledges/ (last accessed December 2013).

Global Fund (Global Fund to Fight AIDS, Tuberculosis and Malaria). 2012. *Donors and contributions*. http://www.theglobalfund.org/en/about/donors/ (last accessed December 2013).

Hotez PJ. 2011. The neglected tropical diseases and the neglected infections of poverty: overview of their common features, global disease burden and distribution, new control tools, and prospects for disease elimination. In Choffnes ER, Relman DA (eds) *The Causes and Impacts of Neglected Tropical and Zoonotic Diseases: Opportunities for Integrated Intervention Strategies*, pp. 221–36. Washington, DC: National Academies Press.

Maskery B, Levin A, DeRoeck D *et al.* 2011. *Oral Cholera Vaccines: An Investment Case*. http://apps.who.int/immunization/sage/SAGE_April_2011_cholera_investment_case.pdf (last accessed December 2013).

Medicines for Malaria Venture. 2009. *Price of Coartem® reduced for the third time in 8 years*. http://www.mmv.org/newsroom/news/price-coartem%C2%AE-reduced-third-time-8-years (last accessed December 2013).

Moran M, Guzman J, Abela-Oversteegen L *et al.* 2011. *Neglected Disease Research and Development: Is Innovation Under Threat?* Sydney: Policy Cures

Moran M, Ropars AL, Guzman J, Diaz J, Garrison C. 2005. *The New Landscape of Neglected Disease Drug Development*. London: London School of Economics and The Wellcome Trust.

Policy Cures. 2011. *Staying the Course? Malaria Research and Development in a Time of Economic Uncertainty*. http://policycures.org/downloads/Malaria%20Research%20and%20Development.pdf (last accessed December 2013).

Policy Cures. 2012. *Saving Lives and Creating Impact: Why Investing in Global Health Research Works*. http://policycures.org/downloads/Saving%20lives%20and%20creating%20impact.pdf (last accessed December 2013).

Ridley DB, Grabowski HG, Moe JL. 2006. Developing drugs for developing countries. *Health Affairs* 25(2), 313–24.

Trouiller P, Olliaro P, Toreele E, Orbinski J, Laing R, Ford N. 2002. Drug development for neglected diseases: a deficient market and a public-health policy failure. *Lancet* 359(9324): 2188–94.

Tufts Center for the Study of Drug Development. 2011. *Drug developers are aggressively changing the way they do R&D*. http://csdd.tufts.edu/news/complete_story/pr_outlook_2011 (last accessed December 2013).

UNITAID. 2012. *Audited Financial Report for the period 2010–2011*. http://www.unitaid.eu/images/budget/Financial%20Statements%202010%202011%20final%20%2028%2003%202012%20with%20auditors%20opinion.pdf (last accessed December 2013).

VisionGain. 2012. *World Vaccines Market 2012–2022*. http://www.visiongain.com/Report/859/World-Vaccines-Market-2012-2022 (last accessed December 2013).

WHO (World Health Organization). 2002. *Review of application for inclusion of a drug in the WHO essential list. Fixed Combination of Artemether and Lumefantrine. Coartem® CDS/RBM, 18 March 2002*. http://archives.who.int/eml/expcom/expcom12/coartem.doc (last accessed December 2013).

WHO (World Health Organization). 2012. *Procurement of artemether-lumefantrine (Coartem®) through WHO*. http://archives.who.int/tbs/access/CoA_website5.pdf (last accessed December 2013).

Chapter 13

The Fight for Global Access to Essential Health Commodities

Manica Balasegaram, Michelle Childs, and James Arkinstall

Abstract

The question of global equity in access to essential health commodities became a political priority and attracted considerable financial resources in the early years of the twenty-first century, largely due to strong international mobilization by civil society. Significant progress was made in reducing the incidence of and morbidity and mortality from major diseases, with a considerable impact made through increased access to medicines. However, at a time when donor support has started to decline, the question of access to essential health commodities has not been resolved. Medicines, diagnostics, and vaccines for many diseases continue to elude people living in the developing world. This lack of access to health commodities has three major causes: the commodities have not been developed for lack of a commercially viable market, they are ill-suited to the needs and conditions in developing countries, or they are priced at unaffordable levels.

Lowering the price of health commodities is therefore essential for developing countries. Price reductions can be achieved by limiting patentability criteria, overcoming patent barriers through lawful means, and resisting trade-related pressures from the pharmaceutical industry and from western governments that negatively impact access to medicines. More fundamentally, there is a need to develop alternative strategies to develop new commodities in a way that responds to developing country priorities and that breaks the link between the cost of research and the price of the final product. This "delinkage" ensures affordability of medical innovation from the outset. A new global convention for essential health research could provide an overarching framework to such strategies. Such a framework could prioritize medical needs over commercial incentives, serve as a tool to raise necessary funds, and steer innovation to ultimately overcome inequity in access to essential health commodities.

The Handbook of Global Health Policy, First Edition. Edited by Garrett W. Brown, Gavin Yamey, and Sarah Wamala.
© 2014 John Wiley & Sons, Ltd. Published 2014 by John Wiley & Sons, Ltd.

Key Points

- Developing countries continue to lack access to essential medicines, diagnostics, and vaccines for tackling infectious and non-communicable diseases.
- The commercial imperative driving medical innovation means that many urgently needed health commodities are left undeveloped and many existing commodities are often unsuitable for use in developing countries or are unaffordable.
- Voluntary or industry-driven means to lower commodity prices have been limited in scope, and more effective measures such as limiting or overcoming intellectual property rights have been fiercely opposed by the pharmaceutical industry and by western governments.
- Alternative models of innovation are needed to develop health commodities that respond to developing country needs and that ensure affordability of the final product from the outset.
- Such approaches, which couple innovation with access, should be coordinated through a global framework on essential research, so that medical priorities can be identified and funds raised and channeled towards areas of greatest need within a normative context that ensures access to the developed products.

Key Policy Implications

- In a context of dwindling donor resources for global health, innovative policy solutions must be found to reduce the price of medicines, diagnostics, and vaccines in developing countries.
- Alternative ways of conducting medical innovation must be supported, so that new life-saving health commodities can be developed to respond to developing country needs in ways that ensure affordability of the final product from the outset.
- Countries should agree to pursue talks towards establishing a global framework for essential health research and development, which could prioritize needs, serve as a tool to raise necessary funds, and steer medical innovation to overcome inequity in access to essential health commodities.

Introduction

The first 10 years of the twenty-first century have been labeled the "golden decade" for global health (von Schoen Angerer *et al.* 2012), or the "decade of health" (Dybul *et al.* 2012), in recognition of the major transformation that took place in the global health landscape. The period was marked by the rising importance of health on international political agendas and huge increases in financial resources targeted at health.

Development assistance for health increased from US$6 billion in 2000 to almost $30 billion in 2010 (IHME 2011). Donor commitments were solidified through the 2002 creation of the Global Fund to Fight AIDS, Tuberculosis and Malaria (the Global Fund), which Kofi Annan, former secretary general of the United Nations, called "a war chest to fight the diseases of poverty" (Annan 2012). The increased focus on global health in recent decades yielded incredible gains, including, for example, a 41% reduction in child mortality from 1990 to 2011 (UNICEF 2012) and a 33% decline in malaria mortality rates in sub-Saharan Africa over the past 10 years (WHO 2011).

The first years of the twenty-first century were also marked by a rapid transformation in the political landscape with regard to access to medicines, spurred by catalytic changes in the response to the AIDS epidemic in developing countries. The preceding decade (1990–2000) had been characterized by explosive growth of this epidemic in developing countries, especially in Africa (WHO 2004), coupled with a devastating lack of access to life-saving antiretroviral treatments (ARVs) that were, by then, broadly accessible in developed countries (Reich *et al.* 2005). In 2000, ARVs were priced at $10,000 per patient per year – out of reach of the vast majority of people living in developing countries (MSF 2001) – yet pharmaceutical firms repeatedly rebuffed efforts to lower prices for these populations (von Schoen Angerer *et al.* 2001). But, in the space of a few years, between 1999 and 2001, the landscape for affordable ARVs was completely transformed.

Civil society groups across the world who had for years been working in isolation – particularly in high-burden countries such as Thailand, India, South Africa, and Brazil – joined together in an international campaign that brought together AIDS activists, consumer groups, and international treatment providers. As a result, access to medicines made international headlines during the 1999 World Trade Organization (WTO) summit in Seattle, where the high price of ARVs to treat HIV/AIDS became a symbol of the world's inequities. Activist efforts were reinforced by the work of patent lawyers, doctors, health economists, and pharmacists who together provided rigorous evidence to inform policy.

The campaign for access to ARVs forced multinational pharmaceutical firms to make ground-breaking concessions. Generic competition triggered massive ARV price reductions that dropped prices by a factor of 10 by the end of 2000 – a watershed moment in the fight against the HIV/AIDS epidemic in developing countries (see Chapter 25). From 2000 to 2006, ongoing generic competition reduced ARV prices even further (Figure 13.1). Massive efforts to implement national HIV/AIDS programs, coupled with unprecedented financial commitments from donors, have since helped to put more than 9.7 million people on ARVs (UNAIDS 2013).

The influence of this campaign for access to ARVs went beyond price reductions for HIV treatments. In November 2001, this movement scored an important victory: amid fierce debates about the negative impact of trade agreements on access to medicines, members of the WTO adopted the Doha Declaration. The declaration affirmed countries' sovereign rights to protect public health when intellectual property stands in the way of access to medicines (WTO 2001). These developments gave rise to a broader access to

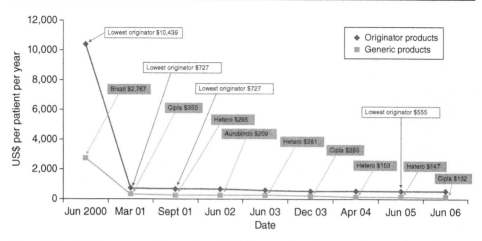

Figure 13.1   The lowest possible generic and originator prices of one year's treatment with stavu-dine/lamivudine/nevirapine. By maintaining artificially high prices, patent-backed monopolies can serve to deny people access to affordable medical tools. Generic competition acts to drive prices down. Source: MSF (2012a).

medicines movement that today advocates on behalf of millions of people who lack access to life-saving medical tools that are needed to prevent, detect, and treat disease.

Nevertheless, after a decade of significant progress in expanding access to treatment and reducing infectious disease incidence and mortality, urgent needs remain and new challenges lie ahead. In particular, many patients in low-income countries (LICs), particularly in the most marginalized and vulnerable communities, have not benefited from the advances of the last decade. Twenty-two million of the world's most vulnerable children fail to receive basic life-saving vaccinations every year (UNICEF/WHO 2012). Ninety percent of those with multidrug-resistant tuberculosis (TB) do not have access to treatment, and the few that do must endure a highly toxic, 2-year treatment regimen that can cost between $3,000 and $5,150 – and has only a one-in-two chance of curing them (Ahuja *et al.* 2012; IUATLD/MSF 2013). Under the 2013 World Health Organization (WHO) guidelines, the HIV treatment coverage in low- and middle-income countries represented only 34% of the 28.6 million people eligible in 2013 (UNAIDS 2013). Access to essential health commodities refers not only on the physical availability of a product (i.e., whether appropriate products have been developed to meet health needs), but also to whether those products are affordable to the populations that need them.

There are many factors in play in this dynamic of inequity. One of the most significant is the fact that today's global health research and development (R&D) priorities and access strategies are more market-driven or donor-driven than they are patient-driven. We begin by examining the current global system for medical innovation, which we argue is failing too many patients. We particularly focus on high commodity prices and the lack of R&D for neglected diseases and neglected populations. We then turn to potential global policy solutions that address high prices and that can tackle the "innovation crisis" so that greater equity in access to essential health commodities may be achieved.

The Medical Innovation System is Failing Many Patients

In the current predominant model that determines medical innovation and access to medical products, companies are incentivized to develop drugs and other medical tools based on the return on investment that the product will offer (WHO 2012). A company today seeks to recoup its R&D costs through sales revenues, so its R&D costs are inevitably "linked" to product prices.

Within this system, the best way to guarantee a return on investment is to control the market: ensure customers can pay a high price, and make sure no one else can sell the same product at a lower price. This kind of market control is achieved through obtaining patent protection and other exclusive rights that can protect products from competition. Patents on medicines, for example, give companies exclusive rights to sell their product at any price the market will bear for a period of time, usually 20 years (WTO 2006).

Consequently, the medical R&D system is driven by commercial incentives, not patient needs, and particularly not the needs of vulnerable and marginalized populations. This system creates three key problems, all of which have the direct consequence of inequity in access to medicines.

The First Problem: Medical Tools are Often Priced Out of Reach

Sustainable affordable pricing of health commodities – best achieved through robust generic competition – is vital to scaling-up access to healthcare in the developing world. But many factors, including increased use of patenting in the developing world and the resulting lack of price-reducing generic competition, mean that the prices of new vaccines, diagnostics, and medicines often remain prohibitively expensive.

Companies routinely price new products out of the reach of patients in developing countries. In these countries, where people usually pay for medical care out of pocket and very seldom have health insurance, the high price of medicines and other interventions can quickly become a question of life and death.

This situation is exacerbated by the fact that international trade rules now require the patenting of medicines in key producing countries like India and Brazil. In recent years, patent laws have been increasingly harmonized across many countries through the WTO's Agreement on Trade-Related Aspects of Intellectual Property Rights (TRIPS), the world's most comprehensive multilateral agreement on intellectual property. TRIPS is slated to be imposed on the least-developed countries (LDCs) in a few years, although the deadline was recently extended to 2021 following negotiations at the WTO. It is unclear, however, whether this new deadline covers pharmaceutical product patents, or whether LDCs will be forced to implement and enforce such patents by 2016 (WTO 2013).

We can already see the effects of increased patenting in the high prices of newer products. For example, newer first-line ARVs, such as raltegravir, which is patented in India and therefore exists only as an originator product, cost many times more than today's ARV regimens. Raltegravir costs at best $675 per year – in India Médecins Sans Frontières (MSF) is paying $1,775 – to which the price of two or more other drugs need to be added to form a complete treatment regimen. Today, the WHO-recommended first-line protocol of three drugs (including tenofovir) costs only $114–139 per year – but ARV treatment costs could obviously explode once these newer ARVs are widely used.

Demand for second-line HIV treatments is growing fast: an estimated 25–30% of people living with HIV in Africa now need second-line ARVs to avoid treatment failure, but only 3% are receiving them (UNAIDS 2012). Yet, as a result of increased patenting, the most affordable second-line HIV regimen today is twice as expensive as the recommended first-line regimen, and the price of a third-line regimen is more than 14 times higher (MSF 2013). Unless these prices are reduced, treatment providers are effectively facing a treatment time bomb, as more and more patients will need to be switched to more expensive regimens (APPG HIV/AIDS 2009).

Affordability is a critical issue in the area of vaccines too. Ten years ago, it cost countries less than $1.50 to buy the main WHO-recommended vaccines to protect a child's life. But today, the lowest price for the WHO-recommended package of vaccines has risen to nearly $40 for countries that are eligible for subsidies negotiated by the GAVI Alliance (GAVI), a public–private partnership that aims to increase access to immunization in poor countries. Many countries that are ineligible for GAVI subsidies, because their gross national income (GNI) per capita is above the $1,570 threshold, pay much more than $40. The skyrocketing prices are due not only to more vaccines being included in immunization programs, but also to new vaccines that cost much more than older traditional vaccines. The two newest vaccines – against rotavirus and pneumococcal disease – now make up almost three quarters of the total cost of vaccinating a child (Figure 13.2) (MSF 2012b).

As countries become wealthier and thus lose their GAVI eligibility, they face even higher vaccine prices. Today, thanks to GAVI subsidies, Honduras pays just $1.43 per child for both the rotavirus and pneumococcal conjugate vaccines. But in 2015, once it "graduates" – meaning it becomes ineligible for GAVI support due to its increased GNI per capita – the country will have to pay $15.60 per child for the two vaccines (MSF 2012b).

The affordability of diagnostics is another major area of concern. For example, viral load monitoring for HIV has been proven, when combined with appropriate programmatic interventions, to improve treatment outcomes by helping people stay on

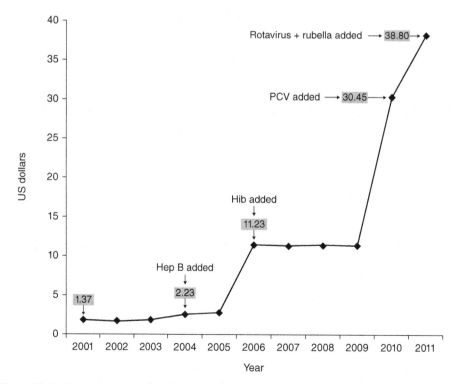

Figure 13.2 Increasing cost of global immunization programs. In recent years, WHO has recommended products with higher unit costs be added to routine immunization protocols globally, significantly raising the price of purchasing a full vaccination course for a child. Two products in particular, the rotavirus vaccine and the pneumococcal conjugate vaccine (PCV), make up the bulk of the cost increase. Source: MSF (2012b).

ARV combinations and stave off resistance for as long as possible (Keiser *et al.* 2011; Sygaloff *et al.* 2011). Access to viral load monitoring can yield important cost savings by avoiding unnecessary or premature switching, based on CD4 testing alone, to more expensive second-line drugs (Lynen *et al.* 2010). Unfortunately, the cost of the equipment today can be in excess of $40,000 (MSF 2012g), and the price of running just one test can range from $20 to $100 (Stevens *et al.* 2010; Wang *et al.* 2010).

Looking ahead, achieving equitable access to medicines in both LICs and middle-income countries (MICs) will also mean tackling non-communicable diseases (NCDs), such as diabetes, cardiovascular disease, and cancers. Many developing countries now face a double burden of NCDs and infectious diseases, and several high profile patent disputes related to treatment of NCDs (e.g., cancer chemotherapy) are under way.

Developing countries are not the only ones to be hit, as ever higher prices for new medical tools strain the healthcare budgets of developed countries too, posing access barriers to increasing numbers of people. New drugs to treat HIV or cancer can cost hundreds of times more than a person's average annual income – Gilead recently announced a new treatment for hepatitis C costing a staggering $84,000 per treatment course. The battle for access increasingly has to be waged in a targeted manner – targeting a drug company's specific drug that is inaccessible in a particular country.

One such battle is underway in India, where Bayer is charging about $66,812 per patient per year – more than $5500 per month – for sorafenib tosylate, used to treat liver and kidney cancers. In order to allow a more affordable version of the drug to be produced, in 2012 India issued a "compulsory license" to compel Bayer to license the patents for sorafenib tosylate to the generic manufacturer Natco in return for a 7% royalty payment. The compulsory license brings the price down by 97%, to a more affordable $175 per month (MSF 2012c). The first use of a compulsory license in India – a mechanism that has been used by both developed and developing countries to meet public health needs – is seen as a prospective watershed for affordable access to patented medicines. But Bayer is fighting the compulsory license in the Indian court system (Arie 2012), and the final outcome – which will set a precedent affecting access to medicines for years to come – remains in the balance.

The Second Problem: Medical Tools to Address "Unprofitable" Diseases are Often Unavailable

The second problem is that the current medical innovation system is structured such that the needs of people who can pay high prices trump the needs of the poor. The result is a severe lack of investment in medical tools to meet the medical needs of patients who cannot afford to pay high prices, or who do not constitute a sizeable or lucrative market, or where a drug needs to be rationed.

A 2002 analysis of new medications developed between 1975 and 1999 found that only 1% were treatments for TB and tropical diseases, despite these diseases causing 11% of the global disease burden (Trouiller *et al.* 2002). In 2012, a new analysis found that, despite important progress in R&D for global health over the past decade, not much had changed. Between 2000 and 2011, only 3.8% of newly approved drugs (excluding vaccines) were for tropical diseases, TB, and other neglected infections, which together account for 10.5% of the global disease burden (Pedrique *et al.* 2013). Much of the progress in the treatment of neglected diseases during this time came about through drug reformulations and repurposing of existing drugs, while only four (1%) of the 336 new medicines (new chemical entities) were for the treatment of neglected diseases. This new survey highlights that the "fatal imbalance" between global disease burden and drug development for some of the world's most devastating illnesses, first identified more than a decade ago, remains a significant barrier to meeting patient needs. Illustrating this trend, it is notable that Pfizer, the world's largest pharmaceutical company, has now completely divested from infectious disease, and AstraZeneca recently announced it was stopping all new research in TB, neglected diseases, and malaria (Clark 2014).

Similarly, a recent survey found that the top 60 research universities in the United States and Canada spend an average of just 3% of their total biomedical research funding on neglected diseases (UAEM 2012). These are publicly funded, public interest institutions that should arguably be addressing health research challenges that are being neglected by others.

This gap between patient needs and the tools that are actually produced is one reason the WHO has classified 17 diseases as "neglected tropical diseases (NTDs)" – diseases that suffer from a lack of investment in diagnostics, treatments, and cures, and that disproportionately affect the world's poorest populations. Box 13.1 highlights just two of these 17 NTDs to illustrate the gap between needs and health commodities.

Box 13.1   The Gap Between Needs and Health Commodities for Two NTDs

- The current drug treatments for the vector-borne parasitic illness Chagas' disease, which causes about 12,500 deaths every year, mostly in rural Latin American populations, are benznidazole and nifurtimox. These drugs were developed more than 40 years ago, they can have significant side effects, and their efficacy may be limited in chronic forms of the disease in adults (MSF 2012d). Thus, there is an urgent need for new drugs for Chagas' disease. There is also an urgent need for a "test of cure" to confirm that the patient is rid of the parasite after treatment (and is therefore no longer at risk of long-term complications). Such a test would also be valuable in measuring the effectiveness of potential new medications.

- New diagnostics and treatments are also needed for kala azar (visceral leishmaniasis, VL), a parasitic disease that infects around 400,000 people each year, and causes about 40,000 annual deaths (MSF 2012e). Diagnosing VL is not easy, given symptoms are often mistaken for other diseases. For example, in East Africa, a negative result from the rapid diagnostic test needs further investigation by another serological test, the diagnostic agglutination test, or by microscopic examination of spleen, bone marrow, or lymph node aspirates. These techniques require technical expertise and laboratories that are seldom available in areas where VL thrives (MSF 2012d). While there are various treatment options, none of them are ideal – especially in the East African region, where the disease presents in a more virulent form. Some of the drugs are highly toxic, or must be given over long periods of time, others require injections or infusions, or are prohibitively expensive.

It is not just the diseases defined as "neglected" by WHO that are lacking adapted tools because of this market failure. Since the 1960s, no new TB drug had come to market until the December 2012 US approval of the drug bedaquiline. TB continues to be an unattractive market for companies, with only 10 drugs in clinical testing, six of which are new chemical entities (Stop TB Partnership 2014).

The most widely available diagnostic method for TB, microscopy, detects less than half of cases, cannot determine whether the bacteria are drug-resistant, and fails to detect the disease in children 93% of the time (NIH 2010; MSF 2012f). The newest tool has not been widely deployed in part due to prohibitive pricing (Pantoja *et al.* 2013), and a simple-to-use and accurate point-of-care diagnostic test for TB is still lacking.

Pediatric diagnostics and formulations across a range of diseases are also absent. Pediatric HIV infection has become rare in wealthy countries, and so, in the absence of a viable commercial market, the needs of HIV-infected children in the developing world have been consistently overlooked. Such neglect has occurred because the "market" of children living with HIV is considered to be too small to incentivize commercial investment. There are about 3.4 million HIV-infected children, but almost all of them live in the developing world (Calmy and Ford 2011).

WHO recommends immediate antiretroviral therapy for all HIV-infected children under 2 years of age. However, the safety and appropriate dosing of some key ARV agents used in adults have not yet been established in children and appropriate formulations simply do not exist. Similarly, there are rising numbers of children who are infected with drug-resistant forms of TB, who are very difficult to diagnose with existing diagnostic tools, and pediatric formulations of the drugs required to treat them are simply not available.

It is critical to note that this distortion of research towards areas of commercial reward rather than medical need also affects patients in wealthy countries. Antibiotic resistance threatens the gains made in treating life-threatening bacterial infections, such as sepsis, pneumonia, dysentery, and hospital-acquired infections (EOHSP 2010). Yet, within the current R&D system, the development of new antibiotics has been neglected. Companies have deemed them unattractive markets because health professionals would necessarily try to reserve and restrict the use of new antibiotics – which would therefore keep sales low. Short treatment courses for acute conditions are also less profitable than chronic conditions that require long-term treatment. As a result, the number of new antibiotics has fallen over recent years, with 16 approved in the United States in the 5 years 1983–87, compared with two between 2008 and 2012 (Boucher *et al.* 2013), with only four big pharmaceutical companies still engaged in antibiotic research.

The Third Problem: Medical Tools are Often Unsuitable for Neglected Populations

As a general rule, the medical R&D pipeline usually involves products that are developed first and foremost for industrialized countries and only in a second stage are rolled out in the developing world. At best, this means there is a lag of several years between the time a patient in a rich country benefits from the fruits of medical innovation and the time that a patient in a LIC receives the same benefit. For example, viral load monitoring is the gold standard in HIV treatment monitoring and regularly used in developed countries (MSF 2012g), yet an MSF survey of treatment protocols in 23 LICs and MICs found that viral load technology is only widely available in four of these countries (MSF/UNAIDS 2012).

Addressing the time lag for developing countries has been one of GAVI's priorities. In the case of pneumococcal vaccines, GAVI established an Advance Market Commitment (AMC) precisely to counter this delay. An AMC is a binding contract between donors, who commit funds to purchase a set volume of products at a set price, and manufacturers, who can then make a risk-free commitment to develop and manufacture the needed product.

The pneumococcal AMC has met with mixed success: two new pneumococcal vaccines, originally developed for industrialized country markets, are being rapidly rolled out in developing countries; however, the cost of the scheme has exacerbated GAVI's financial challenges and created opportunity costs for donors (Berman and Malpani 2011). Additionally, in the case of the pneumococcal AMC, the vaccine was not specifically developed or adapted for developing country needs. Instead, the scheme relies on subsidizing multinational pharmaceutical companies sufficiently for them to increase their production levels to cover developing country market demand, but for products developed with industrialized country markets in mind.

Products being rolled out in developing countries can be unsuitable because of differences in epidemiology between high-income and low-income settings. For example, the two currently available vaccines against rotavirus – an important cause of life-threatening severe diarrhea, particularly in Africa – were developed for industrialized countries. Both vaccines have been shown to have lower efficacy in African countries (Armah *et al.* 2010; Madhi *et al.* 2010; Zaman *et al.* 2010; Cunliffe *et al.* 2012).

Medical tools, such as vaccines, can also be unsuitable because they fail to take into account the resource conditions in developing countries, such as the availability of qualified health staff, the capacity of health systems, and the available laboratory infrastructure. Today, vaccines typically need to be maintained at 2–8°C from the time they leave a factory to when they are administered to a child. Maintaining this cold chain is a considerable challenge, and most developing country governments do not have the means at their disposal to manage the logistics. The two available rotavirus products present a particular logistical challenge – they are extremely bulky, requiring more than three times as much cold chain space as traditional vaccines (WHO 2013).

In addition, today's dosing schedules for vaccines mean that five separate visits to a health facility before a baby's first birthday must take place in order to receive the basic package of immunization. This schedule is prohibitive for caregivers who may have to walk for hours or pay for transportation, stopping work, and leaving their families for extended periods in order to get to the clinic. These challenges point to the need for flexible dosing schedules and alternative technologies that will allow community health workers to easily vaccinate children, such as heat-stable vaccines, needle-free vaccines, and vaccines that can be administered orally (such as the oral polio vaccine) or via inhalation.

Diagnostics provide a similar illustration of the lack of adaptability and the limitations of relying solely on adaptation of existing products to fulfill developing country needs. However much the latest TB diagnostic tool may facilitate diagnosis, it still requires a relatively stable uninterrupted electric supply and a low temperature to function, making it difficult to roll out the machine in peripheral settings. It is also still a sputum-based test, which does not address the difficulties that both people co-infected with HIV and children have in producing adequate sputum samples.

Similarly, for HIV, poor access to viral load testing to date is a result of current test complexity. Most manufacturers offer only very large systems designed for central and reference laboratories. These tests are therefore not suited to district-level settings, even though most HIV-positive patients globally live in remote settings. Because district-level laboratories may be without reliable access to a power supply or highly trained staff, most existing viral load monitoring tools remain ill-suited for use in developing countries.

How to Ensure Better Access to More Appropriate Innovation

In a context of dwindling donor resources for global health, policy solutions must be found to reduce the price of medicines, diagnostics, and vaccines. Generic competition is a cornerstone in ensuring access to health commodities. MSF and other treatment providers rely heavily on affordable generic drugs to treat HIV, TB, malaria, and many other infectious diseases. More than 80% of the ARVs that MSF uses worldwide are generics. More than 80% of ARVs used in developing countries by donor-funded initiatives, such as the Global Fund, are generics manufactured in India (Waning *et al.* 2010). Indeed, India is often called "the pharmacy of the developing world" (Reid-Henry and Lofgren 2012) because of the crucial role that its generic industry has in providing affordable medications. For programs funded by the US President's Emergency Plan for AIDS Relief, the figure is 98% (White House 2011). The fact that thanks to generic competition, medicines became more affordable was a key factor in enabling treatment to be scaled up to the levels seen today.

Next we discuss three different policy approaches to overcoming barriers to affordability: voluntary measures primarily driven by industry, limits on the reach of patents for health commodities, and compulsory licensing and trade deals.

Voluntary Measures

When industry is compelled to respond to access issues in developing countries – usually in response to public pressure – the preferred response is most often to establish product-specific donation programs, or limited defined discount programs. These discount programs are also known as tiered or differential pricing schemes, in which product prices are adapted to different geographic or socioeconomic segments.

Differential pricing allows pharmaceutical companies to demonstrate a commitment to social responsibility by increasing access to specific products, usually in LICs, within carefully controlled parameters designed to protect profitability in other market segments or countries. It also may have some use where generic competition is not, and never can be, an option (Moon *et al.* 2011).

The structure of donation programs and differential pricing schemes can vary greatly and is determined by the manufacturer. The schemes are often limited to specific geographic areas, and long-term sustainability usually depends on the unilateral willingness of the company to continue or renew programs on an ongoing basis. In some cases, the scope is extremely limited and insufficient to address large-scale health problems. For example, the donation program for the current best treatment for VL, liposomal amphotericin B (sold under the brand name Ambisome), addresses less than 5% of the estimated new cases each year (MSF 2011a). In other cases, donation programs can be instrumental in controlling disease. Twenty-five years ago, Merck agreed to provide unlimited quantities of mectizan, a treatment for onchocerciasis (river blindness), in perpetuity for as long as it was needed (Mectizan Donation Program 2013).

Both donation programs and differential pricing schemes are largely targeted towards LICs, and often fail to address needs of patients in MICs, which represent potentially lucrative markets for manufacturers and are therefore often excluded from such programs (Moon *et al.* 2011). Yet today, more than 70% of the world's poorest people – the new "bottom billion" – live in MICs (Sumner 2011). MSF studies on ARV pricing show that several pharmaceutical companies have abandoned standardized HIV drug discounts for patients in MICs (MSF 2013).

GAVI, too, relies on a tiered pricing scheme for vaccine financing, whereby LICs pay a highly subsidized price for vaccines, and economically stronger countries co-finance a higher share of vaccine costs (GAVI 2010). This model has undoubtedly contributed to countries' ability to finance vaccination programs. However, as countries move into the middle-income range and graduate from GAVI subsidies, they will face enormous challenges in paying the full cost burden for vaccines, putting the health of the poorest at risk, as the example of Honduras illustrates.

Tiered pricing schemes and donation programs may sometimes address immediate affordability or access issues, but their impact is necessarily limited by their nature: they are mainly aimed at increasing access to *originator* products (i.e., products manufactured by the patent-holding company). Tiered pricing remains inferior to competition for reliably achieving the lowest sustainable price. Therefore, approaches that promote competition should generally be the default approach (Moon *et al.* 2011).

When looking at voluntary measures designed to enable production of, and increase access to, *generic* versions of patented products, there is a growing trend to implement voluntary licenses. In this scenario, a patent-holding company voluntarily issues a license to a generic manufacturer authorizing them to produce, market and distribute a generic version of a medicine under specific terms and conditions. Such authorization is usually granted in exchange for royalty payments, thus creating a form of controlled competition. Voluntary licenses exist in contrast to compulsory licenses, which are discussed in the next section.

In the HIV/AIDS arena, dozens of ARVs are now being produced under different forms of voluntary licensing agreements between originator and generic producers (Amin 2007). More than fifteen generic companies, primarily based in India or South Africa, have already entered into voluntary license agreements for more than 20 key HIV medicines (MSF 2013).

When voluntary licenses include appropriate terms, conditions, and geographic reach, they can enable generic competition and allow for the sale of generic products in developing countries where patents are in force, improving the affordability and accessibility of medicines (MSF 2013). However, for countries unable to access the generics because of patent barriers or because they are excluded from the scope of voluntary licenses, prices remain consistently high.

Critically, the contractual terms and conditions of voluntary licenses are kept confidential by the manufacturers. However, a review of the little information that is publicly available reveals that these agreements often contain anticompetitive and restrictive terms, and may actually stifle access to medicines by excluding certain countries from their reach (MSF 2013). For example, some clauses limit the sources that can be used to obtain active pharmaceutical ingredients, which are the most expensive components in medicines. This measure can limit the affordability of generic versions of a medication. To date there is no voluntary license that covers *all* developing countries, with most excluding lower middle-income countries and MICs (MSF 2013).

As an alternative to bilateral licensing, the Medicines Patent Pool (MPP), established in 2010, aims to develop voluntary licenses transparently and to manage patents collectively in the interests of public health, as opposed to solely commercial interests. As such, the MPP has the support of MSF and other civil society organizations as the preferred way to manage voluntary licenses. The organization negotiates with patent holders to share their HIV medicines patents with the MPP, and then licenses those patents to generic companies and other producers to facilitate the production of affordable generic medicines well-adapted for use in resource-poor settings. The MPP is working to help overcome intellectual property barriers to facilitate the production of both more affordable medicines and fixed-dose combinations that would otherwise require lengthy negotiations with many different patent holders.

The MPP's first license with a pharmaceutical company was with Gilead, which agreed to license four ARVs, including tenofovir, to the MPP. The license continues to exclude key developing countries and restricts production to India. But, on the positive side, the license provides a termination clause – which means that if the patents end up being rejected or not granted, a company that has signed the license can terminate the agreement and freely manufacture the drug on its own (MSF 2011b). A review of the terms shows that the voluntary licenses which have been signed between originator companies and generic producers outside of the MPP – including earlier licensing agreements on tenofovir signed by Gilead with several generic companies in 2006 – have negotiated less favorable terms.

Limiting and Overcoming Patent Barriers

Supporting policies that can ensure newer and better medicines are made affordable for people in developing countries is a political choice – one that countries committed to in signing the Doha Declaration in 2001. Developing countries can make use of public health safeguards and other legal flexibilities enshrined in TRIPS and reaffirmed in Doha to bring down the cost of medicines. LDCs can use their right not to grant or enforce medicines patents until they graduate beyond LDC status.

Because unrestricted generic competition is far better than voluntary bilateral agreements at stimulating lower prices, efforts to ensure equitable access to medicines should be directed at enabling multiple manufacturers to compete and bring prices down. One strategy is to design flexible patent laws that favor access to medicines, including limiting the reach of patents in cases where public health is at stake. For example, governments should put in place high standards for patentability to ensure that only innovative products are rewarded with patent monopolies. When India was obligated under TRIPS to begin patenting pharmaceuticals, it set high patentability standards to guard against unwarranted patents and to maintain a robust generic industry with a view towards meeting patient needs. Section 3d of India's patent law, for example, excludes the patenting of new forms of existing medicines if these bring no additional therapeutic benefit (Roderick and Pollock 2012). The result is that only medicines that are truly new and innovative are rewarded with patent protection.

Yet the strict limitations that India imposes on patentability repeatedly come under threat. When Swiss pharmaceutical company Novartis applied for a patent in India on its cancer medicine imatinib mesylate, the patent was rejected on the grounds that the medicine was merely a new form of an old medicine, and therefore not patentable under Indian law (Lawyers Collective 2010; Roderick and Pollock 2012). Novartis decided to challenge this decision, and indeed sought to declare Section 3d unconstitutional, or to weaken its interpretation so as to make it meaningless. After 7 years of legal proceedings, the case was finally settled by the Indian Supreme Court, which in April 2013 validated the choice of the Indian government to grant patents only for medical products that represent a genuine advance over older medications.

Another strategy is to oppose patents from being granted in the first place. It is a myth that every patent application that is filed is valid and represents true innovation. Drug companies routinely apply for patents or are granted monopolies on medicines even when such patents or monopolies are not actually deserved. Determining what deserves a patent, and examining patent applications carefully, is therefore essential.

In that regard, patent oppositions are another crucial safeguard for access to medicines, so that undeserved patent applications can be challenged. India's law, for example, allows any interested party to oppose a patent both before it is granted (through a "pre-grant' opposition), or after (through a "post-grant' opposition).

The use of these safeguards in Indian law has resulted in the withdrawal of patent applications on key medicines and in the rejection of patent applications on others, including many critical HIV drugs (MSF 2013). These decisions have allowed generic companies in India to continue to manufacture, supply, and export these HIV medicines to other developing countries. In Brazil, patents have been similarly annulled in 2012 by the federal courts, following oppositions (Intellectual Property Watch 2012a). In October 2012, MSF launched an online resource to support civil society groups in other countries that want to stop unwarranted patents from blocking patients' access to more affordable medicines (Patent Opposition Database 2012).

South Africa is a case in point of excessive patenting and so-called "evergreening," a practice common in developed countries, whereby companies are given successive 20-year patents for making small modifications to existing drugs. In 2008 alone, the South African government granted 2442 pharmaceutical patents, compared with only 278 in Brazil for the 5-year period 2003–2008 (Correa 2011). Stronger patentability criteria and a stronger patent examination system in Brazil account for this difference. Introducing key public health flexibilities into South African patent law could help to promote public health and ensure generic competition by preventing unwarranted patenting. At the time of going to print, the Treatment Action Campaign and MSF are calling on South Africa to amend its patent law to include stricter patentability criteria and a stronger patent review system, and to allow pre- and post-grant oppositions (TAC/MSF 2012), although leaked documents reveal pharmaceutical industry plans to oppose such reforms (Kitamura 2014).

Compulsory Licensing and Trade Deals

When patents are already in place and pose barriers to access to medicines, countries need to find ways to overcome them. Under TRIPS, countries are allowed to exercise their right to override patents in the interest of public health by issuing compulsory licenses to allow generic production and bring down drug costs.

Compulsory licenses enable generic manufacturers to manufacture patented drugs and usually involve royalty payments to the originator company. Several countries have used compulsory licenses to deliver important price reductions on key HIV medicines. In 2007, Thailand issued a compulsory license to bring down the price of lopinavir/ritonavir, and in the same year, Brazil overcame a patent on efavirenz, enabling the government to import a generic version from India at one third of the originator company price ('t Hoen 2009). A compulsory license in Ecuador in 2010 halved the cost of lopinavir/ritonavir to the public health system (Intellectual Property Watch 2010). India (Intellectual Property Watch 2012b) and Indonesia (Public Citizen 2012) each issued their first compulsory licenses in 2012. In India, the move brought down the price of a patented anticancer drug, sorafenib tosylate, from more than $5500 per month to $175 per month – a 97% reduction in price.

Countries should be using these flexibilities routinely – yet the governments that have used them have regularly suffered from retaliation in the form of threats of economic sanctions and other pressures by US and EU governments and companies (MSF 2013). Furthermore, some governments are seeking to incorporate stipulations into regional trade agreements that overturn the public health safeguards in the TRIPS agreement. Several trade agreements currently being negotiated, such as the EU–India free trade agreement and the Trans-Pacific Partnership agreement, include harmful provisions known as "TRIPS-plus" measures that serve to delay generic competition in favor of market protections for patent-holders. Such provisions include preventing pre-grant patent oppositions from happening, lowering patentability requirements, or adding new forms of protection that act like patents to ensure generic competition is impossible (MSF 2012h).

Innovation and Access: Towards a System that Delivers what Patients Need

The examples given above of aggressive western trade policies and pharmaceutical company lawsuits demonstrate that however much the 2001 Doha Declaration was a historic moment that recognized the primacy of health over trade interests, applying the declaration's public health principles in the real world is difficult.

In many industrialized countries, intellectual property rights (IPRs) are hailed as drivers of innovation, economic growth, and entrepreneurship. IPRs are vigorously and aggressively defended by powerful institutions, such as the US and European governments, and by multinational corporations. The argument in favor of IPRs is that strong intellectual property norms are required in order to safeguard R&D. Yet despite ever stronger norms, productivity of US and European pharmaceutical firms is declining (Pammolli *et al.* 2011). Remarkable advances in basic biomedical research have not yielded an increase in the rate of new drug applications or approvals (White House 2012; WHO 2012), let alone delivering products priced affordably or specifically designed to meet the needs of developing countries.

The pharmaceutical industry's response to this innovation crisis is to tighten its grip on intellectual property. But this approach does not stimulate innovation that actually meets patient needs, and must be challenged. More than 10 years on from Doha, this difficulty raises the fundamental question: does the TRIPS Agreement need reviewing? Is TRIPS fit for purpose? Should other multilateral measures also be pursued in order to redefine the rules of the game?

Alternative Approaches

In April 2012, an independent expert group at WHO completed an analysis of the R&D system as it relates to the health needs of developing countries (Røttingen and Chamas 2012). The analysis included a review of two decades of work and research on the persistent gaps in R&D for developing country needs, and assessments of various proposals for better financing and coordination in this realm. The group recommended that R&D mechanisms should be designed in a way that will put patient needs at the forefront (WHO 2012). Part of the expert group's recommendations concerned existing ways of conducting R&D.

The group favored, for example, open knowledge innovation (WHO 2012), whereby the traditional closed in-house R&D process is opened up and there is more open sharing of information with multiple external entities, such as universities and research institutions. This view is in contrast to industry's understanding of open innovation – industry sees open innovation merely as sharing the risk of research by having more people work on a problem but then the use of any research results remains subject to a company's control. Truly open knowledge innovation is subject to the principle that the results should be in the public domain. Examples of open knowledge innovation favored in the expert working group report included open source drug discovery, open access publishing, open "pre-competitive" R&D platforms and equitable licensing of intellectual property.

The group also acknowledged the important role of entities known as product development public–private partnerships (PDPPPs). In some cases, PDPPPs have been able to address the needs of developing country patients and concerns about affordability from the outset, spurred on by incentives other than intellectual property rights. Today, 16 PDPPPs are focused on medical R&D, and they have received more than $2.5 billion in funds in 2007–2011 (Policy Cures 2012). In 2003, MSF helped to set up one such

PDPPP, the Drugs for Neglected Diseases initiative (DNDi). DNDi focuses on delivering new treatments for neglected diseases. It has already delivered improved treatments for malaria, sleeping sickness, VL, and Chagas' disease. It currently has two promising drugs in the pipeline that could eventually deliver what we need for sleeping sickness: a medicine that can be taken orally and handed out at a simple community health post. In partnership with the drug company Sanofi-aventis, DNDi also developed a patent-free malaria treatment that costs just $1 and that has been used by tens of millions of people (DNDi 2008).

Another example is the Meningitis Vaccine Project (MVP), a partnership between PATH and the WHO that resulted in the development of a vaccine against meningitis A (MVP 2011). The product was designed to meet the specific needs of the meningitis belt in sub-Saharan Africa. The vaccine was developed through a technology transfer from the US Food and Drug Administration to a developing country producer, the Serum Institute of India, linked with commitments from the producer to a minimum supply at an affordable price. PATH funded the clinical trials. The new MenAfriVac vaccine was prequalified by WHO in June 2010 and rolled out in countries across the meningitis belt, including by MSF, at an affordable price of less than $0.50 per dose (MVP 2011).

The expert group's report also recommended new R&D mechanisms. Prize funds, for example, bring new resources to a given field of research. Unlike grant funding, which is only able to target one potential research group at a time, prizes allow several promising research proposals to be taken forward, and can pay out at regular milestones on the achievement of results. Thus, several different approaches can be tried simultaneously. At the same time, prizes only pay for results, so if no new health commodity comes to market, resources will not be wasted. Prizes are particularly interesting as they offer an alternative "pull" incentive that could replace the granting of exclusive monopoly rights and enable immediate price-lowering competition. Todays, IPRs are granted to secure high prices through monopolies, but the payment of prizes in exchange for the innovator surrendering its exclusivity rights could be game-changing (KEI 2007). For example, discovering and validating TB biomarkers is a priority research area to advance the development of a simple TB diagnostic (Pai *et al.* 2010) and a prize fund could be particularly useful if targeted to this specific area of research.

A New Global Framework: Could We Achieve a Global R&D Convention?

The expert group also noted that these individual mechanisms would likely be insufficient to meet today's developing country health challenges. The group argued that there is an urgent need for an overarching system to drive and fund innovation in health commodities targeted at patients in developing countries (WHO CEWG 2012). It recommended that WHO Member States begin negotiating a global R&D convention that would put in place systems to steer funding and innovation towards the most urgent patient needs (WHO CEWG 2012). A similar model of a multilateral agreement housed by WHO exists, in the form of the Framework Convention on Tobacco Control, which was created under article 19 of the WHO Constitution and which now has over 160 country signatories (WHO FCTC 2003).

An R&D convention could establish an evidence-based inclusive process that sets priorities for medical R&D, so that innovation could be steered towards developing country needs, which commercially driven R&D is largely failing to address. It could link global health priorities with adequate and sustainable financing, by harnessing the contributions of countries to R&D devoted to meeting the health needs of developing countries and global health R&D priorities. Finally, a global convention could establish norms to ensure the widest possible access to the fruits of R&D, so that the question of affordability of finished products is addressed.

Despite the promise and the potential, the momentum of political discussions at WHO remains uncertain, with many countries seeking to delay substantive negotiations for many years, despite clear recognition of the urgency of the medical needs (*Lancet* 2013). Whether the WHO is the right forum for such negotiations remains to be seen – what is clear is that the need for such a process is ever more apparent (Moon 2014).

Conclusions

After more than a decade of efforts to prioritize global health, the gains and achievements in fighting many diseases are remarkable. Yet progress remains fragile. The fights in securing greater access to affordable HIV medicines kickstarted a global movement for access to medicines, which remains as needed today as it when it emerged over a decade ago.

Faced with ever-evolving health challenges, developing countries should, in line with the Doha Declaration, seek to secure a space for generic competition, which continues to be the most effective way to ensure that essential health commodities remain affordable. These countries should look at limiting patents to true innovations only, at opposing unwarranted patents, and at overcoming patents through lawful means if they pose a barrier to access to medicines.

Despite many successes, it may not be possible to repeat the battles of the past 10 years on a case-by-case, country-by-country, and drug-by-drug basis, as intellectual property norms become ever stronger. The proposal for an R&D convention seeks to address part of this challenge. A more sustainable and fundamental solution is required, one that allows for the question of affordability and access to be dealt with at the same time as the problem of the lack of medical innovation.

Acknowledgment

The authors wish to thank Katy Athersuch and Michelle French for research and contributions to the manuscript.

Key Reading

Knowledge Ecology International. 2007. *The Big Idea: Prizes to Stimulate R&D for new Medicines.* http://www.keionline.org/misc-docs/bigidea-prizes.pdf (last accessed December 2013).

MSF (Médecins Sans Frontières). 2013. *Untangling the Web of Antiretroviral Price Reductions.* http://utw.msfaccess.org (last accessed December 2013).

Patent Opposition Database. http://patentoppositions.org (last accessed December 2013).

't Hoen E. *The Global Politics of Pharmaceutical Monopoly Power.* http://www.msfaccess.org/content/global-politics-pharmaceutical-monopoly-power (last accessed December 2013).

WHO (World Health Organization). 2012. *Research and Development to Meet Health Needs in Developing Countries: Strengthening Global Financing and Coordination.* http://www.who.int/phi/cewg_report/en/index.html (last accessed December 2013).

WHO (World Health Organization). 2013. *Public Health, Innovation, and Intellectual Property Rights.* http://www.who.int/entity/intellectualproperty/report/en/ (last accessed December 2013).

References

Ahuja S, Ashkin D, Avendano M *et al.* 2012. Multidrug resistant pulmonary tuberculosis treatment regimens and patient outcomes: an individual patient data meta-analysis of 9,153 patients. *PLOS Medicine* 9(8), e1001300.

Amin T. 2007. *Voluntary Licensing Practices in the Pharmaceutical Sector: An Acceptable Solution to Improving Access to Affordable Medicines?* Geneva: World Health Organization. http://apps.who.int/medicinedocs/documents/s19793en/s19793en.pdf (last accessed December 2013).

Annan K. 2012. *Ten-year fight for world health: a war chest. Le Monde Diplomatique.* http://mondediplo.com/2012/01/16warchest (last accessed December 2013).

APPG HIV/AIDS (All-Party Parliamentary Group on HIV/AIDS). 2009. *The Treatment Timebomb. The APPG Inquiry into long-term access to HIV treatment in the developing world.* http://www.appghivaids.org.uk/events/timebomb.html (last accessed December 2013).

Arie S. 2012. Bayer challenges India's first compulsory license for generic version of cancer drug. *BMJ* 345, e6015

Armah G, Sow S, Breiman R *et al.* 2010. Efficacy of pentavalent rotavirus vaccine against severe rotavirus gastroenteritis in infants in developing countries in sub-Saharan Africa: a randomised, double-blind, placebo-controlled trial. *Lancet* 376(9741), 606–14.

Berman D, Malpani R. 2011. High time for GAVI to push for lower prices. *Human Vaccines* 7(3), 290.

Boucher HW, Talbot GH, Benjamin DK *et al.* 2013. 10 × '20 Progress – development of new drugs active against Gram-negative bacilli: an update from the Infectious Diseases Society of America. *Clinical Infectious Diseases* doi 10.1093/cid/cit152.

Calmy A, Ford N. 2011. Improving treatment outcomes for HIV in children. *Lancet* 377(9777), 1546–8.

Clark A. 2014. AstraZeneca turns its back on "diseases of the poor." *The Times* January 31. www.thetimes.co.uk/tto/business/industries/health/article 3991082.ece (last accessed February 2014).

Correa C. 2011. *Pharmaceutical innovation, incremental patenting and compulsory licensing.* www.law.fsu.edu/events/documents/Correa.docx (last accessed December 2013).

Cunliffe NA, Witte D, Nqwira BM *et al.* 2012. Efficacy of human rotavirus vaccine RIX4414 in Malawian infants in the first two years of life. *Vaccine* 30(Suppl 1), A36–43.

Drugs for Neglected Diseases Initiative (DNDi). 2008. *ASAQ: fixed-dose combination artesunate/amodiaquine.* http://www.dndi.org/diseases-projects/portfolio/asaq.html (last accessed December 2013).

Dybul M, Piot P, Frenk J. 2012. *Reshaping Global Health. Stanford University Policy Review.* http://www.hoover.org/publications/policy-review/article/118116 (last accessed December 2013).

EOHSP (European Observatory on Health Systems and Policies). 2010. Policies and Incentives for Promoting Innovation in Antibiotic Research. Geneva: World Health Organization. http://www.euro.who.int/__data/assets/pdf_file/0011/120143/E94241.pdf (last accessed December 2013).

GAVI. 2010. *GAVI Alliance Revised Co-financing Policy.* http://www.gavialliance.org/library/gavi-documents/policies/gavi-alliance-revised-co-financing-policy/ (last accessed December 2013).

IHME (Institute for Health Metrics and Evaluation). 2011. *Financing Global Health 2011: Continued Growth as MDG Deadline Approaches.* http://www.healthmetricsandevaluation.org/publications/policy-report/financing-global-health-2011-continued-growth-mdg-deadline-approaches (last accessed December 2013).

Intellectual Property Watch. 2010. *Ecuador grants first compulsory license, for HIV/AIDS drug.* http://www.ip-watch.org/2010/04/22/ecuador-grants-first-compulsory-licence-for-hivaids-drug/ (last accessed December 2013).

Intellectual Property Watch. 2012a. *Brazil HIV drug patent ruling allows generics, sends pipeline process into doubt.* http://www.ip-watch.org/2012/03/21/brazil-hiv-drug-patent-ruling-allows-generics-sends-pipeline-process-into-doubt/ (last accessed December 2013).

Intellectual Property Watch. 2012b. *India grants first compulsory license, for Bayer cancer drug.* http://www.ip-watch.org/2012/03/12/india-grants-first-compulsory-licence-for-bayer-cancer-drug/ (last accessed December 2013).

IUATLD (International Union Against TB and Lung Control)/MSF (Médecins Sans Frontières) Access Campaign. 2013. *DR-TB Drugs Under the Microscope*, 3rd edn. http://www.msfaccess.org/content/dr-tb-drugs-under-microscope3rd-edition (last accessed February 2014).

KEI (Knowledge Ecology International). 2007. *The Big Idea: Prizes to Stimulate R&D for New Medicines.* http://www.keionline.org/misc-docs/bigidea-prizes.pdf (last accessed December 2013).

Keiser O, Chi B, Gsponer T *et al.* 2011. Outcomes of antiretroviral treatment in programmes with and without routine viral load monitoring in Southern Africa. *AIDS* 25, 1761–9.

Kitamura M. 2014. Drug patent threat opens division on how to fight back. *Bloomberg News* January 31. http://www.bloomberg.com/news/2014-01-31/drug-patent-threat-opens-division-on-how-to-fight-back.html (last accessed February 2014).

Lancet. 2013. Editorial: Neglected tropical diseases and priorities. *Lancet* 381, 268.

Lawyers Collective. 2010. *Novartis AG v. Union of India and Others, SLP (Civil) Nos. 20539–20549 of 2009.* http://www.lawyerscollective.org/access-to-medicine/atm-current-cases.html (last accessed December 2013).

Lynen L, Van Griensven J, Elliott J. 2010. Monitoring for treatment failure in patients on first-line antiretroviral treatment in resource-constrained settings. *Current Opinion in HIV and AIDS* 5, 1–5.

Madhi S, Cunliffe N, Steele D *et al.* 2010. Effect of human rotavirus vaccine on severe diarrhea in African infants. *New England Journal of Medicine* 362(4), 289–98.

Mectizan Donation Program. 2013. http://www.mectizan.org/ (last accessed December 2013).

Moon S. 2014. WHO's role in the global health system: what can be learned from global R&D debates? *Public Health* 128(2), 167–72.

Moon S, Jambert E, Childs M, von Schoen-Angerer T. 2011. A win-win solution? A critical analysis of tiered pricing to improve access to medicines in developing countries. *Globalization and Health* 7, 39.

MSF (Médecins Sans Frontières). 2001. *Accessing ARVs: Untangling the Web of Price Reductions for Developing Countries*, 1st edn. utw.msfaccess.org/downloads/documents (last accessed December 2013).

MSF (Médecins Sans Frontières). 2011a. *MSF statement in response to Gilead donation of AmBisome for visceral leishmaniasis.* http://www.msfaccess.org/content/msf-statement-response-gilead-donation-ambisome-visceral-leishmaniasis (last accessed December 2013).

MSF (Médecins Sans Frontières). 2011b. *MSF review of the July 2011 Gilead licences to the Medicines Patent Pool.* http://www.msfaccess.org/content/msf-review-july-2011-gilead-licences-medicines-patent-pool (last accessed December 2013).

MSF (Médecins Sans Frontières). 2012a. *Untangling the Web of Antiretroviral Price Reductions*, 15th edn. http://utw.msfaccess.org/downloads/documents (last accessed December 2013).

MSF (Médecins Sans Frontières). 2012b. *The Right Shot: Extending the reach of affordable and adapted vaccines.* http://www.msfaccess.org/content/rightshot (last accessed December 2013).

MSF (Médecins Sans Frontières). 2012c. *MSF statement on India's dismissal of Bayer's request for a stay on compulsory licence.* http://www.msfaccess.org/content/msf-statement-indias-dismissal-bayers-request-stay-compulsory-licence (last accessed December 2013).

MSF (Médecins Sans Frontières). 2012d. *Fighting Neglect. Finding ways to manage and control visceral leishmaniasis, human African trypanosomiasis and Chagas disease.* http://www.msfaccess.org/our-work/neglected-diseases/article/1855 (last accessed December 2013).

MSF (Médecins Sans Frontières). 2012e. *About kala azar.* http://www.msfaccess.org/our-work/neglected-diseases/article/1517 (last accessed December 2013).

MSF (Médecins Sans Frontières). 2012f. *Standard TB test failing to detect the disease in children 93% of the time.* http://www.msfaccess.org/about-us/media-room/press-releases/standard-tb-test-failing-detect-disease-children-93-time (last accessed December 2013).

MSF (Médecins Sans Frontières). 2012g. *Undetectable: How viral load monitoring can improve HIV treatment in developing countries.* http://www.msfaccess.org/content/undetectable-how-viral-load-monitoring-can-improve-hiv-treatment-developing-countries (last accessed December 2013).

MSF (Médecins Sans Frontières). 2012h. *Submission to the US Trade Representative regarding the 2011 Special 301 Review Process.* http://www.doctorswithoutborders.org/publications/reports/2011/2011Special301MSF_Final.pdf (last accessed December 2013).

MSF (Médecins Sans Frontières). 2013. *Untangling the Web of Antiretroviral Price Reductions,* 16th edn. http://utw.msfaccess.org/downloads/documents (last accessed February 2014).

MSF (Médecins Sans Frontières)/UNAIDS. 2012. *Speed Up Scale-Up: Strategies, Tools and Policies to Get the Best HIV Treatment to More People, Sooner.* http://www.msfaccess.org/content/speed-scale-strategies-tools-and-policies-get-best-hiv-treatment-more-people-sooner (last accessed December 2013).

MVP (Meningitis Vaccine Project). 2011. *Developing a meningococcal A conjugate vaccine.* http://www.meningvax.org/developing-conjugate-vaccine.php (last accessed December 2013).

NIH (National Institutes of Health). 2010. New test detects TB in less than 2 hours. http://www.nih.gov/researchmatters/september2010/09132010tbtest.htm (last accessed December 2013).

Pai M, Minion J, Steingart K, Ramsay A. 2010. New and improved tuberculosis diagnostics: evidence, policy, practice, and impact. *Current Opinion in Pulmonary Medicine* 16(3), 271–84.

Pammolli, N, Magazzini, L, Riccaboni, M. 2011. The productivity crisis in pharmaceutical R&D. *Nature Reviews Drug Discovery* 10, 428–38.

Pantoja A, Fitzpatrick C, Vassall A, Weyer K, Floyd K. 2013. Xpert MTB/RIF for diagnosis of TB and drug-resistant TB: a cost and affordability analysis. *European Respiratory Journal* 42(3), 708–20.

Patent Opposition Database. 2012. http://www.patentoppositions.org (last accessed December 2013).

Pedrique, B, Strub-Wourgaft, N, Some, C et al. 2013. The drug and vaccine landscape for neglected diseases (2000–11): a systematic assessment. *Lancet Global Health* 1(6), e3719. http://www.dndi.org/images/stories/pdf_scientific_pub/2013/LancetGH_NeglectedDiseasesLandscape_2013.pdf (last accessed February 2014).

Policy Cures. 2012. *G-Finder. Neglected disease research and development: a five year review.* http://policycures.org/downloads/GF2012_Report.pdf (last accessed December 2013).

Public Citizen. 2012. *Public Citizen's statement on Indonesia's compulsory licenses.* http://www.citizen.org/PC-statement-on-compulsory-licensing-in-Indonesia (last accessed December 2013).

Reich M, Bery P. 2005. Expanding global access to ARVs: the challenges of prices and patents. In Mayer KH, Pizer HF (eds) *The AIDS Pandemic: Impact on Science and Society*, pp. 324–50. New York: Academic Press.

Reid-Henry S, Lofgren H. 2012. Pharmaceutical companies putting health of world's poor at risk. *Guardian* July 26. http://www.guardian.co.uk/global-development/poverty-matters/2012/jul/26/pharmaceutical-companies-health-worlds-poor-risk (last accessed December 2013).

Roderick P, Pollock AM. 2012. India's patent laws under pressure. *Lancet* 380, e2–4.

Røttingen JA, Chamas C. 2012. A new deal for global health R&D? The recommendations of the Consultative Expert Working Group on Research and Development (CEWG). *PLOS Medicine* 9(5), e1001219.

Stevens W, Scott L, Crowe S. 2010. Quantifying HIV for monitoring antiretroviral therapy in resource-poor settings. *Journal of Infectious Diseases* 201(Suppl 1), S16–26.

Stop TB Partnership, Working Group on New TB Drugs. 2014. *Drug pipeline.* http://www.newtbdrugs.org/pipeline.php (last accessed February 2014).

Sumner A. 2011. *Institute of Development Studies (IDS), Poverty in Middle-Income Countries (commissioned by The Bellagio Initiative: The Future of Philanthropy and Development in the Pursuit of Human Wellbeing)*. http://www.bellagioinitiative.org/wp-content/uploads/2011/10/Bellagio_Sumner.pdf (last accessed December 2013).

Sygaloff K, Hamers R, Wallis C *et al.* 2011. Unnecessary antiretroviral treatment switches and accumulation of HIV resistance mutations; two arguments for viral load monitoring in Africa. *Journal of Acquired Immune Deficiency Syndromes* 58, 23–31.

't Hoen E. 2009. *The Global Politics of Pharmaceutical Monopoly Power*. Ramsey: AMB Publishers. http://www.msfaccess.org/content/global-politics-pharmaceutical-monopoly-power (last accessed December 2013).

TAC (Treatment Action Campaign)/MSF (Médecins Sans Frontières). 2012. *Fix the Patent Laws*. http://www.fixthepatentlaws.org/ (last accessed December 2013).

Trouiller P, Olliaro P, Torreele E, Orbinski J, Laing R, Ford N. 2002. Drug development for neglected diseases: a deficient market and a public-health policy failure. *Lancet* 359(9324), 2188–94

UNAIDS. 2012. *Sidibé, M. Letter to Partners*. http://www.unaids.org/en/media/unaids/contentassets/documents/unaidspublication/2012/UNAIDS_2012_LetterToPartners_en.pdf (last accessed December 2013).

UNAIDS. 2013. *UNAIDS Report on the Global AIDS Epidemic 2013*. http://www.unaids.org/en/media/unaids/contentassets/documents/epidemiology/2013/gr2013/UNAIDS_Global_Report_2013_en.pdf (last accessed February 2014).

UNICEF. 2012. *Levels and Trends in Child Mortality Report 2012: Estimates Developed by the UN Inter-agency Group for Child Mortality Estimation*. http://www.unicef.org/media/files/UNICEF_2012_IGME_child_mortality_report.pdf (last accessed December 2013).

UNICEF/WHO (World Health Organization). 2012. *Progress towards global immunization goals: summary presentations of key indicators*. http://www.who.int/entity/immunization_monitoring/data/SlidesGlobalImmunization.pdf (last accessed December 2013).

UAEM (Universities Allied for Essential Medicines). 2012. *University global health impact report card (preliminary analysis)*. http://essentialmedicine.org/category/content-cloud/uaem-university-global-health-impact-report-card (last accessed December 2013).

Von Schoen Angerer T, Ford N, Arkinstall J. 2012. Access to medicines in resource-limited settings: the end of a golden decade? *Global Advances in Health and Medicine* 1, 52–9. http://www.msfaccess.org/sites/default/files/MSF_assets/Access/Docs/ACCESS_MedJourn_GAHMJ_Golden Decade_ENG.pdf (last accessed December 2013).

Von Schoen Angerer T, Wilson D, Ford N, Kasper T. 2001. Access and activism: the ethics of providing antiretroviral therapy in developing countries. *AIDS* 15, S81–90.

Wang S, Xu F, Demirci U. 2010. Advances in developing HIV-1 viral load assays for resource-limited settings. *Biotechnology Advances* 28(6), 770–81.

Waning, B, Diedrichsen, E, Moon, S. 2010. A lifeline to treatment: the role of Indian generic manufacturers in supplying antiretroviral medicines to developing countries. *Journnal of the International AIDS Society* 13, 35.

White House. 2011. *Office of the Press Secretary. Factsheet: The Beginning of the End of AIDS*. http://www.whitehouse.gov/the-press-office/2011/12/01/fact-sheet-beginning-end-aids (last accessed December 2013).

White House. 2012. *Executive Office of the President, President's Council of Advisors on Science and Technology. Report to the President on Propelling Innovation in Drug Discovery, Development and Evaluation*. http://www.whitehouse.gov/sites/default/files/microsites/ostp/pcast-fda-final.pdf (last accessed December 2013).

WHO FCTC (World Health Organization Framework Convention on Tobacco Control). 2003. *WHO Framework Convention on Tobacco Control*. http://www.who.int/fctc/text_download/en/index.html (last accessed December 2013).

WHO (World Health Organization). 2004. *The World Health Report 2004*. http://www.who.int/whr/2004/en/ (last accessed December 2013).

WHO (World Health Organization). 2011. *Malaria deaths are down but progress remains fragile*. http://www.who.int/mediacentre/news/releases/2011/malaria_report_20111213/en/index.html (last accessed December 2013).

WHO (World Health Organization) CEWG (Consultative Expert Working Group). 2012. *Report of the Consultative Expert Working Group on Research and Development: Financing and Coordination. Research and Development to Meet Health Needs in Developing Countries: Strengthening Global Financing and Coordination (CEWG)*. http://www.who.int/phi/CEWG_Report_5_April_2012.pdf (last accessed December 2013).

WHO (World Health Organization). 2013. *WHO prequalified vaccines*. http://www.who.int/immunization_standards/vaccine_quality/PQ_vaccine_list_en/en/index.html (last accessed December 2013).

WTO (World Trade Organization). 2001. *Doha Declaration on TRIPS agreement and public health*. http://www.wto.org/english/thewto_e/minist_e/min01_e/mindecl_trips_e.htm (last accessed December 2013).

WTO (World Trade Organization). 2006. *Fact Sheet: TRIPS and pharmaceutical patents, obligations and exceptions*. http://www.wto.org/english/tratop_e/trips_e/factsheet_pharm02_e.htm (last accessed December 2013).

WTO (World Trade Organization). 2013. *Responding to Least Developed Countries' Special Needs in Intellectual Property*. http://www.wto.org/english/tratop_e/trips_e/ldc_e.htm (last accessed February 2014).

Zaman K, Dang D, Victor J *et al*. 2010. Efficacy of pentavalent rotavirus vaccine against severe rotavirus gastroenteritis in infants in developing countries in Asia: a randomised, double-blind, placebo-controlled trial. *Lancet* 376(9741), 615–23.

Chapter 14

The Social Determinants of Health

Arne Ruckert and Ronald Labonté

Abstract

The beginning of the twenty-first century has seen the emergence of a global public health discourse that focuses its attention on the ways in which global health is shaped by various social factors and living conditions. These factors have come to be known as the social determinants of health (SDH), and a veritable body of literature has emerged linking such factors through a variety of pathways to health effects and outcomes. This chapter first provides some historical background on SDHs through a discussion of the emergence of the SDH discourse in global health. It highlights the role that different institutions have played in the dissemination of current knowledge about the topic, such as the World Health Organization through its Commission on Social Determinants of Health. The chapter then traces the pathways that link individual SDHs to health outcomes, before assessing the impact of the globalization of finance and production on SDHs. Globalization's most substantial impacts on population health are found to arise from its tendency to increase economic inequality, insecurity, and vulnerability. The chapter concludes with a call for national governments to pay more attention to social determinants in policymaking. Given the interconnectedness of different spheres of social activity and the ways in which SDHs influence each other, intersectoral action through better coordination of government policy across ministries and departments and an assessment of the health consequences of policy initiatives outside the health system are considered necessary ingredients to improve overall population health and reduce health inequities.

The Handbook of Global Health Policy, First Edition. Edited by Garrett W. Brown, Gavin Yamey, and Sarah Wamala.
© 2014 John Wiley & Sons, Ltd. Published 2014 by John Wiley & Sons, Ltd.

Key Points

- The social determinants of health (SDHs) are the daily living conditions in which people are born, grow, and live.
- SDHs shape the health of populations through their inequitable distribution in society.
- The World Health Organization (WHO) Commission on SDHs has recently provided a solid evidence base for the multiple linkages between different SDHs and health inequities.
- Inequalities in power, resources, and money within and between societies have been identified by the WHO as the root cause of health inequities which can be influenced by policy choices.
- Globalization has an inherent tendency to undermine SDHs and deepen health inequities through its differential impacts on populations and their health status.

Key Policy Implications

- Governments need to pay more attention to how living conditions and socioeconomic factors shape population health outcomes.
- Addressing the SDHs requires policy coordination across departments and ministries through intersectoral action.
- Redistributive mechanisms and strong welfare programs are the best policy interventions to reduce health inequities.

Introduction

The beginning of the twenty-first century has seen the emergence of a global public health discourse – what some argue had or should become a global social movement (Friel and Marmot 2011) – concerned with actions on the social determinants of health (SDHs). More intense and evidence-rich attention is being directed towards the part that every-day living conditions play in shaping the unequal distribution of health of individuals and populations (CSDH 2008). Despite significant gains in life expectancy over the last quarter century, many of the socially disadvantaged groups in developed and develop-ing countries continue to have poorer health status than the more affluent members of their society (Marmot 2005). At the same time, gross inequalities in health remain pro-nounced between developed and developing countries, with average life expectancy and child mortality improving more in the richest countries than the poorest (Marmot 2006). Policy or program interventions using an SDH approach starts from the assumption that many of these health *inequalities* are actually health *inequities*, rooted in the wider social structure and processes of social stratification that are not accidents of nature, but unfair outcomes of political and economic choices.

The rise of the social determinants movement can in part be understood in response to neoliberal market-oriented policy reforms, which have exacerbated health inequities within and between nations (De Vogli 2011). In addition, pressures on nation states emanating from economic globalization processes have resulted in the resurfacing of approaches to health that situate health interventions in their global context, recogniz-ing that many of the most pressing health concerns are either transnational in cause or consequence, or can only be solved through collaboration in a global effort (Labonté *et al.* 2011). Economic interconnectedness is increasingly a link in the causal pathways of disease, while conditions of life and work that increase vulnerability to disease and affect access to preventative and curative health services have become inseparable from the global distribution of power, wealth, and resources (CSDH 2008). This means that any attempt to understand global health needs to incorporate elements into its analysis that combine different levels (global, national, and local) with a wide variety of socioe-conomic factors and trends.

In highlighting the analytical potential of an SDH approach, we first provide a brief historical account of how it has come to gain (some) prominence amongst global health policy-makers. We next outline the evidence base for how several SDH shape population health outcomes, before identifying some of the most pronounced global challenges to health equity embedded within SDH pathways. Here, our focus is a selective discussion of some of the policy constraints unleashed by the global integration of production and finance. We conclude by discussing the policy implications of taking an SDH approach to health seriously.

A Brief Genealogy of the SDH Approach

Despite having gained worldwide prominence only recently through the WHO Commis-sion on Social Determinants of Health, the ideas inherent in its approach to health are not wholly new. There is a long public health tradition of concern with the social, economic, and environmental contexts that shape health outcomes. Its origins can be traced back to nineteenth century research and activism on the sources of health inequities that lay within modern capitalism and the health risks and inequities of rapid industrialization (Rosen 1993). The impact of absolute material deprivation – grossly inadequate housing, nutrition, clothing, water, and sanitation – on health has been acknowledged for centuries (Braveman *et al.* 2011). Yet, throughout much of the twentieth century, apart from a resurgence in social analyses of disease following the Great Depression, the focus of health research and health systems has tended to be on single factor models that emphasize clinical solutions to health problems, leading to narrowly defined, technology-based medical and public health interventions. In line with this, the World Health Organization (WHO) and other global health actors predominantly promoted technology-driven, "vertical" campaigns targeting specific diseases, with little regard for the larger social contexts of illness in the first few decades following World War II (Solar and Irwin 2007). However, challenged by the rise of new countries in a decolonizing world, in which the limits of constructing health systems based solely on a biomedical approach were becoming starkly obvious, the WHO and UNICEF hosted an international conference in Alma Ata in 1978. At this meeting a social understanding of health was revived by the seminal Alma Ata Declaration on Primary Health Care (PHC) and the ensuing Health for All movement, which reasserted the need to strengthen health equity by addressing social conditions of ill-health through intersectoral programs and actions. The PHC movement called for a new approach to health, grounded in a holistic social understanding of health and people-centered actions to address health inequalities (Friel and Marmot 2011). If the Alma Ata Declaration was considered an activist clarion call for developing countries, over the same period more socially critical forms of health education and health promotion practice were arising in the wealthier North, bringing the analytical tropes and social values of many of the "new social movements" to the practice of public health (Labonté 1994), and culminating in the Ottawa Charter for Health Promotion (WHO 1986).

The international profile of the social determinants of health was further raised by the publication of the *Black Report* and the *Health Divide* in the UK in the early 1980s (Townsend *et al.* 1988). Both reports demonstrated that, in spite of the post-war welfare state and the establishment of the National Health Service (NHS), health disparities between the rich and poor in the United Kingdom had widened rather than narrowed. While many indices of health had improved in all socioeconomic groups, the improvement had been greater among the more educated and the more affluent. What is more, both reports showed that health differences occurred in a step-wise progression across the socioeconomic spectrum, with professionals displaying the best health and manual laborers the worst (Raphael 2004). The ascendancy of neoliberal economic models and policy during the 1980s, however, created obstacles to policy action on SDH, including suppression in the release of the original *Black Report* by the Conservative government led by Margaret Thatcher. In the health sector, market-oriented reforms, often mandated by international financial institutions as part of loans to indebted developing countries, emphasized efficiency over equity, further reducing disadvantaged social groups' access to healthcare services and undermining health equity goals (Solar and Irwin 2007).

By the late 1990s, SDH was on the agenda of a number of governments, and had found its way into health strategies in a wide range of countries, including in Sweden, New Zealand, Australia, the United Kingdom, the Netherlands, Italy, Scotland, and Wales. Meanwhile, in developing regions, including sub-Saharan Africa, Asia, the Eastern Mediterranean and Latin America, reemerging critical traditions complementing health with the social justice agenda, such as the Latin American social medicine movement (ALAMES) and the People's Health Movement, refined their critiques of market-based, technology-driven healthcare reforms and called for action to tackle the social roots of ill-health (Solar and Irwin 2007: 6). At the same time, an increasingly vocal civil society movement called for greater attention to the social conditions underlying health inequities as market-oriented policies began to fall out of favor globally (Friel and Marmot 2011).

Arguably the biggest boost to global policy attention on the SDH came when the WHO announced in 2003 that it would form a Commission on Social Determinants of Health that would mobilize current knowledge and propose policy actions to remedy inequities in health. The Commission's work focused predominantly on the upstream political, economic, and sociocultural drivers of health and health inequity as well as the intermediate conditions of daily living, and the Commission created nine research networks to summarize current knowledge in each area:

- Women/gender.
- Early child development.
- Urban settings.
- Social exclusion.
- Employment conditions.
- Globalization.
- Health systems.
- Priority public health problems.
- Evidence and measurement.

The final report provided three major conclusions:

1. Inequities in the daily living circumstances in which people are born, grow, live, work, and age cause health inequities within and between countries.
2. These daily living conditions are influenced by inequities in structural drivers (i.e., inequities in resources, power, and money).
3. There is a need to continue to expand the knowledge base surrounding the social determinants of health and to train experts to ensure implementation of the social determinants of health approach (Friel and Marmot 2011).

Some Conceptual Clarifications

Health is a complex phenomenon that is influenced by a wide range of factors, such as personal behavioral choices and knowledge, the physical environment, the level of medical care, living and working conditions, but also social and economic opportunities. Different theoretical understandings of health place different emphases on each of these factors. Traditionally, the focus of most research has been on how immediate individual risk factors rooted in a biomedical understanding and an individualist methodology and ontology can explain differences in health outcomes. In recent years, a new wave of health research has placed emphasis on the more distant and complex drivers of health outcomes, and how these are rooted in social and political inequities (Östlin *et al.* 2011). One way of distinguishing between more immediate and more distant determinants of health is the distinction between upstream and downstream determinants of health. Downstream determinants of health are temporally and spatially close to health effects and hence relatively apparent. Upstream determinants of health are the temporally and spatially removed and structurally embedded causes of health effects that set in motion causal pathways leading to health affects that are less apparent and require a more complex research design. Although these concepts might make intuitive sense, Braveman *et al.* (2011) note that "the causal pathways linking upstream determinants

Table 14.1   Various conceptualizations of the social determinants of health.

Ottawa Charter	Health Canada	World Health Organization
Peace	Income and social status	Social gradient
Shelter	Social support networks	Stress
Education	Education	Early life
Food	Employment and working	Social exclusion
Income	conditions	Work
Stable ecosystem	Physical and social	Unemployment
Sustainable resources	environments	Social support
Social justice	Healthy child development	Addiction
Equity	Health services	Food
	Gender	Transport
	Culture	

Source: WHO (1986); Health Canada (1998); Wilkinson and Marmot (1998).

with downstream determinants, and ultimately with health, are typically long and complex, often involving multiple intervening and potentially interacting factors along the way" (Braveman *et al.* 2011: 383). What is more, different social determinants of health interact with each other and cannot be understood or studied in isolation from each other, which implies that a complex methodological research design is required. Such complexity generally makes it easier to study the more direct and straightforward downstream determinants of health, with a methodological (and ideological) bias towards individual risk factors, such as health behaviors. The SDH approach tries to remedy this by shifting the focus of health research away from individual choices and behavior change strategies to the social "root causes" of ill-health – what became known during the work of the Commission on Social Determinants of Health (CSDH) as "the causes of the causes of the causes" (CSDH 2008).

There is a wide range of conceptualizations of the SDHs that have been developed in both policy circles and academia. However, there is significant overlap in most conceptualizations (as can be seen in Table 14.1). At the risk of simplification, we define the SDHs as the societal factors that through their inequitable distribution in society shape and contribute to the health of populations. Put differently, the SDHs represent the quantity and quality of a variety of both monetary and non-monetary resources a society makes available to its members, which exert important influences upon the health of individuals (Raphael 2011).

Health inequities and the unequal distribution of SDHs emanate from patterns of social stratification – that is, from the systematically unequal distribution of power, prestige, and resources among individuals in society (CSDH 2008). These socioeconomic factors are, in turn, shaped by socioeconomic and political contexts. Such an understanding is captured well in a conceptual framework developed for the CSDH final report (Figure 14.1).

In the subsequent discussion, we focus on a select number of what we consider to be the most impactful SDHs, including income and employment, education, health systems, social protection, the built environment, and social patterns of exclusion.

Evidence Base for the Importance of SDHs

There is a large evidence base from decades of research examining the associations between various social factors and health outcomes. In this research, one of the most

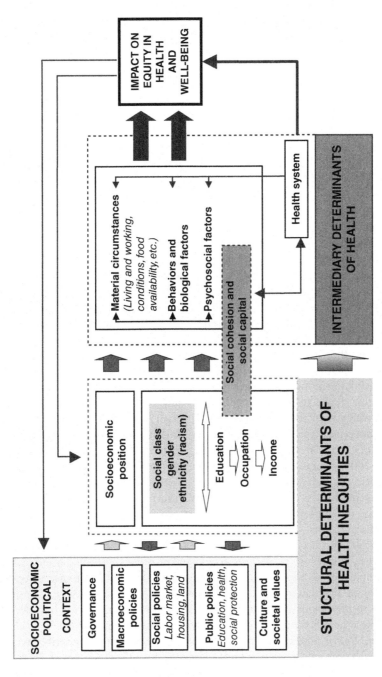

Figure 14.1 Commission on Social Determinants of Health framework of structural and intermediary determinants of health.
Source: Solar and Irwin (2007), reproduced by permission of the World Health Organization.

widely documented links identified is the impact of income on health. Income is widely considered to be the most powerful social predictor of one's health. Studies have documented stepwise socioeconomic gradients in Europe for over 30 years, particularly in the United Kingdom (e.g., Rose and Marmot 1981; Marmot *et al.* 1991), and more recently in the United States (e.g., Pamuk *et al.* 1998; Braveman *et al.* 2010). These studies show that although the most disadvantaged members of society, especially those with below poverty-level incomes or without a high-school diploma, generally experience the worst health, even those with intermediate income appear less healthy than the most affluent and educated members of society (Braveman *et al.* 2011). The multiple pathways by which income impacts health outcomes are still being debated in the literature. The focus in this debate lies on whether income impacts health through a direct effect on the material conditions necessary for biological survival or through an effect on social participation and the opportunity to control life circumstances. The direct impact of income is related to the health benefits of having control over more economic resources, and thus having access to healthier nutrition, housing, or neighborhood conditions, or less stress because of the availability of more resources to cope with daily challenges (Pamuk *et al.* 1998). An important finding is that the fewer goods and services that are provided by the state or by the community, the more important individual income appears to be for health. This implies that in countries with strong social protection mechanisms in place, income is a less dominant upstream determinant of health (Marmot 2002). Growing income inequality is a major concern for proponents of an SDH approach, as it has an inherent tendency to further undermine health equity.

While the literature on the relationship between employment, SDHs, and health outcomes is still in its infancy, there are some important findings that have recently emerged. The WHO's CSDH suggests that employment and working conditions are the origin of many of the other SDHs, as work in its optimal form can provide financial security, social status, self-esteem, social networks and support, personal development, and many other health promoting attributes (CSDH 2008: 72). The physical aspects of work, especially as they relate to occupational health and safety, represent an obvious pathway through which work influences health (Braveman *et al.* 2011). For example, certain jobs that require repetitive movements in physically demanding work environments have been found to be associated with higher risk for musculoskeletal injuries and disorders (O'Neil *et al.* 2001), whereas physically inactive workers are at increased risk for obesity and chronic diseases such as diabetes and heart disease (Warburton *et al.* 2006). What is more, being unemployed is directly associated with various adverse health outcomes, and the link between unemployment, psychosocial stress, and poor health, is quite straightforward. In the published literature, unemployment has been associated with increased self-harm, suicide, and decreased mental health status (Moser *et al.* 1984; Blakely *et al.* 2003). However, workers in precarious arrangements often share similar characteristics with the unemployed, with some evidence suggesting that chronic job insecurity may be more damaging than actual job loss. In fact, dimensions that are typically, but not exclusively, related to precarious work arrangements, such as job insecurity, have long been linked to adverse health outcomes such as psychosocial morbidity (Ferrie *et al.* 2002; Virtanen *et al.* 2005). Studies suggest that workers who are involuntarily involved in temporary work contracts are at an increased risk for mortality (Natti *et al.* 2009). Using cross-sectional data from a Canadian-based questionnaire, Lewchuk *et al.* (2011) point out that insecure employment relationships (where future employment is unknown) are associated with poorer health indicators. What is more, their findings point to a "complex association between less permanent employment and health, where it is the *characteristics of the employment relationship* as much as having or not having permanent employment that are associated with different health outcomes" (Lewchuk *et al.* 2011: 388). This implies that changes in the employment form might be as important as changes to levels of unemployment in understanding challenges to health equity.

Meaningful education has a fundamental role in both personal and social development, and people with higher levels of education tend to be healthier than people with lower educational attainment (Raphael 2011). Educational attainment translates through a number of pathways into better health. For example, it is widely recognized that education can lead to improved health by improving health-related knowledge (Sanders *et al.* 2009). This may be explained in part by literacy, allowing more knowledgeable individuals to make better-informed health-related choices, including about receipt and management of healthcare for themselves and their families (Pignone and DeWalt 2004). However, educational attainment also strongly influences employment opportunities and income, which in turn influence housing, employment, transport, and community participation. In other words, education is strongly correlated with other social determinants of health. For instance, more educated individuals are less likely to experience protracted periods of unemployment, with its associated negative health consequences. Education also directly impacts the income levels of workers, with better educated workers commanding higher wages in the marketplace. Education may also affect health by influencing social and psychological factors. As Braveman *et al.* (2011: 386) note, more education has been associated with greater perceived personal control, which has frequently been linked with better health and health-related behaviors.

Early childhood development has been singled out as a particularly important health determinant related to education, given the importance of early childhood experiences for immediate and long-term biological, psychological, and social effects upon health. On the one hand, early childhood education, or lack thereof, can lead to latency effects (i.e., health effects that exist beyond early childhood) (Lloyd *et al.* 2010). For example, babies with insufficient birth weight tend to experience worse health conditions later in life. On the other hand, pathway effects refer to how risk factors that at one point do not have immediate health effects can have health consequences later in life through a cumulative effect. An example for this is learning ability which does not have any immediate health effect during the childhood years, but rather effects health later in life, for example by impacting educational attainment, employment opportunities, and income levels (Maggi *et al.* 2005).

The ways in which health systems are organized have deep implications for the SDHs, with the WHO noting that "health care systems are a vital determinant of health" (CSDH 2008: 94). Health systems are defined as encompassing all the activities whose primary purpose is to promote, restore, or maintain health (WHO 2000), and are a vital part of the social fabric of any country, providing not only services and influencing health, but also reflecting the dominant social values (Gilson *et al.* 2007). Cross-national epidemiological and econometric analyses demonstrate that health systems, or particular elements within them, can and do promote population health, independent of other factors (Anand and Ravallion 1993; McKee 2002; Anand and Barninghausen 2004). In general, the connections between health system organization and health outcomes are rather straightforward. For example, universal and comprehensive health coverage is associated with better population health, as it effectively protects citizens on lower incomes who could not afford private healthcare insurance. The WHO Knowledge Network on Health systems has identified a range of other characteristics that are as important as universal coverage for improving the performance of health systems:

1. The revitalization of the comprehensive primary healthcare approach, with its focus on proper provision at the local level.
2. Better coordination between government departments and intersectoral action on the social determinants of health.
3. Social empowerment through organizational arrangements that involve population groups and civil society organizations in decisions and actions that identify, address, and allocate resources to health needs (Gilson *et al.* 2007).

Social protection mechanisms have long been identified as representing a crucial element of an approach to health that relies on insights form the SDH literature. While the role of social spending has traditionally been less examined in the SDH literature, a number of recent statistical analyses have found multiple linkages between social spending and health outcomes. For example, social service expenditure has been found to be associated with better health outcomes in a study analyzing such expenditures across the Organisation for Economic Co-operation Development (OECD) countries (Bradley *et al.* 2011). Similar findings were presented by another study that looked at how lower levels of public spending might affect health in OECD countries (Stuckler *et al.* 2010). The statistical model constructed by Stuckler *et al.* shows that each additional $100 increase in social welfare spending has been associated with a 1.19% drop in all-cause mortality in OECD countries (2010: 78). Importantly, the findings are specific to social welfare spending, as there was no observable protective effect associated with higher general government spending. This is not surprising since military, prison, or similar spending would not be expected to have a visible public health effect (Stuckler *et al.* 2010). The WHO similarly suggested in the Commission's final report that redistributive welfare systems impact a range of other social determinants that strongly influence population health, such as poverty and inadequate access to food and housing. According to the WHO, generous universal social protection systems are associated with better population health, including lower excess mortality levels among the older, and lower mortality rates amongst social disadvantaged groups (CSDH 2008). This is why the WHO is calling for the establishment of universal comprehensive social protection policies that support a level of income sufficient for healthy living for all.

The built environment represents another important SDH. In particular, poor housing is frequently associated with poorer health (Dunn 2000). Housing influences health in a variety of ways, for example through the presence of lead and mold, poor heating and draft, inadequate ventilation, and vermin, and other determinants of adverse health effects (Mikkonen and Raphael 2010). Overcrowding enables the speedy transmission of respiratory and other illnesses. What is more, high housing costs can diminish the resources available to support other SDHs. For example, a recent US study showed that affordable housing reduces stress and increases the resources available for better food and healthcare, which in turn can improve overall health and quality of life (Cohen 2007). Neighborhood conditions can also influence health through their physical characteristics, such as water and air quality, access to sanitation, access to nutritious food, and safe places to exercise (Robert Wood Johnson Foundation 2008; Braveman *et al.* 2011). The availability and quality of neighborhood services is yet another way in which neighborhood characteristic shape health outcomes, particularly by affecting income opportunities (Fernandez and Su 2004). This has led the WHO to conclude that neighborhoods that ensure access to basic goods, that are socially cohesive and that are designed to promote good physical health and psychological well-being are essential for promoting population health and achieving health equity (CSDH 2008).

Social exclusion describes the structures and dynamic processes of inequality among groups in society and refers to the inability of certain groups or individuals to participate meaningfully in public and private life, due to structural inequalities in access to social, economic, political, and cultural resources (Galabuzi 2002). These inequalities arise out of oppression related to factors, such as race, class, gender, disability, sexual orientation, immigrant status, and religion. Entrenched societal patterns of social exclusion have been identified as a powerful social determinant of health (Labonté 2002). However, health disadvantages related to social exclusion are not the outcome of intentional discrimination, but are rather rooted in deep-seated societal structures that systematically constrain some individuals' opportunities and resources, for example on the basis of race or ethnic origin. Increasingly, research has begun to confirm the links between the minority status of ethnic, immigrant and racialized groups, and low health status (Bolaria and Bolaria 1994; Adams 1995; Wilkinson 1996; Wilkinson and Marmot 1998; Anderson 2000). A key pathway by which social exclusion impacts health is discrimination in the labor market. Research demonstrates the stratified nature of labor markets across racial lines in Northern America, with racialized groups earning consistently less and being over-represented in flexible non-standard labor arrangements, with associated negative health consequences. Residential segregation based on racial or ethnic origin is another way in which social exclusion can translate into health disadvantages (Braveman *et al.* 2011). This shows how social exclusion intersects with and influences other SDHs in a sustainable manner. In addition to the negative health effects of relative deprivation linked to social exclusion, the actual experience of inequality and the stress associated with dealing with exclusion tend to have pronounced psychological effects and to impact negatively on health (Wilkinson 1996; Kawachi and Kennedy 1997).

Just as there are multiple avenues by which the SDHs influence population health, there is a wide array of factors that shape the SDHs. The following discussion focuses on some of the global forces that have come to be particularly effective in impacting the SDHs, with special attention given to the relationship between contemporary globalization (post-1980) and the SDHs. Addressing the challenges to health posed by globalization demands a consistent willingness to consider influences on public health that operate at the level of social structure and social stratification, with particular attention paid to the differential impacts of globalization processes (Labonté *et al.* 2011).

Globalization of Production and Finance: Undermining SDHs?

As part of the emerging scholarship on the SDHs, a small branch has focused its attention on how global forces and structures are interacting with the SDHs in national and local contexts (e.g., Labonté and Togerson 2005; Labonté and Schrecker 2007a, 2007b, 2007c; Edwards and Di Ruggiero 2011). Over the long term, and with considerable variation at any given income level, richer societies are healthier (Deaton 2003), whereas poverty, however defined, remains one of the most important contributing conditions to ill health. Thus, if globalization could be shown to be reliable and effective in increasing growth rates and reducing poverty, setting aside for the moment the health-negative environmental impacts of such growth, then measures to promote globalization should be embraced for their health benefits (Feachem 2001). The evidence that globalization contributes either to economic growth or to poverty reduction, however, is at best equivocal, depending *inter alia* on how one assesses the extent to which national economies have been integrated into the global marketplace, how poverty is defined, and how many uncertainties about data quality one is willing to live with or overlook (Kawachi and Wamali 2007). Even globalization's enthusiasts concede that there may be substantial numbers of losers within national economies, notably as a consequence of changes in labor markets (World Bank 2007).

What is more, the effects of globalization are almost never uniformly distributed across different groups within society. Due to the differential impact of globalization processes on the life trajectories of individuals, certain population groups have benefitted from globalization-related social changes while others have been left behind. One of globalization's most substantial impacts on population health arises from its tendency to increase economic inequality, insecurity, and vulnerability (Labonté *et al.* 2011). This process operates through three distinct but closely interconnected dynamics: the global integration of production through global value chains, the deregulation and global integration of finance, and the related narrowing of policy space and options for governments.

First, global production has been reorganized across borders through foreign direct investment and outsourcing to independent contractors. This process was facilitated both by technology-driven reductions in transportation and communication costs and the lowering of institutional barriers to trade and investment, in the form of both the World Trade Organization (WTO) regime and a proliferation of bilateral and regional "free trade" treaties. A genuinely global labor market has gradually begun to emerge, although it involves mainly the mobility of capital across national borders in search of lower wages and more flexible working arrangements rather than the mobility of workers themselves (Schrecker 2009a). An important element of this process has been the integration of India, China, and the transition economies of the former Soviet bloc into the global marketplace, roughly doubling the number of workers competing for jobs, which are increasingly independent of geographic location. This has created worldwide downward pressure on wages and undermined healthy working conditions (Freeman 2007). The tendency of globalization to increase economic inequality by way of its effects on labor markets is now conceded even by the World Bank (2007); while the International Monetary Fund (IMF) has recently graced its flagship publication *Finance and Development* with a special issue on inequality, acknowledging that "income inequality has risen over the past quarter-century instead of falling as expected" (Milanovic 2011: 6). One the one hand, this is related to downward pressures on the wages of those whose skills are in abundant supply. On the other hand, those with internationally marketable credentials or skills that are valuable to corporate employers can increasingly command incomes defined by the global marketplace rather than national labor market conditions. Shifts in the share of national income accruing to capital rather than labor, which have been quite pronounced in some countries (IMF 2007), magnify this effect. Given the crucial role that income and working conditions have as SDHs, these developments can, at least partially, explain the lack of significant progress in health indicators over the last quarter century for socially disadvantaged populations.

Second, financial liberalization, as another key pillar of neoliberal globalization, has been negatively impacting the SDHs through a number of pathways. Domestic and international deregulation of financial markets has increased the volume of short-term financial flows and the speed with which investors can move money into – and out of – national economies. Whereas the total value of foreign direct investment (to acquire shares in existing companies or build new facilities) in 2008 was $1.7 trillion, the daily value of foreign exchange transactions on the world's financial markets is currently estimated to be $4.7 trillion (Bech 2012). The effect of this development, again, is to increase economic insecurity and vulnerability. Rapid disinvestment as "hot money" flows out of a country can reduce the value of national currencies by 50% or more and drive millions of people into poverty and economic insecurity, with attendant negative health consequences; such crises occurred in Mexico in 1994–1995, several South Asian countries in 1997–1998, and Argentina in 2001 (Schrecker 2009b). Often, inequality is further increased by the ability of the wealthy to shift their assets abroad in anticipation of a crisis; insecurity is compounded by the public spending cuts necessary to restore the confidence in financial markets and to please foreign portfolio investors. The liberation of financial capital from the regulatory constrains of the nation state have ushered in a new era of market discipline, aptly referred to by some as disciplinary neoliberalism (Gill 1995). Disciplinary neoliberalism refers to the heightened power of capital to discipline both the state and labour in liberalized and market-oriented economies. This is linked to the increasingly free flow of capital and the power associated with the "exit option" for capital (Bakker and Gill 2006: 43). As discussed in more detail later, this limits the policy choices and options of governments that are increasingly making policy not for local constituents, but for globally mobile financiers. However, currently the most potent link between financial liberalization and the SDHs is the global financial crisis, which started in 2007–2008.

The ongoing global financial crisis, the unintended result of the global deregulation of finance, represents the most resilient pathway by which the SDHs have been and will likely continue to be impacted by neoliberal globalization. The most direct connection between the financial crisis and health is the steep decline in overall economic activity that financial crises tend to induce. The opportunity costs of financial crises, understood in terms of lost or forgone output, are much higher than those for normal economic recessions (Gill and Bakker 2011), as financial crises produce far more significant declines in overall economic activity than "normal" recessions (Reinhart and Rogoff 2009). This puts constraints on the government's ability to maintain social, and in particular, healthcare spending and engenders pressures on wages and living conditions, more broadly. This can already be seen in a range of European countries that have dramatically cut back on healthcare spending, including in Bulgaria, Romania, the Czech Republic, Ireland, Latvia, Spain, Greece, and Portugal, in some cases by over 20% (Mladovsky et al. 2012). However, individual health, and especially health equity, is not solely impacted by the levels of health spending. A range of recent studies have found a direct link between social service expenditure and health outcomes. This implies that cutbacks to welfare programs, as currently commonly practiced in response to the financial crisis, will likely undermine population health, even if health spending is maintained at pre-crisis levels. Second, the general decline in economic activity linked to the financial crisis leads to cut-backs in overall government spending, as the crisis response thus far has focused on spending cuts and tax increases. However, tax increases have been mostly socially regressive in nature, such as raising the value added tax (VAT), which have the potential to further undermine SDHs. What is more, lack of economic dynamism translates into job losses and heightened levels of unemployment. The International Labour Organization (ILO) has recently noted that unemployment has reached unprecedented proportions, with more than 200 million unemployed workers, putting global unemployment on the highest level on record (ILO 2011). In addition, previous experiences with economic recessions suggest that the negative distribution of health impacts is likely to be concentrated amongst those who are already socioeconomically deprived or socially excluded (Blakely and McLeod 2009).

Third, the global integration of production and finance has led to a dramatic reduction of policy space for most governments. Policy space can be defined as the freedom, scope, and mechanisms that governments have to choose, design, and implement public policies to fulfill their desired aims (Koivusalo *et al.* 2008). Loss of policy space is related to the ways in which investor decisions can influence the policy-making process, given that under globally integrated financial markets, governments require the confidence of large international institutional investors to fund their operations through sovereign debt markets. This can currently be observed in European sovereign debt markets where governments are forced to dramatically cut back spending in response to rising interest rates. In the realm of health, this implies that even governments committed to improving access to better and more equitable healthcare are reluctant to risk the effects of displeasing financial markets through deficit-induced spending. Governments may also be reluctant to implement policies that might be viewed negatively by sources of foreign direct investment or foreign sovereign bond investors (Labonté *et al.* 2009: 118). This tendency has been intensified with the onset of the financial crisis. Thus, the actual or anticipated reaction of financial markets can limit the social policy options available to national governments, enabling the world's wealthy to impose "implicit conditionalities" (Griffith-Jones and Stallings 1995). For example, concern about redistributive policies that might be adopted by Brazil's Workers' Party (PT), which by 1999 appeared likely to win the 2002 election, led major US financial institutions to warn clients against investing in Brazil. Responding to a process of disinvestment that drove the value of Brazil's currency down by more than 60% relative to the US dollar between January 1999 and July 2002, the PT "chose to suffer low growth, high unemployment and flat levels of social expenditure rather than risk retribution from the global financial actors who constitute 'the markets'," in the words of noted development scholar Peter Evans (2005). This highlights how any serious attempt to address global health through the lens of social determinants must display a willingness to consider the variegated influences of globalization.

Conclusions

This chapter outlines some of the central markers of an SDH approach and suggests that such an approach is well-suited to understanding the pervasive inequities that continue to exist in the international health arena. Yet, despite the consolidation of an impressive knowledge base through the work of the WHO Commission on Social Determinants of Health, most health research remains focused on notions of individual responsibility and lifestyle changes, as though personal choices are solely determined by individual preferences and not embedded within and conditioned by larger social structures and processes of social stratification. The solutions to achieving better health results have long been known, the main question is rather if they are politically feasible, and if politicians are willing to implement policies that counteract the tendency of the global marketplace to magnify economic inequalities and vulnerabilities. To achieve this, states would have to mobilize substantial resources for redistributive purposes, for example, through more progressive forms of taxation, and better regulate the power of corporate actors, especially multinational corporations. Findings from the SDH literature also suggest that states should invest more in social protection regimes and address societal patterns of social exclusion, especially in the labor market. Given the interconnectedness of different spheres of social activity and the ways in which SDHs influence each other, relevant policy instruments to address social determinants are often administratively located outside the purview of the health system and unavailable to health policy-makers. This implies that intersectoral action and an assessment of the health consequences of policy initiatives outside the health system are intricately linked to any effort to improve population health. For example, consideration of the potential impact of macroeconomic policies on population health should be an integral part of the policy development and the health impact assessment process.

However, in many countries, efforts to implement more socially progressive policies are blocked by a range of factors. The ideological predisposition of governments has been shown to impact their willingness to address the social determinants of health. Coburn (2006) highlights how neoliberalism, through its emphasis on the market as the dominant tool for resource allocation, serves to support regressive political and economic forces in society. The policy prescriptions of multilateral agencies, such as the World Bank and the IMF, which have been prescribing macroeconomic adjustments to both developing and, in the context of the global financial crisis, increasingly also to developed countries, are another regressive force impacting the SDHs negatively. The macroeconomic conditionalities imposed on many countries directly undermine health equity goals, for example through promoting the commoditization of public services in an environment of fiscal austerity. This can also currently be seen in a range of European countries where deep cutbacks to health budgets mandated by the IMF are starting to have detrimental health effects (Kentikelenis *et al.* 2011). This means that, more than ever, we need to draw on the valuable insights that the SDH approach has to offer in order to overcome the problematically narrow conceptualizations and understandings of health still dominant in the field of global health today.

Key Reading

Braveman P, Egerter S, Williams DR. 2011. The social determinants of health: coming of age. *Annual Review of Public Health* 32, 381–98.

Commission on Social Determinants of Health. 2008. Closing the Gap in a Generation: Health Equity through Action on the Social Determinants of Health. Geneva: World Health Organization.

Friel S, Marmot MG. 2011. Action on the social determinants of health. *Annual Review of Public Health* 32, 225–36.

Labonté R, Schrecker T. 2007. Globalization and social determinants of health: introduction and methodological background. *Globalization and Health* 3(5).

Marmot MG. 2005. Social determinants of health inequities. *Lancet* 365(9464), 1099–104.

Raphael D. 2011. A discourse analysis of the social determinants of health. *Critical Public Health* 21(2), 221–36.

Wilkinson R, Marmot MG. 1998. *Social Determinants of Health: The Solid Facts*. Copenhagen: World Health Organization.

References

Adams D. 1995. *Health Issues of Women of Color: A Cultural Diversity Perspective*. London: Sage Books.

Anand S, Barnighausen T. 2004. Human resources and health outcomes: cross country econometric study. *Lancet* 364(9445), 1603–9.

Anand S, Ravallion M. 1993. Human development in poor countries: on the role of private incomes and public services. *Journal of Economic Perspectives* 7, 133–50.

Anderson JM. 2000. Gender, race, poverty, health and discourses of health reform in the context of globalization: a post-colonial feminist perspective in policy research. *Nursing Inquiry* 7(4), 220–9.

Bakker I, Gill S. 2006. New constitutionalism and the social reproduction of caring institutions. *Theoretical Medicine and Bioethics* 27(1), 3–57.

Bech M. 2012. FX volume during the financial crisis and now. *BIS Quarterly Review* March, 33–43.

Blakely T, Collings S, Atkinson J. 2003. Unemployment and suicide: New Zealand evidence for a causal association. *Journal of Epidemiology and Community Health* 57, 594–600.

Blakely T, McLeod M. 2009. Will the financial crisis get under the skin and affect our health: learning from the past to predict the future. *Journal of the New Zealand Medical Association* 122(1307), 76–83.

Bolaria SB, Bolaria R. 1994. Immigrant status and health status: Women and racial minority immigrant workers. In Bolaria SB, Bolaria R (eds) *Racial Minorities, Medicine and Health*, pp. 149–68. Halifax: Fernwood Press.

Bradley EH, Elkins BR, Herrin J, Elbel B. 2011. Health and social services expenditures: associations with health outcomes. *BMJ Quality and Safety* 10(1133), 1–6.

Braveman P, Cubbin C, Egerter S, Williams DR, Pamuk E. 2010. Socioeconomic disparities in health in the United States: what the patterns tell us. *American Journal of Public Health* 14, 20–35.

Braveman P, Egerter S, Williams DR. 2011. The social determinants of health: coming of age. *Annual Review of Public Health* 32, 381–98.

Coburn D. 2006. Medical dominance then and now: critical reflections. *Health Sociology Review* 15(5), 432–43.

Cohen R. 2007. *The Positive Impacts of Affordable Housing on Health: A Research Summary*. USA: Center for Housing Policy.

CSDH (Commission on Social Determinants of Health). 2008. *Closing the Gap in a Generation: Health Equity though Action on the Social Determinants of Health*. Geneva: World Health Organization.

Deaton A. 2003. Health, inequality, and economic development. *Journal of Economic Literature* 41, 113–58.

De Vogli R. 2011. Neoliberal globalization and health in a time of economic crisis. *Social Theory and Health* 9, 311–25.

Dunn JR. 2000. Housing and health inequalities: review and prospects for research. *Housing Studies* 15(3), 341–66.

Edwards N, Di Ruggiero E. 2011. Exploring which context matters in the study of health inequities and their mitigation. *Scandinavian Journal of Public Health* 39(6), 43–9.

Evans P. 2005. Neoliberalism as a political opportunity: constraint and innovation in contemporary development strategy. In Gallagher K (ed.) *Putting Development First: The Importance of Policy Space in the WTO and IFIs*, pp. 195–215. London: Zed Books.

Feachem RGA. 2001. Globalisation is good for your health, mostly. *BMJ* 323, 504–6.

Fernandez RM, Su C. 2004. Space in the study of labor markets. *Annual Review of Sociology* 30, 545–69.

Ferrie JE, Shipley M, Stansfeld S, Marmot MG. 2002. Effects of chronic job insecurity and change in job security on self-reported health, minor psychiatric morbidity, physiological measures and health related behaviours in British civil servants: the Whitehall II Study. *Journal of Epidemiology and Community Health* 56, 450–4.

Freeman RB. 2007. The challenge of the growing globalization of labor markets to economic and social policy. In Paus E (ed.) *Global Capitalism Unbound: Winners and Losers from Offshore Outsourcing*, pp. 23–40. Houndmills: Palgrave MacMillan.

Friel S, Marmot MG. 2011. Action on the social determinants of health. *Annual Review of Public Health* 32, 225–36.

Galabuzi GE. 2002. Social inclusion as a determinant of health. Presentation given at the Social Determinants of Health Across the Life-Span Conference, Toronto, November 2002.

Gill S. 1995. Globalization, market civilization, and disciplinary neoliberalism. *Millennium: Journal of International Studies* 24(3), 399–423.

Gill S, Bakker I. 2011. The global crisis and global health. In Benatar S, Brock G (eds) *Global Health and Global Health Ethics*, pp. 221–38. Cambridge: Cambridge University Press.

Gilson L, Doherty J, Loewenson R, Francis V. 2007. *Knowledge Network on Health Systems. WHO Commission on Social Determinants of Health, Final Report June 2007.* http://www.ucl.ac.uk/gheg/whocsdh/knsreports/knshs (last accessed December 2013).

Griffith-Jones S, Stallings B. 1995. New global financial trends: implications for development. In Stallings B (ed.) *Global Change, Regional Response: The New International Context of Development*, pp. 143–73. Cambridge: Cambridge University Press.

ILO (International Labour Organization). 2011. *Global Employment Trends 2011.* Geneva: ILO.

IMF (International Monetary Fund). 2007. *Spillovers and Cycles in the Global Economy: World Economic Outlook.* Washington, DC: IMF.

Kawachi I, Kennedy BP. 1997. Health and social cohesion: why care about income inequality? *BMJ* 314, 1037–40.

Kawachi I, Wamala SP. 2007. Poverty and inequality in a globalizing world. In Kawachi I, Wamala SP. (eds) *Globalisation and Health*, pp. 122–37. Oxford: Oxford University Press.

Kentikelenis A, Karanikolos M, Papanicolas I, Basu S, McKee M, Stuckler D. 2011. Health effects of financial crisis: omens of a Greek tragedy. *Lancet* 378(9801), 1457–8.

Koivusalo M, Schrecker T, Labonté R. 2008. *Globalization and Policy Space. Globalization Knowledge Network, World Health Organization Commission on Social Determinants of Health.* http://www.globalhealthequity.ca/electronic%20library/Globalisation%20and%20policy%20space%20for%20health%20and%20social%20determinants%20of%20health%20Koivusalo%20May%202009.pdf (last accessed December 2013).

Labonté R. 1994. Death of program, birth of metaphor: the development of health promotion in Canada. In O'Neill M, Pederson A, Rootman I (eds) *Health Promotion in Canada*, pp. 72–90. Toronto: WH Saunders.

Labonté R. 2002. Social inclusion/exclusion: dancing the dialectic. Presentation given at the Social Determinants of Health Across the Life-Span Conference, Toronto, November 2002.

Labonté R, Mohindra K, Schrecker T. 2011. The growing impact of globalization for health and public health practice. *Annual Review of Public Health* 32, 263–83.

Labonté R, Schrecker T. 2007a. Globalization and social determinants of health: introduction and methodological background. *Globalization and Health* 3, 5.

Labonté R, Schrecker T. 2007b. Globalization and social determinants of health: the role of the global market place. *Globalization and Health* 3, 6.

Labonté R, Schrecker T. 2007c. Globalization and social determinants of health: promoting health equity in global governance. *Globalization and Health* 3, 7.

Labonté R, Schrecker T, Packer C, Runnels V (eds). 2009. *Globalization and Health: Pathways, Evidence and Policy*, London: Routledge.

Labonté R, Torgerson R. 2005. Interrogating globalization, health, and development: towards a comprehensive framework for research, policy and political action. *Critical Public Health* 15(2), 155–79.

Lewchuk W, Clarke M, De Wolff A. 2011. *Working Without Commitments: The Health Effects of Precarious Employment.* Kingston and Montreal: McGill-Queen's University Press.

Lloyd JE, Li L, Hertzman C. 2010. Early experiences mater: lasting effect of concentrated disadvantage on children's language and cognitive outcome. *Health Place* 16(2), 371–80.

Maggi S, Irwin LG, Siddiqi A, Poureslami I, Hertzman E, Hertzman C. 2005. *Analytic and Strategic Review Paper. Knowledge Network for Early Child Development.* http://www.who.int/social_determinants/resources/ecd.pdf (last accessed December 2013).

Marmot MG. 2002. The influence of income on health: views of an epidemiologist. Does money really matter? Or is it a marker for something else? *Health Affairs* 21(2), 31–46.

Marmot MG. 2005. Social determinants of health inequities. *Lancet* 365(9464), 1099–104.

Marmot MG. 2006. Health in an unequal world. *Clinical Medicine* 6(6), 559–72.

Marmot MG, Stansfeld S, Patel C *et al*. 1991. Health Inequalities among British civil servants: the Whitehall II Study. *Lancet* 337(8754), 1387–93.

McKee M. 2002. What can health services contribute to the reduction of inequalities in health? *Scandinavian Journal of Public Health* 20(59), 54–8.

Mikkonene J, Raphael D. 2010. *The Social Determinants of Health: the Canadian Facts*. http://www.thecanadianfacts.org/The_Canadian_Facts.pdf (last accessed December 2013).

Milanovic B. 2011. More or less: income inequality has risen over the past quarter-century instead of falling as expected. *Finance and Development* 48(3), 6–11.

Mladovsky P, Srivastava D, Cylus J *et al*. 2012. *Health Policy Response to the Financial Crisis and Other Health System Shocks in Europe*. Policy Summary No. 5. Copenhagen: WHO Regional Office for Europe.

Moser K, Fox A, Jones D. 1984. Unemployment and mortality in the OPCS Longitudinal Study. *Lancet* 2(8415), 1324–8.

Natti J, Kinnunen U, Makikangas A, Mauno S. 2009. Type of employment relationship and mortality: prospective study among Finnish employees in 1984–2000. *European Journal of Public Health* 19(2), 150–6.

O'Neil BA, Forsythe ME, Stanish WD. 2001. Chronic occupational repetitive strain injury. *Canadian Family Physician* 47(2), 311–6.

Östlin P, Schrecker T, Sadana R *et al*. 2011. Priorities for research on equity and health: towards an equity-focused health research agenda. *Public Library of Science Medicine* 8(11), 1–6.

Pamuk E, Makuc DM, Heck KE, Reuben C, Lochner K. 1998. *Socioeconomic Status and Health Chartbook. Health, United States, 1998*. Hyattsville, MD: National Center for Health Statistics.

Pignone MP, DeWalt DA. 2004. Literacy and health outcomes: a systematic review of the literature. *Journal of General Internal Medicine* 19, 1228–39.

Raphael D (ed.). 2004. *Social Determinants of Health: Canadian Perspectives*. Toronto: Canadian Scholar's Press.

Raphael D. 2011. A discourse analysis of the social determinants of health. *Critical Public Health* 21(2), 221–36.

Reinhart CM, Rogoff KS. 2009. *This Time is No Different: Eight Centuries of Financial Folly*. Princeton, NJ: Princeton University Press.

Robert Wood Johnson Foundation. 2008. *Where We Live Matters for Our Health: The Links Between Housing and Health. Issue Brief 2: Housing and Health*. http://www.commission onhealth.org/PDF/033756c1-3ee3-4e36-bb0e-557a0c5986c3/Issue%20Brief%202%20Sept% 2008%20-%20Housing%20and%20Health.pdf (last accessed December 2013).

Rose G, Marmot MG. 1981. Social class and coronary heart disease. *British Heart Journal* 45(1), 13–9.

Rosen G. 1993. *A History of Public Health*. Baltimore, MD: Johns Hopkins University Press.

Sanders LM, Federico S, Klass P, Abrams MA, Dreyer B. 2009. Literacy and child health: a systematic review. *Archives of Pediatrics and Adolescent Medicine* 163(2), 131–40.

Schrecker T. 2009a. Labor markets, equity, and social determinants of health. In Labonté R, Schrecker T, Packer C, Runnels V (eds) *Globalization and Health: Pathways, Evidence and Policy*, pp. 81–105. New York: Routledge.

Schrecker T. 2009b. The power of money: global financial markets, national politics, and social determinants of health. In Williams O, Kay A (eds) *Global Health Governance: Crisis, Institutions and Political Economy*, pp. 160–81. Houndmills: Palgrave Macmillan.

Solar O, Irwin A. 2007. *A Conceptual Framework for Action on the Social Determinants of Health*. Discussion Paper, Commission on Social Determinants of Health. http://www.who.int/social_ determinants/resources/csdh_framework_action_05_07.pdf (last accessed December 2013).

Stuckler D, Basu S, McKee M. 2010. Budget crises, health, and social welfare programmes. *BMJ* 341, 77–9.

Townsend P, Davidson N, Whitehead M (eds). 1988. *Inequalities in Health: The Black Report and the Health Divide*. New York: Penguin.

Virtanen M, Kivimäki M, Joensuu M, Virtanen P, Elovainio M, Vahtera J. 2005. Temporary employment and health: a review. *International Journal of Epidemiology* 34(3), 610–22.

Warburton DE, Nicol CW, Bredin SS. 2006. Health benefits of physical activity: the evidence. *Canadian Medical Association Journal* 174, 801–9.

WHO (World Health Organization). 1986. *Ottawa Charter for Health Promotion*. Copenhagen: WHO Europe Office.

WHO (World Health Organization). 2000. *World Health Report: Health Systems Improving Performance*. Geneva: WHO.

Wilkinson R. 1996. *Unhealthy Societies: The Afflictions of Inequality*. New York: Routledge.

Wilkinson R, Marmot MG. 1998. *Social Determinants of Health: The Solid Facts*. Copenhagen: World Health Organization.

World Bank. 2007. *Global Economic Prospects 2007: Managing the Next Wave of Globalization*. Washington, DC: World Bank.

Part IV   Diplomacy, Security, and Humanitarianism

Chapter 15

Arguments for Securitizing Global Health Priorities

Simon Rushton

Abstract

In recent years there have been significant changes in the way policy communities think about and deal with health threats. Security language, concepts, practices, and institutions have become increasingly evident in national and global health policy, the result of decisions by both public health policy-makers and security policy communities to treat health as a security issue. This has raised concerns in some quarters about the potential negative consequences of securitization, yet there are a number of reasons for the security and public health communities to welcome the securitization of health. These include the fact that security actors have a vital contribution to make to the protection of populations from disease; that disease events can have widespread political, social, and economic effects (and that security policy-makers are inevitably concerned about this); that there are areas in which the two policy communities can profitably work together for mutual benefit; and that securitization offers those in public health an opportunity to gain increased attention and resources for otherwise neglected health issues. The chapter proceeds in three parts. It begins by discussing the securitization of health in the post-Cold War period, highlighting the three health issues (pandemic disease, biological weapons, HIV/AIDS) which have most often been addressed in security terms, and identifying some of the policy initiatives that have resulted from a more securitized approach. Drawing on these examples and others, the second section puts forward four arguments in favor of securitizing health. The conclusion assesses these arguments in favor of securitizing health in the light of some of the potential downsides.

The Handbook of Global Health Policy, First Edition. Edited by Garrett W. Brown, Gavin Yamey, and Sarah Wamala.
© 2014 John Wiley & Sons, Ltd. Published 2014 by John Wiley & Sons, Ltd.

Key Points

- Infectious diseases have increasingly been seen as a security threat in the post-Cold War era.
- The securitization of health could have negative consequences, but can also be an opportunity for furthering public health goals.
- Certain health issues, including major pandemics and biological weapons, are almost inevitably a concern to security policy communities and security actors have important parts to play in protecting populations from them.
- There are areas of synergy between health and security priorities in which the two policy communities can mutually benefit from working together.
- Deliberately seeking to securitize a health issue could in some circumstances be a fruitful strategy for those working in public health, but it is a strategy that should be pursued with caution.

Key Policy Implications

- The range of issues over which the security and public health policy communities are required to cooperate has expanded dramatically, and even closer cooperation seems likely to be required in future.
- A small number of health issues are now well-established on the security agenda and the involvement of health professionals in security policy-making is serving to institutionalize this.
- The strategic use of securitization may in some circumstances offer those in public health the chance to get attention and resources for a neglected health issue, but caution is required.

Introduction

Humans always have been, and always will be, vulnerable to disease. History is replete with examples of the devastating consequences that pathogens can have on populations. According to the best estimates we have, the Black Death of 1347–1351, one of the worst natural disasters in European history, killed around 24 million people – approximately one third of the continent's population at that time (Gottfried 1983: 77; Watts 1997: 1). Smallpox famously ravaged the indigenous populations of Central and South America in the sixteenth century (Watts 1997, chapter 3). The estimates of medical historians for the excess mortality caused by the 1918 "Spanish flu" pandemic vary widely, ranging from 20 million to 100 million (Murray *et al.* 2006: 2211), but whatever the true figure, the death toll was unimaginably high, and certainly far higher than the number of deaths resulting from the fighting in World War I. Disease is not, then, a new challenge facing governments. Neither are governments new to the business of attempting to protect their populations and territories from disease. The first quarantine regulations were implemented by the port of Ragusa in 1377 (Gensini *et al.* 2004), and in the centuries since states have employed a variety of different rules and procedures designed to prevent diseases entering their territories or disrupting their international trade relations.

However, there have been significant recent changes in the ways in which policy-makers think about and deal with health threats. Security language, concepts, practices, and institutions have become increasingly evident in national and global health policy, the result of moves by both public health policy-makers and foreign and security policy communities towards treating health as a security issue. Reflecting these developments in the policy world, a good deal of attention in the academic literature has focused on the "securitization of health" – the way in which certain health issues have come to be understood as security threats. In some quarters this securitization process has been welcomed as a means to place health policy in a more prominent agenda position and as a way of creating better responses to health problems. Others, however, have worried about the potentially negative consequences of securitizing health. These worries have included the following concerns:

- That securitization can distort the global health agenda and lead to a narrow and disproportionate focus on certain types of health problem (McInnes and Lee 2006).
- That securitization can undermine the traditional humanitarian orientation of public health (Feldbaum *et al.* 2006).
- That securitization can impact negatively on individual rights – particularly the rights of those infected with illnesses seen as "security threats" (Elbe 2006, 2009).
- That national security-based approaches might undermine the global cooperation necessary to deal with infectious disease threats in a globalized world (Enemark 2009; see also Chapter 16).
- That the national security agendas of the most powerful states may drive global health policy in directions which are not in the best interests of developing states, which suffer from the highest burdens of disease (and which, epidemiologically speaking, are often the "source" of disease threats to the West) (Aldis 2008; Ingram 2008).

That said, weighing the pros and cons of securitizing health is not a simple matter. As Stefan Elbe (2011) rightly noted in *The Lancet*, health professionals face a difficult dilemma in deciding whether or not to "play the global health security card." This chapter does not pretend to offer any solutions to that dilemma. What it attempts to do is to contribute to the ongoing debate by putting forward some of the arguments *in favor* of securitizing global health priorities. This is done not because I believe securitization is necessarily a good thing (in fact my own work (e.g., Rushton 2011) has tended to stress the problems associated with securitizing health and has argued that those working in public health should be circumspect in promoting security-based responses to health). Rather, the pro-securitization arguments are engaged with in order to allow the cons of securitizing health to be carefully weighed against as full an account as possible of the potential pros. Only then can policy-makers and commentators begin to reach more informed judgments about whether the securitization of health is to be welcomed or resisted.

The chapter proceeds in three parts. It begins by briefly discussing the securitization of health over the past two decades, highlighting the three health issues (pandemic disease, biological weapons, HIV/AIDS) that have most preoccupied security policy-makers and identifying some of the policy initiatives which have resulted from those concerns. Drawing on these examples and others, the second section forwards four arguments in favor of securitizing health. Finally, the conclusion returns to address some of the potential negatives of securitizing health in the light of the identified benefits.

Securitization of Infectious Disease in the Post-Cold War World

It has been widely noted that infectious disease has increasingly come to be treated by states as a security threat in the post-Cold War era. Indeed David Fidler (2007: 42) has argued that "the securitisation process is now over. Efforts to approach public health challenges through security concepts have prevailed in a way that constitutes a transformative development for public health governance." Although some have wondered whether this is overstating the case (e.g., Maclean 2008), it is true that there has been a dramatic increase in "security talk" in policy discussions around health in recent years. The rapid growth of the academic literature on health and security reflects this trend. Laurie's Garrett's (1994) *The Coming Plague* was an unusually early (and highly influential) example, but in the early 2000s a steady stream of work began to emerge from scholars within international relations and political science (as well as some from public health) who examined various aspects of the relationship between health and security. Andrew Price-Smith (2001, 2009), David Fidler (2003a, 2003b, 2007), Colin McInnes and Kelley Lee (2003, 2004, 2006), Stefan Elbe (2003, 2009, 2010) and Christian Enemark (2007) amongst others made particularly noteworthy early interventions in the field.

Whilst both the academic and policy discussions have addressed a reasonably wide range of aspects of the health–security link – and have examined health as a threat to human security as well as to the more traditional notions of national/international security, which I focus upon in this chapter – there have been three health issues which have been of particular concern to security policy communities (see Feldbaum and Lee 2004: 22–4).

The first is pandemic disease, in particular the threat of a major flu pandemic or an outbreak of some new or unexpected pathogen (so-called emerging and re-emerging infectious diseases). It is widely accepted that globalization has changed the nature of the infectious disease threat, not least through dramatically increasing the scale and rapidity of international travel and trade as well as promoting other processes such as migration and urbanization that impact upon patterns of disease transmission. The result of these developments is that the impossibility of containing pathogens within state borders has become clearer than ever. As a seminal report from the World Health Organization (WHO) put it, "an outbreak or epidemic in any one part of the world is only a few hours away from becoming an imminent threat somewhere else" (WHO 2007: x). The logic of this is not simply that states are potentially imperiled by public health emergencies that happen in other countries, but also that a collective international response is the only way to ensure what has come to be known as "global health security." SARS is the classic illustration of both the potential for rapid international disease transmission and the danger posed by states failing to cooperate in the face of infectious disease threats. The US National Intelligence Council's investigation into the SARS outbreak (National Intelligence Council 2003) graphically illustrated the way in which a single "superspreader" infecting fellow guests at the Metropole Hotel in Hong Kong led to the disease spreading to Singapore, Vietnam, Ireland, Canada, and the United States within a matter of hours (Figure 15.1). Four thousand cases of SARS were eventually traced back to this one individual. The actions of the People's Republic of China – which initially tried to cover up the outbreak

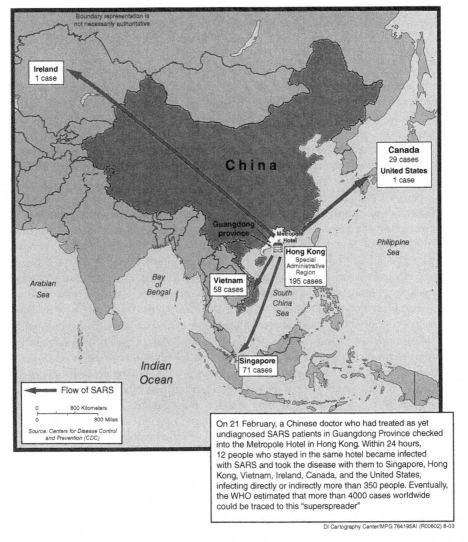

Figure 15.1   Portrait of a superspreader: spread of SARS from the Metropole Hotel in Hong Kong as of March 28, 2003. Source: National Intelligence Council (2003: 10).

and refused to allow the WHO to send investigators into Guangdong province where SARS first emerged – were particularly heavily criticized for having delayed an effective response, contributing to the international spread of the outbreak.

In more recent years these same concerns have been evident in discussions over the threat posed by pandemic influenza as well as slightly less high-profile threats such as "multidrug resistant" and "extensively drug resistant" tuberculosis. Perhaps the most tangible result of this heightened worry over pandemics was the revision of the International Health Regulations (IHRs), which WHO Member States agreed in 2005. These new regulations place states under an obligation to report all disease outbreaks "of international concern" to the WHO within 24 hours in order that the international community is alerted to the threat and so that appropriate measures can be put in place. The new IHRs are much more demanding of governments than the previous set of rules, and were intended to produce a far more effective global surveillance and reporting system than had previously existed. As has been widely noted (e.g., Fidler 2003a), the troubling experience of SARS, and the concerns of states over their future security, played a big part in bringing about the political commitment needed to get a global agreement on the revised regulations.

The second major concern has been that pathogens may be weaponized, either by terrorists or through state-sponsored biological weapons programs, and used against military forces or civilian populations. The attacks of September 11, 2001, and the "anthrax letters" which were posted to media organizations and US senators in the weeks afterwards, revitalized policy-makers' interest in this area – particularly around bioterrorism. This upsurge in interest was seen especially clearly in the United States, but was also evident internationally in the creation of bodies such as the Global Health Security Initiative (GHSI). The GHSI brought together the governments of Canada, France, Germany, Italy, Japan, Mexico, the United Kingdom, and the United States as well as the European Commission in order to develop "a more coordinated approach to improving the health security of citizens, and to better prepare for and respond to acts of terrorism, in the aftermath of September 11, 2001" and to promote "concerted global action to strengthen the public health response to the threat of international biological, chemical and radio-nuclear terrorism" (GHSI 2001). The new level of prioritization being given to concerns about biological weapons was also apparent in the massive increases in biodefense research budgets (much of which has been targeted at developing new and more effective ways of detecting incidents and diagnosing and treating those affected); heightened international intelligence cooperation; and a far greater emphasis on preparedness planning, interagency coordination mechanisms, and simulation exercises.

The third health-related issue that has appeared prominently on security agendas has been HIV/AIDS, the result of a perception that high burdens of HIV and AIDS can have social, political, economic, and military impacts that threaten the stability of heavily affected states. A variety of ways in which AIDS can contribute to state instability have been proposed, including: (i) the "hollowing out" of state institutions as key civil service workers become ill and die (Garrett 2005: 41); (ii) lost productivity producing detrimental economic and social effects (Fox and Kassalow 2001: 1555); (iii) the possibility that large numbers of AIDS orphans may, in some countries, fuel the child soldier problem (Singer 2002: 151); and (iv) that illness and premature death could undermine the effectiveness of the military and security services charged with maintaining order (Ostergard 2002: 342–4).

The linking of health and security is not in itself new. Szreter (2003), indeed, has argued that it is the separation of health and security rather than their coming together which is relatively recent. Yet it is clear that something changed in the 1990s and early 2000s – the security and public health communities increasingly found themselves discussing the same issues, and increasingly found themselves doing so in the same terms. The extent to which (particularly western) security policy communities have added health concerns – in particular infectious diseases – to the range of threats that they routinely concern themselves with is striking. Health threats have become a fixture on security agendas in much of the developed world, changing the way in which security is practiced (Elbe 2010). One clear example of this phenomenon is the *National Risk Register of Civil Emergencies*, which the UK government first published in 2008 and subsequently updated in 2010 and 2012 (Cabinet Office 2012). These reports examined both naturally occurring threats to the United Kingdom as well as malicious ones, rating each on the basis of "relative likelihood" and "relative impact." As in the previous reports, the 2012 update noted that pandemic influenza "remains the most significant civil emergency risk" (Cabinet Office 2012: 6). The potential threat posed by pandemics has assumed a similarly prominent place in US national security policy (e.g., National Intelligence Council 2000; Homeland Security Council 2006). At the global level, the UN Secretary-General's High-Level Panel on Threats, Challenges, and Change pointed to the threat posed by infectious diseases and called for a "new security consensus" that recognized disease as a key contemporary security threat (Secretary-General's High-level Panel on Threats Challenges and Change 2004: 1–2).

The ending of the Cold War, which had dominated security policy-making for decades, is generally credited with opening up space on security agendas for issues such as infectious disease (e.g., Buzan 1997). Yet it is also the case that the concerted efforts of some in the public health community to frame certain health issues in security terms has had an effect. One of the most prominent examples of this was Peter Piot's involvement in bringing HIV/AIDS to the United Nations Security Council in 2000. Piot, a Belgian medic who had worked widely in Africa in the 1970s and 1980s and was UNAIDS's first Executive Director from 1995 to 2008, played a prominent part in the Security Council sessions. Alongside other key players such as US Ambassador to the United Nations (UN) Richard Holbrooke and US Vice-President Al Gore, Piot addressed the Security Council on the social, economic, and security effects of HIV and AIDS in sub-Saharan Africa, his expertise doing much to add credibility to the securitizing claims which were being made. Indeed, advancing the argument that HIV/AIDS is a security issue was one of the leitmotifs of Piot's leadership of UNAIDS, with his official biography noting that he "challenged world leaders to view AIDS in the context of social and economic development as well as security" (UNAIDS n.d.). This was by no means an isolated example of public health figures deploying security arguments to highlight the seriousness of diseases. A 1992 report published by the US Institute of Medicine (Lederberg *et al.* 1992) entitled *Emerging Infections: Microbial Threats to Health in the United States,* which did much to dramatize the threat posed to the United States by infectious diseases and was highly influential in Washington policy circles, is another example. Key global health institutions have also played a role, not least the WHO through its championing of the concept of "global public health security" (e.g., WHO 2007).

Reasons to Welcome the Securitization of Health

The securitization of health has, then, been the product of ideas and initiatives emanating from two policy communities – security and public health – which have historically been only marginally connected. This has now changed, and both have come to see merit in addressing certain health issues in security terms. Yet, as will be discussed below, there can be a variety of motives for supporting securitization, and the two communities may not always be doing so for the same reasons. It is in these divergent motives that some of the potential dangers of securitization emerge. Before returning to these issues, however, this chapter outlines four of the most persuasive reasons for welcoming the securitization of health.

Security Actors can Help Protect Us from the Health Effects of Infectious Diseases

In 1962, Nobel Prize-winning virologist Sir Frank Macfarlane Burnet (in)famously declared that "One can think of the middle of the 20th century as the end of one of the most important social revolutions in history – the virtual elimination of infectious disease as a significant factor in social life" (Burnet 1962). Burnet's statement was, alas, somewhat premature. Although the WHO declared in 1980 that smallpox had been eradicated, that notable success has not been widely replicated elsewhere. Rinderpest, a virus affecting cattle, was declared to have been eradicated in 2010 and a small number of human diseases – polio being the most high profile – are close to eradication. Yet infectious disease still constitutes a major threat to populations in both the developing and (although to a lesser extent) developed worlds.

One of the fundamental purposes of the state is to provide security for its population, so there is clearly a basis for arguing that protection should be afforded against the threat posed by disease as much as against terrorist acts or invading armies (Price-Smith 2001: 118–19). The threat which disease poses to the health of the population, according to this argument, requires the state to take action to protect its citizens. In failing to see pathogens as security threats – and in failing to take action to minimize the risk – a state would be failing its most basic duty. The challenge that states face is providing this security in practice, especially in a globalized world in which people, animals, and goods routinely move across borders, massively increasing the speed at which an outbreak can spread internationally. The question then becomes not *whether* infectious disease should be seen as a security problem, but *what states should do about it*.

Addressing the challenges posed by infectious disease calls for various forms of response at both the national and international level, many of which rest upon well-established security concepts and practices. The most obvious of these are surveillance and preparedness activities, both of which are central to defending populations against infectious disease threats, and both of which are closely aligned to traditional security activities. Whilst public health expertise (and public health institutions) clearly remains central to these efforts, surveillance and intelligence gathering for the detection of potential security threats, preparedness planning, and crisis management are all staples of security. Although the threat posed by disease is different in many respects from military or terrorist threats, in principle the types of response required (such as attempting to detect disease threats where they occur, preparedness activities such as the stockpiling of antiviral medications, and the running of disease outbreak simulations in order to test civil contingency plans) are not so far removed from more traditional security activities. We have increasingly seen security actors fulfilling these roles in relation to infectious diseases alongside their counterparts from public health. As Elbe (2010) has noted, this increasing engagement of security actors with health issues has led to significant changes in the ways in which security is understood and practiced (leading, according to Elbe, to insecurity being redefined as a medical problem), and a far greater level of involvement of medical and public health professionals in formulating national security policy (Elbe 2010: 54–62; see also Chapter 16). This has been important in addressing concerns that security institutions lacked the necessary expertise to deal properly with health threats (e.g., Tucker 2001), but it has also served to cement health's status as a security issue, reducing the risk that it will drop off the agenda in future, and to foster institutionalized cooperation between security and public health agencies. The result is that security policy communities play a key part in protecting their populations from disease threats. Without that contribution, citizens would be in greater danger.

Diseases can Cause Significant Political, Social, and Economic Disruption

Andrew Price-Smith (2009: 20–2) provides a useful summary of the various ways in which disease can be seen as threatening to the state and society – further reasons for taking health seriously as a security threat. These include, amongst others, economic impacts (e.g., through lost productivity, the disruption of foreign trade, and the destabilization of markets); governance impacts (e.g., undermining a government's ability to ensure the provision of essential services and compromising the institutions charged with upholding law and order); and impacts upon a state's international relations (e.g., cross-border migration or the imposition of travel and trade restrictions). It is not hard to see how severe outbreaks of infectious disease could significantly threaten the ability of the state to operate effectively, and the types of measures that are commonly used in response to major outbreaks – measures such as "social distancing," which often involves the closure of schools, transport, and other public institutions – can pose major challenges to the normal functioning of society.

Certainly these problems have been well-recognized in the policy world. The UK's *National Risk Register of Civil Emergencies* (Cabinet Office 2012: 9–10) notes the "significant wider social and economic damage and disruption" that a pandemic would cause, including "significant threats to the continuity of essential services; lower production levels; shortages; and distribution difficulties." The pandemic preparedness plans of many other countries make very similar statements about the potential knock-on effects of a pandemic (e.g., Public Health Agency of Canada 2006; Council of Australian Governments 2011). It is clear in these statements that disease outbreaks are being viewed as potential national emergencies, and therefore as issues of security, for reasons that go beyond the direct impact on population health.

Whilst all of these issues are of ongoing concern to security policy-makers who plan for an influenza pandemic or a major outbreak of some other rapidly transmissible disease, there have been warnings that high HIV prevalence rates in parts of the developing world – especially sub-Saharan Africa – could be even more threatening to states and societies. Indeed, the US intelligence community was concerned about the impact of AIDS on countries in sub-Saharan Africa as early as 1987 (CIA 1987) and this worry spread more widely through Washington policy circles through the 1990s (see McInnes and Rushton 2010: 226–7). By the time it came to be discussed in the UN Security Council in 2000, the argument that AIDS threatened state stability had become well-established. In a powerful opening speech to the Security Council session, US Vice-President Al Gore said that:

> For the nations of sub-Saharan Africa, AIDS is not just a humanitarian crisis. It is a security crisis – because it threatens not just individual citizens, but the very institutions that define and defend the character of a society. This disease weakens workforces and saps economic strength. AIDS strikes at teachers, and denies education to their students. It strikes at the military, and subverts the forces of order and peacekeeping. (Gore 2000)

Given the strikingly high prevalence rates in some states in sub-Saharan Africa in particular, there is a compelling logic to the idea that states could be weakened as a result. Nevertheless, whilst these links were widely accepted in the late 1990s and early 2000s, more recent research has suggested that the links between AIDS and state fragility may in fact be more complex than was previously thought (e.g., Fourie 2007). The analysis undertaken by the AIDS, Security and Conflict Initiative (ASCI), which was published in 2010, for example, noted that "[a]s a long-wave event, the non-linearities and feedback loops in the relationship between HIV and AIDS and state fragility make it extremely difficult to discern any causal links" (de Waal *et al.* 2010: 35).

Notwithstanding these doubts, there is a clear logic to the case that infectious diseases of various kinds can cause political, economic, and social disruption, and for these reasons security institutions are inevitably concerned with mitigating their effects.

There are Synergies between Public Health and Security Priorities

It may well be that there are a number of other benefits to be gained from the security and public health policy communities working more closely and effectively together. For example, it has been argued that the structures, systems, and processes that need to be put in place to defend against naturally occurring disease events can also contribute to efforts to counter chemical, biological, radiological, and nuclear (CBRN) threats. The reverse has also been argued: that investing in biosecurity measures designed primarily to protect against biological weapons can have broader spin-off benefits for public health. In such areas, as Elbe (2011: 220) notes, "the worlds of health and security collide inescapably." There are a number of areas in which these purported synergies have translated into actions designed to address both deliberate and naturally occurring public health emergencies.

To take one example, in the period since the Fifth Review Conference of the Biological and Toxins Weapons Convention (BWC) in 2002, states party to the convention have begun to discuss the apparent synergies between public health infrastructure (e.g., disease surveillance and emergency response capabilities) and the types of surveillance and response capacity required to address biological weapons incidents. Although it remains at an early stage in terms of tangible outcomes, this incorporation of public health into the BWC is a particularly clear example of the securitization of health: for better or worse, public health has started to take on a role in what is effectively an arms control exercise.

Biodefence is another area in which synergies have been claimed. Spending on such research – particularly within the United States – increased exponentially in the wake of the 2001 anthrax attacks. According to *Nature*, approximately US$60 billion was spent on US biodefence programs (including research and development efforts and the stockpiling of vaccines and other medical countermeasures) in the decade from 2001 onwards (Check Hayden 2011). Some have argued that this massive increase – much of which has been spent on scientific research into detecting, diagnosing, and treating pathogens – has had significant knock-on benefits for public health more broadly. Burnett et al. (2005: 371), for example, have argued that "as with all good science, many recent biodefense research discoveries/advances have also directly facilitated our understanding and ability to treat other diseases, including antibiotic resistant bacteria and viruses (such as HIV and SARS)." According to a study by the Center for Biosecurity at the University of Pittsburgh Medical Center, the vast majority of US biodefence funding – $5.78 billion out of a total of $6.42 billion in the financial year 2012 – is indeed directed at programs that "have both biodefense and nonbiodefense goals and applications" (Franco and Sell 2011).

However, some have debated whether such purported "win–wins" are real or illusory. Fidler and Gostin (2007) in particular have called the "synergy thesis" into question, pointing out the continuing "surveillance gap" between developed and developing countries that persists despite the synergy rhetoric. They have also raised other objections to the idea that both the security and public health communities can benefit – including the seemingly inescapable tension between security's privileging of secrecy and health's traditional focus on scientific freedom and open dissemination of findings. It is also unclear whether the real benefits for public health are as significant as the amounts spent on defence measures might suggest. In the biodefence case, a number of commentators have argued that the real effect of this investment in research has been to promote and enrich a "biodefence industrial complex" rather than bringing significant benefits for public health more broadly (Fidler and Gostin 2007). Critics have also called into question whether the money which has been spent has been used effectively (even for biodefence); they have suggested that the prioritization of programs focusing on a narrow range of biological agents has distorted agendas and has diverted attention from other naturally occurring disease threats (Scientists Working Group on Biological and Chemical Weapons 2010); and they have suggested that the huge scale of biodefence research could actually increase rather than reduce the security threat. Given that the anthrax attacks of 2001 were widely (although not yet definitively) linked to Bruce Ivins, a scientist working in the US government biodefence lab at Fort Detrick, there seems to be merit in this latter concern, which reflects more general worries about the potential of life science research to be used for nefarious purposes.

Securitization brings Attention and Resources to Health

Despite these doubts, the idea that securitization can play an important role in bringing attention and resources to otherwise neglected health issues persists. Indeed, within the securitization of health literature this is the reason most commonly put forward in favor of securitization: that it can result in health issues being raised up the political agenda, and can persuade governments to devote attention and resources on a scale which would not otherwise be forthcoming. Reframing something as a security issue can, securitization theorists argue, have the effect of lifting it above "normal politics," making it "so important that it should not be exposed to the normal haggling of politics but should be dealt with decisively by top leaders prior to other issues" (Buzan *et al.* 1998: 29). It can also give public health the ability to access security budgets, offering new avenues for resourcing the fight against disease. This is one explanation for the enthusiasm of many in public health for presenting health issues in security terms. These efforts seem, at least for some health issues, to have borne fruit. As noted above, AIDS, flu, and biological weapons in particular have had a prominent place on global policy agendas over the past decade. Fidler, using the common distinction between "high politics" and "low politics" (where health has traditionally resided) has argued that "the frequency with which health concerns have cropped up in the realm of national and international security, whether the issue is bioterrorism or damage to state capacity caused by communicable diseases, suggests that the pursuit of health capabilities has become important even for the highest of high politics" (Fidler 2005: 183).

The significance of this inclusion on top-tier policy agendas should certainly not be underestimated. The G8, for example, has demonstrated a massively increased level of commitment to global health issues since the turn of the millennium, a commitment that has led to the creation and financing of new institutions such as the Global Fund to Fight

AIDS, Tuberculosis and Malaria and the launching of the Global Health Security Initiative. The US government, which launched the President's Emergency Plan for AIDS Relief (PEPFAR) in 2003 – a program which now claims to directly support treatment for 2.5 million people (PEPFAR 2011) – and the broader Global Health Initiative in 2009, has also paid unprecedented attention (and committed unprecedented amounts of money) to selected global health issues. It remains to be seen whether these commitments will be undermined in future by the ongoing financial crisis (Williams and Rushton 2011), but it is clear that health has rocketed up the political agenda. It is also clear that this has happened during the same period in which the securitization of health has been most clearly seen. It seems certain that the perception of health as a security issue played a part in this (although few would argue that securitization was solely responsible). The links to security rationales are clear in the case of the GHSI, for example, which was founded explicitly to address the challenge of bioterrorism and which has subsequently broadened its remit to include pandemic influenza. It is difficult in general, however, to separate out the independent effects of securitization from other powerful policy drivers. In the case of global health these include a renewed international focus on international development, as reflected in the Millennium Development Goals (MDGs); the commitment of a generation of political leaders – the most high profile of which within the G8 context were Tony Blair and Gordon Brown – to addressing some of the problems facing Africa; and (in the AIDS case in particular) the influence of powerful lobbies – operating from a variety of perspectives on both the left and right of the political spectrum – advocating increased access to antiretroviral medications.

Conclusions

There are, then, a number of arguments to support the securitization of health. First, security actors have a part to play in protecting populations from the health effects of disease threats. Second, the smooth running (and in extreme instances perhaps even the viability) of a state can be threatened by major public health events. Third, some health-related issues – such as those surrounding biological weapons – require the security and public health communities to work together. There remains room for significant improvement in this regard, but the fact that these two policy communities are now better connected and are increasingly "speaking the same language" is a source of encouragement. Finally, there is some evidence that through the strategic use of security arguments, high-level policy-makers can be "taught" to care about issues that have not previously been on their radar, and that this can bring benefits for public health.

But these potential benefits of securitization need to be weighed carefully against some of the possible downsides. Some of these downsides were highlighted in the introduction to this chapter: that public health can become politicized in unhelpful ways (see Chapter 16); that individual rights can be undermined; that global cooperation can be threatened; and that the security interests of powerful states can tend to dominate when it is the developing world that suffers by far the greater burden of disease. At the very least these risks should lead those working in public health to exercise caution in pursuing a strategy of securitization (see Chapter 18). It is also true that securitization can tend to privilege a narrow (and arguably distorted) global health agenda. Not all health challenges can be presented convincingly as security threats, and those which have tend to share certain characteristics: they are infectious diseases; they are (with the arguable exception of AIDS in Africa, which in many places has become an everyday fact of life) unusual and extraordinary events; and they are (again with the arguable exception of AIDS) events where individuals have little control over their exposure (McInnes 2005: 16–17). These health issues are all important, and governments and other actors need to address them. But only a small number of the health threats facing populations across the world fit into these categories. The range of factors that determine health status is vast, including poverty, diet and nutrition, housing, access to potable water, tobacco use, working conditions, and environmental degradation, to name but a few (see Chapter 14). The real danger is that the dominance of the global health agenda (and resource allocation) by a small number of securitized infectious disease threats can leave these myriad other issues in the shade. Whatever benefits securitization may offer, it is not a panacea for the many health problems that humanity faces.

Key Reading

De Waal A, Klot JF, Mahajan M *et al.* 2010. *HIV/AIDS, Security and Conflict: New Realities, New Responses*. New York: SSRC/Netherlands Institute of International Relations.

Elbe S. 2010. *Security and Global Health*. Cambridge: Polity.

Fidler DP. 2007. A pathology of public health securitism: approaching pandemics as security threats. In Cooper AF, Kirton JJ, Schrecker T (eds) *Governing Global Health: Challenge, Response, Innovation*, pp. 41–64. Aldershot: Ashgate.

Garrett L. 1994. *The Coming Plague: Newly Emergent Diseases in a World out of Balance*. New York: Farrar, Straus and Giroux.

Lakoff A, Collier SF (eds). 2008. *Biosecurity Interventions: Global Health and Security in Question*. New York: Columbia University Press.

McInnes C, Lee K. 2006. Health, security and foreign policy. *Review of International Studies* 32(1), 5–23.

Price-Smith AT. 2009. *Contagion and Chaos: Disease, Ecology, and National Security in the Era of Globalization*. Cambridge, MA: MIT Press.

References

Aldis W. 2008. Health security as a public health concept: a critical analysis. *Health Policy and Planning* 23, 369–75.

Burnet M. 1962. *Natural History of Infectious Disease*. Cambridge: Cambridge University Press.

Burnett JC, Panchal RG, Aman MJ, Bavari S. 2005. The rapidly advancing field of biodefense benefits many other, critical public health concerns. *Discovery Medicine* 5(28), 371–7.

Buzan B. 1997. Rethinking security after the Cold War. *Cooperation and Conflict* 32(1), 5–28.

Buzan B, Waever O, de Wilde J. 1998. *Security: A New Framework for Analysis*. Boulder, CO: Lynne Rienner.

Cabinet Office. 2012. *National Risk Register of Civil Emergencies: 2012 Update*. London: HMSO. http://www.cabinetoffice.gov.uk/sites/default/files/resources/CO_NationalRiskRegister_2012_acc.pdf (last accessed December 2013).

Check Hayden E. 2011. Biodefence since 9/11: the price of protection. *Nature* 477, 150–2.

CIA (Central Intelligence Agency). 1987. *Sub-Saharan Africa: Implications of the AIDS pandemic*. SNIE 70/1–87 (approved for release May 2001). Washington, DC: CIA.

Council of Australian Governments. Working Group on Australian Influenza Pandemic Prevention and Preparedness. 2011. *National Action Plan for Human Influenza Pandemic*. http://www.dpmc.gov.au/publications/pandemic/docs/NAP.pdf (last accessed December 2013).

De Waal A, Klot JF, Mahajan M *et al.* 2010. *HIV/AIDS, Security and Conflict: New Realities, New Responses*. New York: SSRC/Netherlands Institute of International Relations.

Elbe S. 2003. *Strategic Implications of HIV/AIDS*. Adelphi Paper No 357. Oxford: International Institute for Strategic Studies/Oxford University Press.

Elbe S. 2006. Should HIV/AIDS be securitized? The ethical dilemmas of linking HIV/AIDS and security. *International Studies Quarterly* 50(1), 119–44.

Elbe S. 2009. *Virus Alert: Security, Governmentality, and the AIDS Pandemic*. New York: Columbia University Press.

Elbe S. 2010. *Security and Global Health*. Cambridge: Polity.

Elbe S. 2011. Should health professionals play the global health security card? *Lancet* 378, 220–1.

Enemark C. 2007. *Disease and Security: Natural Plagues and Biological Weapons in East Asia*. Abingdon: Routledge.

Enemark C. 2009. Is pandemic flu a security threat? *Survival* 51(1), 191–214.

Feldbaum H, Lee K. 2004. Public health and security. In Ingram A (ed.) *Health, Foreign Policy and Security: Towards a Conceptual Framework for Research and Policy*, pp. 19–28. London: Nuffield Trust.

Feldbaum H, Patel P, Sondorp E, Lee K. 2006. Global health and national security: the need for critical engagement. *Medicine, Conflict and Survival* 22(3), 192–8.

Fidler DP. 2003a. *SARS, Governance and the Globalization of Disease*. Basingstoke: Palgrave Macmillan.

Fidler DP. 2003b. Public health and national security in the global age: infectious diseases, bioterrorism, and realpolitik. *George Washington International Law Review* 35, 787–856.

Fidler DP. 2005. Health as foreign policy: between principle and power. *Whitehead Journal of Diplomacy and International Relations* Summer/Fall, 179–94.

Fidler DP. 2007. A pathology of public health securitism: approaching pandemics as security threats. In Cooper AF, Kirton JJ, Schrecker T (eds) *Governing Global Health: Challenge, Response, Innovation*. Aldershot: Ashgate.

Fidler DP, Gostin LO. 2007. *Biosecurity in the Global Age: Biological Weapons, Public Health, and the Rule of Law*. Palo Alto, CA: Stanford University Press.

Fourie P. 2007. The relationship between the AIDS pandemic and state fragility. *Global Change, Peace and Security* 19(3), 281–300.

Fox DM, Kassalow JS. 2001. Making health a priority of US foreign policy. *American Journal of Public Health* 91, 1554–6.

Franco C, Sell TK. 2011. Federal Agency biodefense funding, FY2011–FY2012. *Biosecurity and Bioterrorism* 9(2), 117–37.

Garrett L. 1994. *The Coming Plague: Newly Emergent Diseases in a World out of Balance*. New York: Farrar, Straus and Giroux.

Garrett L. 2005. *HIV and National Security: Where are the Links?* New York: Council on Foreign Relations.

Gensini, GF, Yacoub MH, Conti AA. 2004. The concept of quarantine in history: from plague to SARS. *Journal of Infection* 49, 257–61.

GHSI (Global Health Security Initiative). 2001. *Ministerial statement, Ottawa, November*. http://www.ghsi.ca/english/statementottawanov2001.asp (last accessed December 2013).

Gore A. 2000. Opening statement. *The United Nations Security Council 4087th Meeting, January 10, 2000*. S/PV.4087, p. 6. http://www.securitycouncilreport.org/atf/cf/%7B65BFCF9B-6D27-4E9C-8CD3-CF6E4FF96FF9%7D/CC%20SPV%204087.pdf (last accessed December 2013).

Gottfried RS. 1983. *The Black Death: Natural and Human Disaster in Medieval Europe*. New York: Free Press.

Homeland Security Council. 2006. *National Strategy for Pandemic Influenza: Implementation Plan*. Washington, DC: Homeland Security Council. http://www.flu.gov/planning-preparedness/federal/pandemic-influenza-implementation.pdf (last accessed December 2013).

Ingram A. 2008. Pandemic anxiety and global health security. In Pain R, Smith SJ (eds) *Fear: Critical Geopolitics and Everyday Life*, pp. 75–85. Farnham: Ashgate.

Lederberg J, Shope RE, Oaks S. 1992. *Emerging Infections: Microbial Threats to Health in the United States*. Washington, DC: Institute of Medicine/National Academy Press.

Maclean S. 2008. Microbes, mad cows and militaries: exploring the links between health and security. *Security Dialogue* 39(5), 475–94.

McInnes C. 2005. *Health, Security and the Risk Society*. London: Nuffield Trust.

McInnes C, Lee K. 2003. *Health, Foreign Policy and Security*. London: Nuffield Trust.

McInnes C, Lee K. 2004. A conceptual framework for research and policy. In Ingram A (ed.) *Health, Foreign Policy and Security: Towards a Conceptual Framework for Research and Policy*, pp. 10–18. London: Nuffield Trust.

McInnes C, Lee K. 2006. Health, security and foreign policy. *Review of International Studies* 32(1), 5–23.

McInnes C, Rushton S. 2010. HIV, AIDS and security: where are we now? *International Affairs* 86(1), 225–45.

Murray CJ, Lopez AD, Chin B, Feehan D, Hill KH. 2006. Estimation of potential global pandemic influenza mortality on the basis of vital registry data from the 1918–20 pandemic: a quantitative analysis. *Lancet* 368, 2211–18.

National Intelligence Council. 2000. *The Global Infectious Disease Threat and its Implications for the United States*. NIE 99–17D. http://www.fas.org/irp/threat/nie99-17d.htm (last accessed December 2013).

National Intelligence Council. 2003. *SARS: Down but Still a Threat*. NIC ICA 2003–09. http://www.fas.org/irp/nic/sars.html (last accessed December 2013).

Ostergard RL. 2002. Politics in the hot zone: AIDS and national security in Africa. *Third World Quarterly* 23, 333–50.

PEPFAR (President's Emergency Plan for AIDS Relief). 2011. *Treatment*. http://www.pepfar.gov/about/138312.htm (last accessed December 2013).

Price-Smith AT. 2001. *The Health of Nations: Infectious Disease, Environmental Change, and their Effects on National Security and Development*. Cambridge, MA: MIT Press.

Price-Smith AT. 2009. *Contagion and Chaos: Disease, Ecology and National Security in the Era of Globalization*. Cambridge, MA: MIT Press.

Public Health Agency of Canada. 2006. *Canadian Pandemic Influenza Plan*. http://www.phac-aspc.gc.ca/influenza/plans-eng.php (last accessed December 2013).

Rushton S. 2011. Global health security: security for whom? Security from what? *Political Studies* 59(4), 779–96.

Scientists Working Group on Biological and Chemical Weapons. 2010. Biological threats: a matter of balance. *Bulletin of the Atomic Scientists* February 2. http://thebulletin.org/biological-threats-matter-balance (last accessed December 2013).

Secretary-General's High-level Panel Report on Threats, Challenges and Change. 2004. *A More Secure World: Our Shared Responsibility*. New York: United Nations.

Singer PW. 2002. AIDS and international security. *Survival* 44, 145–58.

Szreter S. 2003. Health and security in historical perspective. In Chen L, Leaning J, Narasimhan V (eds) *Global Health Challenges for Human Security*, pp. 31–52. Cambridge, MA: Harvard University Press.

Tucker JB. 2001. *Improving infectious disease surveillance to combat bioterrorism and natural emerging infections*. Testimony before the Subcommittee on Labor, Health and Human Services, Education, and Related Agencies of the U.S. Senate Committee on Appropriations, October 3. http://cns.miis.edu/archive/cbw/testtuck.htm (last accessed December 2013).

UNAIDS. n.d. *Biography of former UNAIDS Executive Director Dr Peter Piot*. http://www.unaids.org/en/aboutunaids/unaidsleadership/formerexecutivedirectorofunaids/formerunaidsexecutivedirectorpeterpiot/ (last accessed December 2013).

Watts S. 1997. *Epidemics and History: Disease, Power and Imperialism*. New Haven, CT: Yale University Press.

WHO (World Health Organization). 2007. *The World Health Report 2007. Global Public Health Security in the 21st Century: A Safer Future*. Geneva: WHO.

Williams OD, Rushton S. 2011. Are the "good times" over? Looking to the future of global health governance. *Global Health Governance* 5(1), 1–19.

Chapter 16

Viral Sovereignty: The Downside Risks of Securitizing Infectious Disease

Stefan Elbe and Nadine Voelkner

Abstract

This chapter analyzes how the "securitization" of highly pathogenic avian influenza (H5N1) contributed to the rise of a protracted international virus sharing dispute between developing and developed countries. As fear about the threat of a possible human H5N1 pandemic spread across the world, many governments scrambled to stockpile antiviral medications and vaccines – albeit in a context where there was insufficient global supply to meet such a rapid surge in demand. Realizing that they were the likely "losers" in this international race, some developing countries began to openly question the benefits of maintaining existing forms of international health cooperation – especially the common practice of sharing national virus samples with the rest of the international community. Given that such virus samples were also crucial to the high-level pandemic preparedness efforts of the West, the Indonesian government in particular felt emboldened to use international access to its H5N1 virus samples as a diplomatic "bargaining chip" for negotiating better access to vaccines and other benefits for developing countries. The securitized global response to H5N1 thus ended up unexpectedly entangling the longstanding international virus sharing mechanism within a wider set of political disputes, as well as prompting governments to subject existing virus sharing arrangements to much narrower calculations of national interest. In the years ahead these risks to international health cooperation must be balanced with the policy attractions of the global health security agenda.

A version of this chapter was previously published as: Elbe, Stefan. 2010. "Haggling over viruses: the downside risks of securitizing infectious disease." *Health Policy and Planning* 25(6), 476–85, doi 10.10786/598283.

The Handbook of Global Health Policy, First Edition. Edited by Garrett W. Brown, Gavin Yamey, and Sarah Wamala.
© 2014 John Wiley & Sons, Ltd. Published 2014 by John Wiley & Sons, Ltd.

Key Points

- Indonesia's decision in December 2006 to cease sharing its H5N1 virus samples with the international public health community prompted widespread consternation in the West, as well as eliciting considerable support from many developing countries.
- The resulting international virus sharing controversy persisted for many years and became enmeshed in a broader set of complex legal, political, and economic issues that make the disagreement very difficult to resolve.
- Presenting highly pathogenic avian flu as a pressing global security threat contributed to this re-politicization of existing virus sharing mechanisms, and also enabled countries like Indonesia to use access to H5N1 virus samples as a diplomatic bargaining chip for fundamentally reforming the international virus sharing system.
- The securitization of H5N1 rendered international health cooperation a matter of more narrow and calculated national interest, prompting Indonesia to assert its "viral sovereignty" over the virus.
- The international virus sharing dispute shows that a securitized response to infectious disease management has downside risks in terms of complicating international health cooperation.

Key Policy Implications

- A securitized response to infectious disease management can help to mobilize political leadership and resources for the management of emerging and re-emerging infectious diseases.
- A securitized response to infectious disease management can also have unanticipated effects that complicate existing forms of international health cooperation.
- The downside risks associated with a securitized response to global public health will need to be balanced with the evident benefits of the global health security agenda.

Introduction

Amidst pressing international concern that the world was on the cusp of a renewed human influenza pandemic, the Indonesian government took the controversial decision in December 2006 to cease sharing its H5N1 virus samples with the international community. It did so after discovering that the virus samples it had been forwarding freely to the World Health Organization (WHO) through the longstanding Global Influenza Surveillance Network (GISN) were being passed on to pharmaceutical companies in the West, where they were being used to develop lucrative new vaccines. Indonesia pointed out that this violated the WHO's own guidelines, according to which, virus samples should not be distributed outside the WHO network without the prior consent of originating countries (WHO 2005b: 2). Western pharmaceutical companies subsequently also offered those novel vaccines back to the Indonesian government at commercial rates, which Indonesian authorities deemed unaffordable in light of the country's large population of more than 220 million people.

Indonesia's decision to stop this "exploitative" process by withholding its virus samples split opinion within the international community. Many governments and medical researchers in the West expressed consternation and even anger at a decision they claimed was recklessly endangering international public health and global health security. Yet Indonesia's position also won considerable support, especially amongst many developing countries who felt similarly unable to afford vaccines at market rates. The resulting international dispute over virus sharing lasted for many years, and marks one of the most substantial setbacks in international health cooperation of the past decade. The course of events leading up to the international virus sharing dispute is complex, and is also likely to involve a range of factors associated with Indonesian domestic politics, including attempts to locate Indonesia's health policies within wider anti-western struggles and other political reasons (Forster 2009: 47–9). Notwithstanding, this chapter examines the way the initial "securitization" of highly pathogenic avian influenza provoked a chain of events that contributed to the emergence of the international dispute. It argues that the securitized international response to H5N1 had two fateful consequences.

First, the considerable fear of an imminent human pandemic provoked a competitive rush amongst governments around the world (including Indonesia) to secure access to medical countermeasures for reducing the spread of H5N1. Considering the insufficient global supplies to meet that sudden surge in demand, developing countries became acutely aware that a profound conflict of interest exists between developed and developing countries in existing forms of international health cooperation. The international virus sharing mechanism may work well for developed countries that possess their own pharmaceutical manufacturing base, but the material benefits accruing from such cooperation for developing countries are far less evident.

Second, the high-level concern about H5N1 in the West suddenly also rendered the viruses circulating in Indonesia's territorial borders very "valuable." At the time, the West needed unencumbered and legal access to samples of those viruses in order to track the global evolution of the virus and to develop pharmacological treatments against the threat. Without such access, the West would not be able to maintain a set of comprehensive and up-to-date medical interventions to protect their populations – even if they had the manufacturing capacity to do so. Amidst the occasionally frenzied efforts of the West to shore up its defences against the impending H5N1 threat, and the political pressure it consequently put on developing countries where human cases of H5N1 infection were already occurring, the Indonesian government in particular came to realize that it now controlled access to what was in fact a very precious "resource" – and one which it, in turn, could deploy as a diplomatic bargaining chip on the international stage for negotiating greater access to vaccines and other benefits for developing countries.

Both effects of the securitization of H5N1 ultimately made the virus sharing dispute more difficult to resolve: the first embroiled the longstanding international virus sharing mechanism in a much wider set of North–South disputes, whilst the second rendered international health cooperation a matter of more narrow and calculated national interest. A key lesson to emerge from the international virus sharing controversy is therefore that a securitized response to infectious disease management can also have unanticipated consequences in terms of further complicating international health cooperation. In the years ahead the downside risks associated with a securitized response to global public health will need to be balanced against the evident benefits of the global health security agenda – especially in terms of mobilizing political leadership and resources for the management of emerging and re-emerging infectious diseases.

Method

The chapter undertakes a case study analysis of the international response to the emergence of human infections with highly pathogenic avian influenza A viruses of the subtype H5N1 (hereafter simply called H5N1). The study draws upon securitization theory as its conceptual framework, which was initially developed in the non-medical disciplines of international relations and critical security studies (Buzan *et al.* 1998; see Chapter 15). Securitization theory is principally concerned with discerning how issues are responded to differently in national and international policy circles when they become widely perceived or "framed" as pressing existential threats. Crucially, and as a constructivist social theory, securitization theory does not try to establish whether any particular issue "really" constitutes a security threat or not. Instead, it mostly comes into play once an issue has already been securitized, and forms a useful conceptual tool for studying the political consequences of such a securitization process. Based on an extensive analysis of a wide range of different international issues that have become securitized over the past two decades, securitization theory has been able to identify a set of policy advantages and drawbacks that can accrue once issues are securitized. A rapidly evolving literature now documents the securitization of infectious diseases specifically (Elbe 2006; McInnes and Lee 2006; Ingram 2007; Kelle 2007; Davies 2008; Fidler and Gostin 2008; Leboeuf and Broughton 2008; Scoones and Forster 2008).

Taking an interdisciplinary approach and bringing securitization theory to bear directly on the international response to highly pathogenic avian influenza is useful in that H5N1 too became widely perceived as constituting such a pressing existential threat in international policy circles (especially throughout 2005 and 2006). Indeed, H5N1 marks one of the most prominent international health issues to have become securitized over the past decade. The following study analyzes the political consequences in relation to the international virus sharing dispute.

The empirical material for this study on the international politics of virus sharing was drawn from a variety of different sources. Those sources include more than a dozen semi-structured, one-to-one background interviews carried out with key participants in the international virus sharing dispute. The chapter also took into account a range of policy papers, background papers, working papers, and articles on virus sharing generated by international organizations, governments, think tanks, and newspapers (secondary data), as well as scholarly articles and books published on the virus sharing controversy (tertiary data). Those sources were located through library searches, scholarly databases in public health and international relations, internet searches using a commercial search engine, and contacts in the international academic and policy communities.

Results and Discussion

The Securitization of H5N1

The manifestations of the securitization process of H5N1 are too numerous to recount in full; but a few examples will suffice to illustrate the point. Writing in the *New York Times* in 2005, two senators from the US Senate Foreign Relations Committee warned their readers that we usually think about national security threats in terms of nuclear proliferation, rogue states, and terrorism, but that "another kind of threat lurks beyond our shores, one from nature, not humans – an avian flu pandemic. An outbreak could cause millions of deaths, destabilize Southeast Asia (its likely place of origin), and threaten the security of governments around the world" (New York Times 2005). One of the two senators sounding that alarm was – at the time – a junior Democrat from the state of Illinois who would later go on to become President of the United States of America – Barak Obama. In his view H5N1 was not just another infectious disease to be dealt with by routine international public health measures, but a new and grave global threat requiring a much more urgent policy response. That same year, across the Atlantic, the Civil Contingency Secretariat in the United Kingdom echoed that avian flu is "as serious a threat as terrorism" (Lean 2005).

In 2006 the National Security Strategy of the United States (NSS 2006) then directly acknowledged the threat posed by "public health challenges like pandemics (HIV/AIDS, avian influenza) that recognize no borders." The 2006 World Economic Forum held in Davos, Switzerland, similarly identified H5N1 as the primary threat preoccupying global business and political leaders. Noting limited supplies of antiviral drugs, its report warned that in the worst case scenario there could even be "rioting to gain access to scarce supplies of anti-virals and vaccines; a collapse of public order; partial de-urbanization as people flee population centres; the extinction of trust in governments; decimation of specific human skill sets; and forced, large-scale migration, associated with the further collapse of already weak states" (WEF 2006: 9). In retrospect, 2005 and 2006 thus emerge as the two years in which the securitization of highly pathogenic avian influenza reached its highest level in terms of H5N1 being widely perceived as a pressing existential threat demanding an urgent and sustained international response.

That concern with the acute existential threat posed by H5N1 would continue well into 2007 and 2008 – although there is some evidence that the threat perception began to decline in the course of 2008, and attention also rapidly shifted to the emergence of influenza A (H1N1) in the spring of 2009 (World Bank 2008). Yet in 2007, the WHO still referred to avian flu as "the most feared security threat" (WHO 2007: 45), whilst in 2008, pandemic threats remained salient enough to be officially incorporated into the United Kingdom's National Security Strategy – both because of their ability to directly affect the country and because they could potentially undermine international stability (Cabinet Office 2008: 3). That same year the World Bank warned in one of its reports that even though the incidence of human cases of infection was declining in many countries, "the virus remains a substantial threat to global public health security" (World Bank 2008: 10).

It is possible, then, to trace how highly pathogenic avian influenza became "securitized" during the past decade. During this time H5N1 was elevated from a technical public health issue that could be dealt with through the routine procedures of public health institutions and scientific experts, to something perceived as posing a much more existential threat to populations, economic systems, and even political structures. The international response to the threat of H5N1 thus makes an ideal case study for analyzing the kinds of policy advantages and drawbacks that accrue when issues become securitized specifically in the field of global health.

Turning first to the policy advantages, the securitization of H5N1 undoubtedly raised political awareness about the virus around the world, and persuaded policy-makers to formulate a range of pandemic preparedness plans. A survey carried out by the United Nations System Influenza Coordination Unit suggests that over 140 countries developed national pandemic preparedness plans, although their extent varied significantly between countries and many of those plans still remain untested in practice (World Bank 2008: 52). The threat associated with H5N1 has also freed up resources to address the issue – with US$2.7 billion having been pledged globally ($1.5 billion disbursed) for pandemic preparedness efforts (World Bank 2008: 8). A 2008 World Bank report thus found that "the threat posed over the last 5 years has mobilized an unprecedented coming together of the animal health, human health, disaster preparedness and communication sectors to work in a cross discipline, cross sector and cross boundary way" (World Bank 2008: 8). Moreover, such preparations were undoubtedly helpful in making governments feel more prepared when dealing with the outbreak of new human influenza A infections (H1N1) in the course of 2009. All of these developments also confirm a core insight witnessed in relation to a range of other securitization processes, namely that they can have policy benefits in terms of mobilizing resources and garnering greater political attention for important issues (Buzan *et al.* 1998: 29).

Those benefits notwithstanding, however, international efforts to prepare the world for a possible human H5N1 pandemic also encountered at least one very significant setback when the Indonesian government unexpectedly decided that it would no longer share its H5N1 virus samples with the rest of the international community. That move threw a sizeable spanner into the global pandemic preparedness machinery because Indonesia was, in many ways, at the "forefront" of a possible H5N1 pandemic – reporting both the highest number of human cases and deaths of H5N1 infection up to that point in time. Without access to the viruses circulating within Indonesia's territorial borders, it was no longer possible for the international public health community to acquire comprehensive surveillance data about how the virus was evolving, nor to develop stockpiles of up-to-date candidate vaccines based on the more virulent Indonesian virus strands.

With emotions running high on both sides, the stand-off between the West and Indonesia (backed vocally by many other developing countries such as Thailand, Brazil, and India as well as the Third World Network) has become known in the international public health community as the "virus sharing controversy." That dispute lasted several years until a new Pandemic Influenza Preparedness framework was agreed in 2011. As we shall see below, the securitized response to H5N1 contributed to that critical setback in international public health cooperation in at least two ways.

The International Scramble for Antivirals and Vaccines

As bird flu came to be perceived as a pressing global security threat, many governments around the world embarked upon a frenzied race to acquire special medical countermeasures to meet this impending threat. In the case of H5N1 there are actually many different ways in which governments could respond to a possible pandemic, including a range of non-pharmacological interventions such as isolation, quarantine, and contact tracing, through to traveler screening and implementing social distancing measures that minimize public gatherings by closing schools and canceling mass spectator events. In fact, when it comes to seasonal flu, many developing countries do not routinely resort to medical countermeasures such as mass vaccination or prescribing antivirals – an understandable public health strategy in light of competing budgetary pressures and a range of other health issues that also need to be urgently addressed.

Yet given the perceived level of the H5N1 threat, most governments rapidly concluded that confronting H5N1 required more than just the usual public health responses to communicable diseases – not least because the considerable international anxiety around H5N1 created immense domestic pressures for governments to be seen as taking the strongest possible action to protect citizens against a pending pandemic. Following the recommendation of the WHO, many governments decided that in the event of a pandemic the best line of defense would be the extensive use of pharmacological interventions such as antivirals and new vaccines (WHO 2005a: 45). Amongst the considerable anxiety that a human H5N1 pandemic was imminent, antivirals and vaccines quickly became seen as the "magic bullet" or "gold standard" for countries to defend themselves against the looming threat. Not surprisingly, the serious concern about the threat posed by H5N1 ended up stimulating immense international demand for these pharmacological products. Many governments around the world felt that the only way to adequately protect their populations was to take the extraordinary step of proactively stockpiling those medicines (especially antivirals) to ensure availability of supplies for rapid dispersal in the event of a pandemic materializing.

Yet from a global public health perspective, that intense focus on acquiring medical countermeasures had a significant drawback: there was insufficient international manufacturing capacity to meet such a sudden surge in demand. As the WHO report noted, "Demand will unquestionably outstrip supply, particularly at the start of a Pandemic" (WHO 2005a: 46). Put differently, in the event of pandemic transmission of H5N1, there would be countries that would benefit from the protection afforded by pharmacological interventions (or at least do so before the majority of other countries), and those that would have to settle for a more "low-tech" approach probably associated with higher rates of morbidity and mortality.

It was not difficult for several developing countries to deduce that they were likely to be the losers as they were facing a double disadvantage. First, manufacturing capacity – especially in terms of vaccines – was geographically concentrated in developed countries (Australia, Europe, Japan, North America), giving those countries a distinct advantage in terms of securing access to medicines for their populations (WHO 2005a: 47). Second, under market conditions where demand outstrips supply, the factor most likely to determine who would secure those treatments would be price; and here, too, it would be difficult for developing countries to compete with their wealthier counterparts.

Such global inequalities are certainly not new. Many developing countries have long been aware of how the market dynamics of supply and demand have frequently worked to their disadvantage in the area of public health. In many cases such free market conditions do not exist in the first place, because the allocation of medical countermeasures are often agreed between governments and commercial companies through pre-purchase agreements long in advance of a pandemic actually materializing. Moreover, related concerns about global inequalities were already simmering amongst developing countries amidst the extensive changes negotiated to the International Health Regulations, the rise of new international surveillance mechanisms (Calain 2007), and the wider (and controversial) discussions about global health security (Aldis 2008: 373–4). Yet, as the world was confronted with the spectre of an impending H5N1 pandemic, those inequalities crystallized in quite a stark manner. If a pandemic was coming, there would be huge disparities in the medical defenses available to countries around the world.

The realization of that profound inequality provoked deep frustrations about existing forms of global health governance. In fact, some developing countries were so dismayed at the possibility of having to confront an imminent pandemic without access to such medical interventions that they began to openly question the value of maintaining existing forms of international health cooperation, which appeared to mostly benefit developed countries. These frustrations feature particularly prominently in the account of the virus sharing dispute advanced by the Indonesian Health Minister Siti Supari in her book *It's Time for the World to Change* in which she described her experiences and views on the international virus sharing dispute (Supari 2008).[1]

In the book Supari recounts an early but formative encounter with this scarcity problem specifically in relation to antivirals. When, in 2005, she was finally able to find some resources from other government budgets to purchase Tamiflu® for treating early cases of human H5N1 infection that had emerged in Indonesia, she claims that she could not obtain supplies because the medicine was being pre-emptively stockpiled by western countries – which at that point did not even have any cases of human infection with H5N1. She was concerned that it may have proved impossible for Indonesia to acquire the medicines at that time, had it not been for the willingness of Australia and Thailand to share their supplies with Indonesia (Supari 2008: 5–6).

That episode occurred early on in the securitization of H5N1, and the international production of Tamiflu has expanded considerably since that time, including production in generic form. Nevertheless, that early experience with the limited availability of Tamiflu clearly left a lasting impression on Supari, especially in relation to the eventual development of a vaccine, for which production capabilities would initially remain similarly insufficient to meet demand (Supari 2008: 5–6). That fear would become partially realized in 2006 when she was informed by a journalist from the Australian Broadcasting Corporation that an Australian company was trying to develop a vaccine on the basis of the Indonesian strain that it had shared with the international community through the GISN.

This problem of the uneven international distribution of medical countermeasures could not be quickly resolved. A report released in March 2009 by the international management consulting firm Oliver Wyman, which was commissioned by the Bill & Melinda Gates Foundation, estimated that the most likely scenario in the event of a H5N1 pandemic would be an international production capacity of 2.5 billion doses of pandemic vaccine in the first 12 months (after the production strain is received), which would require another 4 years to meet global demand (Oliver Wyman 2009). Moreover, because vaccines usually need to be virus-specific, developed countries too would have to wait several months before the first mass-produced vaccines became available. Nevertheless, these inequalities remain an important and enduring feature of global health governance, much to the dissatisfaction of many developing countries.

So frustrated and disillusioned was the Indonesian government, in particular, that it took the controversial decision in December 2006 to withdraw from the GISN by ceasing to share its H5N1 virus samples with the international community unless the viruses were formally recognized as Indonesian (by signing a formal Material Transfer Agreement), and until greater access to vaccines and other benefits derived from the virus sharing mechanism were secured for developing countries. As Supari put it in a March 2007 speech at the High Level Meeting on Responsible Practices for Sharing Avian Influenza Viruses and Resulting Benefits, "it is time to change the mechanism of the GISN because it is not in favour of the avian flu affected countries" (Supari 2008: 52). Indonesia, in other words, would no longer cooperate with the longstanding virus sharing mechanisms unless the concerns of developing countries about access to vaccines and other benefits were systematically addressed. That crucial decision effectively triggered the international virus sharing dispute.

With the benefit of hindsight, then, it is possible to trace how the securitized response to H5N1 provoked a chain of events that would end up putting substantial new pressure on existing forms of international public health cooperation. The immense fear surrounding H5N1 compelled governments around the world to protect their populations by under-taking emergency defensive measures such as seeking stockpiles of antivirals and new vaccines. Yet, because there is insufficient supply capacity at the international level for meeting this demand, that proved very difficult for developing countries to achieve. The latter quite understandably became disillusioned with the merits of maintaining existing forms of public health cooperation like the international virus sharing mechanism and began openly questioning its legitimacy. From their perspective, those forms of international health cooperation might work well for developed countries that possess their own pharmaceutical manufacturing base, but the material benefits accruing from such cooperation for developing countries are far less evident.

These events also fundamentally changed the prospects of continuing international health cooperation between developed and developing countries. Whereas hitherto the international virus sharing mechanism was largely seen as a routine system of functional public health cooperation between countries, its operation now became a heavily politicized North–South issue that eventually also attracted the support of the 112-member-strong Non-Aligned Movement (in May 2008). By this time the international virus sharing mechanism was no longer just a technical or functional issue between Indonesia and the WHO, but a political contest between developed and developing countries. After operating for more than half a century, the GISN suddenly faced one of its most significant political challenges to date (Brammer et al. 2007: 254–5). This is one way that the securitized global response to H5N1 has unexpectedly ended up politically complicating an important and longstanding mechanism of international health cooperation.

Turning Lethal Viruses into Diplomatic Bargaining Chips

The securitization of H5N1 also encouraged greater and more high-level state involvement in infectious disease management, which ended up complicating international health cooperation further still. This is because some states suddenly began to subject the international virus sharing mechanism to much narrower calculations of national interest, and even attempted to use virus samples as diplomatic bargaining chips for pursuing their national interest.

The Indonesian government in particular recognized that the securitized international response to H5N1, with all of its frenzied pandemic preparedness activities, also offered positive political opportunities for exploiting the virus sharing mechanism in the pursuit of the country's national interest. The Indonesian government knew at least three things. First, all the high-level attention on H5N1 made it clear to the government how pressing a political concern H5N1 was in the West, and how much political pressure there was to protect populations against this threat. Second, because western countries initially had no human cases of H5N1 infection occurring within their own territories, they could only make the vaccines by getting access to viruses from other countries, such as Indonesia (Supari 2008: 10). Virus samples were thus a crucial "resource" for western governments as they scrambled to protect their populations against the prospect of an imminent pandemic. Third, because it was eventually confirmed that the Indonesian virus strand was more virulent than other strands, a vaccine based on the Indonesian strand would be the most desirable in terms of offering protection (Supari 2008: 25–7). Describing her realization that the Indonesian virus was distinct and more virulent (and thus of immense interest to those tracking the evolution of the virus and making vaccines), Supari actually felt "happy" because for Indonesia that now meant "bargaining power!" (Supari 2008: 27). Supari, in other words, realized at this crucial moment that access to Indonesian virus samples could form new diplomatic leverage for the Indonesian government in its attempts to secure greater access to medical countermeasures for Indonesia. The Indonesian health minister described her thinking in the following, candid terms: "I had to change the paradigm. How? I had nothing. My country is not a superpower. I am only a Health Minister with 240 million people to serve. … I had to do something. … the main variable … is the wild virus. So I had to stop the virus sharing with the WHO-CC [World Health Organization Collaborating Centers]" (Supari 2008: 163). As Indonesia began to assert its "viral sovereignty" over H5N1 viruses circulating in its territory, those viruses now became transformed from mere biological materials to key political "bargaining chips" in the diplomatic arsenal of the Indonesian state, which it would use to further its own national interest on the international stage.

Going down this path was a high-risk strategy, of course, in that this would only work as long as the Indonesian government could actually maintain tight control over the viruses circulating in its territories, and prevent outside countries from obtaining virus samples from Indonesia through other channels. Presumably this is part of the reason why Supari would later also express her desire to evict the US Naval Laboratory (NAMRU-2) from the country, which she suspected at the time as being a back channel for virus samples leaving the country. It is probably also for the same reason that, before leaving office, Supari further instructed laboratories and researchers in Indonesia not to accept foreign donations any more, as she feared that those funding streams could be accompanied by other demands from foreign donors. Although the future status of a military facility by a foreign country, or indeed foreign aid, would not normally be seen to fall with the remit of a health minister, these are issues she began to take a very keen interest in, presumably because if viruses were to be transferred out of the country through a military facility or other links, that would seriously – and perhaps fatally – undermine her bargaining position on virus sharing.

Armed with these new "bargaining chips," Supari also felt sufficiently emboldened to hold out for more than just a few concessions made by the West, and to push for a fundamental transformation of the virus sharing mechanism. When, for example, she was approached by the WHO with offers of a laboratory upgrade and as much vaccine as they needed, in February 2007, she turned those offers down. The reason she cites for this decision is that she did not want Indonesia to be dependent upon the charity of other countries, insisting that "by recognizing our right over the viruses, we can obtain whatever we need respectfully, because we own something precious to give" (Supari 2008: 41).

Rather than simply accepting those offers of material support, and resolving the dispute there and then, the Indonesian health minister instead formulated a much stronger demand that made Indonesia's resumption of virus sharing conditional upon a more fundamental reformation of the whole virus sharing mechanism. Her underlying position, which she subsequently advanced at the intergovernmental meeting in November 2007, became: "Number One: Virus Sharing is a sovereign right of a country and not to be com-promised. Number Two: Benefits sharing is a consequence of virus sharing, which instead of a charity from the developed country to the country where the virus originated, it is the right of the latter" (Supari 2008: 116–17). The negotiations around virus sharing therefore could no longer turn simply around reintegrating Indonesia into the GISN, but would have to become about fundamentally transforming the entire virus sharing mech-anism. Even after Supari left office, this position continued to be defended by Indonesian officials (Budianto 2010).

Here too it is possible in retrospect to trace how the securitized response to H5N1 eventually began to put new pressures on the international virus sharing mechanism and international health cooperation. As a result of the much closer and high-level govern-mental attention on H5N1, the entire issue of virus sharing suddenly and unexpectedly became subject to much more narrow calculations of state interest. The Indonesian gov-ernment in particular realized that it was in the United States's national interest to secure and maintain access to these samples, while Indonesia in turn could use the granting of access to these samples as a way of furthering its own national interest of achieving greater benefits from sharing its viruses. That push for a more fundamental transfor-mation of the virus sharing system also raised the political stakes in the dispute further still, and ultimately prolonged the difficult stand-off between the supporters of the GISN mechanism and those states pushing for reform. In that process, the entire virus sharing mechanism became transformed from a largely low-level, habitual, and routine system of functional public health cooperation, to something subjected to much narrower con-siderations of state interest, and would effectively become a bargaining chip in high-level diplomatic negotiations between states pursuing competing national interests. This too forms an important vector through which international health cooperation has, in the end, been complicated by the securitized international response to H5N1.

Conclusions

What wider lessons about the securitization of infectious diseases can be drawn from the case of H5N1? Those lessons need to be teased out with considerable care. Not only is it very difficult to generalize from a single case study, but we have also already noted that there are a variety of different factors involved in the emergence of the international virus sharing dispute – including factors particular to Indonesian politics. It is also note-worthy that besides Indonesia no other country (including those vocally supporting the Indonesian position) has undertaken a similar, formal refusal to share virus samples. Nor, for that matter, has such a refusal manifested itself in the more recent case of the 2009 influenza A (H1N1) pandemic.

That said, there is a wider and important lesson that can be learned from the virus shar-ing episode. Scholars of securitization processes usefully remind us that "one has to weigh the always problematic side effects of applying a mind-set of security against the possible advantages of focus, attention, and mobilization" (Buzan *et al.* 1998: 29). In the case of H5N1 we have seen there were discernible benefits to a securitized response to global health, especially in terms of resources and political mobilization. However, in many ways the more important lesson to emerge from the ongoing international virus sharing dispute, and one that has still not been sufficiently appreciated in international policy circles, is that there can also be unanticipated downside risks associated with responding to health issues in a securitized mode. In the case of H5N1, the securitized international response has had a range of less salient effects in terms of entangling the longstanding virus sharing mechanism in a wider set of non-technical and non-medical disputes in international politics. Indeed, the securitized response to H5N1 ended up inadvertently provoking an intense repoliticization of international virus sharing, where the latter is no longer seen to be of mutual benefit, but as a bargaining chip used by countries like Indonesia to fundamentally reform the virus sharing mechanism.

None of the foregoing analysis implies that things inevitably had to turn out this way, nor to detract from the responsibilities of the key parties involved in the dispute. Nor is it to deny that the prospect of a H5N1 pandemic associated with high human mortality and morbidity rate was indeed a very disquieting prospect. Yet, as an important instance in which a health issue became prominently securitized in international policy circles, the case of H5N1 demonstrates very clearly that a securitized response to infectious diseases can also structure global health debates in ways that are not conducive to achieving higher levels of international health cooperation. That is an important insight and cautionary note worth retaining for the future when it comes to dealing with emerging infectious diseases. After all, one of the most salient features of global health over the past decade has been the tendency by many policy-makers to try and deliberately shift global health from the mold of "low" politics to make it a more pressing concern of "high" politics, by actively seeking the securitization of health through the agenda on global health security.

Acknowledgment

The research conducted for this chapter was supported by a grant from the British Academy (BARDA-47928).

Note

1. We would like to thank Paul Forster from the STEPS Centre in the Institute of Development Studies at the University of Sussex for his assistance in locating a copy of this book.

Key Reading

Aldis W. 2008. Health security as a public health concept: a critical analysis. *Health Policy and Planning* 23(6), 369–75.

Buzan B, Wæver O, de Wilde J. 1998. *Security: A New Framework for Analysis*. Boulder, CO: Lynne Rienner.

Calain P. 2007. From the field side of the binoculars: a different view on global public health surveillance. *Health Policy and Planning* 22, 13–20.

Forster P. 2009. *The Political Economy of Avian Influenza in Indonesia*. STEPS Working Paper No. 17. Brighton: STEPS Centre.

Kamradt-Scott A, Lee K. 2011. The 2011 Pandemic influenza preparedness framework: global health secured or a missed opportunity? *Political Studies* 59, 831–47.

McInnes C, Lee K. 2006. Health, Security and Foreign Policy. *Review of International Studies* 32(1), 5–23.

WHO (World Health Organization). 2007. *A Safer Future: Global Public Health Security in the 21st Century. The World Health Report 2007*. Geneva: WHO.

References

Aldis W. 2008. Health security as a public health concept: a critical analysis. *Health Policy and Planning* 23(6), 369–75.

Brammer L, Postema A, Cox N. 2007. Seasonal and pandemic influenze surveillance. In M'ikanata M, Lynfield R, van Beneden C, de Valk H (eds) *Infectious Disease Surveillance*, pp. 254–64. Oxford: Blackwell.

Budianto L. 2010. RI pushes for fair virus sharing scheme despite Obama visit. *Jakarta Post* February 10.

Buzan B, Wæver O, de Wilde J. 1998. *Security: A New Framework for Analysis*. Boulder, CO: Lynne Rienner.

Cabinet Office. 2008. *The National Security Strategy of the United Kingdom: Security in an Interdependent World*. London: Cabinet Office.

Calain P. 2007. From the field side of the binoculars: a different view on global public health surveillance. *Health Policy and Planning* 22, 13–20.

Davies S. 2008. Securitizing infectious disease. *International Affairs* 84(2), 295–313.

Elbe S. 2006. Should HIV/AIDS be securitized? The ethical dilemmas of linking HIV/AIDS and security. *International Studies Quarterly* 50(1), 119–44.

Fidler D, Gostin L. 2008. *Biosecurity in the Global Age: Biological Weapons, Public Health and the Rule of Law*. Stanford, CA: Stanford University Press.

Forster P. 2009. *The Political Economy of Avian Influenza in Indonesia*. STEPS Working Paper No. 17. Brighton: STEPS Centre.

Ingram A. 2007. HIV/AIDS, security and the geopolitics of US–Nigerian relations. *Review of International Political Economy* 14(3):510-534.

Kelle A. 2007. Securitization of international public health: implications for global health governance and the biological weapons prohibition regime. *Global Governance* 13(2), 217–35.

Lean G. 2005. Bird flu "as grave a threat as terrorism." *Independent* June 26. http://www.independent.co.uk/environment/bird-flu-as-grave-a-threat-as-terrorism-496608.html (last accessed December 2013).

Leboeuf A, Broughton E. 2008. *Securitization of Health and Environmental Issues: Process and Effects. A Research Outline*. Working Paper. Paris: Institut Français des Relations Internationales.

McInnes C, Lee K. 2006. Health, security and foreign policy. *Review of International Studies* 32(1), 5–23.

NSS (National Security Strategy). 2006. *The National Security Strategy of the United States*. Washington, DC: The White House.

New York Times. 2005. Grounding a pandemic. *New York Times* 6 June

Oliver Wyman. 2009. *Influenza Vaccine Strategies for Broad Global Access. Key Findings and Project Methodology.* http://www.oliverwyman.com/media/VAC_infl_publ_rpt_10-07.pdf (last accessed December 2013).

Scoones I, Forster P. 2008. *The International Response to Highly Pathogenic Avian Influenza: Science, Policy and Politics*. STEPS Working Paper No. 10. Brighton: STEPS Centre.

Supari S. 2008. *It's Time for the World to Change*. Jakarta: PT. Sulaksana Watinsa Indonesia.

WEF (World Economic Forum). 2006. *Global Risks 2006*. Geneva: WEF.

WHO (World Health Organization). 2007. *A Safer Future: Global Public Health Security in the 21st Century. The World Health Report 2007*. Geneva: WHO.

WHO (World Health Organization). 2005a. *Avian Influenza: Assessing the Pandemic Threat*. Geneva: WHO.

WHO (World Health Organization). 2005b. *Guidance for the Timely Sharing of Influenza Viruses/Specimens with Potential to Cause Human Influenza Pandemics*. Geneva: WHO.

World Bank. 2008. *Responses to Avian Influenza and State of Pandemic Readiness*. Fourth Global Progress Report. Washington, DC: World Bank.

Chapter 17

The Changing Humanitarian Sector: Repercussions for the Health Sector

François Grünewald and Veronique de Geoffroy

Abstract

Humanitarian aid is one of the most meaningful areas of modern solidarity. In a context of growing needs and the permanent turbulence of our world, with complex conflicts and a multitude of other threats and hazards, the health sector has proven to be a very dynamic component of humanitarian aid and has developed a high level of professionalism and ethics. A rise in humanitarian funding and an explosion in the number of humanitarian actors has led to new coordination mechanisms, such as the cluster system established as part of the humanitarian reform process launched in 2005. Western humanitarian aid is now being confronted with the growing engagement of actors from state institutions, civil society organizations, and the private sector in the South. Humanitarian actors, especially from the health sector, are increasingly involved in the management of new kinds of crises, and confronted with the challenges posed by large-scale disasters (such as the management of mass casualties) and new epidemics. Largely dependent on resources from the public or from states, the humanitarian sector must defend its independence and its capacity to intervene in difficult environments against political encroachments that can hinder access to affected populations. The health sector, for example, must consider how it can work with military emergency deployments while maintaining its humanitarian principles. In the face of increasingly volatile situations and complex issues, the humanitarian community must constantly improve its methods for needs assessment, project design, monitoring of interventions, and impact evaluations. Information technology is becoming increasingly critical. The capacity to anticipate, to proactively prepare for new challenges, and to innovate remains the only solution for the aid sector, including its health component, to remain relevant in the long run.

The Handbook of Global Health Policy, First Edition. Edited by Garrett W. Brown, Gavin Yamey, and Sarah Wamala.
© 2014 John Wiley & Sons, Ltd. Published 2014 by John Wiley & Sons, Ltd.

Key Points

- The nature of humanitarian emergencies has changed in recent years, characterized by a rise in local conflicts and natural disasters, as well as increased blurring of the distinction between man-made and natural disasters.
- The response to such disasters is now being managed by a wide array of humanitarian aid actors, including western, southern, and eastern non-governmental organizations, United Nations organizations, armed forces, and the private sector.
- Responding to the need to ensure greater coordination of these disparate actors, the United Nations Office for the Coordination of Humanitarian Affairs initiated the cluster approach, a mechanism to strengthen partnerships and clarify the division of labor among organizations. This mechanism needs to be continuously improved to cope with regularly emerging new challenges.
- The policy response to a humanitarian crisis must be context-specific: responding to open conflicts in urban settings versus mass refugee situations will require different responses.
- "Pre-disaster" risk management needs to become an integral part of preparedness for future humanitarian intervention.

Key Policy Implications

- Achieving a contextually relevant and effective humanitarian response depends on the inter-play between (i) the objectives of the response (as defined by mortality/morbidity and the expected end state for the local health institutions); (ii) contextual constraints (e.g., the status of the health system prior to the crisis, access to the wounded or sick); and (iii) the technical, financial, and political capacity of health-based aid agencies.
- For large-scale rapid onset disasters, such as earthquakes, in order to analyze the situation and plan an appropriate response, humanitarian policy-makers should distinguish between three different phases: the acute emergency phase, the stabilization phase, and the recovery phase.
- While humanitarian policy-makers should adopt evidence-based practices, they must also support innovation and accept a certain level of risk-taking – in rapidly changing and unpredictable circumstances, risk-averse attitudes can be a major impediment to effective humanitarian action.

Introduction

The landscape of global humanitarian crises and intervention once seemed simple to describe, at least on the surface. Global fault lines, economic and political divisions, and the roots of conflict and social tension were seen through the simple prism of Cold War, Sino-Soviet, and North–South antagonisms. The aid community was relatively small and was dominated by its health and food aid components. In conflict situations, there was the diplomatic International Committee of the Red Cross (ICRC), whose symbol was respected; the United Nations, which was seen as paralyzed by Cold War politics (Ryan 2000); and the risk-taking Médecins Sans Frontières (MSF), who conducted stealthy cross-border operations.

Such simple descriptions no longer hold true. When the Berlin Wall fell, and new states emerged from the collapse of the Eastern bloc, many of the complexities that were previously hidden came to the surface. The early 1990s saw a dramatic increase in the number of civil wars, ethnic confrontations, and local and regional conflicts over resource control (SIPRI 2000), often exacerbated by external powers, and accompanied by a rise in media attention and coverage. New concepts emerged to describe the complexity, such as "unstructured conflicts," defined as conflicts whose determinants do not follow classic, understandable patterns, and "complex political emergencies," which refers to internal wars that are political in nature, with complex origins and a multiplicity of players (Sondorp and Zwi 2002).

Global humanitarian assistance more than doubled between 1990 and 2000, from US$2.1 billion to $5.9 billion (HPG 2002), associated with an explosion in new humanitarian agencies both in the West as well as in developing countries. Many more actors became involved in humanitarian action, such as the military and the private sector. As the landscape of humanitarian action became more crowded, coordination became crucial, over and above the issue of clarification of mandates, roles, and responsibilities. Several mechanisms were developed under an "integration agenda":

1. Integrated missions (i.e., military, political, development, and humanitarian aid brought together under one objective and structure).
2. Strategic frameworks supporting coordination between different actors, such as the framework proposed by the United Nations Office for the Coordination of Humanitarian Affairs (OCHA 2010).
3. The recent "one UN approach," which tries to bring all UN agencies together into single "country teams.
4. The humanitarian reform agenda, with its new sectoral coordination mechanism, known as the cluster system.

In this chapter, we examine the increasing complexity of humanitarian action and the efforts to better coordinate disparate activities, including some of those listed above. We begin by describing the recent landscape of humanitarian crises, including the increasing impacts of natural hazards. Then we examine some of the key actors in humanitarian assistance, many of whom are new to the scene, such as the private sector and a new range of non-governmental organizations (NGOs). This is followed by a description of the current status of humanitarian responses, and the evidence on what works best. We end by laying out some of the challenges and opportunities ahead in preparing for future humanitarian crises, using the humanitarian response to the 2010 Haiti earthquake as a case study to help illustrate key concepts.

The Changing Nature of Humanitarian Crises

Rise of Local Confrontations

The recent era of humanitarian crises has been characterized by a rise in local confrontations. The Cold War's "East–West" confrontation had masked many other local fault lines, such as ethnic divides in Angola, or a divide between the modern urbanized class versus the traditional religious peasantry in Afghanistan. These fault lines re-emerged with great force after the collapse of the Soviet Union. In addition to conflicts based on such re-emerging fault lines, new ethnic or religious conflicts erupted and brought international attention, such as in sub-Saharan Africa (Burundi, the Democratic Republic of the Congo (DRC), Rwanda, Somalia), the Balkans, the North and South Caucasus, East Timor, and the Philippines. In these conflicts, the basic foundations of human rights and international humanitarian law quickly reached their limits.

Many of these conflicts are related to the control of natural resources, such as oil, agricultural land and pastures, and precious stones and metals (Humphreys 2005). In some of the most recent cases, such as conflicts in the eastern part of the DRC, local conflicts have been exacerbated by the presence of underground resources (e.g., minerals, oil). The emergence of religious conflict and the "global war on terror" also created a new geopolitical situation where the difference between military and civilians, and between acts of war and acts of terror, became increasingly blurred (Cunningham 2009).

Increasing Impacts of Natural Hazards

Natural disasters, such as the Asian tsunami, the Sahel drought, and hurricanes in the United States, the Caribbean, and the Philippines, have also been on the rise. Though disasters have become less lethal, due to the actions of the international community in terms of both preparedness and disaster response (CRED 2011), they have caused greater damage to infrastructure and inflicted higher economic losses (World Bank 2011). For example, a recent World Bank report on assessing disaster risks to strengthen financial resilience found that 2011 was "the worst year on record for disasters caused by natural hazards, resulting in an estimated $380 billion in economic losses (World Bank 2012).

Crises are Usually Multifactorial

Humanitarian crises rarely have a single causative factor. In many instances, old root causes, such as conflict over land, collide with recently emerged catalysts, such as control of underground resources. The collision can create an extremely complicated mix in which it is difficult to identify the real dynamics of violence, to foresee the likely evolution, and to determine the real factors that have led to the destitution of a population.

The distinction between man-made and natural disasters has become increasingly blurred. Many "natural" catastrophes take place in conflict zones, such as the 1992 drought in Mozambique, and earthquakes in Afghanistan and Colombia. The real roots of many natural disasters, or at least the magnitude of their impact, often have human causes. A World Bank report on the economic impact of disasters noted that "earthquakes, droughts, floods, and storms are *natural hazards*, but the *unnatural disasters* are deaths and damages that result from human acts of omission and commission" (World Bank 2010). Inequitable land tenure systems leave poor farmers with land on slopes that they inevitably make more fragile. Acute urban poverty increases the likelihood of poor urban dwellers settling in "areas at risk," on flood-exposed river banks or landslide-prone areas. Vulnerability reduces the scope of possible coping mechanisms, while the HIV epidemic drastically affects the resilience of people and societies (Harvey 2004). When a crisis – natural or otherwise – takes place in such debilitated environments, it is no wonder that the community has few coping mechanisms.

Humanitarian Aid Architecture

Thirty years ago, there was just a handful of aid agencies working in crisis zones. Since then the situation has changed dramatically: in Kosovo, more than 200 agencies were competing for money for a territory no bigger than Belgium (Kehler 2004). In Afghanistan, the number of aid actors went from a few dozen during the period of Taliban rule to more than 2000 after 2010 (Grünewald and Binder 2010). After the Haiti earthquake, the number of NGOs jumped from a few dozen to more than 4000 (Grünewald and Renaudin 2010).

Explosion of Western NGOs

In the West, the number of humanitarian NGOs has multiplied by several hundred since the early 1980s (Bagci 2003). In the late 1970s, a wave of NGOs emerged to provide humanitarian assistance to Cambodian and Afghan refugee camps. Further waves followed the end of the Cold War. The growth of NGOs for Somalia, former Yugoslavia, and Rwanda was largely made possible by the increase in money available from donors such as the Humanitarian Aid and Civil Protection department of the European Commission. With this growth of new NGOs, a body of professional administrators emerged, more technocratic than their predecessors. The romanticism of night time cross-border operations faded away and was replaced by the world of the professional humanitarian managers.

This new generation of humanitarian actors continued to grow with the NATO intervention in Kosovo and during the first few years of the post-2001 era in Afghanistan. The last phase took place with the South Asian tsunami of December 2004 and the Haitian earthquake of January 2010. These two key events accelerated the growth of the aid industry, especially of the small health NGOs that were largely inefficient because they were unable to deal with the complexity of the crises and they lacked the relatively important logistic means required to have any meaningful impact.

However, there has been insufficient donor funding to support all of these NGOs. Certain NGOs, such as Equilibre, proved to be too dependent on institutional donors, and disappeared. Others became mere implementing agencies, working at the disposal of institutional donors. A few NGOs, such as MSF, sought financial independence as a way to resist being used as an instrument of the state.

Rise of Southern and Eastern NGOs and Civil Society

There has been incredible growth in the number of local humanitarian NGOs in developing countries, including the Islamic world. This is linked to the growing resources available from international donors. In many crisis-stricken areas, international and national NGOs represent the main source of employment. They are sometimes the organized answer of civil societies to the structural adjustments imposed by international financial institutions; adjustments that have constrained public health spending and put caps on public health wages (Banerji 1999; Kim et al. 2000). Highly qualified medical personnel in many developing countries who have been unable to find government jobs have often been recruited as specialized staff for the aid industry. In places such as Haiti, for instance, the public health system lost hundreds of medical staff to NGOs and UN agencies (Grünewald and Binder 2010; De ville de Goyet *et al.* 2011).

Centrality of the UN Family and a New Approach to Coordination

Just after the Cold War, the UN became increasingly engaged in humanitarian action and its coordination. The creation of the Department for Humanitarian Assistance (DHA) in 1991 and its replacement a few years after by the OCHA put the UN at the centre of aid coordination. Headed by an Under-Secretary General with the title of Emergency Relief

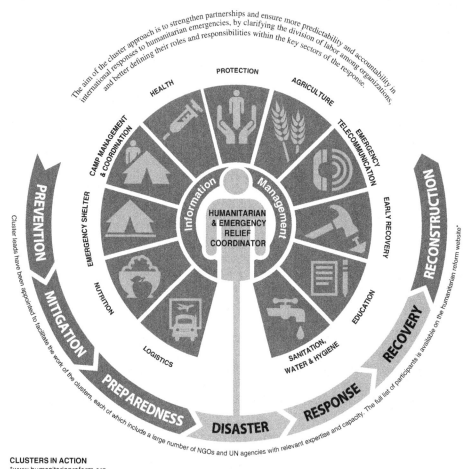

CLUSTERS IN ACTION
*www.humanitarianreform.org

KEY TOOLS
The Global Disaster Alert and Coordination System (GDACS): www.gdacs.org
The Financial Tracking System (FTS): www.reliefweb.int/fts/
The Central Emergency Response Fund (CERF): http://cerf.un.org
The Humanitarian portal ReliefWeb: www.reliefweb.int
Who Does What Where (3W): http://3w.unocha.org
The Consolidated Appeal: http://humanitarianappeal.net
The Inter-Agency Standing Committee: http://humanitarianinfo.org/iasc/

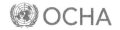

Figure 17.1 The cluster approach. Source: UN (2012), Office for the Coordination of Humanitarian Affairs (OCHA).

Coordinator, OCHA is tasked to support and facilitate coordination within and outside the UN family, in particular via the Inter Agency Standing Committee for Humanitarian Affairs (IASC), which brings together UN agencies, the International Red Cross and Red Crescent Movement, and NGOs.

Having understood that funding for international development was falling, and that institutional visibility was increasingly associated with humanitarian action, most UN agencies created their own "emergency unit." Consequently, OCHA came under pressure to improve the way in which the different UN agencies worked together. One of the milestones in this process of improving coordination was the humanitarian reform launched in 2005. A new mechanism of sector coordination, the cluster approach (Figure 17.1), was introduced as part this reform (UN 2012). OCHA states that the aim of the cluster approach is "to strengthen partnerships and ensure more predictability and accountability in international responses to humanitarian emergencies, by clarifying the division of labour among organisations" (OCHA 2012).

Box 17.1 Benefits and Weaknesses of the Cluster Approach to Humanitarian Assistance

Benefits	*Weaknesses*
• Coverage of humanitarian needs has improved in some thematic areas, including gender-based violence, child protection, disability, water and sanitation, and nutrition.	• Clusters largely exclude national and local actors and often fail to link with, build on, or support existing coordination mechanisms – as a result, the cluster approach weakens national and local ownership and capacities.
• Gaps in assistance are better identified and duplications are reduced, leading to better targeting of assistance and more efficient use of resources.	• The cluster approach can threaten humanitarian principles, especially where cluster members are financially dependent on cluster lead organizations and where cluster lead organizations are part of, or maintain close relationships to, integrated missions, peacekeeping forces, or political actors involved in conflicts.
• Actors are better able to learn through peer review mechanisms and enhanced technical and sometimes normative discussions.	
• Organizations assuming coordination tasks exert more predictable leadership, there is greater clarity concerning leadership roles, and there are more and better trained staff dedicated to coordination.	• Poor cluster management and facilitation in many cases prevents clusters from reaching their full potential; many coordinators are not trained well enough in facilitation techniques, lack a common basic handbook or toolkit and, especially at the sub-national level, often do not have sufficient time dedicated to coordination.
• Stronger partnership between UN agencies and other international humanitarian actors – leading to improved information sharing, greater advocacy power, and enhanced coherence, as cluster members adopt common positions on specific operational questions and support the development and dissemination of local standards.	• Inter-cluster coordination is ineffective in most cases and there is little integration of cross-cutting issues.
• Improved planning for major funding appeals.	

Source: Steet *et al.* (2010).

The cluster approach seeks to make humanitarian assistance more effective by introducing an enhanced system of sectoral coordination (clusters) with designated lead organizations to support each cluster (such as WHO in the health sector, UNICEF for nutrition, and the Food and Agriculture Organization for food security). The lead organizations are accountable to the Emergency Relief Coordinator (UN 2012).

An evaluation of the cluster system conducted in 2009–2010 found that the new system offered both benefits and weaknesses compared with the old way of doing business (Steet *et al.* 2010) (Box 17.1).

In this evaluation (Steet *et al.* 2010) the health cluster was rated relatively well compared to others (Box 17.2).

Box 17.2   Key Findings of a 2010 Evaluation of the Health Cluster

Positive performance of the health cluster

- Involvement with national actors: there is a clear strategy to systematically engage with the national and local health administration.
- Communication to health stakeholders and the public at large: the fact that WHO and the health cluster have a strong commitment to health surveillance results in a dynamic communication strategy.
- Implementation of leadership responsibility: the strong involvement of WHO top management in the cluster has a positive impact on the behavior of WHO representatives in the field.
- Support from the global cluster: this has been very strong from the beginning. The health cluster was the first to produce a cluster handbook. WHO headquarters is systematically and strategically in touch with the field and supporting operations.
- Capacity to interact with the financial components of the reform: health is often seen as a critical life-saving sector and WHO has relatively easy access to the Central Emergency Response Fund (CERF), a unique mechanism to rapidly allocate funds to emergency operations. Health components of the main UN fundraising tool for humanitarian aid (the Consolidated Appeal Process (CAP) and Flash Appeals) are often relatively well covered compared with others.

More varied performance

- WHO is more often playing the role of "advocate of last resort" rather than "provider of last resort." The security constraints on UN agencies affect WHO's capacity to act in the field, whereas institutions such as the ICRC and MSF, which are at best "engaged observers" but not real members in the cluster, can act more freely.
- WHO's capacity to engage with non-cluster members remains limited.

Poor performance

- Accountability to the UN Humanitarian Coordinators (HC): as with many UN agencies, direct accountability is more towards the headquarters and executive board rather than to the HC.

- The health sector does not use participatory approaches, yet it could gain important knowledge on local health practices and specific health issues from such approaches.

Source: Steet *et al.* (2010).

New Role of the Armed Forces

With the end of the Cold War, the combat role of many countries' armed forces lost some of its relevance. The military resources that were freed up by this diminished combat role were in part redirected to peace-keeping operations. These operations have become the military's "visibility and public relations card" and an argument for the military's continued existence (Seybolt 2007).

The engagement of armed forces in crisis management takes many forms, which partly depend on whether or not there is a formal mandate for the military's involvement (Holzgrefe and Keohane 2003). The scope of military humanitarian intervention is very wide, including the deployment of costly logistics and heavy duty equipment in the case of disasters; the establishment of checkpoint controls; the opening of "humanitarian corridors" aimed at allowing safe passage of humanitarian aid into crisis regions, and of refugees out of such regions; and the provision of security for aid workers (Seybolt 2007). However, there is also the risk that these roles can be blurred with other agendas. They can become blurred with economic agendas; for example, in the Balkans, army reservists from different countries were carrying out reconnaissance for private enterprises (Grünewald and De Geoffroy 1999). They can also become blurred with political "state building" agendas, as in Afghanistan, where the Provincial Rehabilitation Teams, made up of a mix of civil and military actors, were created to support the presence of the Afghan State in the provinces (CORDAID 2007), but were often seen as part of the warfare against the insurgency.

Aid and Profit: Growing Involvement of the Private Sector

The private sector has recently attempted to get in on a share of humanitarian funding, as shown by the multiplication of international events such as the Dubai International Humanitarian Aid and Development Conference and Exhibition (DIHAD) or AID EX, which are half commercial fairs, half humanitarian conferences. A variety of factors helps to explain the recent involvement of for-profit companies in humanitarian work. Humanitarian work can be used rather cynically to help boost corporate image or as a corporate team building exercise. Some companies may become involved because they own oil fields or mine precious stones in a crisis zone and so they have a stake in the outcome of the crisis. On a more constructive note, the private sector may sometimes be able to provide the technical or managerial expertise needed in certain operations that may be lacking within humanitarian agencies.

Killing Aid Actors for Political Gains

As discussed further in Chapter 18, one of the most worrying trends in this new world of complexity and turbulence is the increase in deliberate killing of aid actors and humanitarian workers. Of course, casualties among such workers have always happened periodically, but, in most instances, it was because someone was in the wrong place at the wrong time – ambulances were not targeted.

There are two key reasons for the rise in violence against relief workers. First, a large proportion of new violent non-state groups do not see themselves as being party to international humanitarian law (IHL), the law of armed conflict, which prohibits attacks on aid actors. To them IHL is the law of nation states they fight against. The second reason is the perceived role that humanitarian aid plays in the "integrated approach" advocated by the UN and certain governments since the end of the Cold War. The position of the main western powers in relation to NGOs is, "You are either with us or against us." This leaves little room for independence, neutrality, or impartiality, three key principles central to humanitarian action. In a context dominated by the global war on terror, this position leads to aid actors being seen as members of the "warfare system" and therefore as targets for killing (Cunningham 2009).

Adjusting to a Diverse and Fast-Changing World

Assessing Needs and Capacities: Multiple Contexts Require Diverse Responses

Each specific humanitarian context brings about its own specific challenges for health responders (Grünewald 2008). The most difficult situations are open conflicts in urban settings, as seen in the recent conflicts in Libya and Syria, where there are substantial public health needs but humanitarian access is restricted by military operations. Significant numbers of people are wounded in this type of conflict. Managing bullet and shell wounds requires surgeons, anaesthetists, and nurses with a sufficient supply of electricity and blood, and the capacity to provide the required care and maintain basic aseptic conditions. This requires that hospital structures are accessible and that wounded people can be evacuated rapidly.

The experience of ICRC and MSF, as seen in Mogadishu, Grozni (Chechnya), Kabul, or Syria, shows that it is indeed possible to maintain access to a limited number of hospitals, but evacuation systems are by and large deficient during military operations (ICRC 2010). In fact, the key element of their strategy was to ensure that any single opportunity to replenish stocks was used to ensure that a minimal capacity remains in place to cope with difficult times. Often, however, blood was missing.

Large-scale military operations in urban settings have at least three things in common with large-scale disasters:

1. The magnitude of the needs (the wounded are often counted in the thousands).
2. The race against time to get people out of the rubble and to treat those who are wounded in the streets.
3. The fact that these situations immediately require complex triage and treatment (e.g., for crush syndrome, in which massive muscle injury leads to sudden circulatory shock and kidney failure).

The capacity to save wounded people is directly linked to the time required for them to access a suitable treatment. This capacity often requires the ability to stabilize and evacuate patients, but such capacity is missing when cities become active battlefields or are devastated by a large-scale disaster. There may also not be a functioning blood bank. These challenges typically result in a high mortality rate (ICRC 2010). Amputation rates are also high given the high rates of severely infected wounds (De Ville de Goyet *et al.* 2011).

The public health system, which is by and large structured upon a referral system in which patients are first seen at village level health posts and then referred on if needed to larger referral centers in urban settings, is also weakened by wars and disasters. In affected larger towns, especially capital cities, the central reference center, which is normally equipped with functioning acute treatment services, operating theaters, obstetric wards, and laboratories, becomes partly or totally dysfunctional. Equipment is often destroyed, badly maintained, or in short supply. Since the very top of the "reference pyramid" becomes non-functioning, the national health system is unable to fully respond to patient needs.

Humanitarian aid often tries to cover the needs of large populations on the move. These populations either manage to cross an international boundary, becoming refugees and falling under the remit of the UN High Commissioner for Refugees, which can then prove assistance and protection, or they remain within their country and fall into the category of Internally Displaced People (IDP) (Borton *et al.* 2005). IDPs typically are housed in camps, where maintaining sanitation and hygiene and protecting people against harsh climatic conditions can be a challenge. Acute respiratory infection and diarrheal diseases are common and major threats. Some estimates suggest that diarrhea may account for 25–40% of all childhood deaths in conflict situations and as many as 80% of deaths among children under 2 years old (Sharp *et al.* 2002). Kouadio *et al.* (2010) reviewed the literature on measles outbreaks among displaced populations and found 11 documented outbreaks between 1979 and 2005 in Asia and Africa. Measles has a high impact, argue the authors, because of the high population density in IDP camps and because of the low measles vaccination coverage among children. Around two thirds of people affected by humanitarian emergencies, including IDPs and refugees, live in malaria-endemic regions. A recent analysis of malaria in 60 post-emergency refugee sites across nine countries in 2008–2009 found a malaria incidence rate of at least 50 cases per 1000 refugees (Anderson *et al.* 2011). Across all sites, malaria caused 16% of deaths in refugee children under the age of 5 years.

In the past, IDP camps have often been the main targets for public health intervention by aid agencies, and this is still the case for the Turkish and Emirati Red Crescent Societies in the new IDP camps in different parts of Mogadishu, Somalia (Grünewald *et al.* 2011). Yet when health assistance is being provided to IDP camps, there is often a need to extend it to the surrounding population. Indeed, building health infrastructure for IDP camps when the nearby urban population is totally deprived of any access to health services can be unfair and also a source of security problems.

Designing the Appropriate Response

Achieving a contextually relevant and effective humanitarian response depends on the interplay between three factors:

1. The objectives of the response (both in terms of mortality/morbidity and of the expected end state for the local health institutions).
2. The contextual constraints, especially the status of the health system prior to the crisis, access to the wounded or sick, and logistics (e.g., energy and water supply).
3. The technical, financial, and political capacity of the health aid agencies.

The right information is needed at the right time to support decision-making processes, especially information from epidemiological baseline surveys and from analysis of the health impact of the disaster. Improving future humanitarian responses requires professionalism and the capacity to review critically what has worked and what has failed. In the humanitarian sector, this kind of critical analysis has led to previously hidden debates being exposed – debates about providing minimum humanitarian standards of intervention, and about evidence-based versus experience-based decision-making.

In the late 1990s, after the 1994 Rwanda genocide and subsequent cholera crisis in refugees camps in Goma, eastern Zaire, which caused almost 12,000 deaths (Siddique 1994), a group of international NGOs developed a set of standards governing the implementation of relief programs. Known as the Sphere standards, their aim was to improve the quality of humanitarian interventions and to hold humanitarian actors accountable for such improved standards (Sphere 2012). Box 17.3 gives examples of Sphere standards for emergency nutrition interventions (Greekspoor and Collins 2001).

Box 17.3   Examples of Sphere Standards for Emergency Nutrition Interventions

Standard 1: assessment

Before any decisions are made about a program, aid workers must demonstrate understanding of the basic nutritional situation and conditions that may create a risk of malnutrition

Standard 2: response

If nutritional intervention is required, the problems must be clearly described and the strategy for response documented

Standard 3: monitoring and evaluation

The performance and effectiveness of the nutrition program and changes in the context must be monitored and evaluated

Standard 4

The public health risks associated with moderate malnutrition are reduced

Standard 5

Mortality, morbidity, and suffering associated with severe malnutrition are reduced

Source: Greekspoor and Collins (2001).

Although the standards have been generally welcomed, there have also been a series of criticisms about their applicability and relevance (Greekspoor and Collins 2001). A concern raised in 1998 by a group of French NGOs is that these standards apply mainly to relatively clear-cut situations in relief camps and that standardization will prevent relief workers from adapting to more complex situations (Groupe URD 1998; Dufour 2004).

Another fear is that politicians could use the standards to obscure their responsibilities to tackle the underlying causes of emergencies. Finally, the Sphere standards include quantitative indicators of whether the standards have been met – for example, the indicator of whether water standards have been met is that the average water use for drinking, cooking, and personal hygiene in any household is at least 15 liters per person per day (Sphere 2012). Such indicators could foster unrealistic expectations while ignoring constraints.

Adjusting Programs to Fast-Changing Situations

Disaster scenes are fast changing, and flexibility is essential to remain relevant. For large-scale rapid onset disasters, such as earthquakes, in order to analyze the situation and plan the response, it is important to distinguish between three different phases (Grünewald and Binder 2010):

1. *Acute emergency phase,* requiring acute surgery and postoperative care. In this initial phase, treatment needs to be provided to the very large numbers of people with a variety of injuries of all kinds, such as fractures, head injuries, burns, and amputations. The rapid establishment of a health surveillance system is also very important. During this acute phase, there tends to be an influx of international aid, with the rapid establishment of a large number of emergency hospitals on land and at sea as well as several hundred medical staff mobilized in the field.
2. *Stabilization phase,* which involves establishing or re-establishing a healthcare service for the population at large, including those who may have been displaced by the disaster.
3. *Recovery phase,* in which the health sector is restored to its previous level of functioning, including primary and referral treatment and establishing sound health economics.

Preparing for Future Humanitarian Crises

Risk Management: Predicting the Challenges Ahead

As discussed at the start of this chapter, the world is facing a complex array of risks – from climate change to pandemics – which means that humanitarian emergencies are certain to occur in the future. Thus, "pre-disaster" risk management must be an integral part of preparedness for future humanitarian intervention.

In the humanitarian health sector, establishing risk surveillance systems at the community level and upwards is imperative. Table 17.1 gives an example of how risk analysis can help in understanding and preparing for future crises in Haiti (Grünewald and Binder 2010). Some health risks are predictable, such as those in connection with rainy, hurricane, and winter seasons. Others, such as imported epidemics (e.g., cholera in Haiti or emerging diseases such as SARS) or social tensions and violence, are far less predictable and require extremely fine analytical tools largely drawing from political economy (Grünewald *et al.* 2011a).

In addition to the risks presented in Table 17.1, there are the predictable and known ways in which public health needs develop in situations like these. Figure 17.2, developed by Groupe URD, a research and evaluation institute based in France that focuses on improving the quality of disaster management, presents typical ways in which health

Table 17.1   Risk analysis in Haiti.

Risks	Description	Probability	Level of preparedness
Climatic risks	Management of future rains, which will increase health risks (those linked to sanitation, acute respiratory diseases, or vector-borne diseases such as dengue fever)	Very high	Low
	Management of the hurricane season, which theoretically begins in June and usually ends in November. There are fears that the hurricanes will be violent due to perturbations to the El Niño–La Niña system	High	Medium to high
Geologic risks	Management of geologic and geomorphological perturbations linked to shearing, the creation of weak points and the risk of solifluction (slow downhill movement of soil)	High	Low
Seismic risks	Management of seismic aftershocks, which have continued regularly since the earthquake on 12 January 2010 (e.g., a tremor of 4.4 on the Richter scale was felt in Port-au-Prince on 26 January 2010)	Uncertain, but perceived to be high	Low
Sociopolitical risks	Development of insecurity linked to popular discontent, which is then exploited for political ends	Significant, but should not be exaggerated	Medium (taking into account the UN Stabilization Mission in Haiti and the presence of armies from different countries)
Technological risks	Accident of a technological nature (e.g., an oil slick)	Uncertain	Low

problems and needs develop in post-disaster contexts (Grünewald *et al.* 2011b). Water-borne diseases occur early, as do acute psychosocial problems (a second "wave" of delayed psychosocial problems tends to occur several months later). These are followed by a rise in vector-borne diseases and then respiratory diseases. In the post-earthquake period in Haiti, the country has seen a high burden of both respiratory disease (related to the poor living conditions of IDP camps) (Brennan and Nandy 2001) and psychosocial and mental health problems (Safran *et al.* 2011).

There are a number of myths surrounding post-disaster health risks that tend to be propagated in the wake of disasters, sometimes to try to raise money. The WHO has been aggressive in dispelling these myths (De Ville de Goyet 2000, 2004). As described by De Ville de Goyet (Chief of the Emergency Preparedness and Disaster Relief

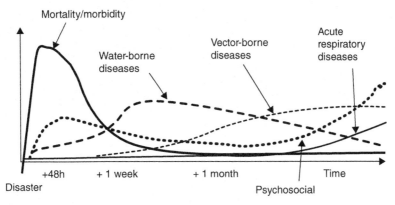

Figure 17.2   Evolution of different health hazards in a post-disaster setting. Source: Groupe URD (1998).

Coordination Programme at the Pan-American Health Organization), these myths include the following:

- Dead bodies are a source of communicable diseases, such as cholera and typhoid fever (De Ville de Goyet 2004).
- "The affected population is helplessly waiting for the Western world" (De Ville de Goyet 2000); most survivors owe their lives to neighbors and local agencies.
- Things return to normal within a few weeks; instead, the effects are prolonged.

Preparedness for future disasters means planning for long-term disabilities, including their medical, psychosocial, and economic consequences. One of the effects of large-scale disasters or conflicts has been to cause a large number of physical and psychological injuries, such as bullet wounds, landmine and shrapnel injuries, or the after-effects of poorly treated gangrene. In a country such as Haiti, which had high unemployment even before the earthquake, a major ongoing challenge is to find work opportunities for such a large number of people with disabilities (Wolbring 2011).

Rethinking Approaches

Old methods of responding to humanitarian disasters seem to have reached their limits and there is a need to explore new and less familiar avenues. In particular, there is a clear need to speed up deployment and ensure a rapid strategic transition from emergency to recovery.

Groupe URD has established a typical timeline for a response to a medium- to large-scale natural disaster, based on numerous evaluations and field studies (Figure 17.3). The thin black arrows in Figure 17.3 show the timing of the key events of a classic response (Grünewald *et al.* 2000). The grey arrows show the sequence of events for the response to the Haiti earthquake. It is clear from the figure that the humanitarian system reacted more quickly than in any previous disaster situations: there was faster deployment of urban search and rescue (USAR) teams, NGOs, and coordination mechanisms. Planning for reconstruction also occurred earlier than in previous crises, as a result of previous studies on the importance of early recovery. Such earlier interventions after the Haiti earthquake

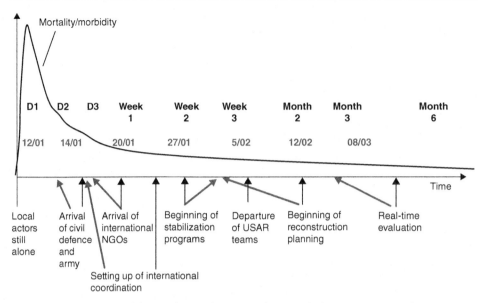

Figure 17.3 Evolution of the timeliness of response: the Haiti deployments compared to past experiences. D, day; NGO, non-governmental organization; USAR, urban search and rescue. Fine black arrows are key events of a classic disaster response; thick grey arrows are key events in response to the Haiti earthquake.

are a positive development, and were a result of acting upon recommendations put forward by evaluations of previous crisis responses (Tsunami Evaluation Coalition 2007). But, as Figure 17.3 also shows, stabilization programs were instituted more slowly than in previous disasters.

Working in Insecure Environments

Since the mid 1990s, hardly a month has gone by without the death of an aid worker or journalist somewhere in the world. These deaths often take place either in contexts linked to rising confrontation between religious fundamentalists and non-religious governments, or in situations of ethnic wars. In these destabilized contexts, the fate of the civilian population is often in great danger. We need to improve our understanding of the link between conflicts, the security of aid workers, and the protection of civilian populations (Rieff 2002). In many contexts, where socioeconomic disparities, growing inequality, and social tensions lead to more burglaries and violence; where illegal trade empires are growing; and where information travels fast and connects violent groups in different parts of the world, aid workers have to be more resilient than ever.

Evaluating the Response

Evaluation is a key tool for both learning and accountability in the humanitarian sector. The evaluation of humanitarian programs, projects, and instruments has become a growing industry in recent years (Hilhorst 2002). But has evaluation actually helped to improve interventions? The answer remains unclear (Hallam 2011). Many evaluation reports remain "on the shelf," without influencing future action.

Nevertheless, there are strategic lessons that can be learned from past evaluations which can go a long way to help rethink the role of health professionals in humanitarian aid. Box 17.4 gives seven key lessons learned from evaluating the humanitarian response to the Haiti earthquake.

Box 17.4 Lessons Learned from Evaluation of the Haiti Earthquake Response

These lessons are based on an evaluation conducted by Groupe URD 1 month after the earthquake (Grünewald and Renaudin 2010).

Strengthen the capacity of national institutions

While health aid organizations, including the WHO, made an effort to strengthen their own tools and working conditions, nothing was done to boost the capacity of national bodies so that they could assume leadership. Yet Haiti's National Ministry of Potable Water and Sanitation (DINEPA) adopted a community-based model that, with adequate support, could continue to have an essential role. It should have been possible to provide support to national bodies, and to strengthen national capacity. The absence of a strategic and systemic analysis of post-earthquake capacities led to a strategy whereby national bodies were neglected.

Do not be too hasty in deciding the humanitarian phase is over: continue to closely monitor the needs of the population

In 2010, tropical rain began to fall during the humanitarian mission, showing the extreme vulnerability of the population. A large proportion of the displaced persons and victims in Port-au-Prince, but also in Léogane, Gressier, and other locations, were still sleeping in shelters made with sheets and rags when the rain began to fall. The situation has improved since then, but very slowly. It is important to ensure that: (a) funds are still available to reduce this vulnerability; and (b) policy-makers do not jump to the conclusion that the emergency relief phase is over, even though it is useful to plan what comes afterwards.

Accelerate access to fast means of transport

One constraint that is systematically present when long distance deployments take place is restricted access to fast means of transport to carry the necessary equipment and logistical support. The mobilization of military assets needed to support civilian operations can be critical to the success of the response. However, this mobilization is also dependent on political decisions, so it is important to maintain a permanent interministerial mechanism to manage crises.

Improve the coordination between search and rescue and disaster medicine/postoperative care

Better coordination is needed between all deployed mechanisms in terms of triage, disaster surgery, and postoperative care (e.g., tents and beds, coordination strategy with local institutions or those supported by other actors).

Provide mental health support to staff, including treatment for post-traumatic stress disorder (PTSD)

Many individuals involved in the first weeks of the response will be affected by these events for the rest of their lives. It is important that they are provided with psychological support and with appropriate treatment if they develop PTSD.

Conduct an economic analysis and formulate a strategy to help rebuild the health system

It is essential to develop mechanisms that will identify and mitigate the possible negative effects that the health emergency response can have on fragile health systems.

Conclusion: Challenges and Opportunities Ahead

The humanitarian sector has undergone major developments in recent years, such as improving its risk management approaches and responding more rapidly to crises. However, the sector will need to remain in a permanent state of alert, as it will continue to face difficult challenges related to new and more complex crises. Confronting complexity with intelligence, turbulence with flexibility, and unpredictability with "multiscenario planning" are not easy tasks. Such challenges often confront the aid community as a whole – the UN, NGOs, and donors – a community that has its own limits in terms of assessment, planning, and resource allocation. In dangerous and fast-changing environments, there is an increased risk that a wrong move will lead to aid workers being killed or access to the affected population being restricted. There is no quick-fix solution for this situation. The humanitarian sector must embrace complexity and turbulence, because from now on they will always be part of the humanitarian landscape. The sector will likely face four key challenges and opportunities in the years ahead.

Improving Humanitarian Operations in Settings of Global Urbanization

The earthquake in Haiti, the fighting in Kabul and Damascus (Grünewald 2013), and the precarious and sometimes explosive situation in the massive slums in Asia and East Africa and the favelas of Brazil underline the complicated nature of development and humanitarian action in cities. Humanitarian intervention in urban settings is complex during the disaster risk reduction stage as well as the acute emergency, stabilization, and reconstruction phases (Boyer 2010). From their Cold War refugee camps and rural guerrilla experience, humanitarian actors are not used to the specific features of urban contexts (Grünewald and Levron 2004). They will need to adjust their operations to deal with factors such as: high population density; the need to manage medical care, logistics, and transport; urban forms of violence; new kinds of relationships with urban authorities and social structures; and the important role of telecommunications (Duijsens 2010; Lucchi 2012).

Applying New Information Technology to Disaster Management

While the famine in Ethiopia in 1985 led to the advent of "show business" humanitarian action and the response to the tsunami in 2004 ushered in the age of donations made via mobile phones, the Haiti crisis of January 2010 was the crisis of Facebook and Twitter, and also the intensive use of satellite images and SMS tools. A range of tools is currently being developed that could aid disaster management (Greenough *et al.* 2011), such as: (i) communications satellites and satellite operators (e.g., TSF, Eurosat, Immersat, and Iridium); (ii) satellites that collect and process images, like those run by the UN Institute for Training and Research (www.unitar.org/unosat/, last accessed December 2013) or by university centres; and (iii) social networks, new SMS tools, and "user generated content," such as content generated by Ushahidi (www.ushahidi.com, last accessed December 2013), an open source project that allows users to crowd-source crisis information to be sent via mobile, and by the Sahana Foundation (http://sahanafoundation.org, last accessed December 2013)), which provides open source software to improve communication in humanitarian crises. These tools will require monitoring at the strategic and technological levels in order to assess their value. Additional opportunities for applying information technology to disaster responses are being offered by Google Street Map and the growing industry of Geographic Information Systems.

Improving Local Disaster Management

Deploying external search and rescue teams is costly and may be less efficient than supporting national efforts. An analysis of the Haiti response by the Pan American Health Organization concluded that "the level of efficiency, in terms of the number of lives saved versus the cost of deploying large teams, was low" (De Ville de Goyet *et al.* 2011). In some cases, it cost an average of $1 million to extricate one person (De Ville de Goyet *et al.* 2011). Everything that can contribute to improving the local response, even if this requires an initial investment, allows both significant gains in terms of effectiveness and of major savings in the long term. National and local civil protection units, prefecture and municipal entities, as well as national Red Cross societies and their many volunteers, need to be given greater support.

Restoring Holistic Humanitarian Principles

To respond to calls for help from those who have lost everything because of war, floods, or lava flow is first and foremost to respect the principles of humanity. Humanitarian action must take a holistic approach: relief activities should strengthen the resilience of a population and its capacity to cope with crises. At a time when the language of consumerism is increasingly being used in the humanitarian field it is important to place the holistic nature of human beings above technical sector-based considerations. Are we responding to demands? Are we meeting needs? Whose needs and whose demands, and identified or collected by whom? Populations affected by crises are increasingly aware of how to respond to NGO questionnaires. Powerful people often know how to manipulate assistance in their favor. The perception of what we want to hear dramatically affects the answers we get and therefore what we establish the demands to be. In this context, where private firms look for new markets, armies search for new mandates, and politicians seek a better image, humanitarian actors must return to the essence of their work with professionalism, humility, decisiveness, political astuteness, and respect for the Hippocratic Oath to do no harm.

Key Reading

Boucher-Saulnier F. 2007. *The Practical Guide to Humanitarian Law*, 2nd edn. Lanham: Rowman and Littlefield.

De Ville de Goyet C, Sarmiento JP, Grünewald F. 2011. *Health Response to the Earthquake in Haiti January 2010: Lessons to be Learnt for the Next Massive Sudden-Onset Disaster.* Washington, DC: PAHO.

Rieff D. 2002. *A Bed for the Night: Humanitarianism in Crisis.* New York: Simon and Schuster.

Seybolt TB. 2007. *Humanitarian Military Interventions: The Conditions for Success and Failure.* Solna: Stockholm International Peace Research Institute/Oxford University Press.

Stockholm International Peace Research Institute. 2000. *SIPRI Yearbook. Armaments, Disarmament and International Security.* Oxford: Oxford University Press.

References

Anderson J, Doocy S, Haskew C, Spiegel P, Moss WJ. 2011. The burden of malaria in post-emergency refugee sites: a retrospective study. *Conflict and Health* 5(1), 17.

Bagci C. 2003. Historical evolution of NGOs: NGO proliferation in the post-Cold War era. *Avrupa Gunlugu* 4, 299–326.

Banerji D. 1999. A fundamental shift in the approach to international health by WHO, UNICEF, and the World Bank. *International Journal of Health Services* 29, 227–59.

Borton J, Buchanan-Smith M, Otto R. 2005. *Support to Internally Displaced Persons-Learning from Evaluations.* SIDA. http://www.oecd.org/countries/eritrea/35093445.pdf (last accessed December 2013).

Boyer B. 2010. *Villes Afghans, Défis Urbains: Les Enjeux de la Reconstruction Post Conflit.* Paris: Karthala/Groupe URD.

Brennan RJ, Nandy R. 2001. Complex humanitarian emergencies: a major global health challenge. *Emergency Medicine (Fremantle WA)* 13(2), 147–56.

CORDAID. 2007. *Principles and Pragmatism: Civil-Military Action in Liberia and Afghanistan.* Utrecht: University of Utrecht.

CRED (Centre for Research on the Epidemiology of Disasters). 2011. *Annual Disaster Statistical Review 2011: Numbers and Trends.* Louvain: CRED/UCL.

Cunningham A. 2009. Somalia case study: shrinking humanitarian space in a collapsed state. Paper presented at the International Humanitarian Conference, Groningen.

De Ville de Goyet C. 2000. Stop propagating disaster myths. *Lancet* 356(9231), 762–4.

De Ville de Goyet C. 2004. Epidemics caused by dead bodies: a disaster myth that does not want to die. *Revista Panamericana Salud Publica* 15(5), 297–9.

De Ville de Goyet C, Sarmiento J, Grünewald F. 2011. *Health Response to the 2010 Haiti Earthquake: Lessons to be Learnt for the Next Massive Sudden Onset Disaster.* Washington: PAHO.

Dufour C, de Geoffroy V, Maury H, Grünewald F. 2004. Rights, standards and quality in a complex humanitarian space: is sphere the right tool? *Disasters* 28(2), 124–41.

Duijsens R. 2010. Humanitarian challenges of urbanization. In *International Review of the Red Cross*, No. 878. http://www.icrc.org/eng/resources/documents/article/review/review-878-p351.htm (last accessed December 2013).

Greekspoor A, Collins S. 2001. Raising standards in emergency relief: how useful are Sphere minimum standards for humanitarian assistance? *BMJ* 323, 740.

Greenough PG, Bateman L, Sorensen BS, Foran M. 2011. Innovations in humanitarian technologies working group: report of the proceedings, Humanitarian Action Summit 2011. *Prehospital and Disaster Medicine* 26(6), 482–6.

Group URD. 1998. *The French Letter Plaisians*. http://www.compasqualite.org/documents/0006_eng_les_dangers_et_incoherences.pdf? (last accessed January 2014).

Grünewald F. 2008. New approaches for need assessments. In: *Humanitarian Response Index*. Madrid: DARA.

Grünewald F. 2013. *Working in Syrian cities at war: humanitarian aid under constraints*. http://www.grotius.fr/working-in-syrian-cities-at-war-humanitarian-aid-under-constraints/ (last accessed December 2013).

Grünewald F, Binder A. 2010. *Real time evaluation for the international response to the Haiti earthquake*. New York/Geneva: Groupe URD/GPPI. http://www.urd.org/IMG/pdf/Haiti-IASC_RTE_final_report_en.pdf (last accessed December 2013).

Grünewald F, Boyer B, Kauffmann D, Patinet J. 2011b. *Real-time evaluation of humanitarian action supported by DG ECHO in Haiti*. Paris: Groupe URD. http://www.urd.org/IMG/pdf/GroupeURD_evaluationECHO-Haiti_final_SA_ANG.pdf (last accessed December 2013).

Grünewald F, de Geoffroy V. 1999. *Kosovo: confusions humanitaires, liberation*. http://www.urd.org/IMG/pdf/publispe_rebonds_armee_entreprises.pdf (last accessed December 2013).

Grünewald F, de Geoffroy V, Lister S. 2000. *NGO Responses to Hurricane Mitch: Evaluations for Accountability and Learning*. HPG Network Paper No. 34. London: Human Practice Network.

Grünewald F, Levron E. 2004. *Villes en Guerre, Guerres en Ville*. Paris: Khartala.

Grünewald F, Renaudin B. 2010. *Real time evaluation of the response to the Haiti earthquake, one month after*. Paris: Groupe URD. http://www.urd.org/IMG/pdf/rapport_DASHaiti.pdf (last accessed December 2013).

Grünewald F, Renaudin B, Raillon C, Maury H, Gadrey J, Hettrich K. 2011a. *Mapping of future unintentional risks: examples of risk and community vulnerability*. Paris: Groupe URD. http://www.urd.org/IMG/pdf/RAPPORT_URD_RISK_NON_INTENTIONNELS_EN.pdf (last accessed December 2013).

Hallam A. 2011. *Harnessing the Power of Evaluation*. ALNAP working paper, London. http://www.alnap.org/pool/files/evaluation-alnap-working-paper.pdf (last accessed December 2013).

Harvey P. 2004. *HIV and Humanitarian Aid*. HPG Report No. 16. London: HPG.

Hilhorst D. 2002. Being good at doing good? Quality and accountability of humanitarian NGOs. *Disasters* 26, 193–212.

Holzgrefe L, Keohane R. 2003. *Humanitarian Intervention: Ethical, Legal and Political Dilemmas*. Cambridge: Cambridge University Press.

HPG (Humanitarian Policy Group). 2002. *Financing international, humanitarian action: a review of key trends*. HPG Briefing Note 4. London: HPG. http://www.odi.org.uk/sites/odi.org.uk/files/odi-assets/publications-opinion-files/365.pdf {last accessed December 2013).

Humphreys M. 2005. Natural resources, conflict, and conflict resolution. *Journal of Conflict Resolution* 49(4), 508–37.

ICRC (International Committee of the Red Cross). 2010. *War Surgery: Working with Limited Resources in Armed Conflict and Other Situations of Violence*. Geneva: ICRC. http://www.icrc.org/eng/assets/files/other/icrc_002_0973.pdf (last accessed December 2013).

Kehler N. 2004. *Coordinating Humanitarian Assistance: A Comparative Analysis of Three Cases*. http://www.ipg.vt.edu/papers/Kehler%20-%20MajorPaper.pdf (last accessed December 2013).

Kim JY, Millen J, Irwin A, Gershman J. 2000. *Dying for Growth: Global Inequality and the Health of the Poor*. Monroe, ME: Common Courage Press.

Kouadio IK, Kamigaki T, Oshitani H. 2010. Measles outbreaks in displaced populations: a review of transmission, morbidity and mortality associated factors. *BMC International Health and Human Rights* 10, 5.

Lucchi E. 2012. Moving from the "why" to the "how": reflections on humanitarian response in urban settings. *Disasters* 36(Suppl 1), S87–104.

OCHA (Office for the Coordination of Humanitarian Affairs). 2010. *OCHA Strategic Framework 2010–2013*. http://ochaonline.un.org/ocha2010/framework.html (last accessed December 2013).

OCHA (Office for the Coordination of Humanitarian Affairs). 2012. *How are disaster relief efforts organized? Cluster approach*. http://business.un.org/en/assets/39c87a78-fec9-402e-a434-2c355f24e4f4.pdf (last accessed December 2013).

Rieff D. 2002. *A Bed for the Night: Humanitarianism in Crisis*. New York: Simon and Schuster.

Ryan S. 2000. *The United Nations and International Politics*. Houndmills: Palgrave Macmillan.

Safran MA, Chorba T, Schreiber M *et al.* 2011. Evaluating mental health after the 2010 Haitian earthquake. *Disaster Medicine and Public Health Preparedness* 5(2), 154–7.

Seybolt T. 2007. *Humanitarian Military Interventions: The Conditions for Success and Failure.* Stockholm: Stockholm International Peace Research Institute.

Sharp TW, Burkle FM Jr, Vaughn AF, Chotani R, Brennan RJ. 2002. Challenges and opportunities for humanitarian relief in Afghanistan. *Clinical Infectious Diseases* 34(Suppl 5), S215–28.

Siddique AK. 1994. Cholera epidemic among Rwandan refugees: experience of ICDDR,B in Goma, Zaire. *Glimpse* 16(5), 3–4.

Sondorp E, Zwi A. 2002. Complex political emergencies. *BMJ* 324, 310–1.

Sphere. 2012. *The Sphere Handbook: Humanitarian Charter and Minimum Standards in Humanitarian Response.* http://www.Spherehandbook.org/ (last accessed December 2013).

Steet J, Grünewald F, Binder A *et al.* 2010. *Cluster Approach Evaluation 2 Synthesis Report.* Inter-Agency Standing Committee.

SIPRI (Stockholm International Peace Research Institute). 2000. *SIPRI Yearbook. Armaments, Disarmament and International Security.* Oxford: Oxford University Press. http://www.sipri.org/yearbook/2000 (last accessed December 2013).

Tsunami Evaluation Coalition. 2007. *Evaluation Report: Tsunami Evaluation Coalition.* http://www.alnap.org/ourwork/tec.aspx (last accessed December 2013).

UN (United Nations). 2012. *Cluster approach.* http://www.unocha.org/what-we-do/coordination-tools/cluster-coordination (last accessed December 2013).

Wolbring G. 2011. Disability, displacement and public health: a vision for Haiti. *Canadian Journal of Public Health* 102(2), 157–9.

World Bank. 2010. *Natural Hazards, Unnatural Disasters: The Economy of Effective Prevention.* Washington, DC: World Bank.

World Bank. 2011. *Kosovo NGO and civil society.* http://go.worldbank.org/H6JVQ8JY50 (last accessed December 2013).

World Bank. 2012. Improving the Assessment of Disaster Risks to Strengthen Financial Resilience: A Special Joint G20 Publication by the Government of Mexico and the World Bank. Washington, DC: Government of Mexico/World Bank. http://www.gfdrr.org/gfdrr/sites/gfdrr.org/files/GFDRR_G20_Low_June13.pdf (last accessed December 2013).

Chapter 18

The Limits of Humanitarian Action

Hugo Slim

Abstract

This chapter looks at the various limits on the effectiveness of humanitarian action in armed conflict and disaster. While the big picture of international humanitarian action is very positive and shows a significant growth in humanitarian finance and coverage in recent years, every humanitarian operation still has to deal with a range of barriers that routinely block total humanitarian success. These barriers are identified as political; organizational; technical; communal; and moral. All barriers combine to different degrees in every international humanitarian operation to reject, skew, confuse, and inhibit humanitarian action. As perennial problems, these difficulties are the natural operating environment for any humanitarian worker. Introducing humanitarian action into armed conflict and disaster will always be a negotiated struggle that is dependent on ideologies, systems, and behavior which are regularly beyond the direct control of medical humanitarian agencies.

The Handbook of Global Health Policy, First Edition. Edited by Garrett W. Brown, Gavin Yamey, and Sarah Wamala.
© 2014 John Wiley & Sons, Ltd. Published 2014 by John Wiley & Sons, Ltd.

Key Points

- Humanitarian action is routinely steeped in the deep politics of global, national, and local interests.
- Effective access to affected populations can be problematic and require negotiation and compromise.
- Leadership of international humanitarian operations is often weak and confused because of inter-state and inter-agency dynamics, so that combined humanitarian resources are seldom coordinated and leveraged to achieve maximum value.
- There is significant knowledge and expertise in humanitarian medicine in UN agencies, national government ministries, and non-governmental organizations, but the struggle remains to build sufficient skills at community level where they are needed most.
- The temporary and restricted nature of emergency medicine creates ethical dilemmas around levels of investment and the sophistication of treatments when an agency's exit is likely at the end of the crisis.

Key Policy Implications

- International humanitarian action is expanding and the need for investment in education, innovation, quality, and capacity in humanitarian medicine is greater than ever.
- Humanitarian public health workers need to know the international legal framework in which they are entitled to operate, and must expect to negotiate their presence on the ground in the context of hard politics.
- All members of the humanitarian health sector need to make special efforts to make the UN's health cluster as effective as possible, as this looks set to remain the main vehicle of coordination in the medium term.

Limits of Humanitarian Action

In an ideal world, the limits of humanitarian action would be set only by the extent of human need in war and disaster. Wherever there is need, there would also be humanitarian action to respond to it and meet it. The two fundamental values of humanitarian action – the principles of humanity and impartiality – declare that every human being who suffers from the effects of war and disaster is entitled to be assisted and protected by humanitarian action.

In the real world, however, there are a great many limits to humanitarian action. The big picture is positive but barriers of various kinds are still the norm in every humanitarian operation. There is more humanitarian aid in the world today than ever before – reaching $16 billion in 2010 – and this aid is spreading further than at any other time in human history (DARA 2011). Anyone in the world facing suffering from armed conflict or disaster stands a good chance of coming into contact with some form of international humanitarian aid. This is remarkable progress. Yet, efforts to extend humanitarian action to meet all human needs still routinely and inevitably bump up against a set of very real limits.

This chapter looks at the range of barriers that prevent the meeting of health needs in armed conflicts and disasters. It identifies a range of limits to global needs-based humanitarian action that prevent effective medical assistance and protection by rejecting, skewing, confusing, or inhibiting it.

Quantitative and Qualitative Limits

Some of the failures to meet needs are essentially quantitative: there are still large numbers of people who could be reached and helped, but are not. Other failures are qualitative: some people who are reached are not helped well enough, leaving their needs partially or inappropriately met. There are also moral limits to the humanitarian project that is bounded by an emergency ethic and struggles over its ethical relationship with longer term development projects of sustainable development and social justice.

External and Internal Barriers

Quantitative and qualitative failures alike can be determined by the politics of wars and disasters. These political contexts can be regarded as "external" limits on humanitarian action that are set by others. There are also very real limits set by affected communities themselves who are not always willing or able to design their own humanitarian strategies or make the most of what is on offer.

Other barriers to effective humanitarian action are more organizational and "internal" to humanitarian agencies or to the operational effectiveness of the humanitarian sector. These limits are set by the failings of humanitarians themselves. There are also barriers that are technological rather than political or organizational. Humanitarian agencies could achieve much more if certain technological innovations were more advanced. There is strong evidence that solid innovation in humanitarian programming leap-frog some barriers to effective humanitarian action. Finally, there are moral limits set by law and principle that only allow humanitarian aid an interim relief role and not a transformative development role.

Five Main Types of Limit

Political Barriers

The most obvious political barrier to humanitarian action is a form of antihumanitarian politics that rejects humanitarian values outright. In an armed conflict, this will typically be a war that is fought with an extreme anticivilian ideology which shows no respect for principles of protection and assistance, but sets out instead to deliberately kill, dispossess, rape, and starve an enemy population (Slim 2007). Such wars are fought in diametric opposition to humanitarian values. Based in political logics of genocide, subjugation, or necessity, such politics makes no place for humanitarian action. Political groups fighting with this logic enter into very little accommodation with humanitarian agencies and give little priority to the health of their enemies. In this kind of politics, humanitarian action is simply rejected. These types of antihumanitarian politics actively violate the humanitarian ethic by sustained and extreme acts of commission.

In a slightly more subtle way, a politics of humanitarian omission also serves to limit humanitarian action. In armed conflicts and disasters, political authorities can be highly selective about who they choose to help, prioritize, and neglect in a population in need. Areas dominated by enemies or insurgents may be kept off limits from significant aid, usually by a strict system of permits and threats that ensures that humanitarian agencies are stalled, deterred, or considerably slowed down. In contrast, areas populated by political supporters can be favored. Aid to these areas can be encouraged and enabled by state and non-state powers that control key gateways. In this kind of politics, humanitarian action is not entirely rejected but is certainly skewed, becoming partial and politically manipulated by acts of omission. In Sri Lanka, the Tamil Tigers and the government both used humanitarian aid strategically and tactically as a military and political resource. The Tamil Tigers tried to force people to stay in their home areas rather than flee so that their troops could hide among them. Later, the Sri Lankan government then used aid resources to create camps for internally displaced people (IDPs) that became effective detainee camps to contain the Tamil population while it was screened for insurgents (Magone *et al.* 2011). The government of Pakistan is the latest in a long line of states being criticized for this kind of partiality, particularly in regard to its recent policy towards flood victims in insurgent areas.

Partiality and "politicization" can also happen at the level of humanitarian donor governments. Humanitarian financing from Organisation for Economic Co-operation and Development (OECD) countries is the most transparent and most accountable of all global humanitarian funding by governments. As a result, it receives the most scrutiny. This scrutiny shows that OECD humanitarian funds also tend to be skewed in support of the main foreign policy objectives of the 23 western governments who make up the OECD. For example, "belligerent donors" fighting counter-insurgency wars and supporting liberal state building in Afghanistan, Iraq, Libya, or Somalia are regularly challenged for investing disproportionate amounts of humanitarian financing in these countries, and their aid is often criticized as "politicized" because of a lack of independence from political objectives (DARA 2011).

Global flows of Islamic humanitarian funding are probably as big or bigger than OECD flows, depending how and where you count them. There are few public data that tracks them but, like OECD financing, these funds are probably skewed in some way too. Islamic budgets tend to focus disproportionately on Muslim emergencies of one sort or another, as in Somalia recently or more routinely in the occupied Palestinian Territories (IRIN 2011; Development Initiatives 2011).

If skewed OECD and Islamic financing is a barrier to globally equitable humanitarian aid flows, local association with western funding can also be a barrier to local humanitarian action. Many UN and non-governmental organization (NGO) workers are convinced that their association with NATO's counter-insurgency (COIN) strategy and its attempts to use humanitarian and development aid to win hearts and minds (WHAM) have put them in grave danger of attacks, so inhibiting their reach. In a conflict that has been framed by all sides as a West–Islamist and imperialist–nationalist struggle, humanitarians have often felt perceived as being on one side, and targeted accordingly. Attacks on medical aid workers have led to a break in humanitarian action from time to time and NGOs, like Médecins Sans Frontières, have left Afghanistan. This violent deterrence of humanitarian action is, of course, not simply the responsibility of NATO's "blurring." It is also the responsibility of the Taliban and others who have attacked, kidnapped, and killed humanitarian workers. But the Taliban do not only deter humanitarian action, they also use it. The Taliban's own WHAM policies have also led them to attract and tolerate NGOs in certain situations (Valente 2011). As in Sri Lanka, this confirms the fact that the restriction and manipulation of humanitarian aid are usually played out by both sides in a war.

Somalia offers another example of this "dual (ab)use" tendency in armed conflicts – (to adapt a phrase from international humanitarian law about dual use facilities). In Afghanistan, humanitarian action has sometimes been compromised for being over-associated with belligerent western governments keen to use lots of aid to reform Afghanistan. In Somalia, however, humanitarians have been actively deterred from using western aid by the US government in case US aid falls into terrorist hands. American legislation against providing any kind of "material support" to prescribed terrorist groups significantly inhibited NGOs from applying for and distributing American food and other aid in Somalia in 2010 and 2011 for fear it would be seen as resourcing Al Shabaab. But the US government was not the only one basing humanitarian policy on political judgments. Al Shabaab made its own analysis of western NGOs and "expelled" the UN World Food Programme (WFP) and several other western NGOs, refusing to work with them because they were allegedly informing on Al Shabaab, fostering secular values and seeking to undermine Sharia Law (Huffington Post 2011). Here, dual abuse meant that NGOs were prevented from operating effectively because they were seen as too close to Al Shabaab by the US government and too close to the West by Al Shabaab. Both suspicions proved to be disastrous barriers to humanitarian action which resulted in unnecessary death rates in the famine that followed. The expulsion of WFP alone led to an immediate 30% drop in food supply into Somalia; and reticent NGO food programming earlier in 2011 meant people were more vulnerable than usual to the drought that followed (Slim 2012a).

The various political barriers to humanitarian action summarized above are usually discussed as problems of "humanitarian access" or "humanitarian space." Both terms seek to encompass the practice of humanitarian agencies getting personal access to affected populations to operate impartially and effectively under humanitarian principles. There has been much discussion of the pressures on humanitarian space in the last few years. Many NGOs at the sharp end of humanitarian negotiations, as well as other commentators, have felt with some passion that the space for principled access to war and disaster-affected people is "shrinking." This misattributed sense of shrinking space is the product of golden age thinking about the humanitarian past and an idealized sense that humanitarian action used to be easier. It did not. Humanitarian reach is currently greater than it has ever been. Perhaps the increasing volume of humanitarian action is what makes it seem harder because normal difficulties are multiplied, but the perennial problems of rejected and skewed humanitarian action remain the same.

A realistic assessment of the inevitable and fairly constant struggle for humanitarian access and space are evident in two important new publications. A new book by MSF (Magone *et al.* 2011) tells the honest tale of MSF's humanitarian negotiations in 12 countries over the last couple of years. These cases make plain that the ability to operate as a humanitarian agency in armed conflict and disaster is never simply a given. It is always a struggle that is negotiated and renegotiated with political power, in which unsatisfactory compromise is more common than outright success (Magone *et al.* 2011). A recent report by the London-based think tank, the Humanitarian Policy Group, supports MSF's experience of political struggle in humanitarian action and also emphasizes the growth in humanitarian space and operation. It notes that increasing pressures are "the result of an expanding humanitarian system that has extended its reach and ambitions into types of conflict and crisis that were previously off-limits" (Collinson and Elhawary 2012).

Health workers in humanitarian operations need to approach these various political barriers with a clear understanding of their rights and duties under international humanitarian law (IHL). Governments and warring parties have a responsibility under international law to consent to, and not to arbitrarily impede, emergency healthcare operations (Barber 2009). All humanitarian health workers need to be aware of the law that protects them and their patients in armed conflicts and disasters. All good humanitarian agencies and NGOs routinely train their staff in IHL and international human rights law, as well as have expert legal advisors in-house. Health workers will need the skill, determination, and patience to use this law to negotiate their presence in an armed conflict and disaster.

Organizational Barriers

External political action obviously limits the extent, content, and effect of humanitarian action in many armed conflicts and disasters. But the so-called "humanitarian system" of the UN, Red Cross, and NGO agencies is also quite capable of self-inflicted limits on its own efficacy by virtue of its fragmentation, competition, bureaucracy, and lack of professionalism.

The continuous quest for "reform" of the UN's "coordinating role" in humanitarian emergencies is a permanent reminder that international humanitarian response is not managed by a single streamlined specialist organization. Nor is it the well-orchestrated and unanimous performance of finely honed collective action. Instead, international humanitarian response is the more challenging task of coalition-building, combining, and aligning multiple interests and diverse organizations around each new emergency. Weiss (2013) has laid bare the inconsistencies, inefficiencies, and impossibilities that create international humanitarian action's inability to work seamlessly to become more than the sum of its unregulated parts. A range of centrifugal forces work against effective international action on the ground: turf wars over different UN agency mandates; the proliferation of independent humanitarian agencies; the expansion of humanitarian activities and sectors; and the broad spectrum of different agency attitudes towards UN authority and coordination. All these make leveraging maximum value and efficiency from international humanitarian resources extremely problematic.

The last 30 years of humanitarian expansion have produced more and more agencies – national and international NGOs – to gather and coordinate. A coordination meeting in a major emergency in the 1980s might have involved 15–20 agencies. Now there may be representatives from 100 organizations crammed into a room. New innovations in humanitarian practice have created new "sectors" like early recovery, security, protection, and telecommunications. These are now added to the more traditional sectors like health, water, sanitation, and shelter to form the "clusters" that are the basis of international coordination. Clusters are led by members of the Inter-Agency Standing Committee (IASC) which is the joint UN and NGO body that provides joint leadership in humanitarian response. Each cluster can have working groups and sub-groups. All of them are "accountable to" the UN's Humanitarian Coordinator (HC) but the HCs themselves are not in charge as such. The emphasis of the cluster system is on reaching agreement on standards and strategy. The drive of a meeting is horizontal towards consensus, not vertical towards direction and control.

This chronic coordinating culture indicates the single greatest weakness in the international system of humanitarian response – the leadership vacuum at the heart of international operations. The various UN agencies all refuse to accept a lead authority with real strategic and decision-making power. NGOs are the same. They will take cover behind UN legitimacy and authority when they need it, but will not always follow it routinely. Like much of international society itself, the dynamics of international humanitarian response is more like an arena than a system. Despite a new "transformative agenda" around UN humanitarian coordination, complete with ideas of "empowered leadership" and "streamlined coordination" (IASC 2012), it seems likely that the essential inter-state and inter-agency politics of humanitarian action will never enable a step change in its strategic effectiveness. The best international operations are those led by inspired and gifted UN leaders whose personality coagulates and drives the system's many players much better than any coordinating arrangements.

Health workers engaged in humanitarian operations need to find the best way to work effectively with the IASC health cluster led by the World Health Organization, and to improve its performance wherever possible (WHO 2012). The Global Health Cluster (GHC) has 38 UN agency and NGO members. It works together to assess, analyze, and improve the effectiveness of emergency health programs at national level. Above all, their task is to ensure that their collective action in any humanitarian response is greater than the sum of their parts. For example, WFP's membership of the GHC is intended to ensure that food aid and nutrition policy and planning is integrated into wider health planning in any emergency. This international coordination arrangement looks set to be the main forum for leading emergency health operations in the medium term. Its efficiency and effectiveness will be a key organizational determinant for optimal health outcomes across complex operations.

The fragmented politics of the inter-agency arena are not the only thing that limits the practical quality of international humanitarian action. Psychological as well as political factors can inhibit effectiveness too in a profession in which the "calling" of emergency action is so crucial. As the ancient tale about a boy and a wolf makes plain, emergencies are notoriously hard to call. When will a drought become a famine? When will a threat become a massacre? When do several massacres become genocide? When is the moment to really spend, and send food, water, planes, and people? When is the right time to shout from the rooftops? Making the right call is as much about personal and group psychology as it is about professional judgment.

Last year's famine in the Horn of Africa was the most recent of many examples of a slow call. Without detailed research, it is hard to unpack the psychological reasons why a range of NGO, UN, and government staff "called it late." Early warning data and the obvious food deficit resulting from WFP's expulsion were clear and serious indicators of likely disaster (Fews Net 2011). Hesitation may have been caused by a seasoned caution.

Many regional experts are aware that they have previously overestimated people's vulnerability in a region where people have regularly proved incredibly resilient. Later good rains have often been just enough to see people through. They did not want to call it, and there be no wolf. Some kind of denial may also have been in play, particularly in US and European capitals where civil servants were being asked to frame the Horn as a key arena of the war on terror rather than a fragile region of drought and poverty. Perhaps diplomats were being rewarded for thinking more about dangerous Islamists than vulnerable pastoralists.

There could also have been an element of groupthink across the Somalia community in particular, which always expects Somalia to be in a terrible state. So, this was just yet another bad year. As such, some aid officials were caught in incremental thinking rather than crisis thinking. This worked in Ethiopia and Kenya, but not in Somalia. Government, UN, and NGO officials were recalibrating across the Horn, pushing estimates of need upwards in a series of constant rises and reappraisals. In Ethiopia, with its impressive government safety net infrastructure this worked well enough and saved many lives. In Kenya, a powerful aid system working with the consent of a weak and disinterested government was able to catch up after a slow start. But, in Somalia, with no strong state, reluctant western donors and a resistant non-state armed group, there was not enough money, resources, or infrastructure to fend off a famine (Slim 2012a). Recalibration did not work and the realization and resourcing of a major crisis came too late.

Political fragmentation in the international humanitarian system may be inevitable but objective scientific thinking around needs can and must be maintained as a mark of humanitarian professionalism by medics, nutritionists, agriculturalists, and political analysts. Calling slow onset emergencies is very hard, but there needs to be a culture in every humanitarian organization – government, UN, Red Cross, and NGO – which encourages people to call early and wrong every now and again, rather than right and late. Groupthink needs to be challenged by dedicated internal critics and questioners. People should be rewarded for being vigilant and not inhibited for fear of being wrong. Their bosses need to back them for "calling" emergencies when there were reasonable grounds to do so.

Technical Barriers

The last 40 years have seen significant and consistent technological development in humanitarian action. Health interventions have improved and the principles and best practices of emergency public health medicine are now well understood. The same goes for other fields of nutrition, shelter, camp planning, emergency social work, and more nascent fields like protection and communications – with all the new emergency aid innovations possible through mobile communications technology like cash transfers and public information.

Technical barriers to life-saving interventions are therefore not created by a core lack of expertise or knowledge. Significant expertise exists in universities, agencies, and in increasing numbers of well-trained professionals. The theory and technical policy-making around health and other emergency disciplines are strong. Instead, the challenge of leveraging and operationalizing this knowledge is where barriers emerge. First, there are real difficulties in disseminating and standardizing sound knowledge and policy across very uneven communities of knowledge and skills. Second, in armed conflicts, medical facilities and health staff are often deliberately targeted for pillage or attack – a problem that is being clearly exposed in the Red Cross Movement's new "Healthcare in Danger" campaign (ICRC 2010). Third, insufficient resources and room for maneuver often means that, even if sufficient knowledge and skills exist, practical capacity is lacking on the ground. There is simply not the kit, salaries, infrastructure, or access to apply technical knowledge on time and across sufficient space. The sad lament of humanitarians is not usually that "we did not know what to do," but that "we were not able to do what we know."

But this is not always the case. The quality of local, national, and international agencies is still uneven. Sometimes humanitarian needs remain unmet because of bad humanitarian practice. Some bad humanitarian work can be the result of a genuine and understandable lack of capacity and resources as explained above. This work is not bad in itself but incomplete. But some bad humanitarian work is just plain bad. Agencies can take on areas of work that are beyond their skills set. An NGO can be badly run, ill-equipped, and ill-staffed simply for no good reason but sheer inefficiency. A single bad member of staff can be a rotten apple that ruins the rest of the work. Some agencies are just not professional enough and this can be a matter of life and death for people, a sort of zip code lottery depending on which NGO you get in your district.

Humanitarian agencies have made a major effort in the last 20 years to self-regulate and improve, most notably through the Code of Conduct (1994) and Sphere Standards (Sphere Project 2011) that set out clear expectations of high quality work. Every agency – big or small – which mandates themselves or is mandated under international law must make professional and technical excellence a core goal. Humanitarian legitimacy is not a given simply by "being there" but must be earned by excellence of various kinds (Slim 2012b).

Humanitarian innovation is now a recognized priority across the humanitarian sector (Slim 2006). New technologies and practices are being actively sought and encouraged by a new humanitarian innovation fund set up by the UK government's Department for International Development, the Swedish government's Ministry of Foreign Affairs and ALNAP (DFID 2010). Humanitarian health professionals need to prioritize innovation and leverage all available funding to do so. New technologies can overcome current technical and practical limits to humanitarian action and, as in every other sector, offer real hope of expanding the quantity and quality of humanitarian response.

The ability to show clear evidence of the impact of various health operations in humanitarian programming is an essential technical priority. Humanitarian medicine has traditionally been better at showing results than many other sectors of humanitarian work. Technical developments in data collection, processing, and interpretation have been significant but, once again, may sometimes falter at field level and in high-pressure phases of relief work. Poor evidence of impact is a major limit to the targeting and improvement of humanitarian health programs. All health workers need to prioritize the collection, interpretation, and application of evidence if humanitarian healthcare is to improve and break new boundaries of high-quality care. Evidence Aid, the new project by the Cochrane Collaboration, is a major contribution to raising standards in humanitarian health projects (Evidence Aid 2012). Their efforts to increase the rigor of health reporting in emergencies and to make available important research results in disaster medicine to guide health workers at field level are gathering important momentum internationally.

Community Barriers

Humanitarian action is structured, perceived, and usually experienced as external intervention – assistance coming from "outside" local communities. In reality, however, and in accordance with best practice, most aid is heavily mediated and controlled by local communities in a variety of ways. Community participation is widely acknowledged as the best and rightful way to share and distribute emergency resources of all kinds. People are usually best placed to identify what they need, how they need it, who needs it, when they need it, and why they need it. Good humanitarian programming works closely with affected and at risk communities, leveraging local knowledge and networks to maximize the value and fairness of aid resources.

This mostly works well enough but local communities are not crammed with a disproportionately high number of experts and angels, nor are they conflict-free and without vested interests and competition around gender, class, and power. In other words, key people in local communities may not always be working to humanitarian principles. As we have seen, local government structures can be partial as much as impartial depending on the political situation or corruption levels. So too can more informal community networks of villages, clans, neighborhoods, and base communities. Elite capture or subversion of aid resources is a risk to humanitarian action at local level. The risk of aid playing into and escalating existing violent conflict in an area is also problematic (Anderson 1999).

International health workers need to be aware of the intricacies and interests of community politics and so design health services that focus on equity and access while leveraging community participation in the best way possible. Health workers cannot understand a community from within a clinic or a hospital but need the close support of community workers and political analysts. The best agencies working in health will usually have strong systems of political analysis integrated into health programming to resist or mitigate capture, and to ensure independence and impartiality.

Moral Limits

Humanitarian action also struggles with a question of moral limits in war and disasters. How far is a humanitarian agency and operation entitled to go in improving people's lives? This may sound like a rather abstract question in the middle of an emergency but it poses very practical operational problems on the ground.

Humanitarian action is tightly bounded under IHL and the Code of Conduct of humanitarian agencies. In essence, these boundaries are set around the principles of relief and neutrality. In the Geneva Conventions, humanitarian agencies are largely restricted to providing "relief" and most relief items that are specifically designated are required to be "essential," as set out in the Fourth Geneva Convention, Articles 23 and 59. The principles of neutrality and impartiality also prevent humanitarian agencies from building up the capacity of one side or another in war in such a way that "a definite advantage may accrue to the military efforts or economy of the enemy," as stated in Article 23, paragraph (c) of the Fourth Geneva Convention.

So, all the talk about developmental relief, early recovery, and the relief–development continuum that is so important to the theory of disaster response, is operationally problematic in armed conflicts. The allocation and investment of relief and development resources affect the balance of power and can develop or free up the capacity of belligerent governments and armed groups. If humanitarian agencies support the development of government health services or temporarily take on the salary bills of clinic staff, this may be good relief and development work, but it may not be essential and it may not be neutral.

If the distinction between relief and development is a hard one to draw on the ground, then deciding when an emergency is over and when it is time to withdraw is another moral difficulty. A good "exit strategy" is always hard to call, particularly in health projects when lives will inevitably depend on the presence of an agency. It is one of the paradoxes of the success of humanitarian aid that public health indicators often go up in protracted armed conflicts – war can be good for public health. The surge in healthcare resources can mean that immunization coverage increases, more staff are trained, and improved outpatient facilities are available (Human Security Report Project 2011). This means that the exit of an international agency and the return of health resources into government hands can risk a return to lower levels of pre-humanitarian health status (see Chapter 14).

Related to exit, there is also the question of how far a humanitarian agency should introduce innovative and expensive drug treatments in war and disaster if they will not be sustainable and available when the agency leaves (see Chapter 24). MSF routinely struggles with this ethical problem of medical excellence and inevitable exit (Laouabdia 2005). Every humanitarian health worker needs to appreciate these and other particular problems associated with medical ethics in humanitarian operations, and bring them for wider discussion in their team and organization (Schopper 2013).

One of the biggest ethical challenges facing humanitarian health workers is the challenge and dilemmas of managing optimal operations in imperfect conditions that are very different from their ordinary rich world working conditions. One of the great shocks for medics in humanitarian work is the extreme problem of triage, limited equipment, and strange cultural preferences that dominate the emergency environment in very poor countries. Recent research with returning expatriate humanitarian workers is beginning to deliver greater understanding of the typical moral problems faced by health workers in poor country emergencies (Schwartz *et al.* 2010; Hunt 2011). These studies show the importance of making humanitarian health workers ethically aware in advance of an emergency mission, and making sure that dilemmas are owned and shared at operational level so that agencies can be accountable to patients and supporters for decisions taken in difficult situations.

Conclusions

This chapter has tried to show the perennial and strategic limits humanitarian health practitioners can expect to face in their work. Some limits are political, others are organizational, technical, and ethical. All are very common. Dealing with them, and occasionally getting past them, comes with the territory of being an international humanitarian worker. Getting stuck and blocked sometimes, unable to design and deliver the perfect health programs that you know could transform people's lives in war and disaster, is how it is. Wishing it were not so and arguing that it should be otherwise is a bit like a pearl diver saying that he or she should not have to get wet. The trick is to swim about in the most efficient and innovative way and find the best possible pearl.

Key Reading

Blakie P, Cannon T, Davis I, Wisner B. 2003. *At Risk: Natural Hazards, People's Vulnerability and Disasters*. London: Routledge.

Bouchet-Saulnier F. 2006. *The Practical Guide to Humanitarian Law*. Oxford and Boulder: Rowman and Littlefield.

Evidence Aid. 2013. http://www.cochrane.org/cochrane-reviews/evidence-aid-project (last accessed December 2013).

Levy BS, Sidel VW (eds). 2008. *War and Public Health*, 2nd edn. Oxford and New York: Oxford University Press.

Magone C, Neuman M, Weissman F (eds). (2011) *Humanitarian Negotiations Revealed*. London: Hurst and Médecins Sans Frontières.

Slim H. 2012. Doing the right thing: relief agencies, moral dilemmas and moral responsibility in political emergencies and war. In *Essays in Humanitarian Action*. Oxford: ELAC and Kindle Books.

References

Anderson M. 1999. *Do No Harm: How Aid Can Support Peace or War*. Boulder and London: Lynne Rienner.

Barber R. 2009. Facilitating humanitarian assistance in international humanitarian law and human rights law. *International Review of the Red Cross* 91(874).

Code of Conduct. 1994. *Code of Conduct for the International Red Cross and Red Crescent Movement and Non-Governmental Organizations (NGOs) in Disaster Relief*. http://www.ifrc.org/en/publications-and-reports/code-of-conduct/ (last accessed December 2013).

Collinson S, Elhawary S. 2012. *Humanitarian Space: A Review of Trends and Issues*. London: Humanitarian Policy Group, ODI.

DARA. 2011. *HRI 2011: The Humanitarian Response Index*. Madrid: DARA.

Development Initiatives. 2011. *Arab Donors and Humanitarian Aid*. donhttp://www.globalhuman itarianassistance.org/report/arab-donors (last accessed December 2013).

DFID (Department for International Development). 2010. Humanitarian Innovation Fund. www.humanitarianinnovation.org (last accessed December 2013).

Evidence Aid. 2012. Evidence Aid. http://www.cochrane.org/cochrane-reviews/evidence-aid-project (last accessed December 2013).

Fews Net. 2011. Fews Net. http://www.fews.net/Pages/default.aspx (last accessed December 2013).

Huffington Post. 2011. Somalia: Al Shabab bans aid groups, including UN agencies. *Huffington Post* November 28. http://www.huffingtonpost.com/2011/11/28/somalia-al-shabab-ban-aid_n_1116522.html (last accessed December 2013).

Human Security Report Project. 2011. *Human Security Report 2009/2010*, chapter 6. Simon Fraser University Canada. New York and London: Oxford University Press.

Hunt M. 2011. Establishing moral bearings: ethics and expatriate health care professionals in humanitarian work. *Disasters* 35(3), 606–22.

IASC (Inter-Agency Standing Committee). 2012. *The Transformative Agenda*. http://www.humanitarianinfo.org/iasc/pageloader.aspx?page=content-template-default&bd=87 (last accessed December 2013).

ICRC (International Committee of the Red Cross). 2010. *Healthcare in Danger: Making the Case*. Geneva: ICRC.

IRIN (Investor Relations Information Network). 2011. *Analysis: Arab and Muslim aid and the West: "two china elephants"*. http://www.irinnews.org/Report/94010/Analysis-Arab-and-Muslim-aid-and-the-West-two-china-elephants (last accessed December 2013).

Laouabdia K. 2005. The medical ambitions of a humanitarian organization. In *My Sweet La Mancha*. Geneva: Médecins Sans Frontières.

Magone C, Neuman M, Weissman F. 2011. *Humanitarian Negotiations Revealed*. London: Hurst.

Schopper D. 2013. Research ethics governance in disaster situations. In O'Mathuna DP, Gordjin B, Clarke M (eds) *Disaster Bioethics*. New York: Springer.

Schwartz L, Sinding C, Hunt M *et al.* 2010. Ethics in humanitarian aid work: learning from the narratives of humanitarian health workers. *AJOB Primary Research* 1(3), 45–54.

Slim H. 2006. Global welfare: a realistic expectation of the international humanitarian system? In Mitchell J (ed.) *ALNAP Review of Humanitarian Action*, pp. 9–34. London: Overseas Development Institute.

Slim H. 2007. *Killing Civilians: Method, Madness and Morality in War*. London and New York: Hurst and Columbia University Press.

Slim H. 2012a. *IASC Real-Time Evaluation of the Humanitarian Response to the Horn of Africa Drought Crisis in Somalia, Ethiopia and Kenya: Synthesis Report*. http://reliefweb.int/sites/reliefweb.int/files/resources/RTE_HoA_SynthesisReport_FINAL.pdf (last accessed December 2013).

Slim H. 2012b. By what authority? NGO legitimacy and accountability. In Slim H (ed.) *Essays in Humanitarian Action*. Oxford: Oxford Institute of Ethics, Law and Conflict.

Sphere Project. 2011. *The Sphere Handbook*. http://www.sphereproject.org/resources/download-publications/?search=1&keywords=&language=English&category=22 (last accessed December 2013).

Valente R. 2011. *Beyond Acceptance: Strategies for NGO Humanitarian Access in Afghanistan*. Kabul: Care.

Weiss TG. 2013. *The Humanitarian Business*. Cambridge: Polity Press.

WHO (World Health Organization). 2012. *About the Global Health Cluster*. http://www.who.int/hac/global_health_cluster/about/en/index.html (last accessed December 2013).

Part V Financing and the Political Economy of Global Health

Chapter 19

The Global Health Financing Architecture and the Millennium Development Goals

Marco Schäferhoff, Christina Schrade, and
Matthew T. Schneider

Abstract

This chapter examines the global health financing architecture through the lens of the health Millennium Development Goals (MDGs), which have a deadline of 2015, and draws lessons learned for a post-MDG framework. It argues that the health MDGs spurred a dramatic increase in global health funding, and catalyzed the emergence of high-profile financing mechanisms, such as the Global Fund to Fight AIDS, Tuberculosis and Malaria. In addition, the health MDGs have contributed to a greater focus on accountability, stimulating the emergence of new global initiatives to better track progress towards the MDGs. Available evidence also indicates that global support for the MDGs and the focused attention on specific goals have yielded demonstrable results.

However, while having three separate health MDGs helps with resource mobilization, this fragmented approach also has drawbacks. The approach encourages the creation of financing silos and the "verticalization" (single disease focus) of programs and initiatives without sufficient integration with broader health systems issues. Furthermore, the health MDGs left important gaps, such as in financing non-communicable diseases and neglected tropical infections, and funding was distributed highly unevenly.

The global community faces a difficult challenge: it needs to keep a focus on the unfinished health MDGs by including them in the post-2015 goals, while incorporating additional issues. Yet donor funding is stagnating because of the global financial crisis and domestic health spending by developing countries has not increased as expected, so raising additional financing for health in the post-2015 era will require innovation and political will.

The Handbook of Global Health Policy, First Edition. Edited by Garrett W. Brown, Gavin Yamey, and Sarah Wamala.
© 2014 John Wiley & Sons, Ltd. Published 2014 by John Wiley & Sons, Ltd.

Key Points

- The Millennium Development Goals (MDGs), with their deadline of 2015, have made a positive impact on global health but progress is uneven.
- The MDGs spurred dramatic growth in global health financing and the creation of new funding initiatives and mechanisms.
- A fragmented approach to achieving the MDGs encouraged the creation of financing silos, mostly targeting MDG 6, and the "verticalization" (single disease focus) of initiatives without sufficient integration with broader health systems issues.
- While the MDGs contributed to greater accountability in how aid for health was raised and spent, more investments are still needed in national health systems strengthening.
- Global health funding is stagnating, raising questions about the prioritization of health issues in a post-2015 framework; the debate is now focused on whether to finish the MDGs or take on new concerns, such as the control of non-communicable diseases.

Key Policy Implications

- The global health community should keep a focus on the unfinished health MDGs by working them into the post-2015 goals; if they lose this focus, the gains that have been achieved to date could be jeopardized.
- Additional funding from traditional donors, domestic sources, and innovative financing mechanisms need to be mobilized to sustain the gains made in global health and to address further health concerns that have moved to the top of the global health agenda.
- Continued efforts are needed to further increase the efficiency and quality of global health spending, through transparent program evaluations, the harmonization of funding across donors, and the alignment of donor and country processes and priorities.

Introduction

In the year 2000, 189 United Nations (UN) Member States signed the Millennium Declaration, which established eight Millennium Development Goals (MDGs) to be achieved by 2015. Three of the eight goals (MDGs 4 to 6) relate directly to health (Box 19.1). Others, including MDG 1 on nutrition and MDG 7 on environmental sustainability (including drinking water and sanitation), are closely related to health.

Box 19.1   The Health MDGs

Goal	Target
MDG 4: Reduce child mortality	**4A:** Reduce by two thirds, between 1990 and 2015, the under-five mortality rate
MDG 5: Improve maternal health	**5A:** Reduce by three quarters, between 1990 and 2015, the maternal mortality ratio
	5B: Achieve, by 2015, universal access to reproductive health
MDG 6: Combat HIV/AIDS, malaria, and other diseases	**6A:** Have halted by 2015 and begun to reverse the spread of HIV/AIDS
	6B: Achieve, by 2010, universal access to treatment for HIV/AIDS
	6C: Have halted by 2015 and begun to reverse the incidence of malaria and other major diseases

---

However, with only two years to go until 2015, discussions about a post-2015 development framework are now gaining significant momentum. Some commentators argue that the new agenda should build on the existing and largely unfinished poverty-related MDGs. Others underline the need to significantly broaden the framework and incorporate Sustainable Development Goals (SDGs) applicable to all countries, which will be developed as a follow-up to the June 2012 Rio+20 Conference (the UN Conference on Sustainable Development).[1] As yet there is also little consensus on which thematic issues should be prioritized or on the role of health in the post-2015 global development framework and beyond.

This chapter examines the global health financing architecture through the lens of the health MDGs. We begin by briefly summarizing progress towards the MDGs and recent trends in global health financing. We then examine key players in the global health financing architecture, including new financing institutions. Next we make the case for increased domestic financing for health, for improvements in the quality and efficiency of global health financing, and for greater accountability in tracking financing resources and results. We end by drawing lessons learned for a post-MDG framework for health.

While it is impossible to ascribe causality, it is likely that the MDGs, as the key framework for addressing global health challenges, have shaped the health financing architecture in a number of ways. We would argue that the health MDGs have spurred three important trends in this architecture. First, the MDGs have provided a focus for mobilizing and targeting substantial additional financial resources for health, contributing to a dramatic increase in global health funding. However, there are now signs that donor funding is stagnating because of the global financial crisis, and this stagnation in turn may influence priority setting and tailoring of global health targets in the post-MDG agenda. Domestic health spending by developing countries has not increased at the expected rate. Second, following the formulation of the MDGs, a range of high-profile financing initiatives and mechanisms, such as the Global Fund to Fight AIDS, Tuberculosis and Malaria (the Global Fund), were established to allocate funding to countries. Some of these mechanisms have introduced new forms of governance and innovative financing approaches. Third, the health MDGs have contributed to a greater focus on accountability. They also spurred the emergence of new global initiatives to better track progress towards the MDGs, particularly towards MDGs 4 and 5.

We also argue that the health MDGs have contributed to two problems. First, while having three separate health MDGs helps with issue-specific advocacy and resource mobilization, this fragmented approach has its drawbacks. It encourages the creation of financing silos and the verticalization of programs and initiatives without sufficient integration with broader health systems issues. Second, the health MDGs leave important gaps (such as their neglect of non-communicable diseases). One key challenge for the post-MDG era will be to address these gaps in the face of existing resource constraints.

Progress Towards the Health MDGs

The MDGs focus on specific, measurable targets, which has the benefit of providing clear goals to the global health community. Available evidence indicates that the global support for the MDGs and the focused attention on specific goals have yielded demonstrable results. However, while significant progress has been made over the past decade towards the health MDGs, results are uneven.

Both the global child mortality rate and the global maternal mortality ratio have declined faster since 2000 than in the previous decade (Lozano et al. 2011). However, despite significant progress, at the current pace the child mortality rate is falling too slowly to reach target 4A of MDG 4 (Box 19.1). Achieving MDG 4 in 2015 would require an annual decline in child mortality of 4.4%, but from 1990 to 2011 the annual decline has been only 2.2% (UN IGME 2011). Even more worrisome is that the neonatal mortality rate is falling much more slowly than the child mortality rate (Schrade et al. 2011).

While the maternal mortality ratio has also fallen, progress towards improving maternal health (i.e., achieving target 5A of MDG 5) has been even slower than progress towards MDG 4. Over a period of 20 years, the maternal mortality ratio fell from 400 per 100,000 live births in 1990 to 210 per 100,000 live births in 2010 (WHO et al. 2012), a rate of decline that is too slow to reach target 5A. Reducing the maternal mortality ratio by three quarters by 2015 appears out of reach for many countries. Progress towards MDG 5B is also insufficient (Countdown 2012).

With regard to MDG 6, the number of newly infected HIV-positive people worldwide fell by 20% over a decade, from 3.2 million in 2001 to 2.5 million in 2011, and in 25 countries the incidence rate among adults fell by more than 50% in the same period (UNAIDS 2012). Significant progress has also been made towards reaching universal access to HIV/AIDS treatment (MDG 6B). In 2002, only about 300,000 people received antiretroviral therapy for HIV/AIDS treatment, but by 2011, 8 million people had access to treatment. However, almost half of all HIV-infected people in low- and middle-income countries still do not have access to this life-saving treatment (UNAIDS 2012).

Globally, the incidence of malaria has fallen by 17% since 2000 (UN 2012a). Reported malaria cases fell by more than 50% between 2000 and 2010 in 43 of the 99 countries with ongoing malaria transmission. In the same timeframe, malaria-specific mortality rates have decreased by 25%. Global tuberculosis incidence rates have been falling since 2002, and current projections suggest that if this trend continues the 1990 death rate from the disease will be halved by 2015 (UN 2012a).

In summary, despite significant progress having been made over the past decade towards MDGs 4 and 5, and also parts of MDG 6, these three goals will likely not be reached by 2015. Moving forward, the global health community should keep a focus on these unfinished MDGs by incorporating them into the post-2015 goals. If they are not kept in sight, the gains that have been made may be lost.

Trends in Global Health Financing

This section provides an overview of key trends in donor funding for global health since the adoption of the MDGs in 2000.

The MDGs Spurred a Substantial Growth in Global Health Financing

Since the MDGs were adopted, development assistance for health (DAH) nearly tripled, from US$10.7 billion in 2000 to $28.2 billion in 2010, an increase of 164% (IHME 2012). While it is difficult to prove that the health MDGs caused this dramatic increase in financing, at a minimum they reinforced positive trends in health financing as they have become the *key reference point for donors* to justify increases in aid (Moss 2010; Schweitzer *et al.* 2012).

Traditional donor governments accounted for the largest share of DAH. Between 2000 and 2010, ten donor governments provided 60% of all DAH: the United States (by far the world's largest donor to global health), the United Kingdom, Japan, France, Germany, the Netherlands, Canada, Norway, Spain, and Sweden. However, even though traditional donors have significantly scaled-up their health aid, only five of the 23 OECD-DAC (Organisation for Economic Co-operation and Development Development Assistance Committee) donor countries are on track to meet their commitment to spent at least 0.7% of their gross national income (GNI) on official development aid (ODA) by 2015. Sweden, Luxembourg, Denmark, and the Netherlands already exceeded the 0.7% target in 2011. The United Kingdom spent 0.56% of its GNI on ODA in 2011, which means that it met the 2010 interim goal of spending 0.51% of GNI in 2010 and it continues to be on track to reach its 0.7% commitment.

Funding by emerging donor countries – countries that were traditionally seen as aid receivers, such as India, Russia, and China – is believed to have risen in recent years (Walz and Ramachandran 2011). However, data on the amount of health funding provided by these emerging donors is still scarce.

Private contributions through foundations have become more important. In particular, the growing relevance of foundations goes back to the increased engagement of the Bill & Melinda Gates Foundation (BMGF) in global health. Funding provided by the BMGF increased 10-fold over about a decade, from $173.2 million in 1999 (1.8% of total DAH) to $1.7 billion in 2010 (6.0% of total DAH). In the 2000–2009 timeframe, the BMGF was the fourth largest funding source of DAH, giving a massive boost to global health programming. It contributed to a renewed dynamism in global health, even if some global health scholars express concerns about the foundation's lack of transparency and accountability, particularly with respect to its priority setting processes (Black *et al.* 2009; McCoy *et al.* 2009).

Despite the dramatic increase in funding for global health, large funding gaps remain. The UN estimates that the additional funding required to achieve the MDGs related to women's and children's health alone was $88 billion for the 2011–2015 period (UN 2010). To accelerate progress towards the health MDGs, innovative financing mechanisms were launched to mobilize additional funding (Taskforce on International Innovative Financing for Health Systems 2009). For example, UNITAID (www.unitaid.eu, last accessed December 2013) has mobilized about $1.1 billion since 2006 through a tax on airline tickets (a "solidarity levy") purchased in UNITAID member countries. UNITAID uses this funding towards achieving MDG 6 (e.g., by financing pediatric antiretroviral drugs). The solidarity levy is one of the financing mechanisms for MDG 6 that has emerged in the past decade (see "Key Players in the Global Health Financing Architecture" section). Another example is the International Finance Facility for Immunisation (IFFIm), which raises financing for the Global Alliance for Vaccines and Immunization (GAVI Alliance or GAVI), a public–private partnership that works to expand immunization coverage in developing countries. IFFIm converts long-term donor pledges into immediately available resources for GAVI by issuing bonds in capital markets. Leveraging funding through IFFIm has made it possible to introduce new and underused vaccines in developing countries, protecting against diseases that cause large numbers of deaths.

However, resources mobilized through innovative financing mechanisms remain modest compared to traditional donor sources (Atun *et al.* 2012). Thus the potential of innovative financing mechanisms has not been fully harnessed to date. One of the instruments currently being discussed, which could potentially raise substantial amounts of funding, is the financial transaction tax (FTT), a levy on monetary transactions. Although the introduction of an FTT could help to finance global health, including in the post-MDG world, key donor countries oppose the introduction of any tax-based mechanisms to finance global health or development more broadly. In 2011, for example, a proposal for an FTT aimed at raising funds for development, promoted by the philanthropist Bill Gates, failed to win the approval of the G20 economies (Wroughton 2011).

The End of the Halcyon Days of Global Health Financing

Most recent evidence indicates that the global financial crisis has affected aid volumes for health. After a decade of growth, the Institute for Health Metrics and Evaluation (IHME) found that DAH peaked in 2010 at $28.2 billion but has flat-lined since then. According to preliminary estimates, DAH amounted to $27.4 billion and $28.0 billion in 2011 and 2012, respectively (IHME 2012).

This plateauing raises a number of key concerns for priority setting and international health targets after 2015. As highlighted above, major financing gaps already existed before the impact of the financial crisis played out. More funding is still required to finance the unfinished MDGs. In addition, important diseases and cross-cutting issues, such as the need to finance health systems, were left out of the MDG framework. While there are now calls to include these diseases and issues more prominently in the post-2015 framework, an important question is how best to design the post-2015 agenda given that funding constraints may become more severe.

Uneven Distribution of Funding across the Health MDGs

The resource distribution across the health MDGs has been uneven up to this point. The largest growth in funding relates to MDG 6, and especially to HIV/AIDS, with funding increases for MDGs 4 and 5 being much more modest. MDG 6 received lots of attention from bilateral donors, in addition to newly dedicated funding channels. Disbursements for HIV/AIDS, tuberculosis, and malaria grew from 5.1% to 34.5% of all DAH between 1990 and 2010 (from $0.3 to $9.7 billion). Funding for HIV/AIDS alone rose from 3.4% to 24.0% of total health aid in this period (from $0.2 to $6.8 billion). Funding to maternal, newborn, and child health (MNCH) increased from $1.2 billion in 1990 to $5.2 billion in 2010. However, the share of MNCH funding out of total DAH fell from 21.2% in 1990 to 18.3% in 2010 (IHME 2012).

Countdown to 2015 (Countdown), an initiative that tracks key global health data related to MNCH, tracks ODA data for MNCH.[2] Countdown estimates that disbursements from 31 key donors for MNCH in developing countries increased from $2.6 billion in 2003 to a record high of $6.51 billion in 2009, but decreased for the first time since 2003 to $6.48 billion in 2010. Of the $6.48 billion spent in 2010, more than two thirds (68.6%) were disbursed to child health, while less than one third (31.4%) was spent on maternal and newborn health. The share of global health funding channeled to maternal health fell from 12.2% in 2003 to 11.4% in 2010, while the share of funding for child health increased from 22.9% to 24.9% (Hsu *et al.* 2012). These data indicate that improving the health of women and children has not been prioritized relative to other areas, most notably MDG 6. Given that there has been the least amount of progress on MDG 5, the fact that maternal health is largely underfunded is a major problem.

Family planning and reproductive health programs vital to the health of women fell off the radar of donors. MDG 5B ("universal access to reproductive health") was only adopted in 2007, as reproductive health goals are politically disputed. The financing trend for reproductive health supports the argument that the MDGs have an impact on the financing levels for specific issues. An analysis of OECD-DAC data shows that commitments to reproductive health grew much more slowly in the 1995–2009 period than total health ODA (Figure 19.1). As a result, the share of health ODA targeting reproductive health fell from 30% to 10.1% in all developing countries over this period. HIV/AIDS

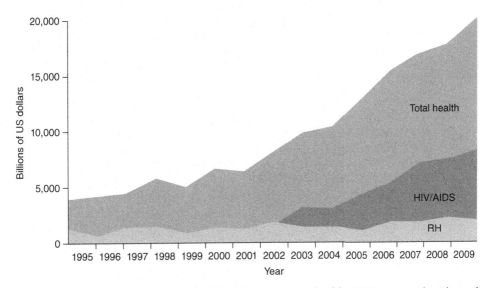

Figure 19.1 Commitments to HIV/AIDS and reproductive health (RH) compared with total health official development aid 1995–2009. Source: data from OECD-DAC Creditor Reporting System.

commitments increased by 20-fold in all developing countries. Aid for family planning in particular fell steadily between 2000 and 2009. According to the OECD-DAC's Creditor Reporting System, as a proportion of total health ODA to all developing countries, funding for family planning fell from 8.3% in 2000 to 2.5% in 2009.

After MDG 5B was adopted in 2005, there was a small increase in annual funding for reproductive health. However, with the target date of the MDGs now in sight, a number of new financing initiatives have been launched in recent years to mobilize funding for reproductive health, as well as for maternal and child health goals.

In September 2010, the UN Secretary-General Ban Ki-moon launched the Global Strategy for Women's and Children's Health (the Global Strategy), which aims to save 16 million lives in the world's 49 lowest income countries by 2015 (UN 2010). The Partnership for Maternal, Newborn, and Child Health (PMNCH), an international alliance of RMNCH (reproductive, maternal, newborn, and child health) organizations, estimates that the Global Strategy has delivered U$18.2–20.6 billion of additional funding commitments to women's and children's health (PMNCH 2012). This figure includes funding previously pledged at the G8 summit in Muskoka, Canada. However, it remains to be seen to what extent donor countries will disburse their Global Strategy commitments in the face of the global financial crisis. A large portion of the additional funds ($5.7–8.1 billion) was also pledged by low-income countries (LICs), which committed to increase their domestic health spending. However, in a survey conducted by the PMNCH (2012), LICs also reported that they require increased financial support from donors to be able to meet their commitments.

Family planning has also been placed back on the development agenda. In July 2012, 17 public and private donors committed $2.6 billion for family planning by 2020 at the London Summit for Family Planning. This commitment did, however, include pledges previously made by donors, including to the Global Strategy.[3]

Finally, in March 2012, the UN launched a Commission on Life-Saving Commodities for Women and Children aimed at improving access to key MNCH commodities (UN 2012b). A new RMNCH Trust Fund is now being established to provide resources for the implementation of the Commission's recommendations. However, it is currently unclear how much new funding will be made available to this trust fund.

Areas Not Covered by the MDGs Receive the Least Financial Attention

The health MDGs also leave important gaps, and health areas not targeted by the MDGs have received less attention. There are no MDG targets for non-communicable diseases (NCDs), including mental health and cancers, or for neglected tropical diseases, although the burden of these diseases in the developing world is large. NCDs, for example, are responsible for most deaths in every region of the world apart from sub-Saharan Africa, but received only $185 million in donor support (1% of total health aid) in 2010 (IHME 2012). The global community has made faster progress in combating communicable causes of deaths than in combating deaths and disability from non-communicable causes.

The MDGs also make no mention of health systems strengthening (HSS), although HSS is essential to improving coverage with key interventions. In particular, the provision of key MNCH interventions depends on functioning health systems, and significant investments are needed to create and maintain health infrastructure and to expand the skilled health workforce. HSS costs related to the health of women and children alone were estimated at an additional $62.4 billion in the 49 poorest countries from 2011 to 2015 (UN 2010).

Targeting and Predictability of Funding Flows

Soon after the MDGs were adopted, it became clear that donors would need to improve the quality of their financing and make it more effective in achieving the MDGs, such as by better geographic targeting and through more predictable funding flows (Radelet 2004).

One recent analysis argues that the MDGs helped in directing ODA to those countries in greatest need (Hailu and Tsukada 2012). This analysis found that, since 2000, ODA was disproportionately allocated to countries that need to make the most progress on the MDGs. Multilateral aid was more "MDG sensitive" than bilateral aid, that is, it was more likely to be targeted towards countries furthest from reaching the MDGs. Hailu and Tsukada's study therefore supports the argument that multilateral aid is better targeted than bilateral aid to the neediest countries.

However, a recent analysis by McCoy and Kinyua (2012) of Global Fund disbursements shows that the Fund could improve its targeting of resources so that it better matches the pattern of global need. A World Bank analysis found that only a third of ODA for reproductive health has targeted countries with the highest maternal mortality ratio and fertility rates (World Bank 2010).

The predictability of ODA can allow for more mid- and long-term planning and goal setting, integrating aid into country budget plans, and creating a stronger relationship between donors and recipients. Funding from donors remains volatile. While there is volatility in global health funding as a whole, volatility appears to be more pronounced in areas receiving comparatively less funding. Countdown to 2015 found that over the 2003–2010 period, several countries experienced sharp fluctuations in aid inflows to MNCH (Hsu *et al.* 2012). The IHME's analysis found even higher volatility in year-to-year funding levels for MNCH, unlike the other focus areas in the IHME 2012 study. The volatility of aid and its short timeframes make it difficult to fund recurrent costs, particularly funding of primary healthcare facilities that are key to achieving maternal and child health goals. And in their 2007 study, Lane and Glassman found that some low- and middle-income countries struggle to cover the volatility in *their own* domestic health funding, let alone in the donor funds that they receive.

Key Players in the Global Health Financing Architecture: the Emergence of New Financing Institutions

Following the adoption of the MDGs, the emergence of large single-issue global health initiatives has changed the way in which international donors provide funding for health. Estimates suggest that over 100 global health initiatives have emerged in the global health sector since the turn of the millennium (WHO/Maximizing Positive Synergies Collaborative Group 2009). Many of these initiatives, including the President's Emergency Plan for AIDS Relief (PEPFAR), the Global Fund, and UNITAID, were explicitly founded to accelerate progress towards the health MDGs. Others, like GAVI, were launched just before the MDGs were adopted, but refer to the MDGs as a key framework of their missions.

Some of these new initiatives introduced new forms of governance to global health. As global health partnerships, GAVI and the Global Fund do not just represent governments, but also civil society, the private sector, and affected communities. The share of DAH channeled through these two major global health partnerships increased from 0.03% ($2.8 million) in 2000 to a projected 17.2% ($4.8 billion) in 2012. At the same time, the share of funding channeled through the World Bank, a traditional multilateral channel for global health, decreased from 18.8% in 1997 to 7.8% in 2012. The share of funding channeled through UNICEF and the UN Population Fund (UNFPA) decreased from 10.2% in 1990 to an estimated 7.7% in 2012. Donor support to the World Health Organization (WHO) as a technical agency rather than a funding channel has also significantly decreased in recent years from 19.2% in 1990 to an estimated 7.3% in 2012 (IHME 2012).

The single-issue initiatives have been successful in both mobilizing and channeling funding to countries. One key innovation was the introduction of performance-based funding (PBF). The Global Fund has implemented PBF at a scale that is unprecedented in global health, and GAVI has also worked with PBF. The single-issue initiatives have also contributed to progress towards the MDGs. GAVI has effectively scaled up vaccination coverage levels, and the Global Fund and PEPFAR have dramatically increased coverage of key HIV/AIDS, TB, and malaria services (Atun *et al.* 2012).

Fragmentation of the Global Health Landscape

While the health MDGs have spurred an increase in global health financing, they also contributed to the promotion of a vertical, disease-specific approach to health issues and to the resulting fragmentation of financing channels. The health MDGs encouraged the creation of financing silos and the verticalization of initiatives without sufficient integration with broader health systems issues, which makes it more difficult to leverage synergies between the health MDGs.

Through the Global Fund and PEPFAR, there is a dedicated and highly focused approach to funding MDG 6. These two organizations provided over 70% of the total international HIV/AIDS funding in 2011 (Kaiser Family Foundation 2012a). The Global Fund is also the largest source of funding for malaria control, accounting for an estimated 40% of total international disbursements to malaria in 2012 (WHO 2012a), and is responsible for 88% of all expected international funding for TB in 2013 (WHO 2012b). This focused approach to channeling funds towards MDG 6 is lacking for MDG 5 and, to some extent for MDG 4. Indeed the slower progress towards MDGs 4 and 5 can be explained in part by the lack of a focused, coordinated approach to mobilizing and channeling resources for reproductive, maternal, and child health, and the associated HSS (Schrade *et al.* 2011).

For MDG 4, there are a number of key financing mechanisms. One important element of MDG 4 – vaccination – is funded through GAVI. The Global Fund has positive "spillover effects" on MDG 4 through funding key child health interventions (e.g., insecticide-treated bed nets to protect against childhood malaria). Child health is, furthermore, a priority for several large bilateral donors (e.g., Canada, the United Kingdom). Some UN organizations, particularly UNICEF, also finance child health interventions (e.g., UNICEF is the largest procurer of childhood diarrhea treatments).

MDG 5 attracts the least attention from global health funders. There is no dedicated large-scale multilateral funding channel for MDG 5, and no donor has emerged to take decisive leadership in the financing of MDG 5. There are a range of funding channels for maternal and reproductive health within the UN system (e.g., UNFPA), but all of them are too small-scale to fill the identified gaps. Interventions surrounding childbirth in particular remain significantly underfinanced. Funding for maternal health has been piecemeal, with many different donors financing services and associated HSS through projects that have often been small-scale and duplicative. In their study of health aid flows, Piva and

Dodd (2009) found that over half of all health projects exceeding $10 million targeted HIV/AIDS, TB, and malaria over the 2002–2006 period, while only 9% of these projects focused on reproductive health and family planning. Many small activities have high transaction costs for countries, and are more likely to suffer from lack of coordination between countries and donors. Large activities are more likely to attract political attention at the country level. It is only in the last few years that the donor community has started to pay attention to MDG 5, especially to reproductive health.

Improvements in maternal and neonatal health also largely depend on HSS, but donors are reluctant to fund HSS as progress is only visible in the long run and is difficult to monitor. While the Global Fund has significantly invested in health and community systems to enable better access to health services, its HSS investments have been largely specific to the three Global Fund target diseases. GAVI's HSS funds have also mainly been used for downstream support to overcome service delivery constraints rather than for large capital investments in infrastructure, the training of new skilled health personnel, or for larger health sector reform.

The World Bank, one of the world's largest multilateral financers of global health, has not stepped up to fill this void in HSS support. Instead, the World Bank has placed a strong focus on communicable diseases, particularly HIV/AIDS, which accounted for 44% of all of the Bank's health, nutrition, and population portfolio in the 2002–2006 period (IEG 2010). World Bank support for HSS has also largely been directed towards middle-income countries, rather than LICs. In 2010, the World Bank released its Reproductive Health Action Plan 2010–2015 (World Bank 2010), which might contribute to a greater focus on MDGs 4 and 5.

Unintended Side Effects Resulting from Fragmentation

Single-issue, vertical initiatives have also been criticized for causing *unintended negative effects* and for causing fragmentation, duplication, and poor coordination of health assistance (Garrett 2007; Biesma *et al.* 2009). A review of the evidence on the effects of vertical HIV initiatives on country health systems found evidence of "distortion of recipient countries' national policies, notably through distracting governments from coordinated efforts to strengthen health systems and re-verticalization of planning, management and monitoring and evaluation systems" (Biesma *et al.* 2009). The sheer number of international actors providing support to a developing country may overwhelm the scarce capacity of its already weak health system. Given these concerns, single-issues initiatives have been urged to reduce their transaction costs, harmonize their procedures with other donors, and align their projects with country systems (Garrett 2007; Biesma *et al.* 2009).

The Need for Domestic Financing

At the start of the second decade in the new millennium, donor funding for health stagnated (IHME 2012). Therefore, the importance of domestic spending on health has never been more important: if donor funding continues to stagnate or declines, the gains that have been made by the MDGs may be nullified without the sustainable support of domestic funds.

The WHO tracks National Health Accounts (NHAs), which compile country-reported spending on health from both domestic and donor funds. However, systematically verifying that these funds were actually spent is nearly impossible and NHAs are often plagued by incomplete reporting. IHME subtracted out its estimates of DAH from NHAs and found that domestic funds for health have continued to rise in LICs since the signing of the MGDs (IHME 2012).

In 2001, 55 African Union Member States signed the Abuja commitment, agreeing to dedicate at least 15% of their domestic budgets to health. Many countries are still a long way from reaching this commitment. By 2011, only two of the 55 African Union Member States, Rwanda and South Africa, were spending at least 15% of their domestic budgets on health (WHO 2011). Nevertheless, domestic spending on health by developing countries increased by 115% between the signing of the MDGs and 2010. During this same time period, DAH increased by 160%.

Lu and colleagues (2010) recently found that with the rapid increase in DAH given to LIC governments, especially in sub-Saharan Africa, some domestic funding for health has been shifted away to other sectors (a phenomenon known as aid displacement). The researchers found that, on average, for every dollar of DAH going to an LIC government, the ministry of finance reduces the amount of government expenditures allocated to the ministry of health (and other agencies that engage in health spending) by about $0.43–1.14. It is arguable that this shift in funding allocation is simply a rational reaction by an LIC government. On receiving an influx of external funds for health, domestic governments find themselves free to invest in other sectors of their economy, such as education and infrastructure.

Critics of international aid responded to the study results by arguing that these shifted funds are often pocketed or spent on building up the military. For example, in an interview with the Associated Press, Philip Stevens, of the International Policy Network, a London-based pro-market think tank that is skeptical about the value of health aid, said: "When an aid official thinks he is helping a low-income African patient avoid charges at a health clinic, in reality, he is paying for a shopping trip to Paris for a government minister and his wife" (Cheng 2010). However, there has been no systematic tracking of these shifted funds and it is possible that they are being diverted to sectors that could benefit health, such as education, water, or sanitation (Ooms et al. 2010). Lu and colleagues themselves acknowledged that these funds could be going to "education, infrastructure development, poverty alleviation, or various other underfinanced programmes that improve health."

Lu and colleagues also found that DAH given to non-governmental sectors working in LICs actually *drives up* health spending by these LIC governments. Based on this finding, the researchers argued that the risks and benefits of expanding DAH to non-governmental sectors should be carefully assessed. Some donors, such as the US government, are channeling an increasing share of DAH through non-governmental organizations (NGOs) (Lu et al. 2010). Rerouting DAH from governments does carry risks – for example, NGOs may perform worse than the government at reaching the rural poor and they may be less efficient at delivering health services.

The IHME's statistically significant finding – that domestic health spending *on average* decreases by about $0.43–1.14 for every dollar of additional DAH given to the government – is at the aggregate level, but not all governments that receive donor funding for health shift domestic funds away from the health sector. Data that IHME publishes on its website show that Malawi actually invested 166% more domestic funding for health between 2000 and 2006, during which time there was a 115% increase in DAH to the government. It is likely that when donors align their priorities with those of the recipient country, development assistance is more effective, and donors have pledged to try and improve such alignment (OECD 2005).

In 2010, domestic funding for health by developing countries totaled $521 billion, compared to the $28.2 billion spent by donors for international aid (IHME 2012). Even with this nearly 20-fold difference in spending, some developing countries, in particular in sub-Saharan Africa, depend solely on DAH for their entire health spending budgets. For example, 97% of life-saving HIV treatment in Tanzania is currently funded by DAH (Kaiser Family Foundation 2012b).

In summary, while domestic financing for health must increase in developing countries to meet health needs, several obstacles remain. Most African Union Member States are still failing to reach the Abuja commitment. DAH may decrease domestic resources for health. Many developing countries are still dependent on DAH for essential health treatments. But moving forward toward the MDGs and beyond, both donor and domestic funds must be leveraged to their full potential to begin to reach all those in need.

Improving the Quality and Efficiency of Global Health Financing

In this world of tightening pocketbooks and prioritizing of domestic spending, maximizing the quality and efficiency of international aid must take precedence. Of course measuring the quality and efficiency of aid is fraught with pitfalls. Ideally, all donors would weight their comparative advantages in certain health fields and the needs of the recipient countries to prioritize their giving, while allowing for complete transparency and evaluation of programs to learn and improve from. However, since these steps have not always been taken when allocating funding in the past or present, imperfect measures of quality and efficiency must be used in the interim.

The quality of aid can be enhanced by improving the predictability and transparency of funding, and also by lessoning the burden on recipient countries that must juggle their own priorities and those of international health donors. The Center for Global Development (CGD) has developed a tool, called the "Quality of Official Development Aid for Health" (Health QuODA), which assesses aid quality using 31 indicators and then ranks donors by the quality of their aid (Birdsall *et al.* 2011). The indicators are grouped into four dimensions that reflect widespread consensus on what constitutes high-quality aid: maximizing efficiency, fostering institutions, reducing burden, and transparency and learning. In the CGD's latest installment of Health QuODA, they found that the top-ranking donors were the Netherlands, the International Development Bank (part of the World Bank), the Global Fund, and the United Kingdom.

Donor agencies and the global health community are realizing the importance of maximizing the efficiency of global funding, and several agencies, foundations, and research groups are examining ways to improve value for money (V4M or VfM) in global health. Such analyses build on the work of the Disease Control Priorities in Developing Countries Project (DCPP), which relates costs to gains for different global health interventions and is more forward-looking than QuODA. The UK's Department for International Development (DFID) has prioritized, from 2012 to 2015, building institutions in partner countries, focusing its programs on results, and using transparency to drive development. The BMGF has funded work on measuring the efficiency and effectiveness (known as "E^2") of health interventions around the world. The CGD heads a V4M Working Group, which works to lay out recommendations for international donors to maximize technical, productive, and allocative efficiencies, with an initial focus on the Global Fund. Some key institutions have taken important steps to modify their funding mechanisms to better align their processes with those of the recipient countries. For example, in its new funding model, the Global Fund will accept national health plans – rather than just narrowly focused HIV, TB, or malaria projects – as funding proposals (Global Fund 2012).

Moving forward, this growing work on maximizing the efficiency and quality of global health financing will play an essential role, with the aim of stretching every last dollar to its full potential in the hope of saving as many lives as possible.

Increased Accountability

The MDGs have contributed to better accountability for global health financing. A key example is the Commission on Information and Accountability for Women's and Children's Health (COIA), which was initiated by the UN Secretary-General to strengthen accountability of funding and progress towards MDGs 4 and 5. The COIA was created in 2010 to make recommendations on global reporting, oversight, and accountability on women's and children's health. *Ten recommendations* developed by the COIA form the basis for monitoring the accountability of all stakeholders for women's and children's health. The recommendations focus on better information for better results, on better tracking of resources, and on better oversight of results and resources, nationally and globally.

In 2011, an independent Expert Review Group was formed to track progress towards the Global Strategy. The group reports annually to the UN Secretary-General on the results and resources related to the Global Strategy and on progress in implementing the Commission's recommendations. It found that five of these recommendations were fulfilled in 2012 (iERG 2012).

The low priority given to maternal and child health until very recently was reflected in the lack of a mechanism to track RMNCH flows. However, donors have now agreed upon an improved system for tracking RMNCH donor funding. To improve the tracking of donor flows for RMNCH, the COIA recommended that, by 2012, donors agreed on how to improve the Creditor Reporting System of the OECD-DAC, which collects data on international aid, to capture RMNCH expenditures in a timely manner. Following these recommendations, in 2013, donors committed to estimating the share of funding that benefits RMNCH. While this system can help to give a more accurate picture of RMNCH financing in future years, compared with the tracking of other health areas, the tracking of RMNCH funding flows remains less precise.

Looking Forward: Lessons Learned and Recommendations

Our analysis of financing for, and progress towards, the health MDGs has shown that important gaps remain, particularly in the fight to reduce maternal and newborn deaths. Unattained goals should be incorporated into the post-2015 agenda. However, a key question is how to finance this post-2015 health agenda. The continued global economic crisis means that increased external financing from traditional donors is unlikely in the near term. Nonetheless, additional funding from traditional donors, new donors (such as Brazil, China, and India), domestic sources, and innovative financing mechanisms need to be mobilized to sustain the gains made in global health and to address further issues that have moved to the top of the global health agenda.

In addition, the efficiency of global health financing must be further improved. Key financers, such as the Global Fund, have taken important steps to "increase the bang for the buck." However, more needs to be done to increase the efficiency and quality of global health spending, through transparent program evaluations, the harmonization of funding across donors, and the alignment of donor and country processes and priorities.

Furthermore, the slow progress on maternal and newborn health needs to be addressed. Several initiatives have recently been launched aimed at addressing gaps and inefficiencies in the architecture to raise and channel funding for reproductive, maternal, and newborn and child health. However, there is still no focused, coordinated approach to mobilizing and channeling resources for the health of women and children, and associated health systems strengthening, and this lack needs to be considered and addressed by policy-makers.

Notes

1. The Resolution adopted by the UN General Assembly at the June 2012 Rio Conference, entitled "The future we want," can be found here: http://www.un.org/ga/search/view_doc.asp?symbol=A/RES/66/288&Lang=E (last accessed December 2013).
2. ODA differs from DAH. ODA only includes public funding that fulfills certain criteria and is provided by OECD-DAC members. DAH also includes funding coming from other donors, including private sources and non-concessional funding from the International Bank for Reconstruction and Development.
3. London Summit for Family Planning: New Financial Commitments by Donors and Private Sector at the London Summit on Family Planning. Available at: http://www.familyplanning2020.org/ (last accessed December 2013).

Key Reading

iERG (Independent Expert Review Group). 2012. *Every Woman, Every Child: From Commitments to Action. The First Report of the Independent Expert Review Group (iERG) on Information and Accountability for Women's and Children's Health.* http://www.who.int/woman_child_accountability/ierg/reports/2012/IERG_report_low_resolution.pdf (last accessed December 2013).

IHME (Institute for Health Metrics and Evaluation). 2012. *Financing Global Health 2012: The End of the Golden Age?* Seattle, WA: IHME.

Jamison DT, Breman JG, Measham AR *et al.* (eds). 2006. *Disease Control Priorities in Developing Countries*, 2nd edn. Washington, DC: World Bank.

Schrade C, Schäferhoff M, Yamey G, Richter E. 2011. *Strengthening the Global Financing Architecture for Reproductive, Maternal, Newborn, and Child Health: Options for Action.* Report commissioned by the Partnership for Maternal, Newborn and Child Health. http://www.who.int/pmnch/knowledge/publications/20111110_rmnch_aid_architecture/en/index.html (last accessed December 2013).

WHO (World Health Organization)/Maximizing Positive Synergies Collaborative Group. 2009. An assessment of interactions between global health initiatives and country health systems. *Lancet* 373, 2137–69.

References

Atun R, Knaul FM, Akachi Y, Frenk J. 2012. Innovative financing for health: what is truly innovative? *Lancet* 2380, 2044–9.

Biesma R, Brugha R, Harmer A, Walsh A, Spicer N, Walt G. 2009. The effects of global HIV/AIDS initiatives on country health systems: a review of the evidence. *Health Policy Planning* 24, 4.

Birdsall N, Kharas H, Perakis R. 2011. *Measuring the Quality of Aid: QuODA*, 2nd edn. Washington, DC: Center for Global Development. http://www.cgdev.org/files/1425642_file_Birdsall_Kharas_Perakis_Busan_QuODA_FINAL.pdf (last accessed December 2013).

Black RE, Bhan MK, Chopra M, Rudan I, Victora CG. 2009. Accelerating the health impact of the Gates Foundation. *Lancet* 373, 1584–5.

Cheng M. 2010. Study: Health aid made some countries cut aid budgets. *Seattle Times* April 9. http://seattletimes.com/html/health/2011563141_apeumedhealthaid.html (last accessed December 2013)

Countdown (Countdown to 2015). 2012. *Building a Future for Women and Children: The 2012 Report.* http://www.countdown2015mnch.org/reports-and-articles/2012-report (last accessed December 2013).

Garrett L. 2007. The challenge of global health. *Foreign Affairs* 86, 1.

Hailu D, Tsukada R. 2012. *Is the Distribution of Foreign Aid MDG-Sensitive?* DESA Working Paper. New York, NY: United Nations.

Hsu J, Pitt C, Greco G, Berman P, Mills A. 2012. Countdown to 2015: changes in official development assistance to maternal, newborn and child health in 2009–10 and assessment of progress since 2003. *Lancet* 380: 1157–68.

IEG (Independent Evaluation Group). 2010. *Evaluation of World Bank Group Support to Health, Nutrition and Population (HNP).* Washington, DC: World Bank.

IEG (Independent Expert Review Group). 2012. *Every Woman, Every Child: From Commitments to Action. The First Report of the Independent Expert Review Group (iERG) on Information and Accountability for Women's and Children's Health.* http://www.who.int/woman_child_accountability/ierg/reports/2012/IERG_report_low_resolution.pdf (last accessed December 2013).

IHME (Institute for Health Metrics and Evaluation). 2012. *Financing Global Health 2012: The End of the Golden Age?* Seattle, WA: IHME.

Kaiser Family Foundation. 2012a. *Financing the Response to AIDS in Low- and Middle-Income Countries: International Assistance from Donor Governments in 2011.* http://www.kff.org/hivaids/upload/7347-08.pdf (last accessed December 2013).

Kaiser Family Foundation. 2012b. *Show Me the Money: Political Commitment, Resources and Pricing.* http://globalhealth.kff.org/~/media/Files/AIDS%202012/072612_THBS01_showme.pdf (last accessed December 2013).

Lane C, Glassman A. 2007. Bigger and better? Scaling up and innovation in health aid. *Health Affairs* 26, 4.

Lozano R, Wang H, Foreman KJ *et al.* 2011. Progress towards Millennium Development Goals 4 and 5 on maternal and child mortality: an updated systematic analysis. *Lancet* 378, 1139–65.

Lu C, Schneider MT, Gubbins P, Leach-Kemon K, Jamison D, Murray CJL. 2010. Public financing of health in developing countries: a cross-national systematic analysis. *Lancet* 375, 1375–87.

McCoy D, Kembhavi G, Patel J, Luintel A. 2009. The Bill and Melinda Gates Foundation's grant-making programme for global health. *Lancet* 373, 1645–53.

McCoy D, Kinyua K. 2012. Allocating scarce resources strategically – an evaluation and discussion of the global fund's pattern of disbursements. *PLOS One* 7(5), e34749. doi 10.1371/journal.pone.0034749.

Moss T. 2010. What next for the Millennium Development Goals? *Global Policy* 1, 2.

OECD (Organisation for Economic Co-operation and Development). 2005. *The Paris Declaration on Aid Effectiveness and the Accra Agenda for Action.* http://www.oecd.org/development/aideffectiveness/34428351.pdf (last accessed December 2013).

Ooms G, Decoster K, Miti K *et al.* 2010. Crowding out: are relations between international health aid and government health funding too complex to be captured in averages only? *Lancet* 375, 1403–5.

PMNCH (Partnership for Maternal, Newborn, and Child Health). 2012. *The PMNCH 2012 Report – Analysing Progress on Commitments to the Global Strategy for Women's and Children's Health.* Geneva: PMNCH.

Piva P, Dodd R. 2009. Where did all the aid go? An in-depth analysis of increased health aid flows over the past 10 years. *Bulletin of the World Health Organization* 87, 930–9.

Radelet S. 2004. *Aid Effectiveness and the Millennium Development Goals*. Center for Global Development (CGD) Working Paper No. 39. Washington, DC: CGD.

Schrade C, Schäferhoff M, Gavin Yamey, and Emil Richter. 2011. *Strengthening the Global Financing Architecture for Reproductive, Maternal, Newborn, and Child Health: Options for Action*. Report commissioned by the Partnership for Maternal, Newborn and Child Health. http://www.who.int/pmnch/knowledge/publications/20111110_rmnch_aid_architecture/en/index.html (last accessed December 2013).

Schweitzer J, Makinen M, Wilson L, Heymann M. 2012. *Post-2015 Health Millenium Development Goals*. Overseas Development Institute Working Paper. http://www.odi.org.uk/publications/6444-millennium-development-goals-mdgs-health-post2015 (last accessed December 2013).

Taskforce on International Innovative Financing for Health Systems. 2009. *More Money for Health, and More Health for the Money: Final Report*. Geneva: International Health Partnership.

UN (United Nations). 2010. *Global Strategy for Women's and Children's Health. Packages of Interventions for Family Planning, Safe Abortion Care, Maternal, Newborn, and Child Health*. Geneva: WHO. http://www.who.int/pmnch/topics/maternal/201009_globalstrategy_wch/en/index.html (last accessed December 2013).

UN (United Nations). 2012a. *Millennium Development Goals Report 2012*. New York: UN.

UN (United Nations). 2012b. *UN Commission on Life-Saving Commodities for Women's and Children's Health. Commissioner's Report*. http://www.unfpa.org/webdav/site/global/shared/images/publications/2012/Final%20UN%20Commission%20Report_14sept2012.pdf (last accessed December 2013).

UN (United Nations) IGME (Inter-agency Group for Child Mortality Estimation). 2011. *Levels and Trends in Child Mortality. Report 2011*. http://www.childinfo.org/files/Child_Mortality_Report_2011.pdf (last accessed December 2013).

UNAIDS. 2012. *Global Report: UNAIDS Report on the Global AIDS Epidemic 2012*. Geneva: UNAIDS. http://www.unaids.org/en/media/unaids/contentassets/documents/epidemiology/2012/gr2012/20121120_UNAIDS_Global_Report_2012_with_annexes_en.pdf (last accessed December 2013).

Walz J, Ramachandran V. 2011. *Brave New World: A Literature Review of Emerging Donors and the Changing Nature of Foreign Assistance*. Center for Global Development (CGD) Working Paper No. 273. Washington, DC: CGD.

World Bank. 2010. *Better Health for Women and Families: The World Bank's Reproductive Health Action Plan 2010–2015*. Washington, DC: World Bank. http://siteresources.worldbank.org/INTPRH/Resources/376374-1261312056980/RHAP_Pub_8-23-10web.pdf (last accessed December 2013).

WHO (World Health Organization). 2011. The Abuja Declaration: Ten Years On. http://www.who.int/healthsystems/publications/Abuja10.pdf (last accessed December 2013).

WHO (World Health Organization). 2012a. *World Malaria Report 2012*. Geneva: WHO.

WHO (World Health Organization). 2012b. *Global Tuberculosis Report 2012*. Geneva: WHO.

WHO (World Health Organization)/Maximizing Positive Synergies Collaborative Group. 2009. An assessment of interactions between global health initiatives and country health systems. *Lancet* 373, 2137–69.

WHO (World Health Organization), UNICEF, UNFPA, World Bank. (2012). *Trends in Maternal Mortality, 1990 to 2010*. http://www.unfpa.org/webdav/site/global/shared/documents/publications/2012/Trends_in_maternal_mortality_A4-1.pdf (last accessed December 2013).

Wroughton L. 2011. *G20 fails to endorse financial transaction tax*. http://www.reuters.com/article/2011/11/04/g20-tax-idUSN1E7A302520111104 (last accessed December 2013).

Chapter 20

Can International Aid Improve Health?

Christopher J. Coyne and Claudia R. Williamson

Abstract

Can international aid improve global health? Many current health indicators suggest that millions of the poor suffer from a lack of basic healthcare. International aid to the health sector has increased fourfold over the last 40 years. However, macro-level cross-country studies argue that health aid is ineffective at improving mortality rates, life expectancy, and a number of other health indicators. Recent micro-level studies have found some evidence of successful health aid interventions. This chapter presents an overview of the current state of health in poor countries and summarizes the findings and conclusions from pre-existing work on health aid. We also explain, using the economic way of thinking, why health aid has not achieved results on a large scale. This relies on analyzing the role of information and incentives in both the donor and recipient countries.

The Handbook of Global Health Policy, First Edition. Edited by Garrett W. Brown, Gavin Yamey, and Sarah Wamala.
© 2014 John Wiley & Sons, Ltd. Published 2014 by John Wiley & Sons, Ltd.

Key Points

- Health aid is increasing over time, while worldwide health trends are also improving.
- Macro-level evidence suggests that aid is ineffective at improving health, but micro-level analysis indicates some success stories.
- To explain this apparent paradox and why health interventions have not achieved widescale success, we utilize the economic way of thinking.
- Perverse incentives and a lack of information on the part of both donors and recipients helps to explain why health aid cannot improve health in a systematic manner.
- The ultimate policy (or group of policies) to improve health relies on achieving sustained economic growth, which increases the availability of quality healthcare for larger numbers of people.

Key Policy Implications

- With any foreign intervention, we must consider the local, pre-existing arrangements and institutions.
- Even if we find a solution that works at a local level, this does not mean that this policy is scalable and will work at the national level or in other countries or contexts.
- Ultimately, policies that support sustainable economic growth is the only way to achieve long-term, systematic improvements in healthcare and global poverty.

Introduction

Can international aid improve global health?[1] Attempting to answer this question is of critical importance as current heath indicators suggest that millions are still without basic care. For example, recent annual data suggest the following:

- About 7.6 million children died in 2010, with 1.7 million dying from vaccine-preventable diseases.
- Approximately 1000 women suffer from pregnancy-related deaths on a daily basis.
- One out of every five children is estimated to be underweight.
- There are approximately 2.6 million new HIV infections yearly, and 8.8 million new tuberculosis cases.[2]

The international aid community has increasingly given more attention to social matters such as health and education since the early 1990s. For example, as shown in Figure 20.1a, aid targeted to the social sector (which includes spending on health) continues to receive a larger share of total allocation compared with the other sectors.[3] Among the different social sectors, as shown in Figure 20.1b, health aid has received a large share of social aid over the past 20 years. Health aid includes assistance to hospitals and clinics, disease and epidemic control, maternal and child care, dental services, services for tuberculosis, vaccination programs, nursing, provision of drugs, public health administration, medical insurance programs, and reproductive health and family planning (OECD-DAC 2012).

These trends make sense given that most of the Millennium Development Goals (MDGs) – the blueprint for donors to meet the needs of the poor – target social outcomes. Specifically, three of the eight MDGs focus on global health outcomes (reducing child mortality, increasing maternal health, and combating HIV/AIDS, malaria and other diseases) with nine of the 21 targets aimed at health-related matters. The international donors support these stated goals as aid specific to the health sector continues to rise over time, in absolute terms and as a share of total aid (Figure 20.2). In 2010 alone, health aid accounted for 6% of total aid and amounted to approximately US$10 billion – four times the amount provided in 1994 (OECD-DAC 2012). From 1971 to 2010, aid has supported over 67,000 different health-related interventions at the project level, with approximately 50,000 of those projects starting since 2000 (Findley et al. 2009).

Before examining the pros and cons of international aid for global health, it will be useful to provide a quick overview of the current status of the foreign aid debate as some of the main tenants in this debate still hold for health aid.

Theory and empirical evidence debate the effectiveness of foreign aid to achieve economic development. Two main camps have emerged: the "public interest" view versus the "public choice" view (Williamson 2008).[4] The public interest view claims that foreign aid can be useful because it can break countries out of a so-called "poverty trap." The most notable economist in the public interest camp is Jeffrey Sachs. Sachs' story (see, for example, The End of Poverty, 2005) is that poor countries are often tropical, landlocked, malaria infested, and barren, making investment targeted toward economic development extremely difficult. Since poor countries cannot afford these investments, they are poor simply because, well, they are poor, resulting in a vicious circle of poverty. Sachs proposes a solution to this perplexing dilemma by arguing that foreign aid can jump-start a country onto a new path – a virtuous circle where countries receive the necessary initial investment in critical areas to make them productive by allowing them to break out of

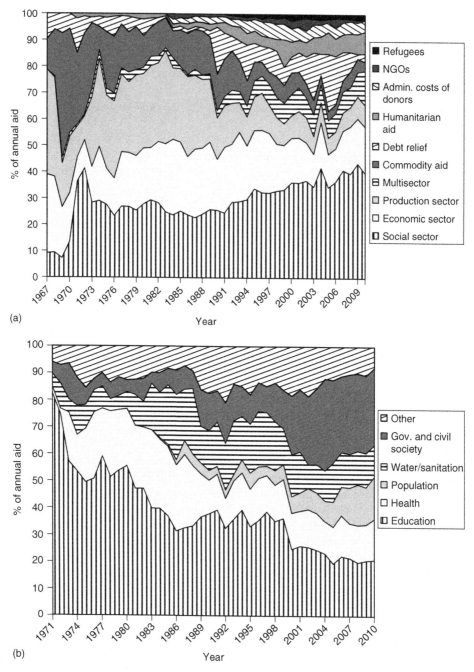

Figure 20.1 (a) Sectoral trends and (b) sectoral social sector trends in the allocation of annual world aid, 1967–2010. Source: data from OECD-DAC Reporting System (2012), International Development Statistics.

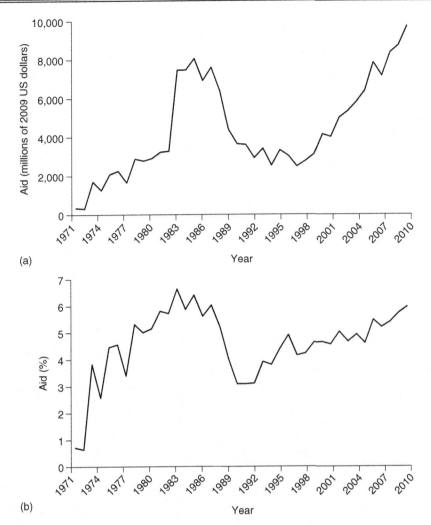

Figure 20.2 (a) Total health aid and (b) health aid share of total aid budget, 1971–2010. Source: data from OECD-DAC Reporting System (2012), International Development Statistics.

the poverty trap. This initial increase in productivity will result in individuals generating enough subsequent income so they themselves can save, leading to future benefits. Sachs calculates the exact amount of foreign aid needed to end poverty by 2025 as being $195 billion per year from 2005 to 2025.

Also supporting the notion that aid should, and can, be used to end poverty are Peter Singer (1972) and Amartya Sen (1999). Part of their arguments hinge on a moral presupposition that we have a duty to help those less well off. Specifically, they argue that poverty handicaps individuals from realizing their full potential. Being poor is not just a lack of money but also a lack a capacity to pursue a flourishing and meaningful life. Sen refers to health as one of the building blocks of development and argues that improvements in health facilities and institutions are fundamental in this process. He stresses that being rich is not a prerequisite for healthcare because even in relatively wealthy societies there can be some individuals who lack the healthcare necessary to pursue a meaningful life.

In contrast to the public interest view, the public choice view holds that foreign assistance goes to governments who may or may not have the public interest in mind. Instead of assuming that the political elite are altruistic and other-regarding in their motives, the public choice approach begins with the assumption that politicians, like those in the private sector, pursue their own interests, which may be narrowly self-interested or broader and other-regarding. Peter Bauer (2000), a proponent of the public choice view, highlights how foreign aid is neither necessary nor sufficient for economic development. In fact, he argues that foreign aid may actually impede growth because it alters incentives in an unfavorable manner (discussed in detail in subsequent sections). Bauer notes that the money intended to help those in need often ends up in the hands of the political elite who may support bad policies and reinforce the predatory policies that are a contributing factor to the existing state of affairs. According to Bauer, the mere existence of developed countries defies the poverty trap argument for foreign aid. After all, at one point all countries were poor, meaning that there was no wealthy country to provide foreign assistance to the first countries that rose from poverty to prosperity. This realization stands in contrast to the standard claim that countries need foreign assistance in order to break out of a vicious circle in order to grow into a virtuous one.

William Easterly (2001, 2006), another proponent of the public choice view, also discusses how foreign aid does not promote growth. He debunks the argument that foreign aid is necessary to make up for the lack of investment in developing countries. Aid, by itself, will not change the incentives to invest in the future and can actually create dependencies that discourage such investments. In addition to highlighting a variety of perverse incentives created by foreign aid, Easterly also discusses how there is a lack of knowledge with the current top-down foreign aid approach, which is similar to Soviet-style central planning. Development is not an engineering or technological problem; instead, it requires constant trial and error and continual searching. Donors rely on the bureaucratic process to try and solve these knowledge problems, a process that often fails to deliver the necessary feedback and monitoring. This is precisely why Easterly emphasizes the importance of "Searchers" over "Planners," since the former refer to those engaged in the process of discovery and experimentation. A large and robust empirical body of work backs up the public choice perspective (Boone 1996; Svensson 1999, 2000; Knack 2001; Brumm 2003; Ovaska 2003; Djankov *et al.* 2006; Powell and Ryan 2006).

Perhaps the aid debate has focused for too long on the big questions such as how to end world poverty. Instead, some aid proponents (for example, Banerjee and Duflo 2011) argue that the discussion should shift toward piecemeal, well-targeted outcomes such as increased vaccinations or providing bed nets. This approach draws a distinction between aid for growth and aid for health. While development is not a purely technological problem, many health-related issues are. We may not know how to solve world poverty, but many global health issues such as preventing certain diseases, preventing deaths related to diarrhea, providing birth control, and treatment for malaria and tuberculosis *are* technical, logistical exercises in moving resources from point A to point B. And many of these solutions have been known for decades. Therefore, health aid should be the "easy" case for aid since health-related issues are concrete problems and the solutions to these problems are (mostly) known.

In this context, a recent article by Skarbek and Leeson (2009) is relevant, where the authors argue that aid can be seen as both as a success and a failure: "Aid can, and in a few cases has, increased a particular output by devoting more resources to its production. In this sense, aid has occasionally had limited success. However, aid cannot, and has not, contributed to the solution of economic problems and therefore economic growth. In this much more important sense, aid has failed" (Skarbek and Leeson 2009: 392). They go on to argue that, at its best, aid can provide more goods and services, but still not find the solutions to the economic problem of poverty. "So, what can aid do? Like other forms of central planning, aid can increase X by devoting additional resources to X's production ... If planners pick a specific outcome, such as more immunizations, aid can provide additional resources to produce immunizations. All of the 'success stories' that aid's advocates highlight are of this nature" (Skarbek and Leeson 2009: 394).

This argument implies that even if aid cannot increase growth and end world poverty, it may be able to ease human suffering *in the mean time*. Although, the best way to alleviate poverty is for a country to achieve sustained economic growth, the question is can aid decrease human suffering while we wait for growth? Until poor countries begin to experience the benefits from more development, health aid may be able to alleviate some of the consequences of extreme poverty. Even in countries that are experiencing high growth rates and increases in standards of living, Boone and Johnson (2009) argue that pockets of poverty still may persist. In principle, health aid may be able to intervene to provide basic care and eliminate the cruelest of suffering for countries stuck in poverty traps and individuals still living in pockets of poverty.

In what follows, we consider the evidence regarding global healthcare outcomes and how these outcomes relate to increased spending on health assistance. We then turn to the economic way of thinking to explain why efforts to provide health assistance to those in need often fail. We conclude with the policy implications of our analysis.

Examining the Evidence

Worldwide trends related to health are improving. For example, Figures 20.3–20.5 illustrate that both the overall death rate and infant mortality are on the decline and life expectancy is increasing. This holds for all income groups.[5]

As stated earlier, health aid is increasing over time as health indicators are improving. Are the two related? Has health aid actually made a difference? Once again it depends on what is described as the end goal. Aggregate studies indicate that health-related aid

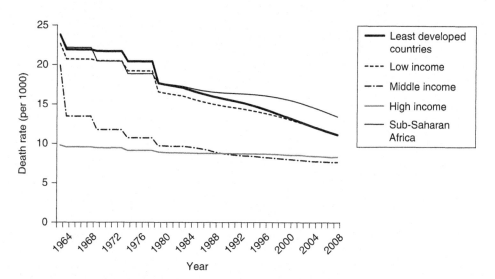

Figure 20.3 Death rate per 1000 population, 1964–2009 (5-year moving average). Source: data from World Bank (2011), World Development Indicators.

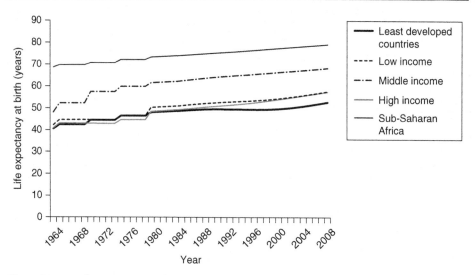

Figure 20.4   Life expectancy at birth in total years, 1964–2009 (5-year moving average). Source: data from World Bank (2011), World Development Indicators.

has no impact on health outcomes. On the contrary, there are micro-level data showing that aid is (somewhat) successful at building hospitals, providing vaccines, and bed nets, for example. We consider each in more detail.

Williamson (2008) examines aid earmarked specifically for the health sector to determine its effect on infant mortality, life expectancy, death rates, and immunizations (diphtheria, pertussis, and tetanus (DPT) and measles). The analysis shows that aid has not had any effect on the five dimensions of health studied. The results support the public choice perspective discussed above, indicating that international aid to the health sector

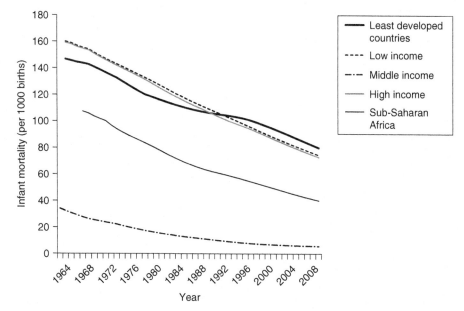

Figure 20.5   Infant mortality per 1000 births, 1964–2010 (5-year moving average). Source: data from World Bank (2011), World Development Indicators.

may be an ineffective policy tool for improving human welfare. In this sense, health is not "special" relative to other forms of development assistance. Just like general aid, which is shown to have an insignificant effect on economic development, aid used specifically for health goals has an insignificant effect on human development.

A follow-up study by Wilson (2011) also finds support for Williamson's conclusion. Wilson uses a new data source, AidData, compiled by Findley *et al.* (2009), to show that development assistance for health does not reduce mortality at the country level. However, economic growth does have a strong negative effect on mortality (as we would suspect). His analysis also supports the notion that health aid effectiveness has not increased over time even though the amount of health aid has increased fourfold. Wilson summarizes his finding as "development assistance for health appears to be *following* success, rather than *causing* it" (Wilson 2011: 2031, italics in original). In other words, economic growth precedes improved health outcomes.

Even though health aid has no discernable effect on county-level aggregate indicators, there are public health programs and projects that might show positive results for specific health outcomes. This is exactly what researchers engaged in randomized controlled trials (RCTs) are attempting to discover. They want to shift the focus away from the "big questions" of what ends poverty towards more narrow ones, such as how to immunize children and increase bed net usage in specific, local contexts.

In *Poor Economics: A Radical Rethinking of the Way to Fight Global Poverty*, Banerjee and Duflo (2011) summarize the last 15 years of research, including hundreds of RCTs, on trying to understand solutions to global poverty. They call health one of the greatest areas of hope but also of great frustration as the solutions to many health-related problems are "low-hanging fruit." However, many of these fruits are left unpicked. Why? As one example illustrates, getting individuals in poor countries to understand "miracle drugs" such as oral rehydration solution (ORS) or chlorine bleach is harder than previously thought: in one Indian town many children die from diarrhea, but ORS, an extremely cheap solution, has not been that effective at saving lives. The reason is that many mothers do not believe that ORS does any good, resulting in the lack of adoption of a solution that is known to be effective.

Banerjee and Duflo summarize this experience, and many others similar to it, as a lack of information and weak beliefs on the part of those suffering from poor health and poverty. The poor often spend valuable resources on healthcare but on the "wrong" healthcare, demanding unnecessary antibiotics or surgeries that come too late to be effective. The poor also tend to believe that the public health system does not work, preferring to use private providers or traditional healers.

This sentiment is also echoed in Samia Waheed Altaf's (2011) book, *So Much Aid, So Little Development: Stories from Pakistan*. Altaf was hired as a technical assistant in the 1990s to the Social Action Program (SAP) in Pakistan. Her journey illuminates how aid actually works and why it fails. She explains that her "own understanding of this situation is that program designs are based on limited conceptual frameworks that reflect a woefully inadequate knowledge of local realities, and thus are inappropriate in the context of national constraints" (Altaf 2011: 3).

Taken together, both the macro- and micro-level studies suggest that even though there are known and cheap cures to many of the health-related issues of the poor, implementing policy that *delivers* effective healthcare has proved to be daunting in practice. The following sections draw on the economic approach to provide insight into the disconnect between the knowledge possessed by those in developed countries regarding healthcare and the effective delivery of these services to those in need.

The Economic Way of Thinking

The puzzle we need to explain is why health-related foreign aid has failed to positively impact health outcomes. Conceptually, the task at hand is clear – donors need to identify those in need of healthcare and then deliver the appropriate assistance. What then explains the failure of health-related aid to improve health outcomes? The economic way of thinking provides insight into this puzzle.

An economic approach is grounded in a few basic, related assumptions. One is that people have ends that they seek to pursue. This just means that each person has certain goals they wish to accomplish. Second, economists assume that people are rational. This does not imply that people are infallible automatons, but rather that they pursue their ends the best way known to them at the time of action. Finally, people respond to incentives, meaning they respond to changes in costs and benefits associated with a course of action.

In addition to these core assumptions, the central economic question is how decisions are to be made regarding the use of scarce resources. Scarcity necessitates choice which, in turn, implies trade-offs since one feasible use of scarce resources must ultimately be chosen over another potential use. The answers to these questions, which constitute the "economic problem," are not given and instead must be discovered in all contexts where scarcity exists, no matter what the desired end – purely humanitarian concerns, maximizing monetary profit, or some other end.

These assumptions and the core economic problem bring into focus the two central issues related to our puzzle regarding health aid and health outcomes. First, the success of health-related aid depends on the existence of the appropriate incentives in the donor and recipient countries. In other words, donors must have an incentive to deliver aid to those most in need, and recipients must have an incentive to use the aid in the matter desired by the donors. Second, both donors and recipients must possess, or obtain, the necessary information to solve the economic problem. Taken together, the incentive and information issues result in a "double-edged sword," which explains why foreign aid is often ineffective (Williamson 2010). If donors and/or recipients lack the appropriate incentives and information, then assistance will fail to have the desired outcome. This applies to health-related assistance just as it applies to foreign aid more broadly. The next two sections explore the role of incentives and information in more detail.

Incentives

As per the public interest view, discussions of foreign aid often implicitly assume benevolence on the part of donor and recipient governments. It is assumed that those involved in delivering health-related aid to those in need put aside their own interests and agendas in order to altruistically assist those in need. This implies that the various parties involved in dispersing and receiving aid utilize the most effective means to achieve the ends of improving health-related outcomes. It is taken for granted that donors are unbiased in their initial decision to donate to certain countries and that recipient government allocate health-related assistance in a manner that accomplishes the desired goals. The public choice view calls this assumption, and the related implications, into question.

The subfield of public choice economics applies the economic way of thinking to non-market decision-making. This includes the entire foreign aid enterprise, which takes place outside the market context. Public choice calls for an extension of the core assumptions laid out previously to both market and non-market decision-making. Often, people have little difficulty applying core economic assumptions to market-related activities, but they assume that people transcend these economics in non-market-related behavior. Public choice economics indicates that this way of thinking is incomplete because people are not transformed from narrowly self-interested individuals into benevolent and other-regarding angels when they move from market to non-market-related activities.

This implies that instead of assuming benevolence on the part of those involved in allocating and distributing health aid, we instead need to focus on the incentives created by the institutions within which these individuals act. Public choice indicates that even though the provision of health-related aid may be motivated by the best of intentions, there are incentives at work which may prevent those desired ends from being achieved. For example, interest groups will seek to influence the actions of both donor and recipient governments to support their agenda even if it is at odds with providing health-related aid to those most in need. Meanwhile, bureaucrats in positions to disperse aid will attempt to influence the process by maximizing their budgets and attempting to create a demand for their services. Finally, elected officials in both donor and recipient countries will seek to pursue their own agendas in the disbursement and allocation of foreign aid. The interaction of these various forces will influence how much health-related aid is disbursed, as well as where and how the aid is allocated. The main result from the public choice model applied to health-related aid is that those involved in the process may fail to facilitate the coordination and cooperation that is necessary to transform spending on healthcare into improved health outcomes.

Donor Incentives

Donor countries and aid agencies face specific incentives when developing policies related to health-related assistance. These incentives emerge from the institutional structures – democratic politics, non-profit government bureaucracy, etc. – within which the pertinent parties act. This subsection explores how the incentives faced by the relevant players – elected officials, special interests, and bureaucrats – shape the effectiveness of health-related aid.

In principle, elected officials within donor governments would cater to the wants of voters. However, a key insight from public choice economics is that individual voters do not have the incentive to become informed about foreign aid policy, let alone the smaller portion dedicated to healthcare, and therefore remain "rationally ignorant" of the specifics of policy. The implication is that in reality individual voters exert little control over health aid. In stark contrast to individual voters, special interest groups within the donor countries do have the incentive to become informed in order to secure large benefits for their members, even if these benefits do not maximize the benefits to those in need in other countries. This logic implies that we should not expect politicians in donor countries to form health-related aid policies that will maximize the value of scarce resources dedicated to improving healthcare from the standpoint of the ultimate consumers – those in need. Instead, domestic political pressures, including lobbying interests, determine policies.

As an example of how domestic politics influences health-related assistance, consider the case of condom production for HIV/AIDS and family planning programs (Dugger 2006). The US Agency for International Development (USAID) has restricted contracts for condom production to US companies, currently manufacturers in Alabama. USAID could buy condoms from Asian manufacturers for half the price, but Alabama Senator Jeff Sessions has continually pushed to ensure that USAID buy condoms from producers in his state. Ultimately, this means that USAID could purchase twice as many condoms – one of the most effective means of slowing the transmission of HIV/AIDS – if domestic special interests did not have to be considered. Domestic producers benefit from producing condoms and elected officials respond to these incentives even though they could increase the number of condoms and potential health-related benefits.

What this example illustrates is that assistance is given based on who wins the political competition through which aid decisions are made. Indeed, an existing literature indicates that donors disburse foreign aid based on political motivation and not necessarily based on the need of the final recipients (see Mosley 1985a, 1985b; Trumbull and Wall 1994). Further, Boone (1996) shows that aid reflects the relatively permanent strategic interests of donors. Taken together, this literature helps to explain why increased spending on health-related assistance does not necessarily result in improved healthcare outcomes.

In addition to special interests, the incentives facing bureaucrats also play a role in influencing health-related aid policy. For example, bureaucrats operate in an environment of negligible feedback from beneficiaries, hard-to-observe outcomes, and low probability that bureaucratic effort will actually translate into favorable outcomes. In response to these incentives, aid bureaucracies have organized themselves "as a cartel of good intentions, suppressing critical feedback and learning from the past, suppressing competitive pressure to deliver results, and suppressing identification of the best channel of resources for different objectives" (Easterly 2002: 247). Numerous layers of bureaucracy are involved in the delivery of assistance. This results in weak incentives for accountability, as there are typically unclear lines of responsibility and ownership over the use of health-related aid. When aid-related projects and initiatives fail, it is rare for a single agency, or a specific bureaucrat within an agency, to be held responsible for failing to achieve the stated outcome.

Bureaucrats in both governments and aid agencies face their own incentives. For example, donors, especially aid agencies, prefer to focus on aid disbursements (i.e., their "burn rate") as the preferred measure of success. Not only are disbursements observable but they are also the agency's budget, and an agency's budget is its source of existence. Without profit and loss, bureaucrats measure success by the size of their discretionary budget, which creates perverse incentives for spending money even if saving for future periods was the preferable course of action. Indeed, bureaucrats face the incentive not only to exhaust their current budget, but also to ask for increases in their annual budget in order to increase the size of the agency. Given these incentives, there is no reason to assume that bureaucrats in donor governments and aid agencies will choose to pursue the most efficient policies and strategies related to improving health outcomes.

We should also note that similar logic applies to non-governmental organizations (NGOs). Werker and Ahmed (2008) provide evidence that NGOs suffer from weaknesses, including inefficient, multilayer decision-making, low-quality service due to a lack of feedback, and agenda control stemming from pressure from national governments, their largest donors. NGOs do not transcend the logic of economics and the importance of incentives in the delivery of health-related assistance.

Recipient Incentives

Recipients refer to those who receive aid from donor governments. This includes the receiving government, individual citizens, and special interest groups within these countries. Recipients of aid face their own incentive structures. Foreign aid disbursements tend to pass through the ruling governments in aid-receiving countries. From an economic standpoint, the central question is: what incentive do these governments have to actually achieve the desired health-related results?

Dysfunctional governments, which are unable to provide healthcare for their citizens, are a key reason that health-related foreign aid is needed in the first place. Corruption poses a major problem for foreign assistance in general because corrupt governments are unlikely to deliver aid in the intended manner. Under this scenario, recipient governments have little to no incentive to achieve the results desired by donors, which further helps to explain why health-related assistance is not necessarily transformed into improved health outcomes.

For example, Easterly (2007b) argues that corrupt governments have an incentive to minimize the productive capability of the poor because of the potential of creating political activism that would threaten the current political regime. Keeping people in poor health is one way to achieve this goal. This is not a new argument, as Bauer (1971) and Friedman (1958) argue that the political elite in recipient countries will tend to distribute aid in an ineffective manner to generate ongoing streams of payments, thus strengthening their relative position of power. Politicians understand that they will benefit from ongoing foreign aid, creating additional incentives to not only misallocate aid but also to seek out an environment that actually attracts it, including keeping citizens in poor health (Brautigram and Knack 2004).

To illustrate the dynamics described above, consider the case of North Korea. The government requested food and health-related assistance from the United Nations (UN) and certain humanitarian NGOs, but restricted their access from over half of the country in order to hide the magnitude of human suffering from outsiders (Orbinski 2008: 306–9). It eventually became evident that by operating in North Korea, the humanitarian organizations were providing credibility to the government, thus reinforcing the status quo that caused the initial suffering. As James Orbinski, the past president of Médecins Sans Frontières (or Doctors Without Borders), writes "By remaining present, silent and without access to the most vulnerable, we were giving the impression that humanitarian action was possible and that the North Korean government respected basic humanitarian principles ... By propping up the regime, aid was not only masking suffering but propping it up" (Orbinski 2008: 308).

In addition to elected officials, special interest and advocacy groups within the recipient country can also distort the allocation of health-related assistance. Consider, for instance, the case of Ethiopia where approximately 60% of health spending is earmarked toward HIV/AIDS initiatives, while less than 1% is allocated toward malaria control (Barder 2009). This allocation is the result of advocacy groups who lobby government agencies and organizations for increased spending on HIV/AIDS prevention. However, a closer look at estimates in Ethiopia indicate that over 65% of the population lives in at-risk areas of malaria and that malaria is responsible for over 25% of deaths in the country. In stark contrast, the HIV/AIDS prevalence rate among adults in Ethiopia is estimated to be 4.4% (WHO 2005). In other words, a reallocation of earmarked funds away from HIV prevention toward malaria prevention could potentially have a higher return in terms of lives saved.

Information

Both donors and recipients must obtain the necessary information to actually target and achieve desired goals. The relevant parties most know what assistance is needed by those who are suffering, and then know how to best allocate assistance to maximize its impact. The problem is that those involved in the aid distribution process often lack access to the relevant information, as it is discontinuous, dispersed across many individuals, and often contained in inarticulate forms. Donors are capable of specifying goals and what they hope to achieve with health-related aid, but they often do not know where aid is required, who it is needed by, in what locations, and in what quantities. Similarly, those suffering in the recipient countries may know what they need and in what quantities, but they may not know who has the aid or how to get it. The broader issue is that in the absence of the appropriate information, health-related assistance will be ineffective even if appropriate incentives exist.

Donors' Information Problem

In order for aid to be effective, donors must be able to gather critical information, requiring the ability to tap into local knowledge. Donors must recognize where assistance is needed, figure out exactly what is needed and who needs it, evaluate whether or not what they are doing is working, and adapt accordingly. These last tasks require some form of evaluation and feedback. As previously discussed, however, donors must rely on a multilayered bureaucratic process to attempt to solve these information problems. This limits the availability of effective feedback information on effective allocation, and reallocation, of health-related resources.

Ideally, there would be some kind of feedback mechanism that would allow donors to obtain and adapt to changing information. In markets, for example, entrepreneurs have access to prices and the profit and loss mechanism to make decisions regarding the reallocation of resource. In bureaucracies, however, no equivalent mechanism exists. Bureaucratic activity is guided by predefined procedures and protocols. Bureaucratic rules serve as a guide for the behavior of bureaucrats, but the rigidity of these rules limits flexibility and adaptability as information and conditions change. Indeed, bureaucratic procedures and protocols create a separation between private knowledge and political knowledge as predefined rules guide behaviors instead of the "on-the-ground" realities and complexities. Further contributing to the weak adaptability of aid bureaucracies is the absence of clear lines of accountability, as well as the fact that the final recipients of health-related aid have very little opportunity to give feedback to the donor agencies. In other words, the ultimate consumers of aid – those in need – have no mechanism of punishing agencies if they fail. This disconnect contributes to the aforementioned separation between the local information and the information used by bureaucrats in making decisions regarding the use of health-related assistance.

Another issue facing donors is the lack of coordination between the various bureaucracies involved in foreign aid, where information needs to be effectively shared within and across these bureaucracies. This can place heavy administrative burdens on those involved in the delivery of health-related assistance. Consider, for instance, that it is estimated that a medical officer in Tanzania spends 50–70% of their time writing reports and missions (Easterly 2007a). When efforts are diverted into purely administrative tasks this reduces the amount of resources that can help to improve the situation of those in need. Donor agencies are constantly calling for more coordination to relieve developing countries of administrative requirements (see, for instance, Commission for Africa 2005; UN Millennium Project 2005), but Easterly (2007a) notes that there is little sign of improvement.

Consider a recent report by Médecins Sans Frontières, which discusses the delivery of humanitarian assistance in Afghanistan. Among other things, the report indicates that the "Lashkargah hospital is piling up with advanced medical equipment – digital x-rays, mobile oxygen generators, scialytic lamps – donated by a range of states including the United States, China, Iran, and India or through the Provincial Reconstruction Teams (PRTs). This equipment is usually dropped off with little explanation and no anticipation of maintenance; most of it sits in boxes, collecting dust, unopened and unused" (MSF 2010: 2).

Along similar lines, a study of drug donations in the post-tsunami Banda Aceh province in Indonesia found that 70% of the drugs had foreign labels that could not be understood by local workers and were therefore unusable. The study also found that 60% of the donated drugs were not relevant to those affected by the tsunami. Further, 25% of the donated drugs had either expired or had no expiration data. In order to store these inappropriate drugs, humanitarian workers had to sacrifice office space and patient rooms. In total, the report noted that approximately 600 tons of medicine had to be destroyed at a cost of $3 million. Adding to the sad irony of this situation is that the Southeast Asia region, where these wasted drugs were sent, produces a significant amount of the generic medicines used in other humanitarian operations! Indeed, there were indications that the indigenous drug suppliers had the ability to cover the existing drug needs.[6] Similar problems with drug donations can be found in numerous other cases as well (Hechmann and Bunde-Birouste 2007).

Whether it is idle equipment or useless drugs, the absence of effective information serves as a hard constraint on the ability of donors to provide effective health services and goods to those in need. Without the appropriate information regarding where assistance is needed, what assistance is needed, and in what quantities, the result will be waste that fails to contribute to improved health outcomes.

Recipients' Information Problem

In addition to the donors, recipients must also possess adequate information about how to achieve the specific goals of health-related aid. Just like donors, recipient governments often lack the ability to tap into the context-specific information that is critical for success. Recipient governments use the same bureaucratic processes that are used in developed countries and, as discussed, this process tends to be ineffective for tapping into the local information necessary for the effective delivery of health-related assistance. With health-related aid provided by donors, recipient governments, which are often corrupt, still must determine who is in need, what is needed, and in what quantities. This may seem like a simple task, but as the evidence provided earlier indicates, health-related aid has failed to be allocated in a manner that has a consistently positive effect on health outcomes.

To illustrate this, consider a report by the World Health Organization (WHO) which noted that "In the Sub-Saharan Africa region … a large proportion (up to 70 per cent) of [health-related] equipment lies idle due to mismanagement of the technology acquisition process, lack of user-training and lack of effective technical support" (WHO 2000: 10). In other words, donors can provide health-related assistance to recipient governments, but the recipients must know how to effectively utilize that assistance for it to be transformed into improved health outcomes. In addition to allocating the assistance to those who need it, recipient governments must also know how to allocate complementary resources (trained medical staff, repair parts, technicians, etc.) in a manner that allows donations to be used effectively. Recipient governments often lack that information.

Conclusions

This chapter has explored the question of whether international aid can improve global health. In contrast to tackling the more complex issue of promoting economic growth, we have focused our analysis on the effectiveness of aid on the more simple task of delivering health to those in need. Theory and the majority of empirical evidence to date suggest that the answer to this question is "No." While RCTs may be a step in the right direction as a means of evaluation, they should not be confused with a panacea of solving global health problems due to the issues outlined. It is also important to emphasize that the provision of healthcare, by itself, does not necessarily translate into the adoption and use of the assistance provided. This leads us back to the question of what aid can and cannot accomplish in practice.

In the health context, aid can potentially build a hospital, set up a fully stocked immunization clinic, and offer free malaria bed nets. In this context, one could say that health aid is a success, if success is defined as providing more of a predefined good or service. However, successfully providing more of a good or service does not necessarily mean that healthcare providers will show up to work in the hospital, that mothers will bring their children to the immunization clinic, or that the nets will actually be used in a manner to reduce malaria risk. This logic begins to explain why small-scale "successes" can be found in the micro-level data but not in the macro-level data, where the overall relationship between aid and health does not exist. It is not that no one has been helped by health aid interventions, but rather that there is no reason to believe that health aid can *systematically* improve outcomes.

Notes

1. For the purpose of this chapter, we define international aid as official development assistance (ODA) from bilateral and multilateral donors, thus excluding non-governmental organizations and private charity.
2. All health statistics are taken from World Health Organization Data and Statistics 2012.
3. The Organisation for Economic Co-operation and Development classifies social sector aid as aid to social infrastructure and services. It is defined as aid that covers efforts to develop the human resource potential and ameliorate living conditions in recipient countries.
4. Public choice refers to the subfield in economics that uses the rational choice framework to highlight sources of government failures. This is further explained in a subsequent section in this chapter.
5. Least developed countries (LDCs) are those countries defined as such by the United Nations.
6. Data on drug donation in Banda Aceh from Pharmaciens Sans Frontiers–Comite International (2006).

Key Reading

Altaf SW. 2011. *So Much Aid, So Little Development: Stories from Pakistan.* Baltimore, MD: Johns Hopkins University Press.

Banerjee AV, Duflo E. 2011. *Poor Economics: A Radical Rethinking of the Way to Fight Global Poverty.* New York: Public Affairs.

Cohen J, Easterly W (eds). 2009. *What Works in Development? Thinking Big and Thinking Small.* Washington, DC: Brookings Institution Press.

Easterly W. 2006. *The White Man's Burden: Why the West's Efforts to Aid the Rest have done So Much Ill and So Little Good*. New York: Penguin Press.

Easterly W. 2008. *Reinventing Foreign Aid*. Cambridge, MA: MIT Press.

Williamson CR. 2008. Foreign aid and human development: the impact of foreign aid to the health sector. *Southern Economic Journal* 75(1), 188–207.

Wilson S. 2011. Chasing success: health sector aid and mortality. *World Development* 39, 2031–43.

References

Altaf SW. 2011. *So Much Aid, So Little Development: Stories from Pakistan*. Baltimore, MD: Johns Hopkins University Press.

Banerjee AV, Duflo E. 2011. *Poor Economics: A Radical Rethinking of the Way to Fight Global Poverty*. New York: Public Affairs.

Barder O. 2009. *The Lethal Effects of Development Advocacy*. http://www.owen.org/blog/2717 (last accessed December 2013).

Bauer PT. 1971. Economic history as theory. *Economica* 38, 163–79.

Bauer PT. 2000. *From Subsistence to Exchange*. Princeton, NJ: Princeton University Press.

Boone P. 1996. Politics and the effectiveness of foreign aid. *European Economic Review* 40, 289–329.

Boone P, Johnson S. 2009. Breaking out of the pocket: do health interventions work? Which ones and in which sense? In Cohen J, Easterly W (eds) *What Works in Development? Thinking Big and Thinking Small*. Washington, DC: Brookings Institution Press.

Brautigam D, Knack S. 2004. Foreign aid, institutions, and governance in sub-Saharan Africa. *Economic Development and Cultural Change* 52, 255–85.

Brumm HJ. 2003. Aid, policies and growth: Bauer was right. *Cato Journal* 23, 167–74.

Commission for Africa. 2005. *Our Common Interest: Report of the Commission for Africa*. London: Commission for Africa.

Djankov S, Montalvo JG, Reynal-Querol M. 2006a. Does foreign aid help? *Cato Journal* 26(1), 1–28.

Dugger CW. 2006. U.S. jobs shape condoms's role in foreign aid. *New York Times* October 29. http://www.nytimes.com/2006/10/29/world/29condoms.html?_r=2 (last accessed December 2013).

Easterly W. 2001. *The Elusive Quest for Growth: Economists' Adventures and Misadventures in the Tropics*. Cambridge, MA: MIT Press.

Easterly W. 2002. The cartel of good intentions. *Journal of Policy Reform* 5(4), 223–50.

Easterly W. 2006. *The White Man's Burden: Why the West's Efforts to Aid the Rest have done So Much Ill and So Little Good*. New York: Penguin Press.

Easterly W. 2007a. Are aid agencies improving? *Economic Policy* 22(52), 633–78.

Easterly W. 2007b. Was development assistance a mistake? *American Economic Review* 97(2), 328–32.

Findley MG, Hawkins D, Hicks RL *et al*. 2009. *AidData: Tracking Development Finance*. Presented at the PLAID Data Vetting Workshop, Washington, DC.

Friedman M. 1958. Foreign economic aid: means and objectives. In Ranis G (ed.) *The United States and the Development Economies*, pp. 250–63. New York: Norton.

Hechmann R, Bunde-Birouste A. 2007. Drug donations in emergencies, the Sri Lankan post-tsunami experience. *Journal of Humanitarian Studies* http://sites.tufts.edu/jha/archives/54 (last accessed December 2013).

Knack S. 2001. Aid dependence and the quality of governance: cross-country empirical tests. *Southern Economic Journal* 68(2), 310–29.

MSF (Médecins Sans Frontières). 2010. *Afghanistan: A Return to Humanitarian Action*. http://www.doctorswithoutborders.org/publications/reports/2010/MSF-Return-to-Humanitarian-Action-4311.pdf (last accessed December 2013).

Mosley P. 1985a. The political economy of foreign aid: a model of the market for a public good. *Economic Development and Cultural Change* 33. 373–93.

Mosley P. 1985b. Towards a predictive model of overseas aid expenditures. *Scottish Journal of Political Economy* 32, 1–19.

OECD-DAC (Organisation for Economic Co-operation and Development Development Assistance Committee) Reporting System. 2012. *International Development Statistics (IDS) online databases*. http://www.oecd.org/dac/stats/idsonline.htm (last accessed December 2013).

Orbinski J. 2008. *An Imperfect Offering: Humanitarian Action for the Twenty-First Century*. New York: Walker and Company.

Ovaska T. 2003. The failure of development aid. *Cato Journal* 23, 175–88.

Pharmaciens Sans Frontiers–Comite International. 2006. *Study on Drug Donations in the Province of Aceh in Indonesia*. apps.who.int/medicinedocs/documents/s17066e/s17066e.pdf (last accessed December 2013).

Powell B, Ryan M. 2006. Does development aid lead to economic freedom? *Journal of Private Enterprise* 22(1), 1–21.

Sachs JD. 2005. *The End of Poverty*. New York: Penguin Press.

Sen A. 1999. *Development as Freedom*. New York: Anchor Books.

Singer P. 1972. Famine, affluence, and morality. *Philosophy and Public Affairs* 1(3), 229–43.

Skarbek DB, Leeson PT. 2009. What can aid do? *Cato Journal* 29(3), 391–7.

Svensson J. 1999. Aid and growth: does democracy matter? *Economics and Politics* 11(3), 275–97.

Svensson J. 2000. Foreign aid and rent-seeking. *Journal of International Economics* 51, 437–61.

Trumbull WN, Wall HJ. 1994. Estimating aid-allocation criteria with panel data. *Economic Journal* 104, 876–82.

UN (United Nations) Millennium Project. 2005. *Investing in Development: A Practical Plan to Achieve the Millennium Development Goals (Main Report)*. New York: UN.

Werker E, Ahmed FZ. 2008. What do nongovernmental organizations do? *Journal of Economic Perspectives* 22(2), 73–92.

Williamson CR. 2008. Foreign aid and human development: the impact of foreign aid to the health sector. *Southern Economic Journal* 75(1), 188–207.

Williamson CR. 2010. Exploring the failures of foreign aid: the role of incentives and information. *Review of Austrian Economics* 23(1), 17–33.

Wilson S. 2011. Chasing success: health sector aid and mortality. *World Development* 39, 2031–43.

World Bank. 2011. *World Development Indicators*. Washington, DC: World Bank.

WHO (World Health Organization). 2000. *Guidelines for Health Care Equipment Donations*. http://www.who.int/hac/techguidance/pht/1_equipment%20donationbuletin82WHO.pdf (last accessed December 2013).

WHO (World Health Organization). 2005. *Ethiopia Strategy Paper*. http://www.who.int/hac/crises/eth/Ethiopia_strategy_document.pdf (last accessed December 2013).

Chapter 21

The Exterritorial Reach of Money: Global Finance and Social Determinants of Health

Ted Schrecker

Abstract

The extent to which global financial markets influence health by way of its social determinants is a neglected area of research. This chapter first describes the "implicit conditionalities" associated with the operation of those markets, and how they limit the policy options available to governments. It then explores two destructive dimensions of the hypermobility of capital: financial crises created by the rapid outflow of foreign investment, and capital flight on the part of domestic elites seeking higher returns, lower risks, and often the opportunity to avoid taxation. The financial crisis that spread across the world in 2008 is identified as underscoring the dangers of economic interconnectedness, imposing as it did major costs on those who had no role in creating the crisis. Evidence linking financial crises with health outcomes is briefly reviewed, and a concluding section explores policy implications.

The Handbook of Global Health Policy, First Edition. Edited by Garrett W. Brown, Gavin Yamey, and Sarah Wamala.
© 2014 John Wiley & Sons, Ltd. Published 2014 by John Wiley & Sons, Ltd.

Key Points

- Financial markets now impose "conditionalities" that limit the ability of governments to reduce health disparities by way of social determinants of health.
- Financial crises resulting from rapid outflows of investment increase poverty, economic inequality, and insecurity in several ways.
- Capital flight on the part of domestic elites starves countries of resources for development and health and magnifies economic inequality.
- The financial crisis of 2008 underscored the dangers of economic interconnectedness by generating major negative consequences for people, at its epicentre and half a world away, who had no role in creating the crisis or control over its outcome.
- Although not always available in a form that meets epidemiological standards of proof, the overall weight of evidence linking the operation of global financial markets to adverse health effects is compelling.

Key Policy Implications

- Global finance is a public health issue, and health researchers and practitioners must acquire sufficient familiarity to participate proactively in key policy debates.
- Low- and middle-income countries must be given more latitude to control capital flows, and multinational cooperation to limit capital flight is needed.
- High-income countries must regulate their domestic financial services industries to avoid repeats of the 2008 crisis.

Introduction

Global Reach (Barnet and Müller 1974) was one of the first books on transnational economic integration (globalization) written for a non-academic audience. Since its appearance in 1974, production has been reorganized across multiple national borders to an extent that would have been difficult to imagine when the book appeared (Dicken 2007). The remarkable essayist Eduardo Galeano has accurately described globalization as "a magic galleon that spirits factories away to poor countries" (Galeano 2000: 166) that compete for foreign direct investment and contract production largely on the basis of low labor costs and flexible employment relations. A comparably far-reaching transformation, the health implications of which have received less attention, involves the influence of financial markets on social determinants of health (see Chapter 14) and on the range of policy options ("policy space;" see Koivusalo *et al.* 2009) available to governments wishing to act on those determinants. This chapter updates and refines an earlier paper (Schrecker 2009) that represented, to my knowledge, the first English-language analysis of health and health policy consequences of the emergence of global financial markets.

To oversimplify somewhat, the emergence of the global financial marketplace in its current form reflects three underlying processes. First, because of advances in information processing and telecommunications, vast sums of money (financial assets) can be moved around the world almost instantaneously. Thus, technological change functions to some extent as an exogenous variable, although the financial services industry was one of the major sources of financing for innovation in this area (Schiller 1999: 13–14). Second, countries within whose borders the dominant financial centers of the late twentieth century were located (namely the United States and the United Kingdom) deregulated the domestic and overseas activities of their financial services industries (Helleiner 1994; Girón and Correa 1999). Third, by the start of the 1980s the precarious state of many low- and middle-income country (LMIC) economies threatened the financial health of institutions in New York and London that had lent heavily to them (Makin 1984: chapters 1, 12). The policy response involved "[a]n alliance of the international financial institutions, the private banks, and the Thatcher–Reagan Kohl governments [that] was willing to use its political and economic power to back its ideological predilections" (Przeworski *et al.* 1995: 5), simultaneously protecting creditor interests and opening up new markets and investment opportunities through trade and investment liberalization. A key strategic element of the response involved "conditionalities" attached to structural adjustment loans for debt rescheduling, with the International Monetary Fund (IMF) in particular insisting on the reduction or elimination of controls on cross-border financial flows (Stiglitz 2004).

Implicit Conditionalities

The critical point for present-day purposes is that financial markets can now impose "implicit conditionalities" (Griffith-Jones and Stallings 1995) on LMIC economies and governments, analogous to – and sometimes in conjunction with – the more explicit dictates of the IMF. As one of the leading researchers on globalization, sociologist Saskia Sassen, has put it: "[T]he global capital market now has the power to discipline national governments ... These markets can now exercise the accountability functions associated with citizenship: they can vote governments' economic policies in or out, they can force governments to take certain measures and not others." Indeed, the markets "have emerged as a sort of global, cross-border economic electorate" (Sassen 2003: 70) whose preferences can override those of national polities. It is therefore important to recognize that markets in this context are a convenient abstraction. Really at issue are the aggregated portfolio choices (decisions about how and where to invest) of asset owners and managers, including not only pension and mutual fund managers, but also hedge funds, private equity firms, and private bankers as well as wealthy individuals, weighted by the resources they command. The asset owners and managers in question operate largely without mechanisms of formal coordination, with the exception of the credit rating agencies (Sinclair 1994) that played an important role in exacerbating the Eurozone crisis of 2011–2012.

Implicit conditionalities operate in several ways, the first of which is specific to government bond markets: investors will demand a higher interest rate (the risk premium) on bonds purchased from governments whose debt they perceive as risky. One instructive example involves Brazil. As it appeared likely that the Workers' Party (PT) would win the 2002 election, investor concern about the effects on domestic inflation and Brazil's budget deficit led major US financial institutions to warn clients against investing in Brazil, with some recommending rapid disinvestment (Santiso 2004). A deputy governor of the Central Bank of Brazil between 2000 and 2003 has described a remarkable correlation between the PT's lead in opinion polls and the risk premium demanded on Brazilian government bonds (Goldfajn 2003). In order to assuage the concerns of foreign investors and avoid a further decline in the value of Brazil's currency, in September 2002 all the presidential candidates agreed on the terms of an IMF lending package most of which would be disbursed after the election, contingent on economic policies that were acceptable to the IMF.

This stabilized the risk premium and avoided an investor stampede, but as a consequence – in the words of noted development scholar Peter Evans – the PT "chose to suffer low growth, high unemployment and flat levels of social expenditure rather than risk retribution" from the markets (Evans 2005; see also Morais and Saad-Filho 2005; Amann and Baer 2006: 221–3; Koelble and Lipuma 2006: 623–5; Paiva 2006). Indeed, the Brazilian government not only kept interest rates high and inflation low, but also ran an even larger primary budget surplus (that is, a surplus before debt service obligations are taken into account) than demanded by the IMF. Over the longer term, this strategy combined with rapidly rising prices for Brazil's commodity exports to permit the PT greater latitude for adopting redistributive policies, including the Bolsa família cash transfer program and an expansion of primary healthcare through the Family Health Strategy (Soares 2011; Victora et al. 2011). In many other cases, the rule stated by one of the most sophisticated observers of bond markets still holds: "[T]hose societies most in need of egalitarian redistribution may have, in terms of external financial market pressures, the most difficulty achieving it" (Mosley 2006: 90; see more generally Mosley 2003). A more emphatic description of how financial markets limit the policy space available to governments was provided by financier George Soros in August 2002: "In the Roman empire, only the Romans voted. In modern global capitalism, only the Americans vote. Not the Brazilians" (Hilton 2002).

The preceding discussion dealt with the market for one kind of investment: government bonds. Markets for other kinds of assets, such as common shares, corporate bonds, and currencies themselves are often more volatile. When investors shift out of several kinds of assets in a particular country at the same time, the results can be devastating. In Mexico in 1994–1995 and several South Asian countries in 1997–1998, such a retreat drove the value of national currencies down by 50% or more, creating a crisis that shrank the economies of Indonesia, South Korea, Laos, and Thailand by 20% or more in a year

(Bhutta *et al.* 2009: 126) and plunging millions of people into poverty and insecurity. At least in the case of the South Asian crisis, speculation by major investment banks and hedge funds – unregulated vehicles for ultra-wealthy private investors – against the Thai baht, played an important role in triggering the crisis. The power dynamics were captured by the then-managing director of the IMF in a speech shortly after the start of the Mexican crisis: "Countries that successfully attract large capital inflows must also bear in mind that their continued access to international capital is far from automatic, and the conditions attached to that access are not guaranteed. The decisive factor here is market perceptions: whether the country's policies are deemed basically sound and its economic future, promising. The corollary is that shifts in the market's perception of these underlying fundamentals can be quite swift, brutal, and destabilizing" (Camdessus 1995). Investor perceptions may or may not in fact be directly related to conditions within a country. Notably, in advance of the events of 2002, Brazil's economy had already been battered and its currency driven down in value by almost 40% between December 1998 and September 1999 as investors reacted to the South Asian crisis and a 1998 Russian debt default by selling off assets throughout the so-called emerging economies, even though actual connections between Brazil's economy and those of South Asia and Russia were minimal (Gruben and Kiser 1999; Goldfajn and Baig 2000; Desai 2003: 136–55).

A full historical account of these and similar crises would situate them with reference to the longer pattern of lending by the high-income countries, which led to successive "debt crises" starting in 1982 (Strange 1998), and to the era of structural adjustment. This historical account would also need to examine the origins of domestic economic mismanagement that often contributed to financial crises, while taking a more nuanced view of the relations between financial market constraints and public policy than is possible here – notably, focusing on how those constraints lend credibility to domestic interests seeking to advance market-orientated policies on the grounds that these are the only ones that "work" in an era of globalization (Fourcade-Gourinchas and Babb 2002; Leiva 2008: chapters 4, 5). For present purposes, it suffices to note that financial crises increase poverty, hardship, and economic inequality in several ways (Halac and Schmukler 2004: 2–3). The distributional effects of increased unemployment, loss of jobs and, in the formal sector, sharp declines in wages for those who remain employed and in labor's share of national income (World Bank 2000: chapter 2; Diwan 2001) are compounded by the fact that employment consistently recovers more slowly than economic output in the aftermath of financial crises (van der Hoeven and Lübker 2006; Walton 2009). This time lag may partly result from the public sector austerity programs and contractionary fiscal policies that governments find necessary to adopt in order to restore the confidence of investors (or the IMF, if has been called on to lend to crisis-hit economies). For example, effects of the 1997–1998 financial crisis on output and employment in Indonesia and Thailand were "exacerbated by the initial insistence of the IMF that governments return a fiscal surplus of 1 percent of GDP" (Hopkins 2006: 354; see also Bullard *et al.* 1998; Desai 2003: 212–41).

Further magnification of economic inequality results from the public bail-outs of financial institutions that commonly follow financial crises. These normally transfer wealth from a broad segment of the population (the national tax base financing the bail-out) to a minority of households with substantial deposits; debtors whose loans are subsequently forgiven; and financial institution shareholders (Halac and Schmukler 2004). In Mexico, by 2003, post-1995 bail-outs had cost the public "[US]$103 billion, or 16 percent of Mexico's GDP in the same year" (Mannsberger and McBride 2007: 328). This took place in a country where only 25% of the population has even a checking account (Skelton 2008), representing what one observer identifies as a recurring pattern of social-ization of financial risk in Mexico (Marois 2011). The cost of the bail-outs was kept from rising even higher only by the sell-off of most of Mexico's commercial banks to foreign firms, which provided a desperately needed infusion of capital.

Capital Flight

Soros' distinction between "the Americans" and "the Brazilians" (i.e., foreign as distinct from domestic investors) may have been accurate as it applied to the specific case he was describing, but it should not be generalized to other contexts. This is largely because of the phenomenon of capital flight: the process in which residents of a country transfer their assets abroad "to evade domestic social control over their assets" in the form of taxation or regulation (Ndikumana and Boyce 1998: 199; see also Beja 2006: 265). The definition of capital flight is contested. Many definitions refer only to illicit (illegal or questionably legal) transfers of assets, in particular for purposes of tax evasion. Illicit transactions are an important element of capital flight, but it must be recognized that large-scale *legal* transfers of financial assets in search of higher returns or lower risks can have comparably destructive consequences (as in the Mexican case cited earlier, to which Mexican investors clearly contributed).

In any event, capital flight is not a new phenomenon, but it has been facilitated by financial liberalization and deregulation and the provision of shelters for flight capital in the financial institutions (and real estate markets) of high-income countries and offshore financial centers. Estimates of the magnitude of capital fight are substantial, although not always directly comparable because of methodological variations. Pastor (1990) esti-mated capital flight from Argentina, Brazil, Chile, Colombia, Mexico, Peru, Uruguay, and Venezuela between 1973 and 1985 at US$151 billlion. Loungani and Mauro (2001) estimated capital flight from Russia post 1994 at $15–20 billion per year, or approxi-mately $100–150 per capita – a figure that is nothing short of astonishing when compared with Russia's post-collapse gross domestic product (GDP)/capita of $1770 in 2000. Beja (2006) estimated the accumulated value of capital flight ("unrecorded" capital flows) plus imputed interest from Indonesia, Malaysia, the Philippines, and Thailand over the period 1970–2000 at $1 trillion. (The imputation of interest, at a conservative rate, reflects the assumption that assets were earning a return after their departure from the origin country.) Perhaps most strikingly given the poverty of sub-Saharan Africa, using simi-lar methods Ndikumana and Boyce (2011b) estimated the value of capital flight from 33 sub-Saharan countries, plus imputed interest, between 1970 and 2008 at $944 billion (in 2008 dollars), with much of this figure related to straightforward looting through mis-appropriation of loans and trade misinvoicing. To put this figure in perspective, compare the annual value of (only partially fulfilled) pledges of additional development assistance to Africa made by the G8 in 2005 – $25 billion – with the estimated $49 billion annual value of capital flight from the region between 2000 and 2008 (Ndikumana 2010).

Capital flight is an important consideration in the context of social determinants of health for several reasons. Capital flight deprives countries of resources that might oth-erwise be made available for their own economic development, and for investing in the health and education of their populations. Although hypothetical and complicated by Russia's deteriorating political institutions, one wonders how much less painful and health-destructive the years after the collapse of the Soviet economy (Field *et al.* 2000; Shkolnikov *et al.* 2004) might have been if newly minted multimillionaires had somehow been prevented from shifting their wealth abroad during the 1990s. The distributional effects of capital flight are inherently regressive: it is by definition available only to a minority of the population – those with liquid assets – and disproportionately only available to a minority of the minority. For example, out of Brazil's population of 195 million, in 2010 an estimated 155,000 were "high net worth individuals" with investable assets of more than $1 million in 2010. In all of Africa (population 1 billion) there were approximately 100,000, with "ultra-high net worth individuals" (investable assets of more than $30 million), constituting an even smaller number (103,000 of the world's nearly 7 billion people) (Capgemini and Merrill Lynch Wealth Management 2011).

Especially pernicious is the relation between capital flight and the external debt that has been a debilitating drain on many LMIC public treasuries since the 1980s, despite successive tranches of partial debt forgiveness (Hurley 2007). Economic historian Thomas Naylor (1987: 370) concluded flatly that "[t]here would be no 'debt crisis' without large-scale capital flight." Debt burdens associated with external borrowing are borne by a country's entire population, directly or in the form of lost services and transfers, as governments give priority to repaying creditors; meanwhile, capital flight enables elites to socialize the cost of accumulating private fortunes (Rodriguez 1987: 136–7; Pastor 1990: 6–7). Pastor estimated that more than 40% of the increase in Latin American debt during the period he studied financed capital flight, and Ndikumana and Boyce (2011a: 64) conclude that "for every dollar of foreign loans to sub-Saharan Africa, *roughly 60 cents flow back out as capital flight in the same year*" (emphasis in original). Comparison with the external debt that continues to be a debilitating drain on many public treasuries is instructive: their estimate of the accumulated value of flight capital from the countries they studied is more than five times the value of those countries' external debts (Ndikumana and Boyce 2011a: 96).

A final consequence of capital flight is that even its anticipation may constrain social policy. John Williamson, who coined the phrase "the Washington consensus" to describe the dominant development policy agenda of the 1980s, observed in 2004 that while "levying heavier taxes on the rich so as to increase social spending that benefits disproportionately the poor" is conceptually attractive in Latin America, where many countries historically have had some of the world's most unequal distributions of income, "it would not be practical to push this very far, because too many of the Latin rich have the option of placing too many of their assets in Miami" (Williamson 2004).

The Crisis of 2008

The financial crisis that spread across the world starting in 2008 was unlike the crises of the previous decades, not only in its scale, but also because it began with a failure of domestic economic policy in the United States. The collapse of the largely unregulated market for securities backed by high-risk US mortgages quickly spread through the highly leveraged US financial services sector (FCIC 2011: xix–xx) and to other high-income countries, revealing what the Bank of England described with masterful understatement as "underappreciated, but potent, interconnections between firms in the global financial system" (Bank of England 2008: 9). The combination of reduced government revenues and heavy borrowing to finance stimulus spending, and the rising cost of social protection, contributed to the subsequent sovereign debt crises that (as of early 2012) threatened several Eurozone economies. The crisis represented the externalization, on an unprecedented global scale, of the cost of accumulating fortunes in the financial services industry, in the same way that a polluting factory externalizes its owners' costs of production. Although on a larger scale, the events of 2008 resembled those described in the previous section of this chapter, in that their costs were mainly borne by relatively vulnerable people, some half a world away and others geographically close to the origins of the crisis, who had no role in creating it or control over its progress.

Only a few impacts can be cited here. Worldwide, an estimated 35 million people were thrown out of work (Calvo 2010). Mexico experienced "arguably the worst year of economic downturn … since the onset of the Great Depression" (Cypher 2010: 51), and a former Under-Secretary General of the United Nations warned of "another lost half-decade of development" in Latin America as a whole (Ocampo 2009: 706). In LMICs, the initial response of social protection systems was described as "limited" and inadequately directed toward the most vulnerable (McCord 2010). A 2011 UNICEF review found that after an initial period of expansionary fiscal policy, many LMICs were considering such austerity measures as limiting or rolling back wages for teachers and health workers, retrenching existing social protection transfers, and increasing consumption taxes on basic goods like food (Ortiz *et al.* 2011). This was true despite evidence that (for instance) the combined effects of the financial crisis and a concurrent spike in food prices were undermining food security, putting households under strain and increasing social exclusion in Bangladesh, Indonesia, Jamaica, Kenya, Nigeria, Yemen, and Zambia, often with disproportionate impacts on women and children (Hossain and McGregor 2011; Samuels *et al.* 2011).

In high-income and transition economies, officially reported unemployment rose by mid- 2011 to 14% in Ireland and 20% in Spain (46% among those under 25) and Latvia, three European countries especially hard hit. In Belarus, Greece, Hungary, Ireland, Latvia, Portugal, and Ukraine, IMF conditionalities and associated austerity measures were in place by mid 2011 – arguably compounding the damage done during the early stages of the crisis by IMF policies that actually worsened output losses (Weisbrot and Montecino 2010). At its epicenter, the crisis produced a largely invisible army of people dispossessed by foreclosure: members of more than 14 million US households, a substantial proportion of them consisting of renters (Sassen 2011); by mid 2011 a record 45 million people were receiving federal government food vouchers (Supplemental Nutrition Assistance, or food stamps) and millions more were eligible (FRAC 2011). Thus, the financial crisis has "brought the war home" to several high-income and transition economies through high levels of unemployment as well as forms of public sector austerity, external influence over domestic policy, and cartographies of inequality more familiar from LMIC contexts. Although the point cannot be explored further here, the effect is likely to be intensification of new patterns of economic inequality associated with three decades of labor market integration.

Evidence on Health Outcomes

The complexity of the connections between macro-scale social processes and individual health outcomes complicates efforts to demonstrate or anticipate health impacts. Some evidence of adverse effects on social determinants of health has been described (see also Chapter 14). In a review of research on health impacts of the less dramatic South Asian financial crisis of 1997–1998, which resulted in one-year reductions in economic output of 20% in some affected economies, Hopkins (2006) described a reversal of past health gains and a deterioration in such indicators as undernutrition, household spending on healthcare, and public spending on health. In 2011, an increase in suicide rates and a decline in self-reported health and in access to health insurance was reported over the very short term in Greece (Kentikelenis *et al.* 2011). The most extreme recent example of an economic crisis with major, clearly documented health impacts is the post-1991 collapse of the former Soviet economy, involving a reduction in economic output of roughly 50%, massive capital flight, official poverty levels of 40%, the disintegration of healthcare and social provision, and a decline of several years in male life expectancy (Field 2000; Field *et al.* 2000; Shkolnikov *et al.* 2004; Leon *et al.* 2009). "In 2004, a Russian boy aged 15 had about a 50–50 chance of surviving to the age of 60; this was much worse than many so-called developing countries, for instance Pakistan, India and Bangladesh" (Vågerö 2010: 26). The most drastic increases were in deaths from violence, cardiovascular disease, and liver disease – proximately related to a drastic increase in alcohol consumption – but alcohol consumption is far from the entire story. Alcohol consumption alone cannot explain increases in undernutrition, diphtheria, and tuberculosis, and should itself be treated as a consequence of economic implosion and social disintegration; further, the stresses associated with those processes are likely to have had a substantial and independent effect on health (Marmot and Bobak 2000).

Financial crises are only one driver of the "disequalizing" dynamics of contemporary globalization (Birdsall 2006). It is therefore useful to consider findings from an innovative econometric exercise aimed at capturing the overall, longer term impact of these dynamics. Using data from 136 countries, Cornia and colleagues (2009) identified a range of social and economic variables with a demonstrated effect on mortality, classifying them as: (i) related to policy choices made in the context of globalization (e.g., income inequality); (ii) endogenous, and therefore unrelated to globalization for purposes of the analysis (the diffusion of medical progress); or (iii) describable as "shocks" (e.g., wars and natural disasters, HIV/AIDS). They then carried out a simulation comparing trends in life expectancy at birth (LEB, an admittedly crude indicator) over the period 1980–2000 with those that would be predicted based on a counterfactual set of assumptions in which trends in all the relevant variables either remained at the 1980 value or continued the trend they followed between 1960 and 1980. Worldwide, globalization post 1980 canceled out most of the progress toward better health that occurred as a consequence of diffusion of medical progress. Regionally, the most conspicuous declines in life expectancy occurred in the transition economies, where globalization accounted for essentially the entire decline, and sub-Saharan Africa, where globalization contributed almost as much as the HIV/AIDS epidemic to a decline of nearly nine years in LEB relative to the counterfactual. Although cautious about inferring direct causation, the authors conclude that "the negative association found between liberalisation-globalisation policies, poor economic performance and unsatisfactory health trends … seems to be robust" (Cornia *et al.* 2009: 58). In other words, even when health gains were achieved, they were often less substantial than they might have been under an alternative set of economic and political conditions in which the gains from growth were distributed more widely, and in some regions the economic and political context has almost certainly contributed to absolute declines in life expectancy.

Assessing the health impact of the workings of financial markets in specific cases unavoidably raises a standard of proof issue. In the case of discrete events like major financial crises, epidemiologists might prefer to set up an elegant (and expensive) longitudinal study of multiple crisis-affected populations, attempt to control for all confounders, and then wait 10 or 20 years in the hope that the casualties, their survivors, or someone will still be interested in the answers. Such a study of how (for instance) capital flight or its anticipation influence public policy would be impossible, raising the prospect that (like Godot) sufficient evidence of destructive consequences for health will never arrive. I regard this approach as ethically irresponsible, rather taking it as given, based on the best available evidence – as did the World Health Organization Commission on Social Determinants of Health (2008) – that events, processes, and policies that create, magnify, or perpetuate poverty and economic insecurity for literally billions of the world's people (cf. Paluzzi and Farmer 2005) are likely to impair their health. Readers who disagree must recognize their disagreement as one that is less about the strength of evidence than about the values that should be brought to bear on policy choices that affect health under conditions of uncertainty, and that such uncertainty may be resolvable, if at all, only by waiting years or decades for the body count (Page 1978; Marmot 2000).

Conclusions and Policy Implications

Generically, the effects of globalized finance on health inequity and the ability of governments to reduce it by way of action on social determinants of health underscore the need for what international relations scholar Richard Falk (1996: 13) has called "a regulatory framework for global market forces that is people-centred rather than capital-driven." The policy space available to LMIC governments in particular is often limited, but it is worth noting (for example) that deterioration in living standards and social determinants of health after the Asian financial crisis appears to have been less severe and shorter lived in Malaysia, which explicitly rejected the neoliberal prescriptions of the IMF in favor of capital controls (Cornia 2006; Hopkins 2006). Thus, it is important to rethink the now-conventional resistance to such measures, and – perhaps even more importantly – to devise effective mechanisms of international cooperation to limit capital flight and repatriate flight capital under conditions ensuring that it will be used for broadly beneficial purposes, rather than simply reappropriated by a new set of elites.

Within the high-income world, policies to reduce the likelihood of repeats of 2008 are not overly complicated: for example, financial institutions must not be allowed to become "too big to fail" (Bank of England 2009: 10; Hoenig 2011; Johnson and Kwak 2011: 153–88). However, the financial services industry invested a great deal in creating and defending the unregulated (but highly profitable) environment that allowed the crises to occur – for example, securing federal legislation in the United States to block state-level efforts to regulate mortgage lending (FCIC 2011: xviii; Immergluck 2011). Indeed, the issuing, securitizing, and selling-on of subprime mortgages that triggered the crisis arguably represents a new economic strategy based on "an efficient mechanism for getting at the savings of households worldwide ... that moves faster than extracting profits from lowering wages" (Sassen 2009: 412; see also Newman 2009). Perhaps predictably, by early 2012 the (still unregulated) US market for mortgage-backed securities was making a comeback (Ahmed 2012).

Specifics of the design of national and supranational institutions to regulate finance are beyond the scope of this chapter, but the issues must not be off limits to health research and advocacy. Given what is known about social determinants of health, it now is (or should be) axiomatic that many of the most important influences on health, and on health disparities, have little or nothing to do with the provision of healthcare and the operation of health ministries or health systems. Rather, they are influenced by the choices of ministries of finance, trade, and social policy; by international institutions like the IMF; and by private actors like bond market investors, credit rating agencies, and the packagers of mortgage-backed securities. Health researchers and practitioners cannot be expected to become expert in these areas, but they should acquire sufficient familiarity with macro-scale social processes, economic and social policy choices, and the human consequences of a global economic policy regime that cedes power to markets to engage proactively in the relevant policy debates. In other words, global finance is a public health issue.

Key Reading

Calhoun C, Derluguian G (eds). 2011. *Business as Usual: The Roots of the Global Financial Meltdown*; the Deepening Crisis: Governance Challenges after Neoliberalism and *After-math: A New Global Economic Order?*, 3 vols. New York: Social Science Research Council and New York University Press.

FCIC (Financial Crisis Inquiry Commission). 2011. *The Financial Crisis Inquiry Report*. Washington, DC: US Government Printing Office. http://www.gpo.gov/fdsys/pkg/GPO-FCIC/pdf/GPO-FCIC.pdf (last accessed December 2013).

Hopkins S. 2006. Economic stability and health status: evidence from East Asia before and after the 1990s economic crisis. *Health Policy* 75, 347–57.

Mosley L. 2003. *Global Capital and National Governments*. Cambridge: Cambridge University Press.

Naylor RT. 1987. *Hot Money: Peekaboo Finance and the Politics of Debt*. Toronto: McClelland and Stewart.

Ndikumana L, Boyce J. 2011. *Africa's Odious Debts: How Foreign Loans and Capital Flight Bled a Continent*. London: Zed Books.

Sassen S. 1996. *Losing Control? Sovereignty in an Age of Globalization*. New York: Columbia University Press.

References

Ahmed A. 2012. *Bonds backed by mortgages regain allure*. Dealbook. http://dealbook.nytimes.com/2012/02/18/bonds-backed-by-mortgages-regain-allure/?hp (last accessed December 2013).

Amann E, Baer W. 2006. Economic orthodoxy versus social development? The dilemmas facing Brazil's labour government. *Oxford Development Studies* 34, 219–241.

Bank of England. 2008. *Financial Stability Report*. Report No. 24. London: Bank of England. http://www.bankofengland.co.uk/publications/fsr/2008/fsrfull0810.pdf (last accessed December 2013).

Bank of England. 2009. *Financial Stability Report*. Report No. 25. London: Bank of England. http://www.bankofengland.co.uk/publications/fsr/2009/fsrfull0906.pdf (last accessed December 2013).

Barnet RJ, Müller RE. 1974. *Global Reach: The Power of the Multinational Corporations*. New York: Touchstone.

Beja EL. 2006. Was capital fleeing Southeast Asia? Estimates from Indonesia, Malaysia, the Philippines, and Thailand. *Asia Pacific Business Review* 12, 261–83.

Bhutta ZA, Bawany FA, Feroze A, Rizvi A, Thapa SJ, Patel M. 2009. Effects of the crises on child nutrition and health in East Asia and the Pacific. *Global Social Policy* 9, 119–43.

Birdsall N. 2006. *The World is Not Flat: Inequality and Injustice in our Global Economy*. WIDER Annual Lecture No. 9. Helsinki: World Institute for Development Economics Research. http://www.wider.unu.edu/publications/annual-lectures/en_GB/AL9/_files/78121127186268214/default/annual-lecture-2005.pdf (last accessed December 2013).

Bullard N, Bello W, Malhotra K. 1998. Taming the tigers: the IMF and the Asian crisis. *Third World Quarterly* 19, 505–56.

Calvo SG. 2010. *The Global Financial Crisis of 2008–10: A View from the Social Sectors*. Human Development Research Paper No. 2010/18. New York: United Nations Development Programme. http://hdr.undp.org/en/reports/global/hdr2010/papers/HDRP_2010_18.pdf (last accessed December 2013).

Camdessus M. 1995. *The IMF and the Challenges of Globalization – The Fund's Evolving Approach to its Constant Mission: The Case of Mexico*. Address at Zurich Economics Society. Washington, DC: International Monetary Fund. http://www.imf.org/external/np/sec/mds/1995/mds9517.htm (last accessed December 2013).

Capgemini and Merrill Lynch Wealth Management. 2011. *World Wealth Report 2011*. New York: Merrill Lynch Global Wealth Management.

Commission on Social Determinants of Health. 2008. *Closing the Gap in a Generation: Health Equity through Action on the Social Determinants of Health (Final Report)*. Geneva: World Health Organization. http://whqlibdoc.who.int/publications/2008/9789241563703_eng.pdf (last accessed December 2013).

Cornia GA. 2006. Harnessing globalisation for children: main findings and policy-programme proposals. In Cornia GA (ed.) *Harnessing Globalisation for Children: A Report to UNICEF*, chapter 1. Florence: UNICEF Innocenti Research Centre. http://www.unicef-irc.org/research/ESP/globalization/ (last accessed December 2013).

Cornia GA., Rosignoli S, Tiberti L. 2009. An empirical investigation of the relation between globalization and health. In Labonté R, Schrecker T, Packer C, Runnels V (eds) *Globalization and Health: Pathways, Evidence and Policy*, pp. 34–62. New York: Routledge.

Cypher JM. 2010. Mexico's economic collapse. *NACLA Report on the Americas* 43(4), 51–3.

Desai P. 2003. *Financial Crisis, Contagion, and Containment: From Asia to Argentina*. Princeton, NJ: Princeton University Press.

Dicken P. 2007. *Global Shift: Reshaping the Global Economic Map in the 21st Century*, 5th edn. New York: Guilford Press.

Diwan I. 2001. *Debt as Sweat: Labor, Financial Crises, and the Globalization of Capital*. Washington, DC: World Bank. http://info.worldbank.org/etools/docs/voddocs/150/332/diwan.pdf (last accessed December 2013).

Evans P. 2005. Neoliberalism as a political opportunity: constraint and innovation in contemporary development strategy. In Gallagher K (ed.) *Putting Development First: The Importance of Policy Space in the WTO and IFIs*, pp. 195–215. London: Zed Books.

Falk R. 1996. An inquiry into the political economy of world order. *New Political Economy* 1, 13–26.

FCIC (Financial Crisis Inquiry Commission). 2011. *The Financial Crisis Inquiry Report*. Washington, DC: US Government Printing Office. http://www.gpo.gov/fdsys/pkg/GPO-FCIC/pdf/GPO-FCIC.pdf (last accessed December 2013).

Field MG. 2000. The health and demographic crisis in post-Soviet Russia: a two-phase development. In Field MG, Twigg JL (eds) *Russia's Torn Safety Nets: Health and Social Welfare during the Transition*, pp. 11–42. New York: St Martin's Press.

Field MG, Kotz DM, Bukhman G. 2000. Neoliberal economic policy, "state desertion," and the Russian health crisis. In Kim JY, Millen JV, Irwin A, Gershman J (eds) *Dying for Growth: Global Inequality and the Health of the Poor*, pp. 155–73. Monroe, ME: Common Courage Press.

Fourcade-Gourinchas M, Babb SL. 2002. The rebirth of the liberal creed: paths to neoliberalism in four countries. *American Journal of Sociology* 108, 533–79.

FRAC (Food Research and Action Center). 2011. *45.1 million Americans received SNAP/Food Stamps in June 2011*. http://frac.org/reports-and-resources/snapfood-stamp-monthly-participation-data/ (last accessed December 2013).

Galeano E. 2000. *Upside Down: A Primer for the Looking glass World*. New York: Picador.

Girón A, Correa E. 1999. Global financial markets: financial deregulation and crises. *International Social Science Journal*, 51, 183–194.

Goldfajn I. 2003. *The Brazilian Crisis, the Role of the IMF and Democratic Governability*. Madrid: Club Madrid. http://archivo.clubmadrid.org/cmadrid/fileadmin/Brazil_paper_Goldfajn_2_revised _Oct_20_2003.pdf (last accessed December 2013).

Goldfajn I, Baig T. 2000. *The Russian Default and the Contagion to Brazil*. Washington, DC: International Monetary Fund.

Griffith-Jones S, Stallings B. 1995. New global financial trends: implications for development. In Stallings B (ed.) *Global Change, Regional Response: The New International Context of Development*, pp. 143–73. Cambridge: Cambridge University Press.

Gruben WC, Kiser S. 1999. Brazil: the first financial crisis of 1999. *Southwest Economy* March/April, 13–14.

Halac M, Schmukler SL. 2004. Distributional effects of crises: the financial channel [with comments]. *Economía* 5, 1–67.

Helleiner E. 1994. Freeing money: why have states been more willing to liberalize capital controls than trade barriers? *Policy Sciences* 27, 299–318.

Hilton I. 2002. Lula, or something worse: with Latin America rejecting neo-liberalism, the US may have to stomach a leftwing president in Brazil. *Guardian* September 20. http://www.theguardian. com/world/2002/sep/20/brazil.comment (last accessed December 2013).

Hoenig T. 2011. *Financial reform: Post crisis?* Address to Women in Housing and Finance, Washington, DC. http://www.kansascityfed.org/publicat/speeches/hoenig-DC-Women-Housing-Finance-2-23-11.pdf (last accessed December 2013).

Hopkins S. 2006. Economic stability and health status: evidence from East Asia before and after the 1990s economic crisis. *Health Policy* 75, 347–57.

Hossain N, McGregor JA. 2011. A "lost generation"? Impacts of complex compound crises on children and young people. *Development Policy Review* 29, 565–84.

Hurley G. 2007. *Multilateral Debt: One Step Forward, How Many Back?* Brussels: European Network on Debt and Development (EURODAD). http://www.jubileescotland.org.uk/ sites/default/files/Eurodad%20-%20Multilateral%20Debt,%20one%20step%20forward,%20 how%20many%20back.pdf (last accessed December 2013).

Immergluck D. 2011. The local wreckage of global capital: the subprime crisis, federal policy and high-foreclosure neighborhoods in the US. *International Journal of Urban and Regional Research* 35, 130–46.

Johnson S, Kwak J. 2011. *13 Bankers: The Wall Street Takeover and the Next Financial Meltdown*. New York: Vintage.

Kentikelenis A, Karanikolos M, Papanicolas I, Basu S, McKee M, Stuckler D. 2011. Health effects of financial crisis: omens of a Greek tragedy. *Lancet* 378, 1457–8.

Koelble T, Lipuma E. 2006. The effects of circulatory capitalism on democratization: Observations from South Africa and Brazil. *Democratization* 13, 605–31.

Koivusalo M, Schrecker T, Labonté R. 2009. Globalization and policy space for health and social determinants of health. In Labonté R, Schrecker T, Packer C, Runnels V (eds) *Globalization and Health: Pathways, Evidence and Policy*, pp. 105–30. New York: Routledge.

Leiva FI. 2008. *Latin American Neostructuralism: The Contradictions of Post-Neoliberal Development*. Minneapolis, MN: University of Minnesota Press.

Leon DA., Shkolnikov VM, McKee M. 2009. Alcohol and Russian mortality: a continuing crisis. *Addiction* 104, 1630–6.

Loungani P, Mauro P. 2001. Capital flight from Russia. *World Economy* 24, 689–706.

Makin JH. 1984. *The Global Debt Crisis: America's Growing Involvement*. New York: Basic Books.

Mannsberger J, McBride JB. 2007. The privatization of the Mexican banking sector in the 1990s: from debacle to disappointment. *International Journal of Emerging Markets* 2, 320–34.

Marmot M. 2000. Inequalities in health: causes and policy implications. In Tarlov A, St Peter A (eds) *The Society and Population Health Reader, Vol. 2: A State and Community Perspective*, pp. 293–309. New York: New Press.

Marmot M, Bobak M. 2000. Psychological and biological mechanisms behind the recent mortality crisis in Central and Eastern Europe. In Cornia GA, Paniccia R (eds) *The Mortality Crisis of Transitional Economies*, pp. 127–48. Oxford: Oxford University Press.

Marois T. 2011. *The Socialization of Financial Risk in Neoliberal Mexico*. Research on Money and Finance Discussion Paper No. 25. London: School of Oriental and African Studies, University of London. http://eprints.soas.ac.uk/11060/1/RMF-25-Marois.pdf (last accessed December 2013).

McCord A. 2010. The impact of the global financial crisis on social protection in developing countries. *International Social Security Review* 63, 31–45.

Morais L, Saad-Filho A. 2005. Lula and the continuity of neoliberalism in Brazil: strategic choice, economic imperative or political schizophrenia? *Historical Materialism* 13, 3–32.

Mosley L. 2003. *Global Capital and National Governments*. Cambridge: Cambridge University Press.

Mosley L. 2006. Constraints, opportunities, and information: financial market–government relations around the world. In Bardhan P, Bowles S, Wallerstein M (eds) *Globalization and Egalitarian Redistribution*, pp. 87–119. New York and Princeton, NJ: Russell Sage Foundation and Princeton University Press.

Naylor RT. 1987. *Hot Money: Peekaboo Finance and the Politics of Debt*. Toronto: McClelland and Stewart.

Ndikumana L. 2010. *Illicit capital flows from Africa – three problems for Africa*. Presented at the United Nations Economic Commission for Africa–African Union Conference of Ministers of Finance, Lilongwe, Malawi, March 29–30. http://www.slideserve.com/kathie/illicit-capital-flows-from-africa-three-problems-for-africa (last accessed December 2013).

Ndikumana L, Boyce JK. 1998. Congo's odious debt: external borrowing and capital flight in Zaire. *Development and Change* 29, 195–217.

Ndikumana L, Boyce JK. 2011a. *Africa's Odious Debts: How Foreign Loans and Capital Flight Bled a Continent*. London: Zed Books.

Ndikumana L, Boyce JK. 2011b. Capital flight from sub-Saharan Africa: linkages with external borrowing and policy options. *International Review of Applied Economics* 25, 149–70.

Newman K. 2009. Post-industrial widgets: capital flows and the production of the urban. *International Journal of Urban and Regional Research* 33, 314–31.

Ocampo JA. 2009. Latin America and the global financial crisis. *Cambridge Journal of Economics* 33, 703–24.

Ortiz I, Chai J, Cummins M. 2011. *Austerity Measures Threaten Children and Poor Households: Recent Evidence in Public Expenditures from 128 Developing Countries*. Social and Economic Policy Working Paper. New York: UNICEF.

Page T. 1978. A generic view of toxic chemicals and similar risks. *Ecology Law Quarterly* 7, 207–44.

Paiva P. 2006. Lula's political economy: changes and challenges. *Annals of the American Academy of Political and Social Science* 606, 196–215.

Paluzzi JE, Farmer PE. 2005. The wrong question. *Development* 48(1), 12–18.

Pastor MJ. 1990. Capital flight from Latin America. *World Development* 18, 1–18.

Przeworski A, Bardhan P, Bresser Pereira LC et al. 1995. *Sustainable Democracy*. Cambridge: Cambridge University Press.

Rodriguez MA. 1987. Consequences of capital flight for Latin American debtor countries. In Lessard DR, Williamson J (eds) *Capital Flight and Third World Debt*, pp. 129–52. Washington, DC: Institute for International Economics.

Samuels F, Gavrilovic M, Harper C, Niño-Zarazúa M. 2011. *Food, finance and fuel: the impacts of the triple F crisis in Nigeria, with a particular focus on women and children*, Background Note. London: Overseas Development Institute. http://www.odi.org.uk/resources/docs/7359.pdf (last accessed December 2013).

Santiso J. 2004. *Wall Street and Emerging Democracies: Financial Markets and the Brazilian Presidential Elections*. AUP Visiting Scholar Working Paper No. 12. Paris: American University of Paris.

Sassen S. 2003. Economic globalization and the redrawing of citizenship. In Friedman J (ed.) *Globalization, the State, and Violence*, pp. 67–86. Walnut Creek,CA: AltaMira Press.

Sassen S. 2009. When local housing becomes an electronic instrument: the global circulation of mortgages – a research note. *International Journal of Urban and Regional Research* 33, 411–26.

Sassen S. 2011. *Beyond social exclusion: new logics of expulsion*. Presented to the 6th Annual Research Conference on Homelessness in Europe: Homelessness, Migration and Demographic Change in Europe, Pisa, Italy [video]. http://www.dailymotion.com/video/xl7upb_saskia-sassen-logics-of-expulsion-a-savage-sorting-of-winners-and-losers_news (last accessed December 2013).

Schiller D. 1999. *Digital Capitalism: Networking the Global Market System*. Cambridge, MA: MIT Press.

Schrecker T. 2009. The power of money: global financial markets, national politics, and social determinants of health. In Williams OD, Kay A (eds) *Global Health Governance: Crisis, Institutions and Political Economy*, pp. 160–81. Houndmills: Palgrave Macmillan.

Shkolnikov VM., Andreev EM, Leon DA, McKee M, Meslé F, Vallin J. 2004. Mortality reversal in Russia: the story so far. *Hygiea Internationalis* 4, 29–80.

Sinclair TJ. 1994. Between state and market: hegemony and institutions of collective action under conditions of international capital mobility. *Policy Sciences* 27, 447–66.

Skelton EC. 2008. Reaching Mexico's unbanked. *Economic Letter: Insights from the Federal Reserve Bank of Dallas* 3, 7.

Soares FV. 2011. Brazil's Bolsa família: a review. *Economic and Political Weekly* 46, 55–60.

Stiglitz JE. 2004. Capital-market liberalization, globalization, and the IMF. *Oxford Review of Economic Policy* 20, 57–71.

Strange S. 1998. The new world of debt. *New Left Review* 230, 91–114.

Vågerö D. 2010. The east–west health divide in Europe: growing and shifting eastwards. *European Review* 18, 1, 23–34.

Van der Hoeven R, Lübker M. 2006. *Financial Openness and Employment: The Need for Coherent International and National Policies*. Working Paper No. 75. Geneva: Policy Integration Department, International Labour Office. http://www.ilo.org/wcmsp5/groups/public/—dgreports/—integration/documents/publication/wcms_079179.pdf (last accessed December 2013).

Victora CG, Barreto ML, do Carmo Leal M *et al.* 2011. Health conditions and health-policy innovations in Brazil: the way forward. *Lancet* 377, 2042–53.

Walton M. 2009. Macroeconomic policy, markets, and poverty reduction. In Bane MJ, Zenteno R (eds) *Poverty and Poverty Alleviation Strategies in North America*, pp. 65–114. Cambridge, MA: Harvard University David Rockefeller Center for Latin American Studies.

Weisbrot M, Montecino J. 2010. *The IMF and Economic Recovery: Is Fund Policy Contributing to Downside Risks?* Washington, DC: Center for Economic Policy Research. http://www.policyarchive.org/handle/10207/bitstreams/95891.pdf (last accessed December 2013).

Williamson J. 2004. *The Washington consensus as policy prescription for development*. World Bank Practitioners for Development Lecture Series. Washington, DC: Institute for International Economics. http://www.iie.com/publications/papers/williamson0204.pdf (last accessed December 2013).

World Bank. 2000. *Global Economic Prospects and the Developing Countries 2000*. Washington, DC: World Bank.

Chapter 22

Trade Rules and Intellectual Property Protection for Pharmaceuticals

Valbona Muzaka

Abstract

Certain trade and intellectual property (IP) rules agreed at the World Trade Organization (WTO), or in bilateral and regional trade agreements, have had an important impact upon access to medicines, especially in the developing world. Most changes in the area of pharmaceutical IP protection were set in motion through the WTO Trade-Related Aspects of Intellectual Property Rights (TRIPS) agreement, which was not negotiated with public health or other social goals in mind. TRIPS and "TRIPS plus" IP pharmaceutical provisions pose significant challenges to expanding affordable access to medicines. Awareness about such detrimental consequences has informed the contests related to IP and access to medicines from the late 1990s onwards. These contests have led to some, albeit qualified, successes, although many issues still remain unresolved. More broadly, most of the problems that present themselves at the intersection of trade rules, IP protection, and pharmaceuticals stem from two seemingly irreconcilable frameworks. The first seeks to fashion trade and IP rules regarding pharmaceuticals as a matter of competitiveness; this framework is central to the United States and European Union (EU) positions. The second seeks to subdue trade and pharmaceutical IP rules to the achievement of public health goals. Any efforts to improve healthcare worldwide would have to include a reassessment of the social purpose of intellectual property rights: in the case of pharmaceuticals, public access to life-saving medicines.

The Handbook of Global Health Policy, First Edition. Edited by Garrett W. Brown, Gavin Yamey, and Sarah Wamala.
© 2014 John Wiley & Sons, Ltd. Published 2014 by John Wiley & Sons, Ltd.

Key Points

- The WTO TRIPS agreement brought about significant changes to pharmaceutical IP protection rules, many of which restrict the availability of affordable medicines worldwide.
- TRIPS was negotiated on behalf of specific commercial interests and not with public health concerns in mind.
- Resistance against expansive pharmaceutical IP protection has achieved only some qualified successes.
- As a result of the powerful interests involved and the high stakes involved, contests over IP and access to medicines are likely to continue in the future.
- Any positive solution for patients worldwide requires a return to IPRs as tools and incentives that are ultimately granted for the benefit of the society.

Key Policy Implications

- A new approach to pharmaceutical IP rule-making is needed – a "freeze, roll-back, and reassess" approach – which would involve freezing all new pharmaceutical "TRIPs-plus" provisions and a roll-back of existing ones to the levels agreed in TRIPS.
- New ways of providing incentives and financing pharmaceutical and medical research and development outside the intellectual property rights (IPRs) system are urgently needed.
- The international community should recapture the social raison d'être of the IPRs system.

Trade Rules and Intellectual Property Protection for Pharmaceuticals

Up until the Agreement on the Trade-Related Aspects of Intellectual Property Rights (TRIPS) was concluded at the World Trade Organization (WTO) in 1994 (Box 22.1), international trade rules and intellectual property (IP) protection rules had for the most part evolved separately. Until the late 1970s, most international trade negotiation rounds had been about tariff reductions. In contrast, various types of intellectual property rights (IPRs) were governed by a number of separate treaties that allowed their respective signatories considerable discretion over IP standard-setting, procedures, and enforcement. Although TRIPS purports to govern only the "trade-related" aspects of IPRs, in effect it is a comprehensive IP treaty. TRIPS mandates all WTO Members (currently there are 153) to establish, protect, and enforce *all* IPRs that were in use in key developed countries by the early 1990s. These IPRs include patents, copyrights, trademarks, geographic indicators, industrial designs, integrated circuits, and trade secrets. By virtue of demanding strong substantive and procedural IP rules in all WTO Members, who, until then, had widely different IP protection standards, TRIPS has brought about substantial changes to how IPRs are governed. Most countries now grant and protect similar types of IPRs regardless of their specific politico-socio-economic contexts, and are legally bound to do so by the WTO's ultra-binding dispute mechanism.

Box 22.1   The WTO TRIPS Agreement

The TRIPS Agreement brought about fundamental changes to the way intellectual property rights are governed. The WTO agreement was negotiated in the Uruguay Round of negotiations (1986–1994) by the members of the WTO. The TRIPS Agreement sets out certain minimum standards regarding the grant, protection, and enforcement of intellectual property rights, from copyrights, to patents, trade secrets, and so on. TRIPS standards and obligations are mandatory and binding on all its signatories The purpose of the TRIPS agreement is to establish a quasi-uniform set of rules that would provide what its promoters – the United States, the European Union, Switzerland, and other key developed countries and IP-reliant business interests – consider "adequate" standards of protection for intellectual property across the world. Member countries reserve the right to go above and beyond – but not below – the provisions of TRIPS, as long as domestic legislation does not controvert the obligations set out in the Agreement.

As IPRs affect the very ways in which societies live, learn, communicate, consume, create, innovate, and develop, the impact of TRIPs goes well beyond the redrafting of domestic IP laws. Amongst others things, changes in trade and pharmaceutical IP rules introduced through TRIPS have had a profound impact upon access to affordable medicines and governments' ability to deal with public health crises, especially in the developing world. To be sure, public health crises, and solutions to them, are complex. Access to affordable medicines is only one of the many constitutive elements, which include addressing poverty and weak public health systems in the developing world. Nevertheless, most developing countries spend a comparatively higher proportion of their *public* healthcare budgets on pharmaceuticals than countries in the developed world. In addition, pharmaceutical expenditures account for as much as 80–90% of *private* household healthcare costs in developing countries (Hammer 2002). Patients in the developing world also face pharmaceutical prices that are often higher than those in the developed world, and certainly higher than their average per capita income (Scherer 2000; Hammer 2002; Gallus 2004). Hence, challenges such as poverty and poorly developed health facilities only serve to make access to affordable pharmaceuticals an even more important and urgent issue.

Given such importance and urgency, this chapter aims to provide an account of how changes in pharmaceutical IP protection rules brought about through TRIPS and certain post-TRIPS developments pose significant challenges to ensuring wide access to affordable medicines across the world. Part of the reason for this state of affairs relates to the fact that TRIPS was not negotiated with public health goals in mind. Rather, it was primarily set in place as a means of entrenching the "competitiveness" of IP-reliant businesses located largely in the developed world, including pharmaceutical business actors. This rationale has been increasingly resisted by a number of developing countries and some civil society groups. Such resistance has led to some, albeit limited, successes, such as the 2001 WTO Doha Declaration on the TRIPS Agreement and Public Health and the 2005 TRIPS amendment. Nevertheless, these efforts have continued to be thwarted by other post-TRIPS developments, such as the negotiation of bilateral preferential trade agreements (PTAs). These post-TRIPS developments have further expanded pharmaceutical IP protection standards. Given the powerful vested interests at stake, even though actors with different interests and positions remain locked in IP-access to medicines contests, it seems implausible that global IP rules for pharmaceuticals will soon be overhauled to better serve public health goals. However, a number of recent initiatives do appear to hold promise for positive changes in the future, but only if all the actors involved pause and reassess the social purpose of IPRs.

Pharmaceutical Patents Before and After TRIPS

Some of the most important TRIPS provisions that impact on public health are those related to pharmaceutical products, such as patent protection (Articles 27, 28, and 33), compulsory licensing (Article 31), protection of pharmaceutical test data (Article 39.3), and parallel importation. One of the most pernicious effects of these provisions taken together is that they hinder or delay the introduction of generic medicines in the market. This hindrance is important because generics are usually priced 40–80% less than patented medicines. Many patients, public health authorities, and programs, both in the developing and in the developed world, are thus priced out of the market.

The entry of generic drugs, and more generally the availability and affordability of pharmaceuticals in a market, are closely related to pharmaceutical patent rights. TRIPS patent provisions were in fact amongst the most controversial of the TRIPS agreement, not least because of the substantial and widespread increase in protection standards they brought about. Provided certain thresholds of novelty, inventiveness, and utility are met for a new drug or molecular entity, all TRIPS signatories must grant a pharmaceutical patent. In turn, this patent grants its holder exclusivity for a period of 20 years, during which only the patent-holder, or its licensees, have the right to produce, use, or sell the drug under patent. Pharmaceutical patents are granted by national patent offices either for a new biomolecular entity or its components (a product patent), or for the process used to produce it (a process patent), and in most cases, for both. It is common for a patented drug to reach the market protected by "patent thickets" of over 100 different patent families (European Commission 2009). This is a conscious strategy on the part of pharmaceutical companies to control competition and markets, which is why patents cover a myriad of biomolecular entities and processes that relate both to new drugs that reach the market and many others that do not.

The current pharmaceutical patent system set in place through TRIPS is not global in the sense that once a patent is granted in one country, it is valid in all countries. Instead, pharmaceutical patents have largely remained territorial in nature, but the obligation to protect pharmaceutical products and processes through patents is now legally binding on all WTO Members. While there is some flexibility with regard to patentability criteria, countries have no option but to grant patents for pharmaceutical product or process innovations. Before TRIPS came into force (in 1995 and 2005 for developed and developing countries, respectively), pharmaceutical patent duration varied greatly among countries. The length of a pharmaceutical patent was significantly shorter than the 20 years currently demanded by TRIPS; indeed, in many developing countries it was as short as 5 years (WHO 2010).

Importantly, many countries did not provide pharmaceutical product patents at all. A study conducted before TRIPs found that of 98 developed and developing countries, 49 excluded pharmaceutical patent protection altogether (WIPO 1988). This exclusion allowed either the production of cheaper generic versions when production facilities existed, or the importation of cheap generic drugs from elsewhere, as a means of ensuring a secure supply of affordable pharmaceuticals. Some countries only provided pharmaceutical process patents, which allowed the production of generic versions of patented drugs provided that a different process to that which had been patented was used. The case of the Indian Patent Act 1970 is often used as an example of such a regime. This Act repealed and replaced the 1911 Act in order to make Indian patent law compatible with Indian developmental objectives. One of the main changes introduced by the 1970 Act was to allow process (but not product) patents in pharmaceutical and agrochemical products. In other words, it allowed the national pharmaceutical industry to develop technical expertise in reverse engineering of existing medicines by modifying the manufacturing process, ushering in one of the most vibrant and successful pharmaceutical generic sector in the world.

The TRIPS Agreement has foreclosed these and other options. Take, for instance, the case of first-line antiretroviral therapies (ARTs). When these drugs initially hit the market in the late 1980s and early 1990s, they were priced at levels as high as US$12,000–14,000 per person per year. Thanks, in large part, to competition from generic companies in countries such as India, these drugs are now available at prices $100–300 per person per year (MSF 2010). However, because of the global pharmaceutical patent system now in place, there is considerably less possibility for generic competition for more effective existing second and/or third-line ARTs and their prices are expected to remain high for the duration of their patents. The patent system is also impeding generic competition for many new patented drugs that treat other, equally important conditions.

To be sure, TRIPS contains a number of flexibilities in the area of pharmaceutical patents, the most relevant of which are those pertaining to compulsory licensing (Article 31). However, although these flexibilities were reconfirmed in the 2001 Doha Declaration and certain compulsory licensing rules were amended in 2005, the more substantial flexibilities of the pre-TRIPS era are now long gone. In sum, TRIPS set in place a pharmaceutical patent system that extends a "one size fits all" model, first developed in the United States and Europe, to across most of the world, where complex legal, social, political, economic, and health conditions prevail.

The extension of this "one size fits all" patent system was not, of course, an unintended or unforeseen consequence of TRIPS rules on pharmaceuticals; it was one of the main aims of the pharmaceutical companies that, alongside other business actors, fought hard to bring about TRIPS. All the provisions in TRIPS that were relevant to pharmaceuticals were inserted at the behest of the pharmaceutical industry in the United States, EU, and Japan and were largely dealt with satisfactorily to their interests (Drahos and Braithwaite 2002; Sell 2003). These companies were instrumental in securing an agreement that essentially locked in their competitive advantage in the pharmaceutical sector (May 2000; Sell 2003), and fenced off lucrative existing and emerging markets. More broadly, TRIPS is an agreement concerned with the global protection and enforcement of the private IP rights of the business actors – high-technology, luxury goods, and entertainment sectors – who during the 1980s framed the lack of uniform IP protection worldwide as "theft" and a non-tariff barrier to free trade (Ryan 1998). Such formulation resonated well with broader material and ideological changes during the late 1970s and 1980s. These changes saw key WTO Members (the United States and EU in particular) increasingly concerned with the competitive positioning in the global markets of their industries, especially of high-tech and service industries in which they had pegged their hopes for continued growth. However, by linking IP protection to competitiveness and trade, TRIPS pays insufficient attention to other crucial links that exist between IP protection and certain public goods, including – but not limited to – public health. The relationship between IP protection and the provision of these other complementary goods is hard enough to balance at the national level. By projecting a narrow and distorted link between IP, trade, and competitiveness, TRIPS has made it even harder to balance IP protection with other competing concerns at the global level.

As TRIPS negotiating history indicates, very little attention was paid to the social purpose and consequences of extending a particular pharmaceutical patent arrangement to the rest of the world. Amongst others, arguments related to the necessity of patent protection to spur innovation and growth were key to justifying TRIPS, as were those that framed the lack of patent protection as "theft" and "piracy." Despite such incriminating language, no independent evidence on the scale of "theft" in pharmaceuticals was used during the negotiations. In any case, charges of "theft" were not legally valid, in so far as some countries' laws did not recognize property over pharmaceutical products and international law allowed such variances. Although a number of developing countries, India and Brazil among them, initially resisted a global IP agreement at the WTO, their resistance was ultimately unsuccessful. They achieved more success through exploiting disagreements between key members (the United States and EU) over issues such as patentability and compulsory licensing (Gorlin 1999). In fact, it is because of these disagreements that TRIPS contained certain flexibilities, in addition to the necessary "wiggle" room and vague language that generally characterizes multilateral agreements.

Hence, neither TRIPS, nor most TRIPS flexibilities, were negotiated with public health concerns in mind, or concerns over how the IP protection it mandated might affect them. Although TRIPS does recognize in principle the need to protect public interest in the area of IP protection (Article 8), measures taken to promote and protect public interest, including public health, must be consistent with TRIPS provisions which, broadly speaking, extend, expand, and strengthen private IPRs (May 2000).

Pharmaceuticals Post-TRIPS and the "IP Access to Medicines" Contests

As we have seen, the WTO TRIPS agreement brought about a sea change in global pharmaceutical rules that, despite the flexibilities, limit governments' hands in improving access to affordable drugs. And further limitations were to come soon after TRIPS was concluded. Having secured a legally binding agreement that locked in their competitive advantage, pharmaceutical business actors and their home countries (mainly the United States, EU, and Switzerland) entered the post-TRIPS period with two missions. The first was to ensure a "proper" and timely implementation of TRIPS. The second was to further expand IP protection in areas dealt with ambiguously in TRIPS, such as parallel imports, defined by the WHO as "imports of a patented or trademarked product from a country where it is already marketed" (WHO 2012), and pharmaceutical data protection. Their efforts found expression simultaneously at the multilateral, bilateral, and unilateral levels: (i) multilaterally, at the WTO through its surveillance and dispute settlement mechanism; (ii) bilaterally, through PTAs; and (iii) through unilateral pressure, particularly from the US Trade Representative (USTR) Office. Together, these efforts resulted in expanding the IP rights afforded to private rights-holders in TRIPS and in further narrowing down the flexibilities and policy space available to governments.

At the WTO, early surveillance work at the TRIPS Council with a view to achieving effective implementation and enforcement of TRIPS was crucial in propagating a restrictive interpretation of TRIPS provisions that limited the flexibilities afforded to governments (Sell 2003). Likewise, technical support to most developing countries was forthcoming primarily in the shape of ready-made draft IPRs laws that generally were not designed to promote the use of TRIPS flexibilities (Drahos 2002). The WTO dispute settlement mechanism was also used strategically by pharmaceutical business and key state actors. These actors brought cases that had good chances of success and represented issues that would set powerful examples and eventually develop the necessary body of precedent on pharmaceutical IPRs.

Among such cases, five were particularly important: the case against India and Pakistan in 1996, against Canada in 1997, against Argentina in 1999, and against Brazil in 2000, all filed either by the United States or the EU (or both) on behalf of complaints raised by their pharmaceutical business actors. Some of these cases were settled bilaterally, with the Canadian and Indian cases being the only ones to go through the WTO dispute settlement procedures, including the Appellate Body in the Indian case. In both the Canadian and Indian cases, the Panel decision arguably adopted a relatively strict interpretation of the disputed TRIPS provisions (Articles 30, 70.8, and 70.9). Together they clearly showed the determination of pharmaceutical business and key state actors to ensure a "proper" and effective enforcement of TRIPS across the world (Matthews 2002; Sell 2003).

In addition to this relentless multilateral pressure to "improve" IP protection for pharmaceuticals post-TRIPS, the USTR also continued to keep the unilateral pressure up under the US Section 301 mechanism as it had done during TRIPS negotiations. This mechanism, a section of the 1974 US Trade Act, grants the US government the right to respond to violations of international trade rules with a range of aggressive measures, such as tariffs (Brown 2010). Indeed, only 1 year after TRIPS entered into force in developed countries, the number of trading partners that came under pressure under Section 301 increased by 25% (USTR 1998). A review of the USTR categorization of countries under Special 301 into the "priority watch list" and "watch list" from 1996 until 2000 indicates that countries such as Canada, Brazil, Chile, Colombia, Costa-Rica, Pakistan, the Philippines, and Thailand made regular entries in the "watch list" each year without fail. Countries such as Argentina, India, Turkey, and Israel saw their IP laws secure them entries into the higher profile "priority watch list" for each year during the same period. Although trade sanctions under Section 301 have not been used routinely by the USTR, the effectiveness of the Special 301 process rests on it pressurising weaker partners to adopt US-like or "TRIPS plus" IP laws so as to avoid further action under the 301 process.

Overall, then, whether within the WTO or outside it, these post-TRIPS strategies adopted by certain state and IP-reliant business actors, particularly the pharmaceutical industry, showed the collective determination of these actors to ensure an implementation of TRIPS that concurred with their interests. This generally meant narrowing down TRIPS flexibilities and expanding private IP rights. However, as these post-TRIPS strategies intensified, so did awareness about and resistance against further encroaching upon TRIPS flexibilities. In the case of pharmaceutical IPRs, resistance came to take a particularly visible form, initially organized in the mid 1990s by non-governmental organizations (NGOs) such as the Consumer Project on Technology (CPTech) and Health Action International (HAI). These NGOs were amongst the first to raise concerns about the impact of IP protection on access to affordable medicines in the developing world (Matthews 2006). Just as IP-reliant business actors had linked IP protection to trade and competitiveness before them, in the late 1990s this NGO network linked strong IP protection for pharmaceuticals with high prices for prescription drugs, restricted access to medicines and unnecessary loss of human health and life. Their "strong IPRs = expensive drugs = loss of health/life" formula provided an alternative framework that resonated particularly well with growing concerns about the unfolding HIV/AIDS crisis. From its relatively contained beginnings in the early 1980s, the crisis had spiraled out of control by the mid 1990s, as had the prices of first-line patented ARTs. What started off as an "access to HIV/AIDS drugs" debate gradually expanded to include access to essential medicines and to public health more generally.

Although other concerns were raised post-TRIPS (e.g., concerns about "life patenting"), there were a number of reasons why contests over pharmaceutical IPRs and access to medicines took precedence over others in the late 1990s. First, public health issues, especially pandemics such as HIV/AIDS, had been attracting considerable concern and attention at the global level throughout the 1990s. This attention was exemplified by the adoption of the UN Millennium Development Goals (MDGs), three of which are explicitly related to health (MDGs 4–6); a series of World Health Assembly resolutions on the need for Member States to respect their public health obligations; and the creation of the Global Fund to Fight AIDS, Tuberculosis and Malaria. Second, the global network of civil society groups working on the broad area of health had a formidable role in raising the profile of the impact of IPRs on access to medicines in the late 1990s. Third, their efforts found fertile ground, not only because of heightened concern over global health issues, but also because of increased awareness about the real scale of TRIPS obligations. This scale was particularly felt by developing countries, many of which shoulder a higher burden of public health crises. Just as important, access to life-saving medicines is a visibly emotive issue, which is partly why the "IPRs-access to medicines debate" became so politicized then and remains so today. As a result, considerable human capital and political will was to be exhausted over this issue alone from the late 1990s onwards, with some effect.

A milestone was reached with the 2001 WTO Doha Declaration on the TRIPS Agreement and Public Health. This declaration was the outcome of a process started in early 2001 when, at the request of the African Group, the TRIPS Council agreed to consider the effects of patents on prices, accessibility, and affordability of pharmaceuticals (Correa 2002). The Doha Declaration eventually recognized the flexibilities provided in the TRIPS Agreement and the right of WTO Members to use them, stating that these flexibilities should be interpreted in a way supportive of public health. The declaration reinforced: (i) the right of the Members to grant compulsory licenses, defined by the WTO as "when a government allows someone else to produce the patented product or process without the consent of the patent owner" (WTO 2006); (ii) the freedom to determine the grounds upon which licenses were granted; and (iii) the freedom to determine the regime of exhaustion of IPRs (closely linked to parallel importing).

Such reaffirmations of flexibilities available to governments to undertake measures to promote public health ran directly against the restrictive interpretation given to the respective provisions until then. Indeed, the language adopted by the Doha Declaration was opposed by some developed countries, particularly the United States, for fear that such language would weaken the commitment to patent protection and TRIPS obligations in general. However, importantly, the Declaration also reiterated the commitment of WTO Members to TRIPS and recognized that such commitment was not in conflict with their right to protect public health. Despite being seen as an achievement of developing countries and health NGOs, the Declaration vindicated simultaneously the positions of pharmaceutical business actors (formulated as "IPRs = research = cures") and NGOs (formulated as "copying = cheap medicines = lives saved"). By explicitly recognizing the significance of IP protection to the development of new medicines and establishing that TRIPS provisions did not prevent public health measures, the Declaration *legitimized* the role of pharmaceutical IPRs and other TRIPS provisions, rather than problematizing them. The Declaration, then, did not challenge the pharmaceutical IPRs mandated by TRIPS, although it did highlight the newly established "IP-access to affordable medicines" framework.

Another milestone was the eventual amendment in 2005 of certain TRIPS provisions relating to compulsory licensing, after long and protracted negotiations at the WTO. The concern that led to the amendment focused on compulsory licensing for countries with insufficient or no pharmaceutical manufacturing capacities, whose options to address public health concerns through compulsory licensing were further reduced by stipulations found in TRIPS Article 31(f). This provision stated that medicines produced under a compulsory license were to be used predominantly for the supply of the domestic market, and not for exports. Not only were countries with no manufacturing capacities limited by their inability to work a compulsory license, but also by their inability to import pharmaceuticals, because other countries that could work a compulsory license were not permitted to issue a compulsory license for export. For over 4 strenuous years, negotiations raged over issues related to the legal form of the solution, which diseases and countries would be eligible to use a possible solution, and what safeguards there would be in place to avoid the "misuse" of such solution (Muzaka 2011).

In the end, an exception was carved out of Article 31(f), which originally limited compulsory licenses to the domestic market. The amended article allows the issuing of compulsory licenses for import and export in the case of a public health crisis in the importing country, but it does so through establishing a mechanism burdened with procedural requirements, designed with a view to protecting the interests of patent-holders. Because of these requirements, many developing countries and health NGOs have considered the 2005 amendment as a step *backwards* from the Doha Declaration. Indeed, the amendment of TRIPS rules to allow compulsory licenses for export have only been only used once, by Rwanda in 2007–2008, reportedly amidst complains over its cumbersome nature (Muzaka 2011).

Despite the 2005 amendment being greeted by the United States and the EU as a means of enhancing access to pharmaceuticals in developing countries, efforts by the latter to deal with their public health concerns through overriding patent rights for pharmaceuticals have not received a sympathetic response. For instance, considerable pressure was placed on Thailand and Brazil by pharmaceutical companies, the USTR and the EU Trade

Commissioner for issuing compulsory licenses on ARTs in 2006 and 2007. In addition to such pressure, the USTR has continued to list several developing countries in its Special 301 "priority watch list" and "watch list" for lack of "effective" patent and data protection for pharmaceuticals while negotiations at the WTO on compulsory licensing and access to medicines were ongoing. But perhaps the most important way in which the 2001 Declaration and 2005 amendment have been undermined is through the spread of PTAs.

PTAs and "TRIPS Plus" Pharmaceutical Standards

In previous section, we saw that a network of civil society groups and some developing countries achieved a victory, albeit a qualified one, in bringing public health concerns in from the cold during the IP-access to medicines contests. Nevertheless, IP-reliant business actors and key developed states, most notably the United States and the EU, continued to successfully spread and expand IP protection standards worldwide through other means.

The US Special 301 procedure, for instance, continued to pressurise other countries to "improve" their pharmaceutical IPRs. Indeed, from 2000 onwards, nearly half of the countries listed in the Special 301 reports were found to have "inadequate" IP protection for pharmaceuticals (GAO 2007). The European Commission, having contemplated the issues at least since 2003, also set up its own version of the US "watch list" in 2006. But perhaps the most important channel has been the PTAs, although bilateral investment treaties have also been used to the same effect (Drahos 2002). Since the late 1990s, the bilateral route has proven to be a particularly effective way of driving IP protection standards upwards. This route has often involved the United States or the EU as key partners and a developing country, the latter all too often willing to accept higher IP standards than TRIPS ("TRIPS plus") in exchange for the seemingly more immediate interest of access to lucrative markets (Okediji 2004). This trend accelerated even further after the 2001 Doha Declaration. Indeed, it was precisely when the IP-access to medicines contests at the multilateral level were at their peak that both the United States and the EU gave a boost to their expansionist IP strategy at home and abroad. The 2002 US Trade Promotion Authority Act (TPA) called for, among other things, any multilateral or bilateral trade agreements to reflect standards of IP protection similar to those found in US laws (US Trade Act 2002 S.2102). Similarly, the Lisbon Agenda for Europe, agreed in 2000, recognized innovation and IP protection as the key to the EU becoming the most competitive and dynamic knowledge-based economy by 2010 (European Council 2000). These developments indicate that both the United States and the EU continued to frame IP protection as a trade and competitiveness issue, despite the many concerns raised over the impact of IPRs on other issue-areas, especially public health, during the same period.

From an increasingly complex set of IP chapters in various PTAs concluded by the United States and EU, it is possible to identify four main "TRIPS plus" provisions that either limit TRIPS flexibilities or go beyond TRIPS with respect to IP protection for pharmaceuticals. These are data exclusivity, compulsory licensing (the key issue during the TRIPS amendment process), patent term extensions, and patentability criteria. It is worth recalling that TRIPS itself leaves it up to each WTO Member to provide protection for pharmaceutical test data submitted to regulatory authorities for marketing approval (data exclusivity) (Article 39:3); determine their own system of IP exhaustion (Article 6) (national exhaustion deems that the IPR has only been exhausted in the nation in which the right holder has first sold the good (but not in other nations), while international exhaustion considers it exhausted on the first sale, wherever it took place); determine the grounds to issue compulsory licenses (Article 31); and define strict criteria for patentability (Article 27). In addition, TRIPS does not obligate members to compensate patent holders for "unreasonable" delays during the marketing approval process by offering patent term extensions. Nor does it make provisions that link the marketing approval of competitors' drugs to the patent status, as is the case in some PTAs.

The issue of data protection has probably been the most important and politicized of them all. Access to original data (e.g., clinical trial data) is crucial for speeding up the entry of generic medicines into the market after patent expiration, or for successfully working a compulsory license during the patent term. These are the very reasons why proprietary pharmaceutical companies have been only too keen to push for restrictive data protection rules in PTA partner countries. While the TRIPS agreement recognizes the importance of data protection, it only requests that data are protected against unfair commercial use. There are a number of options for data protection in practice, but the United States and the EU have adopted what is called an exclusive rights model which protects data against use for 5 and 10 years, respectively. In practice, most parties to US PTAs are introducing pharmaceutical data protection that mirrors the US exclusive right model, whereby access to data is forbidden for 5 years from the date of marketing approval. This is the case with all US PTAs signed from 2000 onwards, with the exception of that with Jordan (2000). The EU PTA with South Korea in 2009 also requires a 5-year exclusivity period (Roffe and Spennemann 2006). Overall, the problem with data protection of the United States/EU type is that it poses a huge obstacle to generic competition and, quite likely, to access to data for compulsory licensing purposes.

While data exclusivity has been the most politicized "TRIPS plus" provision so far, those provisions relating to compulsory licensing are the more interesting, given the prolonged debates over this these provisions at the WTO from 2001 until TRIPS was amended in 2005. As noted above, the existence of data protection can already limit the ability of a generic company to produce a drug under a compulsory license. However, this is not the only way in which options to make effective use of compulsory licenses have been circumvented. For instance, the US PTAs with Jordan (2000), Singapore (2003), Australia (2004), Vietnam, and those initiated in 2003 with the South African Custom Union and the Free Trade Area of the Americas (FTAA) (both stalled) limit the grounds upon which a compulsory license can be granted to cases of anti-trust remedies, national emergencies, or non-commercial use, although neither TRIPS nor the 2001 Doha Declaration specify any such grounds (Morin 2006). Furthermore, the US PTA with Morocco limits the use of TRIPS flexibilities to particular diseases such as HIV/AIDS, malaria, tuberculosis, and other epidemics (Sell 2007), an option that was fiercely and successfully opposed during the TRIPS amendment negotiations.

There are two other ways in which PTAs narrow down TRIPS flexibilities with respect to pharmaceutical patents: patent term extensions and looser patentability criteria. With regard to the former, all US PTAs and that between the European Free Trade Association (EFTA) and Chile request that parties provide extension to the patent term (the length varies between PTAs) when the marketing approval process delays the marketing of a product or process. Further, in all US PTAs cases apart from the US–Jordan PTA, an additional extension of the patent term is also requested for "unreasonable" delays in the patent granting process (Roffe and Spennemann 2006). Similarly, some PTAs require parties to make available patents for new uses of known products. This requirement is the case with the US PTAs with Australia, Bahrain, and Morocco. The result is to allow patent-holders to "evergreen" existing patents by adding another patent term to already known/patent products, and to push the entry of generic versions further away (Roffe and Spennemann 2006).

Interestingly, both the United States and the EU have made references in most of their PTAs to the 2001 Doha Declaration and to their commitment of access to medicines for all, although in a number of cases they have also asserted that the Declaration is in fact limited only to infectious diseases, AIDS, or epidemics (Muzaka 2011). More recently, the United States in particular has resisted the inclusion of references to the 2001 Declaration in negotiations over a potential UN Declaration on Non-Communicable Diseases (Cox 2011). The EU has also come under heavy criticism from public health activists for using its own IP enforcement rules to effect 19 seizures of generic drugs in transit through its ports (in most cases from India or China to other developing countries where these pharmaceuticals are not patented) on account of existing EU patents. India subsequently brought the case to the WTO dispute settlement mechanism in 2010. Although it seems that the EU has agreed in principle to review its rules, its decision remains to be seen, especially in light of ongoing negotiations for an EU–India PTA. It is worth mentioning in passing that during these negotiations India has come under intense pressure from the EU to accept pharmaceutical data exclusivity and additional IP enforcement measures (Menghaney 2011).

More generally, because PTAs' "TRIPS plus" provisions for pharmaceuticals ultimately strengthen the position of the patent-holders and limit or delay access to affordable pharmaceuticals, PTAs threaten to undermine public health gains achieved in multilateral negotiations, such as the 2001 Declaration and the 2005 amendment. One of the functions of PTAs from the perspective of actors with interest in higher and stronger IP protection is to get rid of the "wriggle room" present in most multilateral agreements, which is necessary to secure the consent of all the signatories. From the perspective of these actors, there is considerable "wriggle room" in TRIPS which, incidentally, is what other actors (e.g., NGOs, some developing countries) recognize as TRIPS flexibilities. Hence, it is not surprising that PTAs negotiated between a party who sees strong pharmaceutical IP protection to be in its interests (such as the United States and the EU) and a weaker partner introduce "TRIPS plus" provisions for pharmaceuticals. While not surprising, such a trend is worrying from a public health perspective, in so far as the policy space of governments to deliver on this front is further restricted by such provisions. Moreover, this policy space is also restricted on account of the fact that the implementation of PTAs is a process that involves a continuous oversight from the more advanced partner over actions undertaken by the other party (Biadgleng and Maur 2011).

Looking Ahead – Some Concluding Thoughts

As we have seen, both the United States and the EU, the key state actors pushing forward the current expansionist IP agenda, appear convinced that stronger enforceable IPRs are core to their global competitiveness, a particular way of framing IP that was accepted wholesale from the demands of IP-reliant business actors during the 1980s. Unfortunately, this kind of thinking has been more, rather than less, prominent in the area of pharmaceuticals. Efforts by developing countries to counter this framework by seeking to subdue pharmaceutical IP protection to public health concerns, when not simply rhetorical, have so far had only limited success. Only a handful of better resourced developing countries have been able to take advantage of TRIPS flexibilities, India and Brazil amongst them, and not much advantage has been taken of the 2001 Declaration and the 2005 amendment. Despite the urgency of the issue of worldwide access to affordable medicines, developing countries have not managed to create an effective and unified front, although coalitions between them and civil society groups remain active in IP-access to medicines contests. Ideally, a new approach to pharmaceutical IP rule-making – a "freeze, roll-back, and reassess" approach – would involve freezing all new pharmaceutical "TRIPs-plus" provisions and a roll-back of existing ones to the levels agreed in TRIPS. These steps would need to be followed, necessarily, by a reassessment of TRIPS' impact on access to affordable medicines, and by a very real possibility of refashioning a new and more balanced solution that fully takes into account the social purpose of IPRs. However, in the context of the current state of resistance and powerful vested interests in an expansionist IP agenda, this scenario does not appear very likely in the near future.

Nonetheless, a number of less comprehensive but perhaps more promising developments deserve some attention here. The least reliable of them has been the practice of donations or negotiations of lower prices for certain drugs through specific programs by pharmaceutical companies themselves. This is mainly a piecemeal approach that cannot address the issue of access, not least because the ability to set drug prices (even at zero for donations) is part and parcel of the (quasi) monopolistic position that these companies enjoy thanks to pharmaceutical IPRs, especially patents. A more serious attempt was the creation in 2010 of the Medicines Patent Pool, founded by UNITAID and supported by the WHO, UNADIS, the Global Fund to Fight AIDS, Tuberculosis and Malaria and the G8. The aim of the Pool has been to create a system in which patent-holders could share their patents and license them to generic producers in exchange for modest royalties. So far efforts have focused on HIV/AIDS, and two licenses for ARTs have been agreed – with the US National Institute of Health and with Gilead Sciences. The Gilead deal has been criticized on account of restrictions on compulsory licensing and parallel imports stipulated by the company (Brook 2011). More recently, the Pool has had to deal with Johnson & Johnson's decision not to license its HIV medicines to developing countries via the Pool, although negotiations reportedly continue with other pharmaceutical companies.

Despite the United States' and EU's practice of introducing legally binding "TRIPs-plus" pharmaceutical provisions in their PTAs, during the 2008 World Health Assembly (WHA) they agreed with the need to take into account TRIPS flexibilities and the 2001 Declaration on trade agreements (WHA 2008). So far, this agreement has remained a rhetorical stance. A more promising outcome of the 2008 WHA session was the establishment of an expert working group at the WHO to work on identifying new financing and incentive mechanisms for encouraging research and development (R&D) for conditions that disproportionately affect patients in poorer countries. These mechanisms include ideas such as prize funds, a health impact fund, and new open-source drug development models. Of these, perhaps the most debated proposal at the WHO was that of a prize fund that would use funds raised through taxation or minimum mandatory contributions to allocate yearly prizes for innovative drugs, thus delinking R&D from patents and other pharmaceutical IPRs. Unsurprisingly, it was met with resistance by the pharmaceutical companies reliant on IPRs (Love 2010). Indeed, the final 2010 Report of the expert group came under heavy criticism for being influenced by pharmaceutical companies' interests. In an unusual turn of events, the WHA restarted the process in May 2010, but the result remains yet to be seen.

A final initiative that may be of value is the proposal for a biomedical R&D Treaty, made initially in 2005, and supported by a number of scientists, public health experts, and NGOs. Under this proposed treaty, each country would make a minimum financial contribution to biomedical R&D (including the development of biomedical databases, research tools, pharmaceutical drugs, vaccines, and medical diagnostic tools) on the basis of its national income (Love 2007). Product developers would be paid to carry out the research, with products then being sold at generic prices immediately following their regulatory approval.

Since 2005, many versions of this treaty have been systematically sidelined, especially by countries with an active pharmaceutical sector. According to some reports, prominent foundations active in the area of public health, such as the Bill and Melinda Gates Foundation, also seem to oppose it (Karunakaran 2011), most likely because of the challenge this proposal poses to IPRs on which many of them depend, directly or indirectly. As with other new initiatives mentioned here, the future of the R&D Treaty is uncertain. As we have seen, many of the interests that oppose these initiatives are also actively pursuing the further strengthening and expansion of pharmaceutical IP. In this context, fundamental changes to pharmaceutical IPRs may not be forthcoming in the near future, but even incremental changes would necessarily require an urgent rethink on the part of all actors involved of the social consequences of their IP strategy.

Key Reading

CPTech. http://www.cptech.org/ip/health/ (last accessed December 2013). (Contains a number of studies and reports on IPRs and healthcare, site provided by CPTech.)

Drahos P, Braithwaite, J. 2002. *Informational Feudalism: Who Owns the Knowledge Economy?* London: Earthscan.

ICTSD and UNCTAD. http://www.iprsonline.org/resources/health.htm (last accessed December 2013). (Contains a series of papers published 2001–2007; site maintained by ICTSD and UNCTAD.)

May C. 2000. *A Global Political Economy of Intellectual Property Rights: The New Enclosures?* London: Routledge.

Muzaka V. 2011. *The Politics of Intellectual Property Rights and Access to Medicines.* Basingstoke: Palgrave MacMillan.

Roffe PG, Tansey G, Vivas-Eugui D (eds). 2006. *Negotiating Health: Intellectual Property and Access to Medicines.* London: Earthscan.

Sell SK. 2007. TRIPs-Plus free trade agreements and access to medicines. *Liverpool Law Review*, 28, 41–75.

References

Biadgleng ET, Maur JC. 2011. *The Influence of Preferential Trade Agreements on the Implementation of Intellectual Property Rights in Developing Countries.* Issue Paper No. 33. Geneva: ICTSD-UNCTAD Project on IPRs and Sustainable Development.

Brook B. 2011. Petition to the Medicines Patent Pool Foundation. email to IP-Health List on 13 October. http://lists.keionline.org/pipermail/ip-health_lists.keionline.org/2011-October/001411.html (last accessed February 2014).

Brown S. 2010. For our China trade emergency, dial section 301. *New York Times* October 17. http://www.nytimes.com/2010/10/18/opinion/18brown.html (last accessed December 2013).

Correa CM. 2002. *Implications of the Doha Declaration on the TRIPS Agreement and Public Health.* Geneva: World Health Organization. http://apps.who.int/medicinedocs/en/d/Js2301e/5.html (last accessed December 2013).

Cox K. 2011. Obama Administration wants to eliminate references to Doha Declaration in UN political declaration on non-communicable diseases. email to IP-Health List on 10 September. http://lists.keionline.org/pipermail/ip-health_lists.keionline.org/2011-September/001285.html (last accessed February 2014).

Drahos P. 2002. Developing countries and international intellectual property standard-setting. *Journal of World Intellectual Property* 5, 765–89.

Drahos P, Braithwaite J. 2002. *Informational Feudalism: Who Owns the Knowledge Economy?* London: Earthscan.

European Commission (DG Competition). 2009. *The Pharmaceutical Sector Inquiry Report.* Brussels: European Commission.

European Council. 2000. Lisbon European Council Meeting: Presidency Conclusions. Lisbon, March 23–24, 2000. http://www.europarl.europa.eu/summits/lis1_en.htm (last accessed February 2014).

Gallus N. 2004. The mystery of pharmaceutical parallel trade and developing countries. *Journal of World Intellectual Property* 7(2), 169–83.

GAO (Government Accountability Office). 2007. *Intellectual Property: US Trade Policy Guidance on WTO Declaration on Access to Medicines May Need Clarification.* GAO-07-1198. Washington, DC: US GAO.

Gorlin J. 1999. *An Analysis of the Pharmaceutical-Related Provisions of the WTO TRIPS.* Geneva: Intellectual Property Institute.

Hammer PM. 2002. Differential pricing of essential AIDS drugs: markets, politics and public health. *Journal of Economic Law* 5(4), 883–912.

Karunakaran N. 2011. Dark side of giving: the rise of philanthro-capitalism. *Economic Times* March 25.

Love J. 2007. Measures to enhance access to medical technologies, and new methods of stimulating medical R&D. *UC Davis Law Review* 40(3), 679–715.

Love J. 2010. Why is there resistance to prize funds? email to IP-Health List on 24 May 2010. http://lists.keionline.org/pipermail/ip-health_lists.keionline.org/2010-May/000039.html (last accessed February 2014).

Matthews D. 2002. *Globalising Intellectual Property Rights: the TRIPS Agreement.* London and New York: Routledge.

Matthews D. 2006. *NGOs, Intellectual Property Rights and Multilateral Institutions.* London: Queen Mary Intellectual Property Research Institute.

May C. 2000. *A Global Political Economy of Intellectual Property Rights: The New Enclosures?* London: Routledge.

Menghaney L. 2011. EC pressure in FTA negotiations with India goes up. email to IP-Health List on 25 November. http://lists.keionline.org/pipermail/ip-health_lists.keionline.org/2011-November/001563.html (last accessed February 2014).

Morin JF. 2006. Tripping up TRIPs debates: IP and health in bilateral agreements. *International Journal of Intellectual Property Management* 1(1–2), 37–53.

MSF (Médicins Sans Frontières). 2010. *Untangling the Web of Antiretroviral Price Reductions.* http://utw.msfaccess.org/background/challenges (last accessed December 2013).

Muzaka V. 2011. *The Politics of Intellectual Property Rights and Access to Medicines.* Basingstoke: Palgrave MacMillan.

Okediji R. 2004. Back to bilateralism? Pendulum swings in international intellectual property protection. *University of Ottawa Law and Technology Journal* 1, 125–47.

Roffe P, Spennemann C. 2006. From Paris to Doha: the WTO Doha Declaration on the TRIPs agreement and public health. In Roffe P, Tansey G, Vivas-Eugui D (eds) *Negotiating Health: Intellectual Property and Access to Medicines*, pp. 9–26. London: Earthscan.

Ryan MP. 1998. *Knowledge Diplomacy: Global Competition and the Politics of Intellectual Property.* Washington, DC: Brooking Institution Press.

Scherer FM. 2000. *The Pharmaceutical Industry.* Amsterdam: Elsevier.

Sell SK. 2003. *Private Power, Public Law: the Globalization of Intellectual Property Rights.* Cambridge: Cambridge University Press.

Sell SK. 2007. TRIPs-Plus free trade agreements and access to medicines. *Liverpool Law Review*, 28, 41–75.

USTR (United States Office of the Trade Representative). 1998. *Trade Policy Agenda and 1997 Annual Report of the President of the United States on the Trade Agreements Program.* Washington, DC: USTR.

WHA (World Health Assembly). 2008. Global Strategy and Plan of Action on Public Health, Innovation and Intellectual Property of the Sixty-first World Health Assembly (24 May 2008), WHA 61.21, element 5.2c.

WHO (World Health Organization). 2010. *Intellectual property protection: impact on public health.* http://www.who.int/medicines/areas/policy/AccesstoMedicinesIPP.pdf (last accessed December 2013).

WHO (World Health Organization). 2012. *Glossary of globalization, trade and health terms: parallel imports.* http://www.who.int/trade/glossary/story070/en/index.html (last accessed December 2013).

WIPO (World Intellectual Property Organization). 1988. *Existence, Scope and Form of Generally Internationally Accepted and Applied Standards/Norms for the Protection of Intellectual Property.* Issued as GATT Document MTN.GNG/NG11/W/24/Rev1.

WTO (World Trade Organization). 2006. *Compulsory licensing of pharmaceuticals and TRIPS.* http://www.wto.org/english/tratop_e/trips_e/public_health_faq_e.htm (last accessed December 2013).

Chapter 23

The Health Systems Agenda: Prospects for the Diagonal Approach

Julio Frenk, Octavio Gómez-Dantés, and Felicia M. Knaul

Abstract

The increasing pluralism that has populated the global health landscape, coupled with the accountability pressure represented by the Millennium Development Goals, has fueled a renewed concern for health systems. There is consensus on the idea that agreed goals will only be met and health outcomes improved if health systems are strengthened. However, there is less agreement on *how* to strengthen such systems. The recent attention to health systems has also reignited the debate on some of the dichotomies that have persisted for decades in the global health field: prevention versus treatment, primary versus specialized care, vertical versus horizontal strategies, and social determinants of health versus health services.

This chapter has two aims: to provide a conceptual basis to advance our understanding of health systems and to help settle the disputes between vertical and horizontal approaches to improving health through the construction of a "diagonal" perspective. Its central message is that in order to meet the challenges of the present century we need to offer comprehensive responses and move beyond false dichotomies towards integration. The first part of the chapter is devoted to a discussion of the meaning of health systems. The chapter then revisits the debate around vertical and horizontal approaches to healthcare and discusses the main features of the diagonal approach and exemplifies the use of this approach by addressing the issue of child mortality in Mexico. The chapter concludes with a reflection of the strengths and potential limits of the diagonal perspective.

The Handbook of Global Health Policy, First Edition. Edited by Garrett W. Brown, Gavin Yamey, and Sarah Wamala.
© 2014 John Wiley & Sons, Ltd. Published 2014 by John Wiley & Sons, Ltd.

Key Points

- Additional funding for health can only be effective if national and local health systems are strengthened.
- We need to have a clear idea of what health systems are meant to achieve in order to identify what needs to be strengthened.
- Initiatives to strengthen health systems should aim at improving not only the health conditions of populations and their distribution, but also the system's responsiveness and its level of financial protection.
- These initiatives should also move beyond just the delivery of services to include stewardship, financing, and resource generation.
- In order to meet the complex challenges of the present century we need to offer comprehensive responses and move beyond false dichotomies (vertical versus horizontal) towards integration.

Key Policy Implications

- Present global health challenges demand a "diagonal approach," which explicitly prioritizes certain interventions to strengthen the overall structure and functions of health systems.
- An additional advantage of the diagonal approach is that these priorities can be used to address the needs of the worst off, turning them into entitlements that empower vulnerable populations.
- Major global actors need to act upon the evidence that present global health challenges have strong economic, environmental, political, behavioral, and cultural determinants which demand comprehensive strategies.

Introduction

The concern for the way in which we confront threats, risks, and harms to our health is a central part of the human experience. Every society develops some form of response to disease. For most of history, this response had been limited to the household and carried out by the family nucleus. Alongside the continuing role of the household and family in caring for the sick, the twentieth century has witnessed the explosive emergence of a variety of institutions with the specialized function of looking after the health of individuals and communities.

Today, the different sets of organizations we conventionally call the health system have become a dominant feature of the social fabric in all but the most marginalized corners of the planet. It is estimated that health systems worldwide absorb around 10% of the world economy – about US$6 trillion (WHO 2010, 2012). Of course, there are huge global differences in domestic spending on such systems, and in patients' access to them. For example, while the United States spends $7000 per person on health annually, the Democratic Republic of Congo barely spends $13 per person per year (WHO 2011a).

When we speak of the health revolution of the twentieth century, we typically refer to the spectacular decline in mortality and the dramatic shift in the dominant causes of ill-health, such as the shift from communicable to non-communicable diseases (NCDs). Equally spectacular and dramatic has been the rise of health systems that now permeate all corners of human activity and which have become increasingly complex. During the relatively short period of time since World War II, the social arrangements for dealing with health have been transformed radically. Nowadays, most people come into contact – whether regular or sporadic – with a huge variety of health professionals, organizations, and technologies that specialize in healthcare. A growing proportion of people are born, die, and spend considerable periods of their lives in health-related institutions.

Today, health systems simultaneously take on at least seven multiple roles and meanings. First, a wide variety of different health systems institutions – encompassing an expanding set of complex organizations with distinctive authority structures – have taken over functions previously carried out by the individual and family. Second, such health systems are a source of income and employment for an array of professionals, managers, and technicians, who function within an elaborate division of labor. Third, they are a channel for mobilizing, exchanging, and redistributing large sums of money, both public and private. Fourth, health systems are a focus for technological innovation and a prime site where the common citizen comes into personal contact with science. Fifth, the health system is a vigorous sector of the economy, with important effects on macroeconomic variables such as productivity, inflation, aggregate demand, employment, and competitiveness. Sixth, health systems are an arena for political struggle among parties, interest groups, and social movements. Finally, they represent a set of cultural meanings for interpreting fundamental aspects of human experience, such as birth and death, pain and suffering, normality and deviance, and are a space where many of the key ethical questions of our times are framed and sometimes answered.

Like so many aspects of global health, interest in health systems has gone through cycles of activity and neglect, depending on the dominant winds in the complex process of agenda setting. Around World War II, debate in developed countries centered on the expansion of social insurance, while the establishment of modern ministries of health and other essential institutions was paramount in developing countries, many of which were just achieving independence. Primary healthcare occupied center stage in the late 1970s and early 1980s (WHO 1978; Passmore 1979). Throughout the 1990s, health system reform was a topic of debate (Gwatkin 2001).

Now, in the first part of the twenty-first century, the increasing pluralism that has populated the global health landscape, with 175 different entities, coupled with the accountability pressure represented by the Millennium Development Goals (MDGs), has fueled a renewed concern for health systems. There is broad consensus on the idea that agreed goals will only be met and health outcomes improved if health systems are strengthened (Travis *et al.* 2004). However, there is less agreement on *how* to strengthen such systems. The recent attention to health systems has also reignited the debate on some of the dichotomies that have persisted for decades: prevention versus treatment, infections versus NCDs, primary versus specialized care, vertical versus horizontal strategies, and social determinants of health versus health services.

This chapter, which builds on our previous work on health systems reform and strengthening (Frenk 1994, 2010; Frenk and Gómez-Dantés 2011; Knaul and Frenk 2011), has two aims. The first is to provide a conceptual basis to advance our understanding of health systems. The second is to help settle the disputes between vertical and horizontal approaches to improving health through the construction of a "diagonal" perspective. Our central message is that in order to meet the complex challenges of the present century we need to offer comprehensive responses to them and move beyond false dichotomies towards integration.

The first part of the chapter is devoted to a discussion of the meaning of health systems. The chapter then revisits the debate around vertical and horizontal approaches to healthcare and discusses the main features of the diagonal approach. We apply some of the lessons on the use of this approach to addressing child mortality in Mexico. The chapter concludes with a brief reflection of the strengths and potential limits of the diagonal perspective.

A Conceptual Base for Health Systems

There is growing recognition that additional funding for health, which has been mostly directed to specific diseases, can only be effective if national and local health systems are strengthened (Travis *et al.* 2004). However, we need to have a clear idea of what health systems are meant to achieve in order to identify what needs to be strengthened. In a virtuous circle, better health system performance and results will eventually secure further funding for health.

A poor understanding of the goals and functions of these systems still prevails in the global health field. Three common misconceptions are particularly prevalent, which see the health system as a black box, as a black hole, or as a laundry list (Frenk 2010).

The view of the health system as a "black box" is based on the belief that things are too complicated and we do not know what works, so we should simply put technologies and other inputs in place and then outputs will somehow automatically result. This is a misconception because we have built a sufficient body of knowledge to be able to open the black box and thus devise specific interventions to improve the performance of the health system. As discussed in Chapter 7, there is a growing body of scientific evidence on what works in different settings, which has in turn sparked an emerging evidence-based global health "movement."

The view of the health system as a "black hole" proposes that no amount of money will suffice to achieve the desired results: health systems will suck up huge resources with little pay-off. Yet this is also a misperception, because we know that some systems are much more efficient in achieving better results with limited resources.

Finally, the "laundry list" view proposes that the health system is just a laundry list of different organizations or persons that participate in producing health services, with no requirement that such components be coordinated or integrated. This is a misperception – lack of coordination is one of the reasons for the slow progress in achieving the health MDGs. The international health community has now aligned upon a set of core principles: the Paris Declaration on Aid Effectiveness, aimed at improving integration and coordination (OECD 2005).

We need to expand our view on health systems. We have previously proposed four directions for a more comprehensive view (Frenk 2010). First, we should think of the health *system* not only in terms of its component elements or building blocks (human resources, hospitals, primary care centers, technologies) but also in terms of their interrelations.

Second, in this view we should include not only the institutions of the health system (the supply side), but also the population (the demand side). The population is not simply an external beneficiary of the system, but is integral to it in a dynamic way. Box 23.1 shows the five roles that the population has in the health system.

Box 23.1   The Population's Five Roles in the Health System

1. *Patients*: this is the role most commonly attributed to populations in the health field.
2. *Consumers*: with specific expectations about the way in which they will be treated.
3. *Taxpayers*: who are the ultimate source of health financing.
4. *Citizens*: who may demand access to care as a right.
5. *Co-producers of health*: through care seeking, compliance with prescriptions, and behaviors that may promote or harm one's own health or the health of others.

Source: adapted from Frenk (2010).

A third expanded view refers to the health system's goals. We have traditionally held a narrow view, defining the goal of a health system as simply improving the overall *level* of health. However, we must go beyond this view, looking also at the *distribution* of health, which gives equity a central place in assessing a health system (Murray and Frenk 2000). We must also include other goals that are intrinsically valued beyond the improvement of health: protecting patients and families from financial consequences of disease, and responding to their need for dignity and satisfaction.

Finally, we should expand our view of the functions that a health system must perform, beyond the direct provision or delivery of clinical or public health services. While this is an essential function, health systems must perform other enabling functions, such as stewardship, financing, and resource generation. Key resources include facilities, technologies, information, and, most important of all, the health workforce.

What we have just summarized is a framework that formed the basis for the *World Health Report 2000* on health system performance (WHO 2000). This framework contains a simple logic that allows us to enlarge our understanding of health systems so that we may improve them. Specifying the goals allows us to assess the performance of a health system by measuring how well each of the goals is achieved, given the level of health expenditure and the social determinants of health. Such determinants can be measured by indicators such as income per capita or educational level. In turn, analysis of the way the functions are carried out allows us to explain variations in performance.

In summary, initiatives to strengthen health systems should aim at improving not only the health conditions of populations and their distribution, but also the system's responsiveness and its level of financial protection. These initiatives should also move beyond the delivery of services to include stewardship, financing, and resource generation.

The Diagonal Approach

In addition to a poor understanding of what a health system should achieve, international health in the twentieth century was characterized by a divide between vertical and horizontal strategies for health improvement (Frenk and Gómez-Dantés 2011). Besides strengthening their functions and expanding their goals, health systems in the twenty-first century would benefit from settling this dispute by adopting what has been called the "diagonal approach" (Sepúlveda 2006).

Vertical programs in the health field focus on specific diseases (e.g., diarrheal diseases, malaria, tuberculosis, HIV/AIDS) or health conditions (e.g., pregnancy and delivery) and frequently on only one aspect of care, such as prevention or early detection. Frequently, they also use financing, human resources, information, and delivery mechanisms that are managed separately from the rest of the system. These programs, which tend to be donor-driven, rarely interact with other components of the health system.

In contrast, the horizontal approach to healthcare refers to resource-sharing across disease and population groups. It usually includes efforts to strengthen health systems as a whole or address system-wide constraints, such as shortages of trained healthcare workers or inadequate health facilities or health information systems.

Vertical programs, with their highly focused attention to specific challenges in developing countries, have been accused of creating "islands of sufficiency in a swamp of insufficiency" (Ooms *et al.* 2008). "HIV-positive mothers [in developing countries]," says Garrett, "are given drugs to hold their infection at bay and prevent passage of the virus to their babies but still cannot obtain even the most rudimentary of obstetric and gynecological care" (Garrett 2007). These programs have also been criticized for ignoring the determinants of health, privileging technical-oriented interventions and neglecting those diseases that demand complex interventions and extensive long-term investments (Unger and Killingsworth 1986; Newell 1988).

However, horizontal approaches to healthcare have also been criticized – for example, for being too broad and idealistic, and also for lacking a clear definition of priorities (Walsh and Warren 1979). Critics of the horizontal perspective have argued that spreading the scarce resources of health systems in developing countries too thinly inevitably leads to generalized insufficiency (Ooms *et al.* 2008).

Evidence suggests that, in practice, few programs are purely vertical or horizontal (Atun *et al.* 2010). In any case, these two perspectives can be integrated through the "diagonal approach," which explicitly prioritizes certain interventions to strengthen the overall structure and function of health systems. Instead of focusing exclusively on single disease targets or addressing generic health system constraints, diagonal interventions tackle disease-specific priorities while addressing the gaps within a system. An additional advantage of this diagonal approach is that these priorities can be used to address the needs of the worst off, turning them into entitlements that empower vulnerable populations.

The diagonal approach takes advantage of complementary interventions and optimizes use of resources (Knaul *et al.* 2012). Providing coverage for a specific intervention for one disease can promote expanded coverage for other diseases and population groups. The introduction of regulatory measures to guarantee safe blood in the context of an HIV/AIDS program, for example, improves the quality of this health input for all patients, including women with obstetric emergencies. Inputs to guarantee an adequate cold chain, such as a reliable source of electricity and a refrigerator, benefit the overall operation of a health unit. In their initial phases, mostly devoted to prevention, HIV/AIDS initiatives often function as vertical programs operated by community health workers. However, eventually they demand access to trained personnel, who can be used to provide other types of health services, as well as access to laboratory units, which can offer support to a broad network of health posts.

The diagonal approach also favors the integration not only of disease-specific programs and health systems strengthening initiatives, but also of other sectors whose activities are related to health. Such integration, which addresses the false dilemma between health services and social determinants of health, is particularly relevant to the control of NCDs since many of their risk factors (e.g., smoking, obesity, alcohol) go beyond the limits of the health field.

Solid health systems, with clear priorities and strong inter-sectoral linkages, will be able to address the multiple, diverse, and complex needs of real people. They will also be able to meet both the demands related to the current MDGs and the needs generated by the emerging burden of chronic diseases, which are increasingly dominating the health profile of all but the poorest countries (Farmer *et al.* 2010).

The recent literature on the diagonal approach demonstrates how vaccination programs can be integrated with large-scale antipoverty interventions to expand coverage within health system strengthening initiatives (Sepúlveda *et al.* 2006). Other research has focused on the opportunities to integrate cancer care and control in ways that strengthen health systems, particularly in promoting early detection of breast cancer through maternal and reproductive health initiatives (Knaul *et al.* 2009). Indeed, a host of interventions for the prevention, diagnosis, and treatment of cancer can generate synergies for managing other chronic illness and for strengthening health systems. Improving access to pain control medications has been put forward as yet another example of an opportunity to implement the diagonal approach, as these interventions would benefit many patients and would also serve to strengthen platforms for surgery. Efforts in prevention and early detection of women's cancers can provide important impetus to the empowerment of women (Knaul *et al.* 2012). There are several global initiatives focused on NCDs which are contemplating major integrations into primary healthcare (WHO 2002, 2011b). In addition, the Maximizing Positive Synergies Academic Consortium has identified the benefits of reinforcing links between disease-specific global initiatives and health system strengthening (WHO Maximizing Positive Synergies Collaborative Group 2009). The 2010 *Lancet* Series on NCDs points out that when broader needs and benefits have been identified as goals from the outset, disease-specific investments have contributed to health system strengthening and population health improvements (Samb *et al.* 2010). An example is Rwanda, where HIV/AIDS investments have been channeled into health systems strengthening (Price *et al.* 2009).

In summary, the diagonal approach provides a comprehensive framework that addresses requirements for targeted approaches that correspond to specific diseases or populations, but also provides opportunities for strengthening health systems and other health-related sectors. This approach can generate overall improvements that expand access to interventions for various diseases and population groups.

The Diagonal Approach in Practice: Lessons from Mexico

Mexico is on track to achieving MDG 4: reducing the 1990 child mortality rate by two thirds no later than 2015 (OECD 2010). This progress is the result of the consistent implementation of policies that combined specific disease programs to tackle common infections, malnutrition, and maternal mortality, with health system strengthening initiatives (Frenk *et al.* 2003). A major health reform implemented in the past decade further expanded the benefits of these endeavors.

Efforts to strengthen the provision of personal health services started in 1979 with the creation of a program to enlarge the network of health posts in rural areas. In its initial phase, this program built over 3000 ambulatory units and 64 rural hospitals (Soberón 2006). A decade later, a program to expand access to public healthcare in poor urban areas was also launched (Rodríguez-Domínguez 2006).

In the early 1990s, with federal resources and a loan from the World Bank, a program to strengthen health services for the uninsured population was implemented to improve and expand healthcare facilities in the four poorest states of the country and to upgrade the management capabilities of the Ministry of Health (Gómez-Dantés *et al.* 1999).

Finally, in 1996, the Program for the Extension of Coverage was created to provide 12 essential interventions to poor populations on a regular basis (Secretaría de Salud 1996):

1. Basic household sanitary measures.
2. Family planning services.
3. Prenatal, perinatal, and postnatal care.
4. Nutrition and growth surveillance.
5. Immunization.
6. Treatment of diarrhea.
7. Treatment of common parasitic diseases.
8. Treatment of acute respiratory infections.
9. Prevention and treatment of tuberculosis.
10. Prevention and control of hypertension and diabetes.
11. Initial treatment of injuries.
12. Community training for health promotion.

This program was designed with the explicit idea that adequate provision of services to address priority diseases (diarrhea, respiratory infections, tuberculosis, hypertension, and diabetes) required ample human resources and access to a relatively broad range of health inputs.

The efforts to strengthen health services developed in the last two decades of the past century were complemented with several community-based interventions whose main objective was to reduce the burden of malnutrition and common infections in children (including diarrheal diseases and respiratory infections). Two of these public health interventions are described below: diarrheal disease control and a program aimed at achieving universal immunization.

In 1984, as part of the National Program to Control Diarrheal Diseases, oral rehydration therapy (ORT) was introduced in public facilities (Fajardo-Ortiz 2002). Community measures to control these diseases followed, including surveillance of the municipal chlorination of drinking water, promotion of breastfeeding, and training of mothers in the use of ORT in cases of diarrhea and in the early detection of alarm signs of dehydration.

In the 1990s, important improvements in access to water and sanitation in Mexico were achieved, a clear example of the type of inter-sectoral integration needed to address major determinants of health. Between 1990 and 2008, the percentage of the population with access to improved sanitation facilities increased from 66% to 85%, while access to improved drinking water sources increased from 85% to 94% (WHO and UNICEF 2010). These measures produced a decline in diarrhea mortality in children under 5 from 11.5 per 1000 live births in 1985 to only 1.6 in 2000 (Sepúlveda et al. 2006).

A second major public health measure adopted in this period was the introduction, in 1991, of the Universal Immunization Program (UIP). This program was implemented in response to a measles epidemic, the results of a national vaccination survey showing low vaccination coverage, and the commitments made by Mexico in the 1990 World Summit for Children (Valdespino-Gómez and García-García 2004). The program initially offered six vaccines, which were traditionally applied during Mexico's National Health Weeks, a strategy established in 1993 to promote childhood vaccination. This delivery strategy was used to offer not only vaccines, but also to promote the use of oral rehydration salts and distribute mega-doses of oral vitamin A and the antihelminthic drug albendazole. The impacts of the UIP were dramatic: the last cases of polio and diphtheria were notified in 1990 and 1991, respectively, while the last case of autochthonous measles was reported in 1996 (Santos 2002).

An important complement to these initiatives was the implementation, in 1997, of a conditional cash transfer program called *Progresa* (later renamed *Oportunidades*) intended to enhance basic capabilities of families living in extreme poverty. Conditional cash transfers provide cash payments to poor households on the condition that they meet certain conditions, usually related to childhood health and education. This program, which is still active and benefiting over 5 million households, has had proven benefits in the health and nutritional status of children, especially poor indigenous children (Rivera et al. 2004, González de Cossio et al. 2009).

The impact of these initiatives, implemented between 1980 and 2000, upon child survival was unprecedented. However, additional policy innovations had to be designed in order to guarantee the sustainability of these efforts, meet the health-related MDGs, and address the emerging challenges associated with the rise of NCDs.

Mexican Health Reform

Even though a Constitutional amendment establishing the right to the protection of health was passed in Mexico in 1983, not all Mexicans had been able to exercise this right. Those working in the formal sector of the economy and their families – about half of the population – enjoyed the health benefits of social insurance. The other half (around 50 million) was left without access to any form of social protection in health and was forced to use the services of the Ministry of Health, which were delivered on a public charity basis, or the services offered by private providers.

Several analyses conducted in the 1990s showed that the Mexican population was mobilizing huge amounts of resources out-of-pocket to pay for health services, exposing families to ruinous financial episodes. In fact, in 2000, nearly 3 million Mexican households suffered catastrophic health expenditures (Secretaría de Salud 2001). This reality was exposed in the international comparative analysis of fair financing developed by the World Health Organization as part of the *World Health Report 2000*, where Mexico performed poorly (WHO 2002).

The results of this international report and other local analyses were used to promote a legislative reform that established the System for Social Protection in Health in 2004. This system is increasing public resources for health to provide health insurance through a new scheme, *Seguro Popular,* to all those ineligible for social security.

Seguro Popular guarantees access to two sets of benefits:

1. A package of more than 270 essential interventions, which includes all services offered in ambulatory units and general hospitals of the Ministry of Health.
2. A package of 57 costly interventions, which includes neonatal intensive care, bone marrow transplant, and treatment for cancer in children and teenagers, cervical and breast cancer, and HIV/AIDS (Comisión Nacional de Protección Social en Salud 2009, 2011).

By the end of 2011, 52 million people were enrolled in the new insurance program (Comisión Nacional de Protección Social en Salud 2011).

Specific public health instruments to address the backlog of common infections and the emerging challenges were also developed:

*   A protected fund for community health services targeting health promotion and disease prevention interventions which allowed for a major expansion of the basic immunization scheme (which now includes vaccines against 12 diseases) and a complete immunization coverage of 95% in children under 1 and 98% in children under 5.
*   Additional public health investments to enhance human security through: (i) epidemiological surveillance; and (ii) improved preparedness, to respond to emergencies, natural disasters, and many of the threats related to globalization, including potential pandemics.
*   A major reorganization leading to the establishment of a new public health agency charged with protection against health risks through: (i) food safety; (ii) definition of environmental standards; (iii) promotion of occupational safety and prevention of work-related injury; (iv) regulation of the pharmaceutical industry; and (v) control of hazardous substances, such as alcohol and tobacco.

The reform was also forced to define priorities, which are important not only in terms of resource allocation, but also to garner public support. Every reform needs "flagship initiatives" to focus attention on its specific benefits. From the outset, the Ministry of Health decided that one of these flagship initiatives, Fair Start in Life (*Arranque Parejo en la Vida* (APV)), would address the health problems associated with MDG 4 (the goal of reducing child mortality) and MDG 5 (the goal of improving maternal health).

The maternal component of APV included measures to strengthen healthcare networks and the supply of drugs and other inputs, most notably safe blood. Efforts were also made to improve the identification of high-risk pregnancies, increase the percentage of institutional deliveries, and guarantee the timely diagnosis and treatment of obstetric emergencies. The neonatal component of this initiative included the administration of folic acid to pregnant women for the prevention of neural tube defects, preventive neonatal screening

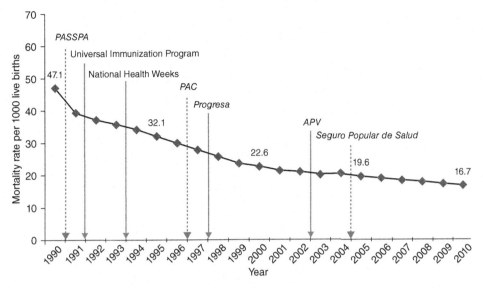

Figure 23.1 Specific health initiatives and under-5 mortality rate in Mexico, 1990–2010.

of congenital metabolic diseases, and strict adherence to the vaccination scheme for this age group.

These measures produced an increase in effective coverage of antenatal care and births attended by skilled health workers; improvements in immunization coverage; and, most importantly, a significant acceleration in the rate of decline of maternal and neonatal mortality (Lozano *et al.* 2006). Between 2001 and 2006, neonatal mortality fell by over 15%, the highest decline in the last 25 years (Secretaría de Salud 2007).

The continuous efforts to expand social protection in health and guarantee access to interventions to address the burden associated with child mortality explain the positive recent evolution of under-5 mortality rate in Mexico. This rate fell from 47.1 per 1000 live deaths in 1990 to 16.7 in 2010 (Figure 23.1). Projections developed by the National Population Council indicate that Mexico will meet the MDG 4 target (15.7 per 1000 live births) ahead of time.

Mexico's impressive progress on MDG 4 offers at least three important lessons for other countries. First, this success was the product of the combined implementation of health system strengthening efforts *and* disease-oriented interventions, which proves again that the dilemma between choosing horizontal and vertical approaches to health-care is a false one.

Second, improvements in child mortality were also dependent on the construction of an evidence base for policy design, policy-making, and policy evaluation. Most of the initiatives implemented in this period were supported by evidence generated by national health and nutritional surveys, and various analyses developed by academic institutions, such as the National Institute of Public Health (which was established in 1987) and global health organizations, such as WHO.

Finally, we cannot underestimate the importance of stable leadership within the Ministry of Health. The story of Mexico in this regard is probably unique: since the 1940s, most ministers have served an entire term of office and many of them have preserved and even expanded policies from preceding administrations when proved effective. This was certainly the case in the past five administrations, which cover a period of 30 years.

Conclusions

The evidence presented in this chapter, including the case study of Mexico's progress in achieving MDG 4, shows that the "diagonal approach" provides a pathway to address global health challenges.

For decades the international health community was trapped in a discussion of the allegedly opposing virtues of vertical and horizontal health programs. However, experience shows that most health challenges can be addressed through the integration of disease-oriented interventions and health system strengthening initiatives (Knaul and Frenk 2011; Knaul *et al.* 2012). Such integration also implies a strong coordination with other sectors involved in health-related activities (e.g., education, housing, agriculture, water, and sanitation). The ties with these other sectors, in fact, allow the ministries of health to act on the broader determinants of health, expanding the scope of action of diagonal approaches. Inter-sectoral relationships were critical in the efforts against diarrheal diseases and will be crucial in confronting the risks related to the emerging NCDs, many of which require interventions in policy domains beyond health.

This process of integration will also benefit from a better understanding of the role of health systems. An important conclusion in this regard is that when thinking about health system strengthening, the global health community should consider not only the delivery of services, but also the financing, stewardship, and resource generating functions. The expansion of the water and sanitation infrastructure in the 1980s and 1990s in Mexico shows the importance of strengthening the stewardship role of the Ministry of Health. An empowered health authority can convince officials in charge of urban infrastructure to mobilize resources of other sectors to meet the health needs of the population.

The global health community should also recognize the need to expand the goals of health systems to include not only the improvement of health conditions, but also the responsiveness of the system and its capacity to provide financial protection. The recent Mexican reform proves that the expansion of social protection in health helps to achieve goals related to specific diseases and population groups, while also protecting families against the financial consequences of health events.

A final conclusion is that the limits of the diagonal approach are not related to its intrinsic features, most of which are being increasingly recognized as useful by many global health actors. Its implementation limits are mostly related to the still widespread belief in the virtues of vertical interventions. It is time to act decisively and creatively to implement the comprehensive strategies demanded by the complex challenges of our times.

Key Reading

Atun R, de Jongh T, Secci F, Ohri K, Adeyi O. 2010. A systematic review of the evidence on integration of targeted health interventions into health systems. *Health Policy and Planning* 25, 1–14.

Knaul FM, Alleyne G, Piot P, *et al.* 2012. Health system strengthening and cancer: a diagonal response to the challenge of chronicity. In Knaul FM, Gralow JL, Atun R, Bhadelia A (eds) *Closing the Cancer Divide: A Blueprint to Expand Access in Low and Middle Income Countries*, pp. 95–122. Boston, MA: Harvard University Press.

Ooms G, Van Damme W, Baker BK, Zeitz, Schrecker T. 2009. The 'diagonal' approach to Global Fund financing: a cure for the broader malaise of health systems? *Globalization and Health* 4, 6.

Price JE, Leslie JA, Welsh M, Binagwaho A. 2009. Integrating HIV clinical services into primary care in Rwanda: a measure of quantitative effects. *AIDS Care* 21, 608–14.

Sepúlveda J, Bustreo F, Tapia R *et al.* 2006. Improvement of child survival in Mexico: the diagonal approach. *Lancet* 368, 2017–27.

Travis P, Bennett S, Haines A *et al.* 2004. Overcoming health-systems constraints to achieve the Millennium Development Goals. *Lancet* 364, 900–6.

References

Atun R, de Jongh T, Secci F, Ohri K, Adeyi O. 2010. A systematic review of the evidence on integration of targeted health interventions into health systems. *Health Policy and Planning* 25, 1–14.

Comisión Nacional de Protección Social en Salud. 2009. *Fondo de Protección contra Gastos Catastróficos.* http://www.seguro-popular.gob.mx/index.php?option=com_content&view=article&id=89&Itemid=124 (last accessed February 2012).

Comisión Nacional de Protección Social en Salud. 2011. *Informe de Resultados 2011.* http://www.seguro-popular.gob.mx/images/contenidos/Informes_Resultados/Informe_Resultados_2011.pdf (last accessed December 2013).

Fajardo-Ortiz G. 2002. De 1982 a 2001: Tiempos de reformas y nuevos avances. In Fajardo-Ortiz G, Carrillo AM, Neri-Vela R. (eds) *Perspectiva Histórica de Atención a la Salud en México 1902–2002*, pp. 101–23. Mexico City: PAHO, UNAM, Sociedad Mexicana de Historia y Filosofía de la Medicina.

Farmer P, Frenk J, Knaul FM *et al.* 2010. Expansion of cancer care and control in countries of low and middle income: a call to action. *Lancet* 376(9747), 1186–93.

Frenk J. 1994. Dimensions of health system reform. *Health Policy* 27, 19–34.

Frenk J. 2010. The global health system: strengthening national health systems as the next step for global progress. *PLOS Medicine* 7(1), e1000089.

Frenk J, Gómez-Dantés O. 2011. Extending the right to health care and improving child survival in Mexico. In Selendy JMH (ed.) *Water and Sanitation-related Diseases and the Environment*, pp. 475–79. Hoboken, NJ: Wiley-Blackwell.

Frenk J, Sepúlveda J, Gómez-Dantés O, Knaul F. 2003. Evidence-based health policy: three generations of reform in Mexico. *Lancet* 362, 1667–71.

Garrett L. 2007. The challenge of global health. *Foreign Affairs* 86, 14–38.

Gómez-Dantés O, Garrido-Latorre F, López-Moreno S, Villa B, López-Cervantes M. 1999. Evaluación de un programa de salud para población no asegurada. *Saúde Publica* 33, 401–12.

González de Cossio T, Rivera J, González-Castell D, Unar-Munguía M, Monterrubio E. 2009. Child malnutrition in Mexico in the last two decades: prevalence using the new WHO 2006 growth standards. *Salud Publica de Mexico* 51(Suppl 4), S494–506.

Gwatkin DR. 2001. The need for equity-oriented health sector reforms. *International Journal of Epidemiology* 30, 720–3.

Knaul FM, Bustreo F, Ha E, Langer A. 2009. Breast cancer: Why link early detection to reproductive health interventions in developing countries? *Salud Publica de Mexico* 51(Suppl 2), S220–7.

Knaul FM, Frenk J. 2011. Strengthening health systems to address new challenge diseases (NCDs). *Harvard Public Health Review*, Fall.

Knaul FM, Alleyne G, Piot P *et al.* 2012. Health system strengthening and cancer: a diagonal response to the challenge of chronicity. In Knaul FM, Gralow JL, Atun R, Bhadelia A (eds) *Closing the Cancer Divide: A Blueprint to Expand Access in Low and Middle Income Countries*, pp. 95–122. Boston, MA: Harvard University Press.

Lozano R, Soliz P, Gakidou E *et al.* 2006. Benchmarking of performance of Mexican states with effective coverage. *Lancet* 368, 1729–41.

Murray CJL, Frenk J. 2000. A framework for assessing the performance of health systems. *Bulletin of the World Health Organization* 78, 717–31.

Newell K. 1988. Selective primary health care: the counter revolution. *Social Science and Medicine* 93, 147–9.

OECD (Overseas Development and Co-operation Institute). (2010). *Millennium Development Goals Report Card: Measuring Progress Across Countries*. London, UK: Overseas Development Institute.

Ooms G, Van Damme W, Baker BK, Zeitz P, Schrecker T. 2008. The "diagonal" approach to Global Fund financing: a cure for the broader malaise of health systems? *Globalization and Health* 4, 6.

Passmore R. 1979. The declaration of Alma-Ata and the future of primary care. *Lancet* 2, 1005–8.

Price JE, Leslie JA, Welsh M, Binagwaho. 2009. Integrating HIV clinical services into primary care in Rwanda: a measure of quantitative effects. *AIDS Care* 21, 608–14.

Rivera J, Sotres-Alvarez D, Habicht JP, Shamah T, Villalpando S. 2004. Impact of the Mexican Program for Education, Health, and Nutrition (*Progresa*) on rates of growth and anemia in infants and young children: a randomized effectiveness study. *JAMA* 219, 2563–70.

Rodríguez-Domínguez J. 2006. Salud para todos. Atención primaria de la salud. In: Urbina-Fuentes M, Moguel-Ancheita A, Muñiz-Martelon ME, Solís-Urdaibay JA. (eds) *La Experiencia Mexicana en Salud Pública. Oportunidad y Rumbo para el Tercer Milenio*, pp. 577–94. Mexico City: Fondo de Cultura Económica.

Samb B, Desai N, Nishtar S *et al.* 2010. Prevention and management of chronic disease: a litmus test for health systems strengthening in low-income and middle-income countries. *Lancet* 376, 1785–97.

Santos JI. 2002. El Programa Nacional de Vacunación: orgullo de México. *Revista de la Facultad de Medicina de la UNAM* 45, 142–53.

Secretaría de Salud. 1996. *Programa de Ampliación de Cobertura: Lineamientos de operación*. Mexico City: Secretaría de Salud.

Secretaría de Salud. 2001. *Programa Nacional de Salud 2001–2006. La democratización de la salud en México. Hacia un sistema universal de salud*, p. 57. Mexico City: Secretaría de Salud.

Secretaría de Salud. 2007. *Salud: México 2006. Información para la Rendición de Cuentas*, p. 19. Mexico City: Secretaría de Salud.

Sepúlveda J. 2006. Foreword. In: Jamison DT, Breman JG, Measham AR *et al.* (eds) *Disease Control Priorities in Developing Countries*, 2nd edn, pp. xiii–xv. New York: Oxford University Press for the World Bank.

Sepúlveda J, Bustreo F, Tapia R *et al.* 2006. Improvement of child survival in Mexico: the diagonal approach. *Lancet* 368, 2017–27.

Soberón G. 2006. Desarrollo de las políticas públicas. In: Urbina-Fuentes M, Moguel-Ancheita A, Muñiz-Martelon ME, Solís-Urdaibay JA (eds) *La Experiencia Mexicana en Salud Pública. Oportunidad y Rumbo para el Tercer Milenio*, pp. 543–66. Mexico City: Fondo de Cultura Económica.

Travis P, Bennett S, Haines A *et al.* 2004. Overcoming health-systems constraints to achieve the Millennium Development Goals. *Lancet* 364, 900–6.

Unger J, Killingsworth J. 1986. Selective primary health care: a critical review of methods and results. *Social Science and Medicine* 22, 1001–100.

Valdespino-Gómez JL, García-García ML. 2004. 30 Aniversario del Programa Nacional de Vacunación contra sarampión en México. Los grandes beneficios y los riesgos potenciales. *Gaceta Médica de Mexico* 140, 639–41.

Walsh J, Warren K. 1979. Selective primary health care: an interim strategy for disease control in developing countries. *New England Journal of Medicine* 301, 967–74.

WHO (World Health Organization). 1978. *Primary Health Care: Report of the International Conference on Primary Health Care. Alma-Ata, USSR, 6–12 September 1978*. Geneva: WHO.

WHO (World Health Organization). 2000. *World Health Report 2000. Health Systems: Improving Performance*. Geneva: WHO.

WHO (World Health Organization). 2002. *Non-Communicable Diseases and Mental Health. Innovative Care for Chronic Conditions. Global Report*. Geneva: WHO.

WHO (World Health Organization). 2010. *World Health Report: Health Systems Financing: the Path to Universal Coverage.* Geneva: WHO. http://www.who.int/whr/2010/en/index.html (last accessed December 2013).

WHO (World Health Organization). 2011a. *World Health Statistics 2011.* Geneva: WHO.

WHO (World Health Organization). 2011b. *Global Status Report on Non-Communicable Diseases 2010.* Geneva: WHO.

WHO (World Health Organization). 2012. *Global Health Observatory.* Geneva. WHO. http://www.who.int/gho/health_financing/en/index.html (last accessed December 2013).

WHO (World Health Organization) Maximizing Positive Synergies Collaborative Group. 2009. An assessment of interactions between global initiatives and country health systems. *Lancet* 373, 2137–69.

WHO (World Health Organization) and UNICEF. 2010. *Progress on Sanitation and Drinking Water: 2010 Update.* Geneva: WHO.

Chapter 24

Will Effective Health Delivery Platforms be Built in Low-Income Countries?

Gorik Ooms, Peter S. Hill, and Yibeltal Assefa

Abstract

Recent estimates indicate that building effective health delivery platforms in low-income countries would cost more than these countries could afford. Low-income countries must rely on international assistance, and therefore global health policies are crucial in determining the future of such delivery platforms. The first decade of the twenty-first century was marked by a substantial increase in development assistance for health (DAH) and by donors committing to align such assistance with the priorities of countries needing assistance. However, most of the additional DAH was allocated to infectious disease control, arguably serving the interests of the countries giving the assistance. Nevertheless, some low-income countries with strong health sector development programs, such as Ethiopia, have been able to take advantage of the international community's willingness to control infectious disease to build stronger and more effective health delivery platforms. Organizations created for global infectious disease control, such as the Global Fund to Fight AIDS, Tuberculosis and Malaria, acknowledge the importance of strong health delivery platforms, although they remain hesitant about their own role in supporting those platforms. Given that the international community will probably always prioritize infectious disease control, the "diagonal approach" – using disease control priorities to drive the building of effective health delivery platforms – should be explored. There are other lessons to be learned from the first decade of the "global health revolution." These include the importance of casting premature and avoidable deaths as human rights violations, and of accepting dependence on international assistance as a problem to be managed with appropriate mechanisms rather than a problem to be avoided.

The Handbook of Global Health Policy, First Edition. Edited by Garrett W. Brown, Gavin Yamey, and Sarah Wamala.
© 2014 John Wiley & Sons, Ltd. Published 2014 by John Wiley & Sons, Ltd.

Key Points

- The "global health revolution" of the first decade of the twenty-first century was in fact a global infectious disease control revolution.
- Casting premature and avoidable deaths as human rights violations helped to provoke the AIDS response, which may be a useful lesson for concerted efforts to build effective health delivery platforms in low-income countries.
- Efforts to achieve universal access to HIV prevention and treatment have relied upon a willingness to accept dependence on international assistance for decades to come, and to consider such dependence as a problem to be managed with appropriate mechanisms rather than a problem to be avoided.
- Such a willingness has not yet been embraced by advocates for effective health delivery platforms.
- Fear of the HIV/AIDS epidemic as a security threat to wealthier countries is another element of the global AIDS response, one that cannot be used for concerted efforts to build effective health delivery platforms in low-income countries.
- Countries with strong health sector development programs have been able to leverage the international community's willingness to control infectious disease to build stronger and more effective health delivery platforms, but this "diagonal approach" has its limits.

Key Policy Implications

Organizations striving for effective health delivery platforms in low-income countries should:

- Acknowledge that international assistance will be needed during decades to come, and consider this a problem to be managed rather than avoided.
- Undertake a principled fight for the acknowledgment of all premature deaths as human rights violations.
- Adopt a pragmatic attitude towards the international community's willingness to control infectious disease.

Introduction

Although health delivery platforms exist in all countries of the world, there is great variation in how *effective* they are in providing "universal health coverage" as defined by the World Health Organization (WHO 2010). In this chapter, we focus on the challenge facing low-income countries in strengthening – or improving the effectiveness of – their health systems. We do not include middle-income countries in our analysis, because we assume that most middle-income countries are financially independent enough to determine their own health systems. In contrast, low-income countries depend financially on international assistance, and therefore health system strengthening in these countries relies to a large extent on policy choices made at the global level.

There is no consensus within the global health policy community on what constitutes ideal health delivery platforms or health systems, or how to build these. The report of the first working group of the Taskforce on Innovative International Financing for Health Systems outlined two quite different approaches. The first approach, developed by the WHO, aims for health centers staffed with "classic" health workers: physicians, nurses, and midwives (Taskforce on Innovative International Financing for Health Systems 2009). The second approach, developed by the World Bank, UNICEF, United Nations Population Fund (UNFPA), and the Partnership for Maternal, Newborn and Child Health, aims for more health posts and basically trained community health workers (Taskforce on Innovative International Financing for Health Systems 2009). Both approaches face a shortage of financial resources in low-income countries – far beyond the capacity of domestic resources – even if they differ on how additional resources would best be used. Assuming that effective health delivery platforms require elements of both approaches, and that decisions about the ideal mix are best left to the health authorities of the concerned countries, the key question becomes: will sufficient, sufficiently reliable, and sufficiently flexible international assistance become available for effective health delivery platforms in low-income countries?

If global health has, during the previous decade, benefitted from an unprecedented increase in international assistance, much of the additional assistance has come with limitations on how these funds can be used. The 2005 Paris Principles for Aid Effectiveness laid out a "roadmap," with 13 targets for improving the quality of aid and its alignment with the priorities of developing countries, which include strengthening their health systems. Yet a recent review, conducted by the Organisation for Economic Co-operation and Development (OECD), suggests that only the target of coordinating technical cooperation has been met by international donors (OECD 2011). In this chapter we examine what happened to the additional funding for global health from an international political economy perspective. How was it spent? Why were the Paris Principles largely ignored? How can we do better at steering the funds towards building effective national health delivery platforms?

First Decade of the "Global Health Revolution": Where Did All the International Assistance Go?

During the first decade of the twenty-first century, with global health prominent on the international political agenda (Fidler 2005), DAH increased substantially (IHME 2010). According to Fidler, this was nothing less than a global health revolution (Fidler 2005). In the same decade, the international community agreed that the efficacy and efficiency of international assistance increases greatly if the countries receiving it are allowed to spend it in accordance with their own priorities (OECD 2005). One would therefore expect that most of the additional DAH was "unearmarked."

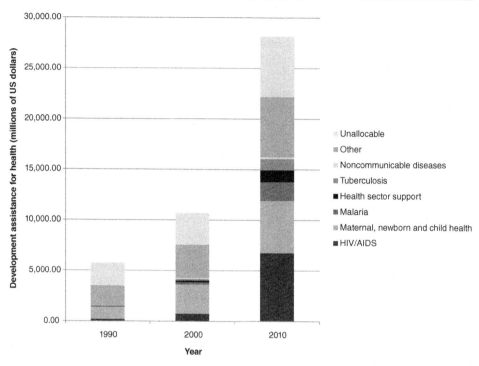

Figure 24.1   The large rise in development assistance for health over the last decade was largely fueled by increased spending on HIV/AIDS, TB, and malaria. Source: data from the IHME.

Yet evidence from the Institute for Health Metrics and Evaluation (IHME) suggests otherwise. The IHME's Financing Global Health 2012 report contained data on DAH 1990–2010, adding preliminary estimates for 2011 and 2012 (IHME 2012). The report disaggregates DAH into six specific categories – HIV/AIDS; maternal, newborn and child health; malaria; health sector support; tuberculosis (TB); and non-communicable diseases – while the rest is allocated to the category "other" or considered "unallocable" (which refers to health aid for which there is no information on the disease focus of this aid). The total amount of international assistance for health was $10.7 billion in 2000 which increased to $28.2 billion in 2010 (in percentages, DAH in 2012 reached 264% of its 2000 level; Figure 24.1). Development assistance to fight HIV/AIDS multiplied by over a factor 9. International assistance to fight TB and malaria multiplied by a factor of 8 (Table 24.1). Development assistance for health sector support in 2010 reached 812% of its 2000 level.

Some will interpret these estimates as evidence that in the fight against HIV/AIDS, TB, and malaria, previously underfunded health systems will have "collaterally" received a great boost (Avila *et al.* 2009). Others believe that the relatively small increase in international assistance for maternal, newborn, and child health is evidence that the international community is mostly interested in efforts to contain infectious disease (Schrade *et al.* 2011). They remain suspicious that the additional international assistance for health sector support was intended to support health delivery platforms unevenly, namely to make sure they would focus on containing infectious disease (Marchal *et al.* 2009). Finally, there are pragmatists, such as Oomman *et al.* (2008), who recognize that the prioritization of infectious disease control by donor countries is an inevitable political reality, but who advocate "seizing the opportunity" for building stronger health delivery platforms. We examine this pragmatic view in the rest of the chapter.

Table 24.1   Between 2000 and 2010, development assistance for health multiplied by a factor 2.6. For development assistance to fight HIV/AIDS, the factor was 9.2; for maternal, newborn, and child health, it was only 1.8.

	Development assistance for health, in millions of US dollars		Development assistance for health in 2010, as a factor of development assistance for health in 2000
	2000	*2010*	
HIV/AIDS	735.26	6,757.36	9.19
Maternal, newborn, and child health	2,899.21	5,166.81	1.78
Malaria	229.52	1,856.67	8.08
Health sector support	145.37	1,180.90	8.12
Tuberculosis	152.55	1,095.13	7.17
Non-communicable diseases	112.22	185.14	1.64
Other	3,293.34	5,945.69	1.80
Unallocable	3,113.54	5,972.06	1.91
Total	10,681.01	28,159.76	2.64

Source: data from the Institute for Health Metrics and Evaluation.

Why was Development Assistance for Health Allocated to Infectious Disease Control?

To test the premise that it is inevitable that the countries providing DAH will prioritize infectious disease control, we need to analyze why the fights against HIV/AIDS, TB, and malaria received such unprecedented levels of international assistance.

First Hypothesis: The "Securitization" of Global Health

The increase in development assistance to fight HIV/AIDS, TB, and malaria coincided with what some have called the "securitization" of global health (a theme discussed in detail in Chapters 15 and 16) (McInnes 2009). In January 2000, the US National Intelligence Council stated: "As a major hub of global travel, immigration, and commerce, along with having a large civilian and military presence and wide-ranging interests overseas, the United States will remain at risk from global infectious disease outbreaks, or even a bioterrorist incident using infectious disease microbes" (National Intelligence Council 2000). The main focus of this report was the HIV/AIDS epidemic and its long-term consequences. Although recent findings suggest that the HIV/AIDS epidemic does not constitute a security threat, the fear that was being expressed back in 2000 did influence the global response (de Waal 2010). McInnes (2009) therefore argues that "it is not 'health' that has been securitised, but rather a limited range of health issues."

Second Hypothesis: Exceptional Activism, Rooted in a Human Rights Approach

Several authors link the unprecedented increase in international assistance to fight HIV/AIDS with exceptional activism (Ingram 2009), rooted in a human rights approach (Forman 2011). AIDS activists succeeded in spreading the idea that every person needing AIDS treatment and dying without receiving it, because they are too poor or they live in a country that is too poor, constitutes a human rights violation. As Forman (2011) argues, the "broader policy consensus that cost-effectiveness demanded a brutal triage in which prevention of HIV/AIDS was funded instead of treatment" was transformed, and "[t]he transformation of this status quo came through effective rights-based advocacy by social movements" (this theme is discussed further in Chapter 25).

However, if rights-based advocacy explains the global HIV/AIDS response, we would expect such advocacy to *also* be effective in other areas of global health. The Declaration of Alma-Ata was all about "primary health care" – a kind of health delivery platform – and was firmly rooted in the right to health, and yet it failed to generate similar levels of international assistance (WHO 1978). Safe motherhood activism was also rooted in human rights (Gruskin *et al.* 2008), but was not as successful as AIDS activism. There must be other factors at work.

Third Hypothesis: Avoiding the "Fatal Attraction" of Cheaper Solutions

Freedman (2011) argues that integrating HIV/AIDS and maternal health services will lead to an "organizational culture clash." Comparing with "the can-do style that has characterized the rapid, well-resourced deployment of HIV services over the last few years," she suggests that maternal health policy reflects "trepidation about services requiring a level of systemic capacity that donors are generally loathe to support – such as emergency obstetric care."

Even if we are willing to accept Freedman's thesis at face value, it has only limited explanatory power. Unless we accept that safe motherhood and primary healthcare activists are intrinsically inclined to accept false solutions, while AIDS activists are natural born "can-doers," the observation only leads to further questions. Could it be that AIDS activists adopted a can-do style simply because they had the international financial resources that allowed them to do so? Then why did they succeed in attracting these resources, while safe motherhood and primary healthcare activists did not?

When it comes to "donors" – if international assistance is about realizing the right to health, "donors" are international duty-bearers – what they really dislike is supporting efforts that will rely indefinitely on their continued support. Pavignani and Columbo (2009) have observed that donors, when faced with protracted crises, "are reluctant to accept the dire fact that a country ravaged by a long-lasting conflict and lacking basic resources and capacity is unsustainable and will remain so for a long time." Such an observation is arguably also true about donor attitudes towards those countries that are not ravaged by conflict, but are simply too poor to finance effective health delivery platforms. Financing effective health delivery platforms, emergency obstetric care, and HIV/AIDS treatment *all raise the same dilemma*: in most low-income countries, such financing is impossible without continued international community support over decades.

Why then have donors been willing to support HIV/AIDS treatment, while remaining reluctant to support comprehensive primary healthcare and emergency obstetric care? Shiffman and Smith (2007) document the longstanding divisions among safe motherhood activists over the issue of emergency obstetric care. Their qualitative study, involving 23 interviews with individuals centrally involved in the development of the global safe motherhood initiative (including most of its founders), had two key findings. First, despite the lack of impact of community-based strategies of the 1970s and 1980s, such as antenatal risk screening and training of traditional birth attendants, some activists continued to support such strategies, arguing that the need for access to emergency obstetric care was "exaggerated." Second, the 2006 *Lancet* series on maternal survival succeeded in building consensus around the need for both attendance by midwives in health centers *and* emergency obstetric care. But this consensus was incomplete: some maternal health advocates continue to question low-income countries' capacity to address the health systems implications of a comprehensive maternal health strategy, and continue to retreat to options within the current reach of low-income countries. Likewise, the Declaration of Alma-Ata was ambivalent on the role of international assistance: primary healthcare should be provided "at a cost that the community and country can afford to maintain at every stage of their development in the spirit of self-reliance and self-determination" (WHO 1978).

The global HIV/AIDS policy community managed to decisively overcome such trepidation. They initially engaged in a debate on whether HIV prevention should be prioritized over antiretroviral treatment – with some arguing that using all available resources for prevention would save more lives in the long run. However, those advocating prioritizing prevention over treatment were ultimately marginalized. For example, within weeks of the publication of an article in which they advocated prevention over treatment (Marseille *et al.* 2002a), Marseille *et al.* conceded that "[t]he cruel choice that should be confronted between prevention and treatment exists mainly because of the failure of wealthy nations, and in part developing countries themselves, to respond effectively to the worldwide pandemic", and that "[t]he era of underfunding and harsh choices has to end quickly, to be replaced by a world in which prevention and treatment both receive their proper support" (Marseille *et al.* 2002b). For the global HIV/AIDS policy community, there was no defendable middle ground: it was either providing treatment or abandoning those already infected to a certain death. For safe motherhood and primary healthcare activists, there still is the "fatal attraction" of cheaper solutions. Despite the cumulative evidence of maternal deaths from the lack of emergency obstetric care, there remains the perverse hope that for those women yet to die from these same causes, "low-cost, simple methods to predict and prevent obstetric complications" (Freedman 2011) will save them.

Fourth Hypothesis: Creation of a Brand New Financing Tool

Considering the hypotheses above, it appears as if the creation of the Global Fund to Fght AIDS, Tuberculosis and Malaria (the Global Fund) was a *consequence* of the international community's willingness to increase support dramatically for the fight against HIV/AIDS, tuberculosis and malaria, rather than a cause. We argue that the three real causes of increased support are as follow:

1. HIV/AIDS, TB, and malaria are infectious diseases and their containment serves the interests of the wealthier countries providing international assistance.
2. AIDS activists maintain their unequivocal commitment to the essentiality of HIV/AIDS treatment in low-income countries, even though such treatment relies on *sustained* international assistance, which donors have traditionally been reluctant to support.
3. Advocates and implementers of the global AIDS response were exceptionally outspoken and rooted their demands in a human rights approach.

Could it be that the consequence (the creation of the Global Fund) reinforced the causes, thus creating a self-amplifying dynamic? There is evidence that such reinforcement has occurred, as discussed below.

If infectious disease control serves the interests of all countries, rich and poor, then international efforts to control infectious disease will provoke "free riding" behavior (a situation in which some countries fail to pay for such disease control efforts, hoping to derive the benefits for free). The US Congress condition that caps American contributions to the Global Fund at 33% of total contributions from all donors aims to prevent such free riding, encouraging other wealthy countries to share the financial burden, rather than simply benefit without contributing (Henry J. Kaiser Family Foundation 2010). Thus, the creation of the Global Fund may have helped to overcome the problem of collective action, as it allowed wealthier countries to increase pressure on each other.

Policy community cohesion, "the degree of coalescence among the network of individuals and organisations that are centrally involved with the issue at the global level" (Shiffman and Smith 2007), is important, but can rapidly fall apart if the policy on which consensus had been reached becomes unfeasible. In many low-income countries, the provision of antiretroviral treatment became possible with the creation of the Global Fund, and the Global Fund's existence provides the financial perspective that allows the policy community cohesion to continue. In November 2011, the Global Fund Board decided to cancel its 11th Round or call for proposals, and created a Transitional Funding Mechanism, because it did not receive enough funding to be able to finance new proposals (Global Fund to Fight AIDS, Tuberculosis and Malaria 2011). The Transitional Funding Mechanism will not finance the scaling up of HIV/AIDS treatment (Global Fund to Fight AIDS, Tuberculosis and Malaria 2012), and it remains to be seen whether the Global Fund will ever be in a position again to support universal access to HIV/AIDS treatment and prevention. We cannot predict how the financial difficulties facing the Global Fund will affect policy community cohesion. For the purposes of our discussion on consequences reinforcing causes, what matters is that the existence of the Global Fund was not only a consequence of policy community cohesion, but also a cause.

Finally, since the creation of the Global Fund, AIDS activists have advocated and lobbied for "burden sharing" between wealthier states (France *et al.* 2002). Spelling out how relatively little it would cost to individual high-income countries to "fully fund the Global Fund" allowed such activists to illustrate the nature of the human rights violation. For less than 2 cents out of every $100 of income produced in high-income countries, HIV treatment and prevention can be provided to *everyone* who needs it. Thus, the Global Fund is both a consequence *and* a cause of rights-based advocacy.

Preliminary Conclusion: An Opportunity for Integrating Infectious Disease Control with Health Systems Strengthening

If our second, third, and fourth hypotheses are valid, then this would mean that there is an opportunity to leverage the international community's willingness to control infectious disease towards building stronger and more effective health delivery platforms.

We can imagine a "Global Fund for Health" (Ooms and Hammonds 2008; Cometto *et al.* 2009) which would provide international co-financing of effective health delivery platforms, providing comprehensive primary healthcare, and encompassing infectious disease control and emergency obstetric care. Such a fund would promote policy community cohesion, and it would illustrate how most premature deaths in low-income countries are related to the unwillingness of the international community to consider health as a real human right. So far, however, most primary healthcare and safe motherhood activists have not embraced this option, while AIDS activists worry that "[w]ithout the necessary additional funding, this proposition will just water down the Global Fund's current ability to deliver effectively and make an impact" (Bermejo 2009).

A Global Fund for Health would, we believe, combine rights-based advocacy for effective health delivery platforms, unequivocal support for a minimum level of health-promoting efforts available to all humans, and a practical solution to make it all possible. However, it is difficult to imagine how such advocacy for effective health delivery platforms would appeal to the security paradigm (hypothesis one). Arhin-Tenkorang and Conceição (2003) studied some of the potential adverse effects upon industrialized nations of the high disease burden of the developing world, such as the spread of infectious diseases and the reduction in investment and trade opportunities. They argue that "*Globalization risks losing its legitimacy*, because disease-stricken people in developing countries are likely to feel disenfranchised and abandoned. Directly or through their advocates, they may question why the asymmetries in addressing health challenges are so dramatic." This is a valid argument, but we do not think that policy-makers in wealthier countries equate the risk of citizens in the poor world developing a grudge against the rich world with the threat of infectious diseases crossing borders. Therefore we tend to agree with Oomman *et al.*'s first premise: it does seem inevitable that the countries providing international assistance will always prioritize infectious disease control, at least to some extent.

Infectious Disease Control Programs Building Health Delivery Platforms: Diagonal Approach, Bottom-Up and Top-Down

The pragmatists' second premise is that international assistance for infectious disease control programs creates opportunities for building stronger health delivery platforms. We examine this premise in two ways:

1. How Ethiopia used development assistance for infectious disease control to build stronger health delivery platforms.
2. How the Global Fund has moved back and forth on the issue of supporting health delivery platforms.

Both can be considered as examples of the "diagonal" approach, or a "strategy in which we use explicit intervention priorities to drive the required improvements into the health system, dealing with such generic issues as human resource development, financing, facility planning, drug supply, rational prescription, and quality assurance" (Frenk 2006). This approach is discussed in Chapter 23.

Bottom-Up: The "Diagonal" Approach Applied in Ethiopia

Ethiopia successfully used the opportunities provided by the global AIDS response to strengthen and expand its health system. The cornerstone of this success was the Health Sector Development Program (HSDP), or more precisely the successive HSDPs, of which the first started in 1997. These national programs introduced important reforms, such as the Health Extension Program that aims to ensure primary healthcare coverage and to institutionalize community health services, thus going far beyond infectious disease control (Sebathu 2008). The priorities of the current HSDP IV (2010/2011 to 2014/2015) are directly aligned with all the health-related Millennium Development Goals (MDGs) and focus on high-impact interventions needed to scale-up coverage of key health services (Ministry of Health of the Federal Democratic Republic of Ethiopia 2010). The global AIDS response offered financial resources and expertise, mainly from the Global Fund, the US President's Emergency Program For AIDS Relief (PEPFAR), and the World Bank Multi-Sectoral HIV/AIDS Program (MAP).

If Ethiopia's partners in the AIDS response agreed to co-finance efforts that went far beyond infectious disease control, it was probably because the government of Ethiopia and the Ministry of Health were able to offer a strategy that offered the partners what they were looking for, and more.

An essential element of the Ethiopian HSDP was a new model of decentralized health-care delivery. This model was essential to making HIV counseling and testing and AIDS treatment more accessible. Ethiopia trained health officers and community-based health extension workers, who also contributed to a significant increase in coverage of primary care services and social mobilization (Assefa *et al.* 2009). This approach was part of the AIDS response, but much more than just a response to AIDS. With funding and expertise from the international partners in the AIDS response, a new cadre of monitoring and evaluation specialists was trained and deployed, to work on monitoring and evaluation for both the AIDS response *and* the broader health system.

Significant progress was made in expanding health facilities in Ethiopia, from 3544 in 2004 to 17,300 in 2010. Again, the international partners in the AIDS response had a crucial role, as these additional facilities were needed for the AIDS response, but the result is that the coverage of primary health service has doubled. Partners in the AIDS response support the National Laboratory Master Plan that promises to also benefit patients with non-communicable diseases, through improved integration of services, and harmonization of procurement, management systems, and referrals. Financing from the AIDS response has been used to strengthen the Pharmaceutical Fund and Supply Agency capacity, to purchase warehouses and trucks, and to build cold storage rooms that will benefit the whole health system.

The case of Ethiopia shows that international partners in the AIDS response are not demanding that each and every dollar can be traced and identified as used for AIDS or other infectious disease control. If it makes sense from an infectious disease control perspective to invest in health systems with a wider purpose, international partners in the AIDS response are flexible enough to support that.

However, the diagonal approach has limits. Health worker posts are essential recurrent expenditures that cannot be linked easily with infectious disease control. This explains why the Minister of Health of Ethiopia, Dr Tedros Adhanom Ghebreyesus, when he was chair of the Global Fund Board, explicitly argued that the Global Fund's mandate should be expanded (Morris 2010).

Yet, with the Global Fund Board cancelling its 11th Round because it did not have adequate funding at hand to finance the expected new proposals (Global Fund to Fight AIDS, Tuberculosis and Malaria 2011), expanding the mandate of the Global Fund under these circumstances is arguably impossible. Somewhat counter-intuitively perhaps, one could argue that this is *exactly* the right time to have the discussion and to push for a well-considered decision on whether or not to expand the Fund's mandate.

Ethiopia is one of the few countries that succeeded in negotiating a "compact" with the International Health Partnerships Plus Related Initiatives (IHP+). IHP+ was launched in 2007 to harmonize donor funding commitments and improve the way that international health agencies, donors, and low-income countries work together to develop and implement national health plans. While such a compact is expected to greatly improve the alignment of international assistance with Ethiopia's priorities, it does not come with commitments to increase international financial assistance (IHP+Results 2011). Ethiopia's Ministry of Health was counting on the participation of the Global Fund in the Health Systems Funding Platform, a joint initiative with GAVI Alliance and the World Bank, to mobilize and harmonize financing in a way that held the promise of more flexible support for health systems. Not only has the future of the platform become uncertain (the Global Fund has suspended its participation in the platform), but we also fear that the current flexibility will be reduced. The same Global Fund Board meeting that cancelled Round 11 also agreed to implement the recommendations of the Report of the High Level Independent Review Panel on Fiduciary Controls and Oversight Mechanisms

(2011), which was established to examine alleged mismanagement issues but which went beyond that task. One of the recommendations was that "[t]he Global Fund must be much more assertive about where and how its money is deployed; it should take a more global look at the disease burden and better determine who needs the money most." A "more assertive" attitude may also be a less flexible attitude.

Top-Down: The Health Systems Funding Platform

The turn of the millennium was marked by anxiety about the global impact of HIV/AIDS, TB, and malaria, and, implicitly, by a strong critique of the current multilateral approach to disease control (Brown and Barnes 2009). The 2000 G8 meeting committed members to raising additional resources "beyond traditional approaches" to combat these threats to economic growth (G8 2000). The solution, a "global fund, dedicated to the battle against HIV/AIDS and other infectious diseases" (Annan 2001), was to be independent of the United Nations, and function non-politically as a financial institution rather than an implementing agency. But the focused commitment – on HIV/AIDS, tuberculosis, and malaria – was clear.

However, the environment in which the "non-political" Global Fund to fight AIDS, Tuberculosis and Malaria was created was intensely political; a product of its time. It bypassed the World Bank, UNAIDS, WHO and built on the successful precedent of the Global Alliance for Vaccines and Immunization (GAVI) as a global public–private partnership (Brugha et al. 2002. It secured funding interests from the Bill & Melinda Gates Foundation, influential wealthier countries, and key non-government organizations. The new Global Fund's commitment to innovation in this fight against infectious diseases, the public–private partnership, the engagement of civil society globally and locally, and the new transparency in operations, temporarily eclipsed some other tensions among diverse stakeholders (such as the appropriateness of launching yet another global health initiative using a vertical approach). Yet, within three years, commentators were pointing to the need to address health systems issues if sustainable population-wide infectious disease control interventions were to be achieved (Travis et al. 2004; Brugha 2005).

In 2005, the GAVI Alliance opened a "window" for health systems strengthening, aimed at addressing systemic obstacles obstructing achievement of immunization targets (Galichet et al. 2010). Despite challenges, the initiative was largely successful (Naimoli 2009). In 2005, the Global Fund replicated GAVI's health systems initiative with its own health systems window to Round 5, despite apprehension that this window might dilute the Global Fund's core mandate. However, the applications submitted were considered "quite poor – lacking operational detail, real budgets and adequate justifications for the activities proposed" (Shakow 2006), and only three health systems grants were awarded. The Global Fund Technical Review Panel recommended the health systems window be discontinued, arguing that systemic change was not achievable within the constraints of the Global Fund's current structure, with 2–3-year funding cycles, and the Global Fund's lack of country presence (Global Fund to Fight AIDS, Tuberculosis and Malaria 2005). A review of health workforce issues at the Global Fund underlined the tension between effectively engaging its three target diseases and attempting to influence broader health systems outcomes (Dräger et al. 2006). Subsequent health system efforts were integrated as components of other Global Fund applications, and attention shifted towards measuring health systems contributions of Global Fund programs, then estimated at up to half of Global Fund funding commitments (Feachem and Sabot 2006). The seeming indiscriminate inclusion of all "health system-related" components in this metric did little to reassure those advocating a more "horizontal" health systems strengthening approach, particularly where those components related specifically to the disease programs (Marchal *et al.* 2009). For advocates of a more targeted mandate, this scale of health systems funding was disquieting.

Three years after the reaffirmation of the Global Fund's focused mandate in 2006, the Global Fund joined the GAVI Alliance in its assertive challenge to the 2009 Taskforce on Innovative International Financing for Health Systems: "It is time to take a comprehensive approach with the necessary support from key donors to refocus on all of the health-related MDGs as a renewed commitment to meeting the basic health service delivery needs in poor countries. We are willing and keen to do this" (Lob-Levyt and Kazatchkine 2009). The shift reflected a change in leadership and context – Michel Kazatchkine was now Executive Director of the Global Fund; Julian Lob-Levyt, an experienced health systems advocate, was the Chief Executive Office at the GAVI Alliance; the International Financing Facility for Immunization offered substantial new funding; and health systems strengthening was again a focus for global development (WHO 2007; Reich *et al.* 2008).

Yet the Health Systems Funding Platform recommended by the Taskforce has been slow to integrate its three partners, with their different governance structures and mandates, distinctive application, approval, and financing processes, and persisting caution within the boards in a changing economic climate (Hill *et al.* 2011). Harmonization of existing health systems components of GAVI Alliance and Global Fund grants has been productive. However, the so-called "Common Funding Application" is not truly "common": contributions sought from each of the partners to be identified in the application still require the separate approval of each of these partners, following the processes of each partner's established practice, and signed off by each partner's respective board. Furthermore, the cancellation of Global Fund's Round 11 has suspended collaboration of the Global Fund in the Platform, and both Global Fund and GAVI Alliance have subsequently reconstructed their health systems support structures so that health systems activities are more tightly linked to their mandated programs. Although both have continued their collaborations on harmonization through the International Health Partnership Plus, there is little enthusiasm to see the Health Systems Funding Platform resuscitated. The subservience of health systems support to infectious disease control has again been underscored (Global Fund to Fight AIDS, Tuberculosis and Malaria 2011).

Conclusions

In the introduction, we formulated the key question: will sufficient, sufficiently reliable and sufficiently flexible international assistance become available for effective health delivery platforms in low-income countries? We have addressed this question by analyzing the evolution of DAH in the first decade of the twenty-first century – or the decade of the "global health revolution" (Fidler 2005) and of *alleged* alignment of international assistance with national priorities (OECD 2005). We find that the global health revolution is not about alignment with the priorities of low-income countries at all, but mostly about infectious disease control. Trying to be useful to people who want effective health delivery platforms in low-income countries, we verified the "pragmatists' view," according to which prioritization of infectious disease control in international assistance is inevitable, but nonetheless creates opportunities for health delivery platforms (Oomman *et al.* 2008).

The global AIDS response benefited from AIDS being an infectious disease, which threatened wealthier countries, and from these wealthier countries desiring to keep the epidemic in check. These features cannot be replicated in some kind of "global health delivery platform revolution." However, advocates for comprehensive primary healthcare or health delivery platforms can learn lessons from AIDS activism:

- The importance of presenting premature deaths as human rights violations.
- The importance of policy community cohesion and of a shared willingness to consider dependence on international assistance as a problem to be managed rather than as a problem to be avoided.
- The need for a financing mechanism that: (a) shows how modest the effort required from the international community is (and thus allows presentation of premature deaths as human rights violations); and (b) provides a sufficiently reliable perspective on available resources for policy community cohesion to be built.

Infectious disease control efforts create opportunities for comprehensive primary healthcare or health delivery platforms. Countries can present their comprehensive health sector development programs as essential for effective disease control; the chances are that their international infectious disease control partners will embrace and support comprehensive health sector development programs. International organizations created for infectious disease control realize that they must support comprehensive programs. The so-called "diagonal" approach is alive but reaching its limits. The Global Fund's cancellation of Round 11, in combination with its acceptance of a recommendation about being "assertive about where and how its money is deployed" (High-Level Independent Review Panel on Fiduciary Controls and Oversight Mechanisms 2011), probably signals that it will have to be more focused on infectious disease control.

In trying to be useful to everyone who wants comprehensive primary healthcare and effective health delivery platforms in low-income countries, we recommend a combination of principle and pragmatism. We recommend a principled fight for the acknowledgment of all premature deaths as human rights violations, and a pragmatic attitude towards the international community's willingness to control infectious disease. So far, we seem to have the opposite: a principled fight that squabbles over narrow attempts to control infectious disease, and yet no pragmatic plan that confronts the reality that most premature deaths are avoidable and constitute human rights violations.

Key Reading

Assefa Y, Jerene D, Lulseged S, Ooms G, Van Damme W. 2009. Rapid scale-up of antiretroviral treatment in Ethiopia: successes and system-wide effects. *PLOS Medicine* 6(4), e1000056.

Forman L. 2011. Global AIDS Funding and the re-emergence of AIDS 'Exceptionalism'. *Social Medicine* 6(1), 45–51.

Freedman LP. 2011. Integrating HIV and maternal health services: will organizational culture clash sow the seeds of a new and improved implementation practice? *Journal of Acquired Immune Deficiency Syndrome* 57(Suppl 2), S80–2.

Hill PS, Vermeiren P, Miti K, Ooms G, Van Damme W. 2011. The Health Systems Funding Platform: Is this where we thought we were going? *Globalization and Health* 7, 16.

McInnes C. 2009. National Security and Global Health Governance. In Kay A, Williams OD (eds) *Global Health Governance: Crisis, Institutions and Political Economy*, pp. 225–45. Basingstoke: Palgrave MacMillan.

WHO (World Health Organization). 2010. *The World Health Report: Health Systems Financing: The Path to Universal Coverage*. Geneva: WHO. http://whqlibdoc.who.int/whr/2010/9789241564021_eng.pdf (last accessed December 2013).

References

Annan K. 2001. *Secretary General proposes Global Fund for Fight Against HIV/AIDS and Other Infectious Diseases at African Leaders Summit.* United Nations Press Release SG/SM/779/REV.1, April. http://www.un.org/News/Press/docs/2001/SGSM7779R1.doc.htm (last accessed December 2013).

Arhin-Tenkoran D, Conceição P. 2003. Beyond communicable disease control: health in the age of globalization. In Kaul I, Conceição P, Le Goulven K, Mendoza RU (eds). *Providing Global Public Goods: Managing Globalization.* New York: Oxford University Press.

Assefa Y, Jerene D, Lulseged S, Ooms G, Van Damme W. 2009. Rapid scale-up of antiretroviral treatment in Ethiopia: successes and system-wide effects. *PLOS Medicine* 6(4), e1000056.

Avila C, Menser N, McGreevey W. 2009. HIV and AIDS Programs: How they support health system strengthening. AIDS2031 Working Paper No. 18. Washington, DC: Results for Development Institute. http://www.aids2031.org/pdfs/hiv%20and%20aids%20programs%20-%20how%20they%20support%20health%20system%20strengthening_18.pdf (last accessed December 2013).

Bermejo A. 2009. Towards a global fund for the health MDGs? *Lancet* 373(9681), 2110.

Brown GW, Barnes A. 2009. The Global Fund to Fight AIDS, Tuberculosis and Malaria: expertise, accountability and depoliticisation of global health governance. Paper presented at the International Studies Association (ISA) Annual Convention, New York. http://citation.allacademic.com/meta/p_mla_apa_research_citation/3/1/3/4/4/pages313441/p313441-1.php (last accessed December 2013).

Brugha R, Starling M, Walt G. 2002. GAVI, the first steps: lessons for the Global Fund. *Lancet* 359(9304), 435–8.

Brugha R. 2005. The Global Fund at three years: flying in crowded air space. *Tropical Medicine and International Health* 10(7), 623–6.

Cometto G, Ooms G, Starrs A, Zeitz P. 2009. A global fund for the health MDGs? *Lancet* 373(9674), 1500–2.

de Waal A. 2010. Reframing governance, security and conflict in the light of HIV/AIDS: a synthesis of findings from the AIDS, security and conflict initiative. *Social Science and Medicine* 70(2010), 114–120.

Dräger S, Gedik G, Dal Poz MR. 2006. Health workforce issues and the Global Fund to fight AIDS, Tuberculosis and Malaria: an analytic review. *Human Resources for Health* 4, 23.

Feachem R, Sabot O. 2006. An examination of the Global Fund at 5 years. *Lancet* 368(9534), 537–40.

Fidler DP. 2005. Health as foreign policy: between principle and power. *Whitehead Journal of Diplomacy and International Relations* 7(1), 179–94.

Forman L. 2011. Global AIDS Funding and the re-emergence of AIDS 'Exceptionalism'. *Social Medicine* 6(1), 45–51.

France T, Ooms G, Rivers B. 2002. The Global Fund to Fight AIDS, Tuberculosis and Malaria: which countries owe, and how much? *IAPAC Monthly* 8(5), 138.

Freedman LP. 2011. Integrating HIV and maternal health services: will organizational culture clash sow the seeds of a new and improved implementation practice? *Journal of Acquired Immune Deficiency Syndrome* 57(Suppl 2), S80–2.

Frenk J. 2006. Bridging the divide: comprehensive reform to improve health in Mexico. Lecture for WHO Commission on Social Determinants of Health, in Nairobi, 29 June. http://www.who.int/social_determinants/resources/frenk.pdf (last accessed December 2013).

G8. 2000. *G8 Communiqué Okinawa.* http://www.g8.utoronto.ca/summit/2000okinawa/finalcom.htm (last accessed December 2013).

Galichet B, Goeman L, Hill PS *et al.* 2010. Linking programmes and systems: lessons from the GAVI Health Systems Strengthening window. *Tropical Medicine and International Health* 15(2), 208–15.

Global Fund to Fight AIDS, Tuberculosis and Malaria. 2005. *Report of the Technical Review Panel and the Secretariat on Round Five Proposals.* GF/B11/6 Eleventh Board Meeting. Geneva, 28–30

September. http://www.theglobalfund.org/documents/board/11/gfb116.pdf (last accessed December 2013).

Global Fund to Fight AIDS, Tuberculosis and Malaria. 2011. *Global Fund Board establishes a Transitional Funding Mechanism to replace Round 11 and revises the application and approval process for renewals.* Geneva: The Global Fund. http://www.theglobalfund.org/en/mediacenter/announcements/2011-12-01_Global_Fund_Board_establishes_a_Transitional_Funding_Mechanism/ (last accessed December 2013).

Global Fund to Fight AIDS, Tuberculosis and Malaria. 2012. *Transitional Funding Mechanism (TFM). Information Note.* Geneva: The Global Fund. http://www.theglobalfund.org/en/application/infonotes/ (last accessed December 2013).

Gruskin S, Cottingham J, Martin Hilber A, Kismodi E, Lincetto O, Roseman MJ. 2008. Using human rights to improve maternal and neonatal health: history, connections and a proposed practical approach. *Bulletin of the World Health Organization* 86(8), 589–93.

Henry J. Kaiser Family Foundation. 2010. *The US and the Global Fund to fight AIDS, Tuberculosis and Malaria. Menlo Park: Henry J. Kaiser Family Foundation.* http://www.kff.org/globalhealth/upload/8003-02.pdf (last accessed December 2013).

High-Level Independent Review Panel on Fiduciary Controls and Oversight Mechanisms of the Global Fund to Fight AIDS, Tuberculosis and Malaria. 2011 *Turning the Page from Emergency to Sustainability.* http://www.theglobalfund.org/en/highlevelpanel/report/ (last accessed December 2013).

Hill PS, Vermeiren P, Miti K, Ooms G, Van Damme W. 2011. The Health Systems Funding Platform: Is this where we thought we were going? *Globalization and Health* 7, 16.

IHP+Results. 2011. *Strengthening accountability to achieve the health MDGs.* http://ihpresults.net/wp-content/uploads/2011/02/IHP+Results-2010-Performance-Report-w-cover_EN.pdf   (last accessed December 2013).

Ingram A. 2009. The international political economy of global responses to HIV/AIDS. In Kay A, Williams OD (eds) *Global Health Governance: Crisis, Institutions and Political Economy.* Basingstoke: Palgrave MacMillan.

IHME (Institute for Health Metrics and Evaluation). 2012. *Financing Global Health 2012: The End of the Golden Age?* http://www.healthmetricsandevaluation.org/publications/policy-report/financing-global-health-2012-end-golden-age (last accessed December 2013).

Lob-Levyt J, Kazatchkine M. 2009. *Letter to the Honorable Gordon Brown, Prime Minister of the United Kingdom and Mr Robert Zoellick, President of the World Bank.* http://www.internationalhealthpartnership.net/pdf/IHP%20Update%2013/Task Force/london%20meeting/new/GAVI%20and%20GFATM%20letter.pdf (last accessed December 2013).

Marchal B., Cavalli A., Kegels G. 2009. Global health actors claim to support health system strengthening: is this reality or rhetoric? *PLOS Medicine* 6(4), 2100059.

Marseille E, Hofmann PB, Kahn JG. 2002a. HIV prevention before HAART in sub-Saharan Africa. *Lancet* 359(9320), 1851–6.

Marseille E, Hofmann PB, Kahn JG. 2002b. HIV prevention and treatment. *Lancet* 360(9326), 87–8.

McInnes C. 2009. National security and global health governance. In Kay A, Williams OD (eds) *Global Health Governance: Crisis, Institutions and Political Economy.* Basingstoke: Palgrave MacMillan.

Ministry of Health of the Federal Democratic Republic of Ethiopia. 2010. *Health Sector Development Program IV 2010/11 – 2014/15.* http://phe-ethiopia.org/admin/uploads/attachment-721-HSDP%20IV%20Final%20Draft%2011Octoberr%202010.pdf (last accessed December 2013).

Morris K. 2010. Profile: Tedros Adhanom Ghebreyesus – a Global Fund for the health MDGs. *Lancet* 375(9724), 1429.

Naimoli JF. 2009. Global health partnerships in practice: taking stock of the GAVI Alliance's new investment in health systems strengthening. *International Journal of Health Planning and Management* 24(1), 3–25.

National Intelligence Council. 2000. *The Global Infectious Disease Threat and its Implications for the United States. National Intelligence Estimate.* http://www.cfr.org/public-health-threats-

and-pandemics/national-intelligence-estimate-global-infectious-disease-threat-its-implications-united-states/p18334 (last accessed December 2013).

OECD (Organisation for Economic Co-operation and Development). 2005. *The Paris Declaration on Aid Effectiveness and the Accra Agenda for Action*. Paris: OECD Publishing. http://www.oecd.org/dac/effectiveness/parisdeclarationandaccraagendaforaction.htm (last accessed December 2013).

OECD (Organisation for Economic Co-operation and Development). 2011. *Aid Effectiveness 2005–2010: Progress in implementing the Paris Declaration*. Paris: OECD Publishing. http://www.oecd.org/dac/effectiveness/48742718.pdf (last accessed December 2013).

Oomman N, Bernstein M, Rosenzweig S. 2008. *Seizing the Opportunity on AIDS and Health Systems*. Washington, DC: Center for Global Development. http://www.cgdev.org/content/publications/detail/16459/ (last accessed December 2013).

Ooms G, Hammonds R. 2008. Correcting globalisation in health: transnational entitlements versus the ethical imperative of reducing aid-dependency. *Public Health Ethics* 1(2), 154–70.

Pavignani E, Colombo A. 2009. *Analysing Disrupted Health Sectors: A Modular Manual*. Geneva: World Health Organization. http://www.who.int/hac/techguidance/tools/disrupted_sectors/adhsm_en.pdf (last accessed December 2013).

Reich MR, Takemi K, Roberts MJ, Hsiao WC. 2008. Global action on health systems: a proposal for the Toyako G8 summit. *Lancet* 371(9615), 865–9.

Sebathu A. 2008. *The implementation of Ethiopia's Health Extension Program: an overview*. http://ppdafrica.org/docs/ethiopiahep.pdf (last accessed December 2013).

Schrade C, Schäferhoff M, Yamey G. Richter E. 2011. *Strengthening the Global Financing Architecture for Reproductive, Maternal, Newborn, and Child Health: Options for Action*. Geneva: Partnership for Maternal, Newborn and Child Health. http://globalhealthsciences.ucsf.edu/sites/default/files/content/ghg/e2pi-options-for-improving-rmnch.pdf (last accessed December 2013).

Shakow A. 2006. *Global Fund-World Bank HIV/AIDS Programs Comparative Advantage Study*. Washington, DC: The World Bank; Geneva: The Global Fund to Fight AIDS, Tuberculosis and Malaria. http://siteresources.worldbank.org/INTHIVAIDS/Resources/375798-1103037153392/GFWBReportFinalVersion.pdf (last accessed December 2013).

Shiffman J, Smith S. 2007. Generation of political priority for global health initiatives: a framework and case study of maternal mortality. *Lancet* 370(9595), 1370–9.

Taskforce on Innovative International Financing for Health Systems. 2009. Working Group 1 Technical Background Report (World Health Organization). Geneva: World Health Organization; Washington, DC: World Bank. http://www.internationalhealthpartnership.net/en/about-ihp/past-events/high-level-taskforce-for-innovative-international-financing-of-health-systems/ (last accessed February 2014).

Travis P, Bennett S, Haines A *et al*. 2004. Overcoming health-systems constraints to achieve the Millennium Development Goals. *Lancet* 364(9437), 900–6.

WHO (World Health Organization). 1978. *Declaration of Alma-Ata. International Conference on Primary Health Care, Alma-Ata, USSR, 6–12 September 1978*. http://www.who.int/publications/almaata_declaration_en.pdf (last accessed December 2013).

WHO (World Health Organization). 2007. *Everybody's Business: Strengthening Health Systems to Improve Health Outcomes: WHO's Framework for Action*. Geneva: WHO. http://www.who.int/healthsystems/strategy/everybodys_business.pdf (last accessed December 2013).

WHO (World Health Organization). 2010. *The World Health Report: Health Systems Financing: The Path to Universal Coverage*. Geneva: WHO. http://whqlibdoc.who.int/whr/2010/9789241564021_eng.pdf (last accessed December 2013).

Part VI   Health Rights and Partnerships

A Rights-Based Approach to Global Health Policy: What Contribution can Human Rights Make to Achieving Equity?

Lisa Forman

Abstract

This chapter explores the contribution of human rights to the achievement of global health equity. In doing so, it outlines the international human rights legal framework relevant to health, explores critiques and limitations of this framework, and turns to explore the potential contribution of human rights to global health equity. The chapter looks at specific mechanisms and illustrative case studies, including traditional human rights measures, such as litigation, social movement and advocacy, and innovative human rights mechanisms, such as rights-based approaches and indicators.

The Handbook of Global Health Policy, First Edition. Edited by Garrett W. Brown, Gavin Yamey, and Sarah Wamala.
© 2014 John Wiley & Sons, Ltd. Published 2014 by John Wiley & Sons, Ltd.

Key Points

- International human rights law offers a potentially powerful tool for achieving global health equity.
- Social actors are increasingly using human rights to successfully claim access to health services.
- Human rights advocacy can effectively advance equity.
- Innovative rights applications can guide standard public and global health policy towards greater equity.
- Additional research is needed to strengthen the contribution of human rights to global health.
- The right to health specifies individual entitlements and state duties to ensure adequate healthcare and underlying determinants (water, housing, sanitation, food).

Key Policy Implications

- The right to health offers a guiding framework for global health equity.
- International human rights law offers social actors potentially powerful norms and mechanisms.
- States are bound by both domestic and global duties regarding health equity.

Introduction

What contribution can human rights make to the achievement of global health equity? In particular, can the right to health in international human rights law assist in remediating global disparities in health and healthcare? These questions are increasingly relevant given growing attention to the way in which the right to health can advance both the social determinants of health (United Nations 2011) and health equity at the domestic level (Yamin and Gloppen 2011), provide a normative and legal framework for global health diplomacy (Gagnon and Labonté 2011), and respond to globalization (Schrecker 2011). The potential for human rights to contribute to health equity is illustrated in successful advocacy for access to antiretroviral (ARV) drugs in sub-Saharan Africa. Such potential is also seen in the growing use of human rights-based domestic litigation by social actors in low- and middle-income countries (LMICs) to claim health needs. Moreover, supranational human rights law systems offer additional monitoring and accountability mechanisms that can guide health equity.

Despite these promising ways in which the right to health can be leveraged, human rights and the right to health in particular are also limited in addressing key structural determinants of global health inequity. These determinants include inadequate domestic and international allocations to health, neoliberal international trade laws that deprioritize domestic health spending and commodify essential health needs, and economic recessions and crises that are gutting northern aid commitments to global health.

Given such limitations, this chapter explores both the strengths and weaknesses of human rights in advancing global health equity. It begins by outlining the international human rights legal framework relevant to health and exploring critiques and limitations of this framework. It then turns to explore the potential contribution of human rights to global health equity, outlining traditional human rights measures, such as litigation, social movement, and advocacy, and innovative human rights mechanisms, such as rights-based approaches, rights-based indicators, and impact assessment. Finally, it outlines a research agenda on global health and human rights to respond to key weaknesses in the international law framework.

The Right to Health in International Human Rights Law

The genesis of the human right to health is rooted in the intertwined emergence of the United Nations (UN) and international human rights law after 1945. As the Allies met through 1945 and 1946 to determine the scope and content of the founding *Charter of the United Nations* (UN 1945), they were successfully pressed by Latin American and Asian delegates and a consortium of mostly US-based non-governmental organizations (NGOs) to include a position on individual rights (Glendon 2002: 14–19). The Charter accordingly established that one of the UN's founding purposes was to "achieve international cooperation … in promoting and encouraging respect for human rights and for fundamental freedoms for all without distinction as to race, sex, language, or religion" (UN 1945: article 1.3). This responsibility was institutionalized in the Charter's directive for the Economic and Social Council (a principal organ of the UN along with the General Assembly and Security Council) to establish a commission on human rights (UN 1945: article 68). In 1946, the newly established UN Commission on Human Rights decided that its first project would be to write a bill of human rights (Glendon 2002: 31–2). Two years later the now iconic *Universal Declaration of Human Rights* (UDHR) (UN 1948) was adopted by the UN General Assembly, providing the first international iteration of human rights, incorporating economic, social, and cultural rights (such as rights to an adequate standard of living, social security, work, education, and participation in cultural life) and civil and political rights (such as rights to be free from torture, equality before the law, free expression, movement, and association).

This conception of human rights as encompassing both social and civil entitlements is rooted in two historical trends. First, earlier western iterations of civil rights (including the British Bill of Rights of 1689, the US Declaration of Independence of 1776, and the French Declaration of the Rights of Man of 1789) emphasized freedom and government responsibility to protect man's natural liberties (Glendon 2002: xvii). Second, continental European notions of rights emerged, encompassing equality and fraternity and imposing duties on the state to protect the poor (Glendon 2002: xvii). These latter notions of rights evolved into social rights, which were synthesized with civil rights in newly independent Latin American countries, and adopted to the exclusion of civil rights by the Soviet Union (Glendon 2002: xvii–xviii). The synthesis of social and civil rights found expression in Franklin D. Roosevelt's influential "Four Freedoms Speech" in 1941, which laid the groundwork for the UDHR by identifying freedom of speech and belief and freedom from fear and want as the essential freedoms necessary to create a secure world (Roosevelt 1941). The combination of social and civil rights became institutionalized within emerging international human rights law as the notion of the indivisibility, interrelated, and interdependent nature of all human rights (World Conference on Human Rights 1993). Yet the geopolitical forces of the Cold War effectively divided civil and social rights for western and eastern blocs, with social rights misconceived in the West as exclusively associated with communism, and similar misconceptions in the East seeing civil rights as dependent on capitalism for their realization. This historical backdrop accounts to some extent for the persistent (and historically inaccurate) characterization of social rights, such as the right to health, as socialist, and civil rights (and sometimes human rights in totality) as liberal and/or capitalist.

Since 1948, the modern international human rights law system has rapidly evolved, producing nine core human rights treaties, many UN institutions, and at least a hundred human rights declarations, resolutions, conferences, and programs of action. Regional analogs of the international human rights law system have developed in Africa, the Americas, and Europe. The speed of these developments has seen international human rights law become the fastest growing field in international law (Mutua 2001).

Development of the Right to Health Within the United Nations

The UN Charter includes the first formal articulation of state duties concerning health, stating that one of the UN's objectives is to promote "solutions of international economic, social, health, and related problems" (UN 1945: article 55). In pursuance of this objective, in 1946 the *Constitution of the World Health Organization* (WHO Constitution) established the WHO as a specialized UN agency with the objective of attaining "by all peoples … the highest possible level of health" (UN 1946: article 1). The WHO Constitution was the first international document to articulate an individual's right to health, recognizing that "the enjoyment of the highest attainable standard of health is a fundamental right of every human being without distinction of race, religion, political belief, economic or social condition" (UN 1946: preamble). The Constitution also recognized that governments have a responsibility "for the health of their peoples which can be fulfilled only by the provision of adequate health and social measures" (UN 1946: preamble). However, the Constitution did not define what might constitute "adequate" measures. The lack of guidance on how adequate health measures could reasonably be expected to fulfill the highest attainable standard of health was complicated further by the Constitution's expansive definition of health as "a state of complete physical, mental and social well-being and not merely the absence of disease or infirmity" (UN 1946: preamble).

The right to health was further developed in the UDHR, which recognizes that "everyone has the right to a standard of living adequate for the health and well-being of himself and of his family, including food, clothing, housing and medical care and necessary social services" (UN 1948: article 25.1). The inclusion of medical care within the minimum socioeconomic conditions necessary for health advances the definition of health by providing potential *parameters* for achieving the highest attainable standard of health (Forman and Bomze 2012). Nonetheless, the combination of health with other social rights fails to provide any textual explanation of what might be needed to ensure health (Toebes 1999: 40). While the UDHR was meant to act as "a common standard of achievement" and not as a binding human rights treaty (UN 1946: preamble), it is widely understood to have become customary international law, imposing obligations that apply to all states globally for realization (UN 1968: article 2; Sohn 1982: 16; International Law Association 1994: 525–69).

The UN's original intention to codify the UDHR through the creation of one new treaty was routed by the ideological conflicts of the Cold War. Instead the UDHR was codified in two distinct international human rights treaties: the *International Covenant on Economic, Social and Cultural Rights* (ICESCR) (UN 1976a) and the *International Covenant on Civil and Political Rights* (ICCPR) (UN 1976b). Together with the UDHR, these instruments form what is known as the International Bill of Rights. The Cold War conflicts also slowed the process down considerably, so that it took almost 30 years before these two treaties became operational.

The ICESCR provides the most authoritative formulation of the right to health in international law. Box 25.1 details article 12, which deals with the right to health where states recognize the right to the highest attainable standard of health and undertake to take steps to achieve this right. However, the duties articulated in article 12 are significantly undercut by article 2 of the ICESCR where states agree:

> … to take steps, individually and through international assistance and cooperation, especially economic and technical, to the maximum of [their] available resources, to achieve progressively the full realization of Covenant rights by all appropriate means, including particularly legislation.

This limitation of state duties to progressively realize the right to health within available resources constrains the expansive promise of a right to the highest attainable standard of health. Certainly for states ratifying this treaty, there was little clarity on the scope and content of this circumscribed duty towards health, a task that fell to subsequent human rights instruments and interpretations.

Box 25.1 Article 12 of the ICESCR

- Article 12 recognizes everyone's right to the enjoyment of the highest attainable standard of physical and mental health.
- It prescribes specific steps for states to take in order to fully realize this right, including to:
  - reduce the stillbirth rate and infant mortality;
  - improve all aspects of environmental and industrial hygiene;
  - prevent, treat, and control epidemic, endemic, occupational, and other diseases; and
  - create conditions that assure medical services and attention to all in the event of sickness.

After the ICESCR, additional human rights treaties were drafted to provide explicit protection to vulnerable groups such as racial minorities, women, children, and people with disabilities. Several of these treaties incorporate rights to health as applied to their focus populations, thereby incrementally developing the scope and content of the right to health. The *International Convention on the Elimination of All Forms of Racial Discrimination* (ICERD) obligates state parties to guarantee everyone's right to public health and medical care in the context of general measures to prohibit racial discrimination (UN 1969: article 5.e.iv). This Convention not only identifies medical care as an individual entitlement but also suggests a collective right to public health. The *Convention on the Elimination of All Forms of Discrimination Against Women* (CEDAW) similarly expands on the right to health (UN 1979). The CEDAW demands that state parties undertake measures to ensure women's equal access to healthcare services, particularly appropriate services for "pregnancy, confinement and the post-natal period, granting free services where necessary, as well as adequate nutrition during pregnancy and lactation" (UN 1979: article 12.1–2). Although this Convention has a narrower focus than either the ICESCR or ICERD, since it refers only to healthcare services and not to underlying health determinants (Toebes 1999: 55), it does fill a significant gap in the right to health, which previously did not specifically address women's reproductive rights.

The *Convention on the Rights of the Child* (CRC) contains the most extensive identification of specific state obligations regarding health (UN 1989), and is distinctive since 193 countries have ratified it, giving it an effectively universal reach (only the United States and Somalia have not ratified it). In the CRC, states recognize children's right to the highest attainable standard of health and to facilities for the treatment of illness and rehabilitation of health, and commit to strive to ensure that no child is deprived of his or her right to access such healthcare services (UN 1989: article 24.1). States undertake specifically to reduce infant and child mortality, combat disease and malnutrition within primary healthcare, ensure appropriate pre- and postnatal healthcare for mothers, ensure access to education on child health, and develop preventive healthcare guidance and family planning (UN 1989: article 24.2).

The newest international human rights treaty is the *Convention on the Rights of Persons with Disabilities* (CRPD), which aims to protect people with disabilities from a variety of social and political obstacles that may impair their full and equal participation in society (UN 2008). The Convention includes a number of articles that directly or indirectly concern health, including the right of people with disabilities to access health facilities (UN 2008: article 9) and their "right to the enjoyment of the highest attainable standard of health without discrimination on the basis of disability" (UN 2008: article 25). Notably, the treaty introduces a new human right related to health – namely, the right of people with disabilities to habilitation and rehabilitation, which obligates states to take steps to ensure that people with disabilities achieve maximum independence and full physical, mental, social, and vocational abilities (UN 2008: article 26).

Right to Health in Regional Human Rights Treaties

The right to health is also recognized in each of the three regional human rights systems that developed alongside and after the creation of the UN and drafting of the International Bill of Rights. The *African (Banjul) Charter on Human and Peoples' Rights* (1981) provides for every individual's right to enjoy the "best attainable state of physical and mental health," with states undertaking to take the necessary measures to protect the health of their people and to ensure that they receive medical attention when they are sick (OAU 1986: article 16).

The *African Charter on the Rights and Welfare of the Child* (1999) specifies every child's right to enjoy the best attainable state of physical, mental, and spiritual health. States agree to undertake a range of measures, including ensuring the provision of necessary medical assistance and healthcare to all (OAU 1999: article 14).

In Europe, health rights are contained in the *European Social Charter* where states undertake to realize two health rights. The first is the right to protection of health, which includes taking appropriate measures to remove causes of ill health, providing advisory and educational facilities for health promotion, and preventing epidemic, endemic, and other diseases (Council of Europe 1965: article 11). The second is the right to social and medical assistance, which includes ensuring adequate assistance and care to people without adequate resources (Council of Europe 1965: article 13).

In the Inter-American system, the *Protocol of San Salvador* provides that "everyone shall have the right to health, understood to mean the enjoyment of the highest level of physical, mental and social well-being." Such a right includes access to primary healthcare; health services for all individuals within a state's jurisdiction; universal immunization against the principal infectious diseases; prevention and treatment of endemic, occupational, and other diseases; health education; and the satisfaction of health needs of the highest risk groups and of those whose poverty makes them the most vulnerable (OAS 1999: article 10).

While there is no regional human rights system in Asia, in 1998 over two hundred NGOs from the region drafted a "people's charter" of Asian human rights, which includes several health-related provisions (Asian Human Rights Commission 1998: articles 3.2, 7.1, 9.3). In the Middle East, the *Cairo Declaration on Human Rights in Islam* provides that "everyone shall have the right to medical and social care, and to all public amenities provided by society and the State within the limits of their available resources" (World Conference on Human Rights 1993: article 17).

Contribution of International Health Conferences

Understanding of the right to health was advanced further through international health conferences focused on clarifying entitlements and developing governmental duties. In 1978 the International Conference on Primary Health Care issued the ground-breaking *Declaration of Alma-Ata*, which declared primary healthcare the principal vehicle for achieving health for all by the year 2000 (International Conference on Primary Health Care 1978). The declaration's emphasis on primary healthcare as "essential health care" played an influential role in the later elaboration by the UN Committee on Economic, Social, and Cultural Rights (CESCR) of core governmental duties to provide essential elements of healthcare (discussed in the next section).

The 1986 *Ottawa Charter for Health Promotion* expanded on the social conditions that influence and determine health to include "peace, shelter, education, food, income, a stable eco-system, sustainable resources, social justice, and equity" (First International Conference on Health Promotion 1986: 1). Accordingly, the Charter proposes that actions on health include intersectoral policy development, individual and community empowerment, and restructuring health services towards preventative rather than curative services. Subsequent international health conferences reinforced and expanded this emphasis on primary healthcare and the social determinants of health. At the 1994 International Conference on Population and Development (ICPD) held in Cairo, 179 states agreed to achieve a number of health-related goals by 2004, marked for the first time by global indicators (UN 1994: chapter VII, objective 8.3). At the 1995 Fourth World Conference on Women held in Beijing, 189 states endorsed the *Beijing Declaration and Platform for Action*. The declaration advanced key definitions later applied to the international human right to health, including state commitments to increase women's access to appropriate, affordable, and quality healthcare and services (UN 1995).

General Comment 14 on the Right to the Highest Attainable Standard of Health

The most significant advancement in the interpretation of the international right to health came in 2000 with a general comment written by the CESCR, a group of independent experts tasked with monitoring state implementation of the ICESCR (UN 2000). General Comment 14 extensively interprets the normative scope of the right to health and identifies state obligations and correlative violations. The Comment makes several important conceptual advances, including identifying entitlements, essential elements of the right to health, and states' core obligations, as well as general duties to respect, protect, and fulfill the right to health.

The Committee explicitly draws from international conferences – including Alma-Ata, ICPD, and Beijing – in specifying these essential elements and minimum core obligations. It interprets the right to health as an inclusive right that includes the rights to both healthcare and the underlying determinants of health (including food, housing, access to water and adequate sanitation, safe working conditions, and a healthy environment) (UN 2000: para. 4). The Committee recognizes that while the highest attainable standard of health and the health system will vary from country to country depending on national resources, the right must contain certain essential elements irrespective of a country's developmental levels (UN 2000: paras 1, 12). These essential elements include that healthcare facilities, goods, and services, and the social determinants of health are available, accessible, acceptable, and of good quality (AAAQ) (UN 2000: para. 12). These elements provide important practical guidance to states on what might constitute adequate compliance with this right.

Allied to the concept of essential elements is the identification of core obligations with which a state party cannot "under any circumstances whatsoever, justify … noncompliance" (UN 2000: para. 47). These duties are intended to ensure that states cannot cite progressive realization within available resources to deny any level of healthcare, including in particular those necessary to address the essential health needs of the most vulnerable. States' core obligations are to "ensure the satisfaction of, at the very least, minimum essential levels of each of the rights," including:

- Non-discriminatory access to health facilities, goods, and services.
- Access to minimum essential food.
- Access to basic shelter, housing, and sanitation and an adequate supply of safe and potable water.
- Essential drugs as defined by the WHO.
- Equitable distribution of all health facilities, goods, and services.
- Adopting and implementing a national public health strategy and plan of action addressing the health concerns of the whole population, with particular attention to vulnerable or marginalized groups. (UN 2000: para. 43)

General Comment 14 also indicates that states hold obligations of comparable priority to minimum core duties, including to take measures to prevent, treat, and control epidemic and endemic diseases, and ensure reproductive, maternal (prenatal as well as postnatal), and child healthcare (UN 2000: paras 44.a, 44.b).

The Committee interprets progressive realization to require states to take immediate action towards realizing the right to health, including guaranteeing the non-discriminatory exercise of rights and by taking deliberate, concrete, and targeted steps towards full realization (UN 2000: para. 31). This means that while states can justify some healthcare deficiencies, they cannot justify the failure to work towards rectifying them. The intent of these clarifications is to provide states with greater guidance in fulfilling their duties of progressive realization regarding the right to health, and to counter any perceptions that progressive realization enables a state to indefinitely delay taking action (Forman and Bomze 2012).

General Comment 14 provides detailed interpretations of state obligations to respect, protect, and fulfill the right to health (UN 2000: para. 33). *Respecting* the right to health requires governments not to interfere with this right, including through policies that are discriminatory or that are likely to cause unnecessary morbidity and preventable mortality (UN 2000: paras 34, 50). *Protecting* the right to health requires states to take measures to ensure equal access to health services provided by third parties, including controlling the marketing of health goods and services by third parties (UN 2000: para. 35). State obligations to *fulfill* the right to health arise "when individuals or a group are unable, for reasons beyond their control, to realize that right themselves by means at their disposal" (UN 2000: para. 37). The Committee emphasizes the importance of distinguishing between non-compliance arising from unwillingness rather than inability when determining whether particular actions constitute violations of the right to health (UN 2000: para. 47). The Committee's interpretation explicitly extends to state action internationally, with states required to respect the right to health in other countries, and to protect the right by preventing third parties from violating it elsewhere if states can influence them by legal or political means (UN 2000: para. 39). In particular, "depending on the availability of resources, States should facilitate access to essential health facilities, goods and services in other countries, where possible and provide the necessary aid when required" (UN 2000: para. 39).

The UN Special Rapporteur on the Right to the Highest Attainable Standard of Physical and Mental Health

An analogously important development came in 2002 when the UN Human Rights Council (which replaced the UN Commission on Human Rights) appointed a Special Rapporteur on the Right to Health with the mandate of promoting the development and realization of this right globally. The position was initially filled by Paul Hunt, a New Zealand law professor in England, and is currently occupied by Anand Grover, an Indian lawyer and HIV/AIDS activist. The Special Rapporteur on the Right to Health has three main objectives: (i) to promote the right to health as a fundamental human right; (ii) clarify specific elements and its general content; and (iii) identify good practices at the community, national, and international levels for operationalizing the right to health (University of Essex Human Rights Centre 2008).

The Special Rapporteur fulfills this mandate by undertaking country missions and other visits, transmitting communications with governments regarding alleged violations of the right to health, and submitting annual reports to both the Human Rights

Council and the General Assembly. These reports detail activities performed under the mandate and include information on particular issues relevant to the right to health, such as poverty, international trade, health systems, mental health, access to medicines, neglected diseases, HIV/AIDS, maternal mortality, indicators, and sexual and reproductive health. Country missions to date include Peru (2004), Uganda (2005, 2007), Israel (2006), Lebanon (2006), Colombia (2007), India (2007), Sweden (2007), Australia (2009), and Guatemala (2010). The Special Rapporteur has also completed missions to international organizations and non-state actors that play a role in the realization of the right to health, including the World Trade Organization (2003), the World Bank (2007), the International Monetary Fund (2007), and GlaxoSmithKline (2008). These latter missions are particularly significant since they expand international human rights law beyond its state-centric orientation, which traditionally has limited application to non-state actors such as international organizations and corporations. The establishment of the Special Rapporteur procedure has provided an important platform for advancing the priority of the right to health within international law and the global political arena. It has also contributed to the development of new right-to-health tools, such as human rights indicators (Backman *et al.* 2008), discussed further in the section "Rights-Based Policy and Tools".

Critiques and Weaknesses of Human Rights and Right to Health

Human rights in general are subject to extensive critiques regarding their universality and efficacy. The right to health in particular is denounced for being overly individualistic and legally unenforceable, state-centric, weakly enforceable beyond domestic borders, and damaging to population health outcomes (DeCock *et al.* 2002; Gostin 2007; Easterly 2009). These critiques take place against longer standing criticisms of rights inflation, targeted in particular at social rights, which are argued to be inappropriately legal rights within international human rights law (Cranston 1973). While some of these critiques of the right to health are poorly supported factually, and are undercut by emerging interpretation and enforcement, others are more cogent in outlining weaknesses that limit the potential force of these rights when it comes to global health policy (Gostin 2007). These critiques are explored in this section, as are efforts to remediate some of these weaknesses.

Rights Inflation

The argument of rights inflation suggests that adding rights such as health to the pantheon of accepted human rights will devalue all human rights (Cranston 1973; Orend 2002; Griffin 2010). Certainly if rights language was used to cover *every* possible case, the risk, as Paul Farmer put it, is that "obscene inequalities of risk would be drowned in a rising tide of petty complaint" (Farmer 2003: 231). However, this risk does not seem to apply in the context of global health inequity, given that its primary focus is on claims by poor and vulnerable populations in LMICs to primary healthcare, safe water and sanitation, nutritious food, and adequate housing. These kinds of essential human needs are far from being petty complaints. Given that, in a global health context, the right to health cannot feasibly be seen as petty, the "rights inflation" argument instead targets the legitimacy of the right to health as a social right (Cranston 1973). Arguments against social rights, such as the right to health, generally rely on characterizations of civil rights as negative rights that are relatively resource free and require little state action to realize, in opposition to social rights which are positive rights that require considerable resources and state action to realize. However, this argument has been undermined in social rights commentaries that show the considerable costs and action required to realize civil rights (Hunt 1996; Holmes and Sunstein 2000). In addition, as the preceding sections imply, the dramatic growth in treaties and institutions on the right to health suggest that arguments that the right to health should not be recognized as a legal right are today largely irrelevant.

Vagueness/Formulation

More valid criticisms focus on the international law formulation of a right to the "highest attainable standard of health." The vagueness of this latter phrase and what it means practically for state action has resulted in considerable opposition to the idea of a right to health, even among international human rights experts. Such experts have argued that it makes more sense to talk about a right to *healthcare* rather than a right to health, since health is something that lies outside our control (Kass 1975, in Toebes 1999: 17). These challenges are exacerbated by the limitation of state duties to progressively realize this right to health within available resources. Certainly General Comment 14 has gone a long way in clarifying the entitlements and duties under this right, which resolves some of the vagueness/formulation arguments and provides policy-makers and courts with clearer guidance for realizing this right. This is not to suggest, however, that General Comment 14 is sufficient to resolve all remaining questions about scope and context, including in particular the content of the minimum core. More legal, political, and academic interpretation is needed to give greater specificity to the right in these respects.

Ineffective/Damaging

Other critics argue that that even with all this legal codification and ratification, at best the right to health is ineffective, at worst counterproductive and even dangerous. While the argument of inefficacy is posed against international human rights law in general (Shand-Watson 1999; Kennedy 2002), the ratification of human rights treaties is argued to have limited impact on improved population health (Palmer *et al.* 2009). The right to health is also critiqued for being overly individualistic, which is argued to subvert both population health outcomes (de Cock *et al.* 2002) and democratic allocations of limited resources (Goodman 2005; Easterly 2009).

Despite state failures to recognize many international human rights (including protection against genocide), these rights have nonetheless played important roles in dismounting deeply entrenched regimes and policies such as colonialism and apartheid (Klotz 1995; Black 1999; Reus-Smit 2001). Similarly, domestic rights-based struggles for gender and racial equality have in many places produced universal suffrage and the eradication of legally entrenched gender and racial discrimination.

In addition, empirical research has shown, in contrast to Palmer and colleagues' findings, that ratification *can* have legally significant outcomes, including in relation to the right to health. Such positive effects were found in a 2006 study that explored access to medicines litigation, which found that in countries where cases were successful, the consistent variables were that the country had ratified the Social Rights Covenant and that it had entrenched the right to health in its domestic constitution (Hogerzeil *et al.* 2006). This outcome suggests that there are important downstream legal consequences from ratification, particularly where individuals and social actors can access independent judiciaries willing to enforce these rights, and whose orders are implemented by governments. Moreover the argument that the right to health is overly individualistic to the detriment of public resources and health is undercut by the judicial approach in countries such as South Africa, discussed in the section "Domestic Litigation." While it is true that the right to health imposes individual entitlements, it clearly also imposes state duties that benefit the collective: individual rights to health are relatively meaningless without a corresponding health system to enable its fulfillment (Forman and Bomze 2012).

Deficiencies of International Law

More cogent critiques point to the structural limitations of international legal formulations of the right to health to appropriately respond to global health inequities. These limitations include insufficient development of this right in relation to resource limitations, weak application beyond domestic borders, and state-centric application that excludes powerful non-state actors such as transnational corporations and international organizations (Gostin 2007). Indeed, international law scholars are turning their efforts to remediate these aspects of international human rights law, including through the prospective creation of a framework convention on global health that will codify global health duties (Gostin 2007; Gostin *et al.* 2011). This convention represents a potentially tectonic shift in human rights approaches to global health. Currently, the international responsibilities of states to respect, protect, and fulfill the right to health in *other* countries are weakly specified – this convention would harden these responsibilities. It would also create a new international legal regime for the right to health in relation to global health.

However, the landscape of international law is littered with "hard" norms that are weakly specified and poorly enforced. The convention faces three crucial questions. Will it deepen commitments to global health or disperse them in unenforceable ways? What are its implications for existing bodies of international human rights law on health? And, as a "top-down" human rights mechanism, how will it interact with the "bottom-up" actors and processes that are key to human rights-driven change? This last question is particularly apposite given growing recognition that law alone is a poor causal mechanism for advancing transformative human rights change, and that social action is key to such outcomes (Koh 1997; Risse *et al.* 1999; Finnemore and Sikkink 2001). Indeed, social action is increasingly understood to be intimately intertwined with the production of international law (Baxi 2002; Rajagopal 2003; Siegel 2004).

Contribution of Human Rights to Global Health Equity

The following section explores traditional human rights mechanisms such as international and regional procedures, domestic litigation, and social movement and advocacy. In the latter context, it also explores the normative/rhetorical framing that human rights offer to social campaigns around health. The section then turns to explore new human rights mechanisms, including rights-based approaches, rights-based indicators, and rights-based impact assessment.

International and Regional Human Rights Procedures

State reporting and individual complaints are the two primary mechanisms within the international human rights treaty system for monitoring and encouraging state accountability for their compliance with ratified treaties, while each of the three regional human rights systems offer mechanisms to deal with individual complaints of violations of the right to health. The two mechanisms are explored below.

Treaty reporting   Treaty reporting is the primary way that human rights treaty bodies monitor governments' compliance with their treaty obligations. On treaty ratification, states agree to submit regular reports that update the treaty's monitoring committee
on the state's progress in complying with its obligations. The committee then publishes
"concluding observations" that identify concerns about non-compliance and recommend
action to enable improved implementation. Reporting is neither adversarial nor adjudica-
tive, but rather is intended to operate as a "constructive dialogue" to assist governments
(Alston 1997: 20). Indeed, there is a relatively low incidence in concluding observations
of violations, and a high incidence of recommendations concerning progressive steps to be
taken (Lyon 2003: 37). However, where committees note their "concern" about particular
acts or omissions by the state, as they often do, this is generally indicative of a treaty violation (Alston 1997). This provides important support for domestic and regional judicial
interpretations of state violations of comparable rights protections, and gives additional
support to individual complaints before the treaty bodies. The institutional aspiration
behind the state reporting system is to significantly assist in the domestic realization of
human rights, by: (i) provoking states to comprehensively review compliance; (ii) providing a platform for a national dialog on human rights; and (iii) enabling international
scrutiny of state accountability for human rights (UN High Commissioner for Human
Rights 2006: para. 5).

There is relatively high compliance with state reporting (around 70% submission of
due reports in 2006), although there is considerable variation in report quality, with only
39% of reports submitted complying with reporting guidelines (UN High Commissioner
for Human Rights 2006: 19, para. 24). The reporting system is also hamstrung by inadequate follow-up procedures beyond the annual reports (UN High Commissioner for
Human Rights 2006: para 26).

Individual complaints   Several international human rights treaties (including those
relating to disability, civil rights, torture, women's rights, migrant workers, and racial
discrimination) allow individual complaints alleging the violation of treaty rights to be
lodged against states at the relevant treaty committee. Approximately 10,000 individual
complaints are received annually, whereas far lower numbers are actually heard before
the committees (Viljoen 2004: 65). For example, Cole (2011) estimated that, between
1976 and 2007, the Human Rights Committee (by far the most active of human rights
committees able to hear individual complaints) filed 1813 communications, registering
655 final views (80% of which found violations). In contrast, in 2006 the Committee
against Torture had 288 overall registered cases, versus 35 registered cases for the Committee on the Elimination of Racial Discrimination (UN High Commissioner for Human
Rights 2006: 29).

There is presently no individual complaints mechanism under the ICESCR. An
optional protocol to initiate this procedure at the CESCR has been under discussion at the
UN since 1996. Once operational, it will allow state parties to the ICESCR to recognize
the Committee's competence to consider individual complaints. As of late March 2012,
while 39 countries had signed the protocol, only eight had ratified it (Argentina, Bolivia,
Ecuador, El Salvador, Mongolia, Slovakia, and Spain) (United Nations Treaty Collection
2012). Ten ratifications are necessary to bring the protocol into effect. Once operational,
the optional protocol will provide an important international mechanism for assuring
accountability with the right to health and further developing its normative content.

While decisions of UN human rights treaty bodies are not legally binding, they can
and often have resulted in relief for individual complainants. For example, in *Sandra*

Lovelace v. Canada (1984), Sandra Lovelace Nicolas lodged a complaint with the Human Rights Committee alleging that the Canadian government had violated her rights under the ICCPR given the legal requirement that women lose their aboriginal status when marrying a non-aboriginal man (a consequence which was not applied to aboriginal men). The Human Rights Committee's decision found Canada to be in violation of the ICCPR, and resulted in the Canadian government's amendment of the law in question to eliminate its gender discrimination and restore aboriginal status to women previously affected. In addition, a comprehensive survey conducted by the International Law Association (2004: para. 175) found that individual communication decisions have become a commonly cited interpretive source in national courts and international tribunals. Most of these references are to the Human Rights Committee, perhaps reflecting the relative volume of its decisions, its long period of operation, and the relatively high public awareness of the Committee (International Law Association 2004: para. 177). However, these references are decisive in only a small minority of such decisions (International Law Association 2004: para. 179).

Regional Human Rights Mechanisms

Regional human rights bodies, such as the European Court of Human Rights, the Inter-American Commission on Human Rights, the Inter-American Court of Human Rights, the African Commission on Human and People's Rights, and the African Court on Human and Peoples' Rights, offer important additional supranational venues for lodging claims against violations of the right to health. In both the European and inter-American systems, decisions are legally binding and offer oral hearings, appointed legal counsel, and detailed remedies (Bayefsky 2002: 173–4). The African system introduced an African Court on Human and People's Rights in 2006 with the capacity to issue advisory opinions and binding judgments. These bodies also frequently refer to the output of the UN human rights treaty bodies (International Law Association 2004: 29–34).

The earlier African Commission on Human and People's Rights has heard several health-related cases. It found violations of the African Charter's right to health in relation to the Democratic Republic of the Congo (then Zairean) government's failure to provide safe drinking water, electricity, and medicines (*Free Legal Assistance Group and Others v. Zaire* 1995) and the Malawian government's failure to provide medical treatment and other adequate living conditions to prisoners (*Malawi African Association and Others v. Mauritania* 2000). In 2000, the Commission found that the Nigerian government had violated a number of the Ogoni people's rights, including the right to health, by failing to prevent pollution and ecological degradation and to monitor oil activities by the national petroleum company, which was a majority shareholder in a consortium with Shell Petroleum (*Social and Economic Rights Action Centre and the Centre for Economic and Social Rights v. Nigeria* 2001).

The Inter-American human rights system has been used extensively by people living with HIV/AIDS to claim access to treatment on the basis of the rights to health and life. In the 2001 case of *Jorge Odir Miranda Cortez et al. v. El Salvador* (2000), people living with HIV/AIDS successfully sought an interim order from the Inter-American Commission on Human Rights for El Salvador's government to provide ARVs on an interim basis while the merits of their claim were being assessed. As a result, the El Salvadoran Supreme Court ordered the Salvadoran Social Security Institute to provide Cortez with ARV drugs, so that it was no longer necessary to proceed with the complaint before the Inter-American Commission (UNAIDS and Canadian HIV/AIDS Legal Network 2006: 71). Notably, the government introduced legislation the same year affirming the right of every person living with HIV/AIDS to "health care, medical, surgical and psychological treatment," and took preventative measures to impede the infection's progress, which have been attributed to the influence of the interim order of the Commission and the order of the Supreme Court (UNAIDS and Canadian HIV/AIDS Legal Network 2006: 71).

Domestic Litigation

National court decisions remain the most well-known and formally binding methods of enforcing the right to health. There has been a significant increase globally in litigation based on the right to health, including in LMICs (Hogerzeil *et al.* 2006; Gauri and Brinks 2008; Gloppen 2008; Yamin and Gloppen 2011). This increase is attributable to many factors, including growing ratification of the ICESCR and domestic entrenchments of the right to health (Hogerzeil *et al.* 2006). Exploration of successful litigation shows that these rights have played an important role in relation to access to ARV drugs for people with HIV/AIDS; prisoners' rights to healthcare services; access to generic drugs; battles over reproductive rights; and efforts to secure social determinants of health, including water, food, and a healthy environment (Yamin and Gloppen 2011: 2). Yet evidence on the impacts of this litigation on health outcomes is mixed.

One of the best examples of a positive impact of domestic litigation is from South Africa, where the Constitutional Court upheld civil society claims under constitutional and international protections of rights to health and life for the government to provide medicines to prevent mother-to-child transmission (MTCT) of HIV (*Minister of Health and Another v. Treatment Action Campaign and Others* 2002). As a result of the case, today a national MTCT program provides medicines in over 96% of government clinics (Statistics South Africa 2010: 5). Similarly successful litigation in Latin America illustrates how respect for and promotion of human rights can lead to both improved access to healthcare and increased budgetary allocations for health (Singh *et al.* 2007). For example, in *Mariela Viceconte v. Ministry of Health and Social Welfare* (1998), an Argentinian court held that the government was liable to provide adequate access to preventative vaccines to 3.5 million people living in an area affected by hemorrhagic fever. The court ruled that the government was legally obliged to intervene despite the government's argument that it lacked an adequate vaccine supply, making the ministers of health and the economy personally liable for producing vaccines within a given time schedule. As a result of the case, Argentina's government developed a plan to deliver basic medicines to those in need within five years of the ruling (Singh *et al.* 2007: 525).

Yet domestic litigation has not always had such positive outcomes. In Colombia, for example, there have been overwhelming numbers of health rights claims lodged under the *tutela* system (an informal and fast-track petition procedure without precedential value) introduced in 1991 alongside constitutional reform (Lamprea 2014). Between 1999 and 2010, 869,604 right to health claims were lodged through the tutela (out of a total 2,725,361 tutela claims) (Lamprea 2014). These claims give Colombia the highest per capita rate of right to health litigation in the world (3289 claims for each 1 million individuals, versus 206, 109, 29, 0.3, and 0.2 respectively for Brazil, Costa Rica, Argentina, South Africa, and India) (Moestad *et al.* 2011: 282). These cases are viewed as having detrimental impacts on existing inequities, giving generous concessions to individual claims without consideration of their impacts if generalized (Yamin *et al.* 2011; Lamprea 2014). Nonetheless, there is concurrence that these massive rates of right to health litigation were not *creative* of the problems per se, but rather *responsive* to deeper institutional dysfunction and inequity arising out of a 1991 health sector reform process (Yamin *et al.* 2011; Lamprea 2014).

In response to both the high rates of litigation and continuing inequity, in 2008, the Colombia Constitutional Court issued a landmark judgment (T-760/08) that ordered both institutional reform to reduce tutela rates as well as extensive restructuring of Colombia's health system (Yamin and Parra-Vera 2009; Lamprea 2014). Certainly the Colombian experience suggests that "successful" cases that favor individual or group claimants at the expense of collective interests may not be conducive to good public health. It nonetheless underscores the important role of courts in advocating for health equity within the policy process. However, as the South African case on perinatal HIV transmission attests, individual and group claims *can* benefit collective health interests and potentially assist in reducing systematic disparities in healthcare access (Forman 2011).

Rights-Based Advocacy

Beyond its function in supporting litigation at the domestic and supranational levels, international human rights law offers a strong buttress to advocacy for global health equity, contributing a normative specificity and analytic framework grounded in binding law. The potential is to affect a paradigmatic shift from viewing health as a charitable and/or superfluous component of budgetary allocations to one implicating binding legal and moral duties. Clearly, however, not all claims will have this power.

The HIV/AIDS treatment advocacy campaigns of the last decade provide a powerful example of the strengths and weaknesses of rights-based advocacy. Throughout the 2000s, global civil society actors used rights-based strategies, including litigation and advocacy, to challenge refusals by the pharmaceutical industry, their host governments, and international institutions to advance access to affordable ARV drugs in sub-Saharan Africa (the epicenter of the global HIV/AIDS pandemic). These efforts not only achieved a dramatic global reduction in the price of ARV drugs, but saw corporations, governments, and international organizations shift towards advocating universal access to ARV dugs (Forman 2011). As a result, access to ARV drugs in sub-Saharan Africa has increased from under 1% to over 40% in eight years, with almost 5.31 million people currently accessing drug treatment (WHO *et al.* 2011). Increased access to ARV drugs is producing tremendous health impacts in the region, including a 19% decline in AIDS-related deaths between 2004 and 2009 (Girard *et al.* 2010), declines in overall death rates since 2005 (UN Programme for HIV/AIDS and WHO 2007; UN Programme for HIV/AIDS 2010), and a 17% decrease in new HIV infections from 2001 to 2008 (UN Programme for HIV/AIDS 2010).

Yet this access is largely reliant on international funding. This dependency was brought to stark light when the Global Fund to Fight AIDS, Tuberculosis and Malaria (the Global Fund) cancelled its 2012 funding round (Round 11, which was supposed to fund new-country proposals up to at least 2014), given funding cuts by northern donors (Globe and Mail 2011). As a result, the scale up of ARV drugs in sub-Saharan Africa has stalled at 40%, and current levels of access have an uncertain future (Global Fund 2011). The experiences of HIV/AIDS medicines therefore suggests that gains produced by rights-based campaigns may be subject to regression with relative impunity, reinforcing the dependency of less-developed countries on northern funding and exacerbating their economic, political, and epidemiological vulnerabilities (Forman 2013). The policy implications of the cancellation of Round 11 by the Global Fund are further discussed by Ooms and colleagues in Chapter 24.

Rights-Based Policy and Tools

Rights can work more systematically to advance health equity than the intermittent incidence and narrow scope of litigation or even issue-based advocacy may permit (Forman 2011). In recognition of the limited scope and impact of traditional human rights measures, such as litigation and advocacy, human rights scholars have developed rights-based versions of public and global health policies, programs, and tools that seek to proactively operationalize the conceptual framework and duties of the right to health. Certainly, the existence of a domestically entrenched health right can itself motivate or at least assist in justifying equity-seeking health programs. For example, in South Africa, a proposed National Health Insurance (NHI) system that seeks to redress persistent gross inequities between the public and private health sectors is explicitly guided by human rights principles, including the constitutional health right (South African Department of Health 2011: para. 52).

Rights-based approaches seek to concretize political commitments to health equity by: (i) mandating the incorporation of core human rights principles (such as non-discrimination, participation, and accountability); (b) demanding a focus on poor and marginalized groups; and (iii) requiring explicit reference to international human rights instruments (WHO and UN Office of the High Commissioner of Human Rights 2010). Indeed human rights scholars argue that in the same way that the right to a fair trial has advanced well-functioning court systems, the right to health has a particular contribution to make to promoting policies that advance health equity (Backman *et al.* 2008: 15). A recent study by Backman and colleagues (2008) examined data from 194 countries, as well as related law, scholarship, and health indicators, to identify the right-to-health features of health systems. The authors proposed 72 indicators that reflect these features (Box 25.2 gives examples of such indicators). The hope is that if policy-makers use indicators such as these, the outcome will be more equitable and accountable health policies.

Box 25.2 Indicators of the "Right to Health Features" of a Health System

Backman *et al.* (2008) have proposed 72 indicators, which include:

- Whether a state recognizes the right to health through treaty ratification or domestic constitutionalization.
- Whether the state has a comprehensive national health plan encompassing public and private sectors.
- Whether there is a legal requirement for including the participation of marginalized groups in developing the national health plan.
- Whether per capita government expenditure on health is greater than the minimum required for a basic effective public health system.
- How total government spending on health compares with total government spending on military expenditure as percentages of gross domestic product.

A Way Forward: Defining a Research Agenda for Global Health and Human Rights

The international human rights law framework offers important strategies, standards, and tools to policy-makers and social actors alike who are invested in the achievement of health equity. Yet the human rights framework is structurally limited in key respects when it comes to addressing major determinants of global health inequity. Such determinants include neoliberal international trade laws that de-prioritize domestic health spending, and economic recessions and crises that are gutting northern aid commitments to global health. The existing right to health framework is also insufficiently developed in terms of the extent to which resource limitations and progressive realization can impact on access to essential health needs. Other key deficiencies include weak application beyond domestic borders, state-centric application that excludes powerful non-state actors such as transnational corporations and international organizations, and weak or non-existent international enforcement.

The challenge for researchers and activists alike is to develop research, scholarship, and strategies capable of responding to and resolving some of these weaknesses. Future research could include:

- Defining the minimum core of the right to health to define essential health needs not subject to resource limitations.
- Ensuring increased ratification of health-related treaties (ICESCR, CEDAW, CRPD, and ICERD).
- Ensuring increased domestic constitutionalization/codification of rights to health.
- Encouraging ratification of the ICESCR optional protocol.
- Codifying international right to health duties.
- Developing the application of international human rights law to non-state actors.

Conclusions

The right to health in international law offers a potentially powerful set of norms, tools, and strategies to social and political actors for advancing health equity. Individual rights to claim accessible and affordable healthcare and public health services – including water, sanitation, food, and access to housing – may produce individual and population health outcomes that ultimately reduce health inequities within and between countries. These capacities may provide the basis for advancing broader health equity initiatives with collective implications. Such capacities may also help us advance towards a new legal framework that works in tandem with existing human rights law to concretize international responsibilities in relation to essential health needs and to build the human rights contribution to advancing health equity globally.

Key Reading

Backman G, Hunt P, Khosla R *et al.* 2008. Health systems and the right to health an assessment of 194 countries. *Lancet* 372(9655), 2047–85.

Beyrer C, Pizer HF (eds). 2007. *Public Health and Human Rights: Evidence-Based Approaches*. Baltimore, MD: Johns Hopkins University Press.

Forman L, Bomze S. 2012. International human rights law and the right to health: an overview of legal standards and accountability mechanisms. In Backman G, Fitchett J (eds) *The Right to Health: Theory and Practice*, pp. 33–72. Lund: Studentliteratur AB.

Hunt P. 2006. The human right to the highest attainable standard of health: new opportunities and challenges. *Transactions of the Royal Society of Tropical Medicine and Hygiene* 100, 603–7.

Mann J, Gruskin S, Grodin MA, Annas GJ (eds). 1999. *Health and Human Rights: A Reader*. New York: Routledge.

Meier BM, Cabrera OA, Ayala A, Gostin LO. 2012. Bridging international law and rights-based litigation: mapping health-related rights through the development of the Global Health and Human Rights Database. *Health and Human Rights* 14(1), 1–16.

Yamin AE, Gloppen S. 2011. *Litigating Health Rights: Can Courts Bring More Justice to Health?* Cambridge MA: Harvard University Press.

References

Alston, P. 1997. The Purposes of Reporting. In United Nations (ed.) *Manual on Human Rights Reporting*. UN Doc. HR/PUB/91/1 (Rev. 1), pp. 19–24. Geneva: United Nations.

Asian Human Rights Commission. 1998. *Asian Human Rights Charter: A People's Charter*. Declared in Kwangju, South Korea, on May 17, 1998.

Backman G, Hunt P, Khosla R *et al.* 2008. Health systems and the right to health an assessment of 194 countries. *Lancet* 372(9655), 2047–85.

Baxi U. 2002. *The Future of Human Rights*. Oxford: Oxford University Press.

Bayefsky AF. 2002. *How to Complain to the UN Human Rights Treaty System*. Ardsley Park, NY: Transnational Publishers.

Black D. 1999. The long and winding road: international norms and domestic political change in South Africa. In Risse T, Ropp SC, Sikkink K (eds) *The Power of Human Rights: International Norms and Domestic Change*, p. 78. Cambridge: Cambridge University Press.

Cole WM. 2011. Individuals v. states: the correlates of Human Rights Committee rulings, 1979–2007. *Social Science Research* 40(3), 985–1000.

Council of Europe. 1965. *European Social Charter*. 529 U.N.T.S. 89, entered into force February 26, 1965.

Cranston M. 1973. *What are Human Rights?* London: Bodley Head.

DeCock KM, Mbori-Ngacha D, Marum E. 2002. Shadow on the continent: public health and HIV/AIDS in Africa in the 21st century. *Lancet* 360, 67.

Easterly W. 2009. Human rights are the wrong basis for healthcare. *Financial Times*, October 12.

Farmer P. 2003. *Pathologies of Power: Health, Human Rights, and the New War on the Poor*. (Berkeley, CA: University of California Press.

Finnemore M, Sikkink K. 2001. Taking stock: the constructivist research program in international relations and comparative politics. *Annual Review of Political Science* 4, 391–416.

First International Conference on Health Promotion. 1986. *Ottawa Charter for Health Promotion*. WHO/HPR/HEP/95.121, November 21, 1986, Ottawa, Canada.

Forman L. 2011. Making the case for human rights in global health education, research and policy. *Canadian Journal of Public Health* 102(3), 207–9.

Forman L. 2013. What contribution have human rights approaches made to reducing AIDS-related vulnerability in sub-Saharan Africa? Exploring the case-study of access to antiretrovirals. *Global Health Promotion* 20(1), 57–63.

Forman L, Bomze S. 2012. International human rights law and the right to health: an overview of legal standards and accountability mechanisms. In Backman G, Fitchett J (eds) *The Right to Health: Theory and Practice*, pp. 33–72. Lund: Studentliteratur AB.

Free Legal Assistance Group and Others v Zaire. 1995. AHRLR 74 (ACHPR 1995).

Gagnon ML, Labonté R. 2011. Human rights in global health diplomacy: a critical assessment. *Journal of Human Rights* 10(2), 189–213.

Gauri V, Brinks DM. 2008. *Courting Social Justice: Judicial Enforcement of Social and Economic Rights in the Developing World*. New York: Cambridge University Press.

Girard F, Ford F, Montaner J, Cahn P, Katabira E. 2010. Universal access in the fight against HIV/AIDS. *Science* 329(5988), 147–9.

Glendon MA. 2002. *A World Made New: Eleanor Roosevelt and the Universal Declaration of Human Rights*. New York: Random House.

Global Fund to Fight AIDS, Tuberculosis and Malaria. 2011. *Transitional Funding Mechanism (TFM) Information Note*, December 12. http://www.theglobalfund.org/documents/tfm/TFM_Request_InfoNote_en (last accessed December 2013).

Globe and Mail. 2011. Economic crisis hits health aid that has helped millions as donors cut back. *Globe and Mail* November 23.

Gloppen S. 2008. Litigation as a strategy to hold governments accountable for implementing the right to health. *Health and Human Rights* 10(2), 21–36.

Goodman T. 2005. Is there a right to health? *Journal of Medicine and Philosophy* 30, 643–62.

Gostin LO. 2007. A proposal for a framework convention on global health. *Journal of International Economic Law* 10(4), 89–1008.

Gostin LO, Friedman EA, Ooms G *et al.* 2011. The Joint Action and Learning Initiative: Towards a Global Agreement on National and Global Responsibilities for Health. *PLOS Medicine* 8(5), e1001031.

Griffin J. 2010. On human rights. *Legal Studies* 30(1), 151–60.

Hogerzeil HV, Samson M, Casanovas JV, Rahmani-Ocora L. 2006. Is access to essential medicines as part of the fulfillment of the right to health enforceable through the courts? *Lancet* 368(9532), 305.

Holmes S, Sunstein CR. 2000. *The Cost of Rights*. New York: W.H. Norton.

Hunt P. 1996. *Reclaiming Social Rights: International and Comparative Perspectives*. Aldershot: Dartmouth Publishing Company.

International Conference on Primary Health Care. 1978. *Declaration of Alma-Ata*. Alma-Ata, USSR, September 6–12, 1978.

International Law Association. 1994. Final report on the status of the Universal Declaration of Human Rights in national and international law. In *Report of the 66th Conference, Buenos Aires, Argentina, 14–20 August 1994*. London: International Law Association.

International Law Association. 2004. Final report on the impact of findings of the United Nations Human Rights Treaty Bodies. Berlin Conference, International Human Rights Law and Practice Section.

Jorge Odir Miranda Cortez et al. v. El Salvador. 2000. Case 12.249, Report No. 29/01, Inter-American Commission on Human Rights, Annual Report 2000, OEA/Ser./L/V/II.111, Doc. 20 Rev. 200.

Kennedy D. 2002. The international human rights movement: part of the problem? *Harvard Human Rights Journal* 15, 101.

Klotz A. 1995. *Norms in International Relations: The Struggle Against Apartheid*. Ithaca, NY: Cornell University Press.

Koh HH. 1997. Why do nations obey international law? *Yale Law Journal* 106(8), 2599–659.

Lamprea E. 2014. Colombia's right to health litigation in a context of health care reform. In Gross A, Flood C (eds) *The Right to Health in a Globalized World*, forthcoming.

Lyon B. 2003. *Discourse in Development: A Post-Colonial Theory 'Agenda' for the UN Committee on Economic, Social and Cultural Rights*. Villanova Public Law and Legal Theory Working Paper Series, Working Paper No. 2003–9. Philadelphia, PA: Villanova University School of Law.

Malawi African Association and Others v. Mauritania. 2000. AHRLR 149 (ACHPR 2000) Communication 155/96.

Mariela Viceconte v. Ministry of Health and Social Welfare. 1998. Case No. 31.777/96 (1998), Argentina.

Minister of Health and Another v. Treatment Action Campaign and Others, 2002. South African Constitutional Court, (2002) 5 S.Afr.L.R. 721.

Moestad O, Rakner L, Motta Ferraz OL. 2011. Assessing the impact of health rights litigation: a comparative analysis of Argentina, Brazil, Colombia, Costa Rica, India and South Africa. In Yamin AE, Gloppen S (eds) *Litigating Health Rights: Can Courts Bring More Justice to Health?*, pp. 273–303. Cambridge MA: Harvard University Press.

Mutua MW. 2001. Book review and note: *Theory and Reality in the International Protection of Human Rights*, by J. Shand Watson. *American Journal of International Law* 95(1), 255–6.

OAS (Organization of American States). 1999. *Additional Protocol to the American Convention on Human Rights in the Area of Economic, Social and Cultural Rights, "Protocol of San Salvador."* OAS Treaty Series No. 69 (1988), entered into force November 16, 1999.

OAU (Organization of African Unity). 1986. *African (Banjul) Charter on Human and Peoples' Rights*. Adopted June 27, 1981, OAU Doc. CAB/LEG/67/3 rev. 5, 21 I.L.M. 58 (1982), entered into force October 21, 1986.

OAU (Organization of African Unity). 1999. *African Charter on the Rights and Welfare of the Child*. OAU Doc. CAB/LEG/24.9/49 (1990), entered into force November 29, 1999.

Orend B. 2002. *Human Rights: Concept and Context*. Peterborough: Broadview Press.

Palmer A, Tomkinson J, Phung C et al. 2009. Does ratification of human-rights treaties have effects on population health? *Lancet* 373(9679), 1987.

Rajagopal B. 2003. *International Law from Below: Development, Social Movements and Third World Resistance*. Cambridge: Cambridge University Press.

Reus-Smit C. 2001. Human rights and the social construction of sovereignty. *Review of International Studies* 27, 519–38.

Risse T, Ropp SC, Sikkink K (eds). 1999. *The Power of Human Rights: International Norms and Domestic Change*. Cambridge: Cambridge University Press.

Roosevelt FD. 1941. *Four Freedoms Speech*. http://www.fdrlibrary.marist.edu/pdfs/ffreadingcopy.pdf (last accessed December 2013).

Sandra Lovelace v. Canada. 1984. Communication No. 24/1977, U.N. Doc. CCPR/C/OP/1 at 10.

Schrecker T. 2011. The health case for economic and social rights against the global marketplace. *Journal of Human Rights* 10(2), 151–77.

Shand-Watson J. 1999. *Theory and Reality in the International Protection of Human Rights*. Ardsley, NY: Transnational Publishers.

Siegel RB. 2004. The jurisgenerative role of social movements in United States constitutional law. Paper presented to the Latin American Seminar on Constitutional and Political Theory 2004 on The Limits of Democracy, June 2004 [unpublished]. On file with author.

Singh JA, Govender M, Mills EJ. 2007. Do human rights matter to health? *Lancet* 370(4), 521–7.

Social and Economic Rights Action Centre and the Centre for Economic and Social Rights v. Nigeria. 2001. ACHPR Communication No. 155/96.

Sohn L. 1982. The new international law: protection of the rights of individuals rather than states. *American University Law Review* 32(1), 1–16.

South African Department of Health. 2011. *National Health Act (61/2003): Policy on National Health Insurance*. Government Gazette Notice No. 657, August 12.

Statistics South Africa, 2010. *Mid-year Population Estimates 2010*. http://www.statssa.gov.za/publications/P0302/P03022010.pdf (last accessed December 2013).

Toebes BCA. 1999. *The Right to Health as a Human Right in International Law*. Antwerp: Intersentia.

UN (United Nations). 1945. *Charter of the United Nations*. June 26, 1945, 59 Stat. 1031, entered into force October 24, 1945.

UN (United Nations). 1946. *Constitution of the World Health Organization*. Signed June 22, 1946.

UN (United Nations). 1948. *Universal Declaration of Human Rights*. G.A. Res. 217A (III), U.N. Doc A/810 at 71 (1948).

UN (United Nations). 1968. *Proclamation of Teheran, Final Act of the International Conference on Human Rights, Teheran, 22 April to 13 May 1968*. U.N. Doc. A/CONF. 32/41 at 3 (1968).

UN (United Nations). 1969. *International Convention on the Elimination of All Forms of Racial Discrimination*. G.A. Res. 2106 (XX), Annex, 20 U.N. GAOR Supp. (No. 14) at 47, U.N. Doc. A/6014 (1966), 660 U.N.T.S. 195, entered into force January 4, 1969.

UN (United Nations). 1976a. *International Covenant on Economic, Social and Cultural Rights*. G.A. Res. 2200A (XXI), 21 U.N. GAOR Supp. (No. 16) at 49, U.N. Doc. A/6316 (1966), 993 U.N.T.S. 3, entered into force January 3, 1976.

UN (United Nations). 1976b. *International Covenant on Civil and Political Rights*. G.A. Res. 2200A (XXI), 21 U.N. GAOR Supp. (No. 16) at 52, U.N. Doc. A/6316 (1966), 999 U.N.T.S. 171, entered into force March 23, 1976.

UN (United Nations). 1979. *Convention on the Elimination of All Forms of Discrimination Against Women*. G.A. Res. 34/180, 34 U.N. GAOR Supp. (No. 46) at 193, U.N. Doc. A/34/46 (1979), entered into force September 3, 1981.

UN (United Nations). 1989. *Convention on the Rights of the Child*. G.A. Res. 44/25, Annex, 44 U.N. GAOR Supp. (No. 49) at 167, U.N. Doc. A/44/49 (1989), entered into force September 2, 1990.

UN (United Nations). 1994. *International Conference on Population and Development, Programme of Action, 5–13 September 1994*. U.N. Doc. A/CONF.171/13 (1995).

UN (United Nations). 1995. *Beijing Declaration and Platform for Action, Fourth World Conference on Women, 4–15 September 1995*. U.N. Doc. A/CONF.177/20 & Add.1 (1995).

UN (United Nations) 2000. *General Comment No. 14 (2000): The Right to the Highest Attainable Standard of Health (Article 12 of the International Covenant on Economic, Social and Cultural Rights)*. U.N. Doc. E/C.12/2000/4, August 11, 2000.

UN (United Nations). 2008. *Convention on the Rights of Persons with Disabilities*. G.A. Res. 61/106, Annex I, U.N. GAOR, 61st Sess., Supp. No. 49, at 65, U.N. Doc. A/61/49 (2006), entered into force May 3, 2008.

UN (United Nations). 2011. *Rio Political Declaration on Social Determinants of Health*. Rio de Janeiro.

UN (United Nations) High Commissioner for Human Rights. 2006. *Concept Paper on the High Commissioner's Proposal for a Unified Standing Treaty Body: Report by the Secretariat*. U.N. Doc. HRI/MC/2006/2, March 22, 2006.

UN (United Nations) Programme for HIV/AIDS. 2010. *Global Report: UNAIDS Report on the Global AIDS Epidemic 2010*. http://www.unaids.org/globalreport/global_report.htm (last accessed December 2013).

UN (United Nations) Programme for HIV/AIDS, WHO (World Health Organization). 2007. *AIDS epidemic update: December 2007*. http://www.who.int/hiv/pub/epidemiology/epiupdate2007/en/ (last accessed December 2013).

UNAIDS, Canadian HIV/AIDS Legal Network. 2006. *Courting Rights: Case Studies in Litigating the Human Rights of People Living with HIV*. Geneva: UNAIDS.

United Nations Treaty Collection. 2012. *Status of Human Rights Treaties*. http://treaties.un.org/Pages/ViewDetails.aspx?src=TREATY&mtdsg_no=IV-3-a&chapter=4&lang=en (last accessed December 2013).

University of Essex Human Rights Centre. 2008. *An Introduction to the Work of the Special Rapporteur*. http://www.essex.ac.uk/hrc/research/projects/rth/rapporteur.aspx (last accessed December 2013).

Viljoen F. 2004. Fact-finding by UN Human Rights Complaints Bodies – analysis and suggested reforms. *Max Planck Yearbook of United Nations Law* 8(1), 49–100.

WHO (World Health Organization), UN (United Nations) Office of the High Commissioner of Human Rights. 2010. *A Human Rights-Based Approach to Health*. http://www.who.int/hhr/news/hrba_to_health2.pdf (last accessed December 2013).

WHO (World Health Organization), UN (United Nations) Programme for HIV/AIDS, UN Children's Fund. 2011. *Progress Report 2011: Global HIV/AIDS Response: Epidemic Update and Health Sector Progress Towards Universal Access*. http://www.who.int/hiv/pub/progress_report2011/en/index.html (last accessed December 2013).

World Conference on Human Rights. 1993. *Cairo Declaration on Human Rights in Islam, 5 August 1990.* U.N. GAOR, World Conference on Human Rights, 4th Sess., Agenda Item 5, U.N. Doc. A/CONF.157/PC/62/Add.18 (1993).

Yamin AE, Gloppen S. 2011. *Litigating Health Rights: Can Courts Bring More Justice to Health?* Cambridge, MA: Harvard University Press.

Yamin AE, Parra-Vera O. 2009. How do courts set health policy? The case of the Colombian Constitutional Court. *PLOS Medicine* 6(2), 148–50.

Yamin AE, Parra-Vera O, Gianella C. 2011. Colombia. Judicial protection of the right to health: an elusive promise? In Yamin AE, Gloppen S (eds) *Litigating Health Rights: Can Courts Bring More Justice to Health?*, pp. 103–31. Cambridge, MA: Harvard University Press.

Chapter 26

From Aid to Accompaniment: Rules of the Road for Development Assistance

Vanessa Kerry, Agnes Binagwaho, Jonathan Weigel, and Paul Farmer

Abstract

Foreign assistance needs new rules of the road. Traditional aid modalities have proven too often inefficient and inequitable. This chapter proposes an *accompaniment* approach in which international development agencies transfer more resources and authority to the national and local institutions of their intended beneficiaries in the form of lasting partnerships. We identify eight principles of accompaniment: (1) support institutions that the poor identify as representing their interests; (2) when possible, fund public institutions to do their job; (3) make job creation a benchmark of success; (4) buy and hire locally; (5) co-invest with governments to build strong workforces and civil services; (6) work with governments to provide capital to the poor; (7) support regulation of non-state service providers; and (8) apply evidence-based standards of care. We consider each of these principles, giving "real world" examples, and suggest the accompaniment approach as a compelling way to help the poor break the cycle of poverty and disease.

The Handbook of Global Health Policy, First Edition. Edited by Garrett W. Brown, Gavin Yamey, and Sarah Wamala.
© 2014 John Wiley & Sons, Ltd. Published 2014 by John Wiley & Sons, Ltd.

Key Points

- Current aid modalities are beset by problems: funds do not reach their intended beneficiaries, initiatives are fragmented and inefficient, and local institutions are often excluded.
- Failures of policy and foreign aid are often failures of implementation.
- Donors cite corruption and lack of absorptive capacity as two reasons why they are reluctant to invest directly in governments.
- Such reluctance can be a self-fulfilling prophecy: by bypassing local and national institutions, aid efforts at best miss an opportunity to shore up systems of accountability and efficient, equitable delivery, and at worst undermine the very systems they seek to help.
- Accompaniment, based on the eight principles discussed in this chapter, offers an alternate approach that seeks to bolster local and national capacity through long-term partnerships.
- By guiding interventions to address both the biological and social determinants of health, an accompaniment approach can help break the cycle of poverty and disease.

Key Policy Implications

- Donors and aid policy-makers should put a premium on identifying and over-coming barriers to the *delivery* of health and development programs.
- To minimize the unintended and sometimes harmful consequences of foreign aid – including internal brain drain, weakened public-sector capacity, and patchy service delivery – donors should design aid programs within national priorities and in close consultation with national priorities while building meaningful partnerships with local organizations.
- Employing the principles of accompaniment will require lengthening donor timelines – deliverables, measurements, and outcomes should be defined in terms of longer term priorities such as building efficient and equitable systems of health-care delivery.
- Donors should re-evaluate their incentive structures to reward staff for their commitment to localized aid.

Introduction

In her chapter, "A Rights-Based Approach To Global Health Policy," Lisa Forman outlines the landscape of human rights and global health policy (see Chapter 25). A rights-based approach begins with the assertion that access to healthcare is a human right, and then designs health programs and health systems accordingly. Realizing the right to healthcare within a population usually means, in practice, a concern for distributive justice for the poor, who are most commonly denied the fruits of modern medicine and public health (Farmer 2008). It also often means tackling large-scale social forces – the "social determinants of health" – that pattern the burden of disease and access to care around the globe. Poverty and inequality are among the strongest predictors of ill health in developing and developed countries alike. The heavy burden of disease in vulnerable populations often perpetuates poverty: one study examining why households in rural India, Uganda, and elsewhere fall into poverty found that ill health was the leading cause of impoverishment (Krishna 2010). Another study found that, among Zambian households that lost their breadwinners to AIDS, two thirds suffered precipitous economic decline (Nampanya-Serpell 2000; UN Development Programme 2002).

Human rights declarations, such as the 1948 Universal Declaration of Human Rights, create standards to which all societies and nation-states can and should aspire. In practice, however, rights declarations are enforced more fully when accompanied by the provision of services and the protection of freedoms. Who ought to protect such rights? In the absence of effective systems of policing human rights abuses, transnational public–private partnerships can help provide certain services (such as healthcare). Such partnerships, and the financial resources that undergird them, begin at the policy-makers' table. Public policy can serve as a bridge between principles, such as healthcare as a human right, and practice. At the global level, for example, the President's Emergency Plan for AIDS Relief (PEPFAR) and the Global Fund to Fight AIDS, Tuberculosis and Malaria (the Global Fund) have together put more than 7 million people with HIV/AIDS on antiretroviral treatment (Joint UN Programme on HIV/AIDS 2010). At country level, in Rwanda, pro-poor policy-making has helped scale up access to HIV/AIDS treatment and care. In 2003, fewer than 500 people with HIV/AIDS had access to treatment in both the public and private sectors; as of November 2011, Rwanda's public-sector health system provided care and treatment to nearly 100,000 people with the disease (Ministry of Health, Rwanda 2011).

On the other hand, policies can at times also unwittingly perpetuate inequities in access to healthcare, education, and other entitlements deemed as human rights. Structural Adjustment Programs, peddled by the International Monetary Fund and World Bank in the 1980s and 1990s, offered credit to developing country governments if they made market-based reforms, including cutting social sector spending. Structural adjustment sought to make health systems – and debt-ridden governments, in general – more efficient by shifting the burden of delivering healthcare onto private providers. In a number of countries, however, this policy inadvertently undermined access to care among poor populations, who can rarely afford to pay for health services (Kim *et al.* 2000). Furthermore, in most countries, such policies had little success in stimulating economic growth; some studies have documented a net *outflow* of resources from Africa during the structural adjustment era (Schoepf *et al.* 2000). Effects of these policies – run-down health infrastructure, thin public-sector health workforces – linger today. Policy failures in global health and development are perhaps more common at the country level (Case Study 26.1).

Case Study 26.1   Policy Failure in Global Development: The Case of Haiti

Haiti's history is rich with examples of development policy failures. The Peligré Dam, built on the Artibonite River in Haiti's Central Plateau in the 1950s, was hailed as a landmark development project; it was, at the time, the largest buttress dam in the world. But, with little warning, the project displaced thousands of people living upstream, most of whom later gathered in a squatter settlement on higher, less arable land where it was more difficult to farm and make a living (Farmer 1992). Impoverishment and ill health became the norm. Meanwhile, the region's residents did not receive electricity from the dam until the 1990s. (It primarily powered elite neighborhoods in the capital city, Port-au-Prince.)

And we need not look back to the 1950s for examples of policy failures in Haiti. Despite some US$4.01 billion of official development assistance (ODA) allocated after the January 2010 earthquake – in addition to another $2.4 billion in humanitarian aid – only 10% of the total $6.4 billion was provided directly to the Haitian authorities (UN OSE 2012).

It is easy to produce a list of grievances with development assistance (the "aid debate" is discussed in Chapter 20), which in total increased from US$54 billion to $129 billion from 2000 to 2010 (Ellmers 2011: 8). A growing literature – what one commentator called "the groaning bookshelf" (Gourevitch 2010) – critiques the machinery of foreign aid, and calls for substantial reform. The current system often fails to effectively deliver resources and services to its intended beneficiaries, much less stimulate economic growth. During the famine in Darfur and Ethiopia in the 1980s, well-funded international relief efforts only met 10–12% of victims' basic needs (de Waal 1991). Few low-income, fragile, or conflict-affected countries, which are together home to 1.5 billion people, have achieved any of the United Nations (UN) Millennium Development Goals (MDGs) despite more than $50 billion in development assistance annually since 2000 (UN Development Programme 2010). Consumed by large overhead expenses of aid agencies – which sometimes spend more on salaries and transport costs than on the delivery of services – too little aid money reaches its target recipients (Bolton 2008; Easterly and Pfutze 2008: 19).

Fragmentation of aid at the country- and sector-level further impairs overall aid effectiveness (High Level Forum on Harmonization 2003). Awarding aid contracts to foreign companies and non-governmental organizations (NGOs) – the status quo in the business of aid – can unwittingly undermine public-sector service delivery. In the health sector, for example, NGOs often offer higher salaries than their public-sector counterparts, thereby pulling health professionals from beleaguered public hospitals and clinics; without coordination, such efforts are unlikely to provide health services equitably and efficiently (Killick 2004). In fragile states, about 80% of development assistance bypasses government systems (UN OSE 2012), and only about 4% of goods and services are procured locally (OECD 2011a: 11–17; UN OSE 2012).

Most of these failings of foreign assistance hamper the effectiveness of global health aid in particular. Even during the past decade of expanding global health budgets and successful programs to combat major infectious diseases, most low-income countries lack healthcare systems capable of delivering quality and timely care to all those who need it. Poor coordination is a particularly intractable problem in global health. Foreign support is often earmarked for specific diseases deemed priorities by donors, which may not reflect the true burden of disease in a particular context. Unless different disease-specific initiatives are integrated, they often have little effect on overall health system strengthening (see Chapters 23, 24) (WHO 2004). Disjointed efforts are wasteful and usually inequitable. Maternal and child health, the focus of MDGs 4 and 5, has been one casualty of inefficacious global health aid: 27 countries made little or no progress in reducing childhood deaths between 1990 and 2006 (UN 2008), not to mention building or rebuilding health systems.

From Aid to Accompaniment

Better aid policies – new rules of the road – might strengthen health systems in developing countries. Raising the standard of care in resource-poor settings requires shoring up derelict health infrastructure, improving supply chains, and expanding training programs for doctors, nurses, community health workers, and other health personnel. It also requires tackling the social determinants of health, including poverty, inequality, lack of access to clean water and healthful foods, and environmental risk factors.

But better policy will do little on its own. Most policies are not bad policies. The problem is *delivery*: providing services and opportunities – safeguarding rights – to those who need them most. In this chapter, we contend that the greatest failures of policy and foreign assistance usually result from failures of delivery. An *accompaniment* approach, we suggest, offers some degree of insurance against such failures.

In a mundane sense, accompaniment means walking alongside another. As an approach to global health and development policy, it signifies a perhaps more humble and certainly more long-term mode of foreign "assistance" and "aid": supporting the poor on the road toward well-being, prosperity, peace, and – indeed – aid independence. It begins with listening to and learning from one's intended beneficiaries, and working alongside them until they deem a task completed. Accompaniment is thus both a strategy and a basic orientation to the business of foreign assistance. The following eight principles sketch how aid might move toward accompaniment.

Principle 1: Support Institutions that the Poor Identify as Representing their Interests

The poor endure the local aid context and have learned from it; they have watched past development projects succeed or fail. They often know which development opportunities exist, and what combination of institutions – public and private, local and international – will be more likely to deliver aid effectively (Farmer and Gastineau Campos 2003). Accompaniment hinges on finding good partners, and the poor are necessary consultants for that task. Donors and foreign aid outfits should therefore work closely with their national counterparts and intended beneficiaries well before formulating policies and writing contracts.

Principle 2: When Possible, Fund Public Institutions to do their Job

In Haiti, Rwanda, and elsewhere, we have found that many of the world's poorest people see the provision of basic services as a responsibility of the government. After the 2010 earthquake in Haiti, during a project called "Voices of the Voiceless," interviewers fanned out across the country to ask the rural and urban poor about the country's reconstruction and development strategy. To the best of our knowledge, this was one of the few attempts to bring the perspectives of the poor to bear on policy discussions about Haiti's future after the earthquake. Not surprisingly, respondents expressed concern that the recovery effort was detached from the needs and interests of the poor majority (Farmer 2011). They also called on "trustworthy authorities" to manage aid responsibly and for "the state to be the state" (Farmer 2011). Although the rural and urban poor experience first-hand the failure of the Haitian government to provide basic services to its citizens, they still called for public-sector programs to improve healthcare, education, and employment opportunities. We have observed similar expectations about the role of the government in global health and development in Rwanda, Peru, Russia, and elsewhere.

There is growing consensus among official circles that if health systems are to reach the poor on a large scale and over the long term, governments must play a leading role. The 2005 Paris Declaration on Aid Effectiveness and the 2008 Accra Agenda for Action, which have been signed by over 160 nations and international organizations (including a number of major funders of foreign aid initiatives), both outlined a significant role for the public sector in managing health and development assistance (OECD 2008b).

Why support public institutions in global health and development work? First, governments are the only institutions capable of enshrining – and providing – healthcare as a *right*, as opposed to a commodity. International covenants such as the Universal Declaration of Human Rights might declare a right to healthcare in principle, but they can do little in the way of delivering health services. Only governments can guarantee that all of their citizens, especially the poor and otherwise vulnerable, have access to the healthcare necessary to live full lives in good health. Most private health systems, which treat healthcare as a commodity that is bought and sold, are beset by market failures in resource-poor settings. When private providers lack consumers – the status quo in impoverished places where few can afford to pay for health services – they almost always relocate to markets capable of recouping costs (Pogge 2005; Sachs 2005). This relocation explains the concentration of private providers in wealthy, urban areas, and the absence of private providers in poor, rural areas. Whenever healthcare is rationed by the price mechanism of the market – as a commodity, not a right – poor people will, by definition, fall through the cracks.

Second, governments are more *accountable* to their citizens than are non-state healthcare providers. NGOs, for example, are dependent on and accountable to their funders. If a major donor withdraws support for HIV/AIDS programs that provide contraceptives to commercial sex workers, NGOs may be forced to cut such services, even if the population they serve will be worse off as a result. PEPFAR, for example, does not in principle support programs that engage with commercial sex workers, who are highly vulnerable to HIV infection. This policy reflects domestic political pressures in the United States that construe, or misconstrue, sex work not as a product of structural violence – poverty, gender disparities, urbanization – but of choice (Dietrich 2007; Piot *et al.* 2009; Charumilind *et al.* 2011). Governments, on the other hand, are less vulnerable to the whims of donors; they can design programs according to evidence and local needs instead of the fads *du jour* of global health. They are therefore charged with providing a broad *scope* of health services instead of specific interventions supported by donors. Governments are also expected to provide services for their citizens over the long term, beyond the ebb and flow of donor or foreign aid. They are thus often more *sustainable* than private-sector efforts.

Moreover, governments are often best positioned to provide services on a large, or indeed national, *scale*, such that vulnerable populations including the rural poor are not left out. There are latent economies of scale in healthcare delivery (Porter and Teisberg 2006; Porter 2009, 2010): based on our experiences, the best health systems are community-based, clinic-enriched, and hospital-linked. Building such tiered networks of care demands a robust supply chain, an efficient flow of resources and personnel, and swift referral capacity. Efforts to strengthen each component of an effective health system are synergistic when brought to scale (Porter 2010). Governments, by dint of their national mandate, are poised to harness these efficiencies.

Finally, governments can *coordinate* and *integrate* the efforts of diverse health providers to ensure that care is delivered efficiently and equitably throughout a given country. Without nationwide delivery strategies, private-sector healthcare providers often cluster in wealthy urban areas, as noted, and forfeit the economies of scale that come with collaboration. For example, thousands of NGOs work in Haiti; with better coordination, as Prime Minister Laurent Lamothe called for, such efforts might amount to more than the sum of their parts (Bolstad and Charles 2012). By integrating public and private healthcare efforts, governments can foster more efficient and equitable health systems.

Nonetheless, the status quo in the business of foreign aid remains: priority is given to foreign contractors and NGOs. In 2010, only 10% of aid to fragile states was channeled as general budget support; the rest bypassed public systems (UN OSE 2012). In addition to forfeiting advantages of partnering with the public sector, relying exclusively on private institutions as partners in global health and development work can unwittingly undermine public-sector capacity. As noted by economist Paul Collier and others, the proliferation of NGOs in a number of poor countries has effectively drained the public sector of resources and skilled personnel (Collier 2007: 99–123). Well-trained doctors often choose to work for NGOs because they offer higher salaries than do public-sector facilities. Parallel public and private delivery systems are difficult to coordinate and thus often lead to patchy access to care, especially among the poor.

Why do foreign aid agencies tend to eschew working with governments in developing countries? In the 1970s, development agencies and international banks often made loans to poor countries in support of anti-poverty programs. When dozens of countries defaulted on their debt in the early 1980s, however, the development discourse changed its tune. Structural adjustment – austerity, privatization, liberalization – became the order of the day; such underlying skepticism toward developing-country governments is detectable to this day. Meanwhile, stories of excessive spending and corruption were (and are) common. According to economist Bill Easterly, 41% of the government revenue of Paul Biya, President of Cameroon since 1982, is siphoned off from foreign aid (Easterly 2006: 157). In addition to ineptitude and corruption, two more often-cited reasons for donors' reluctance to invest directly in governments are the lack of "absorptive capacity" – the infrastructure and personnel to utilize donated resources efficiently – and the uncertainty of political cycles (ODI 2004).

However, based on the experiences of a growing number of organizations that have adopted an accompaniment approach, such concerns are exaggerated, and the benefits of working in the public sector outweigh the real and imagined costs. For example, Partners In Health has for 25 years been working to provide high-quality health services to the destitute sick in Haiti's rural reaches; today, the organization also works in a dozen other countries, including Peru, Rwanda, Lesotho, Kazakhstan, and the United States. In almost every setting, excellent public-sector partners are found – especially at the district level – with whom ranking health challenges, from HIV/AIDS to cancer to maternal health are tackled, while also seeking to strengthen health systems in general (Walton *et al.* 2004). Donors concerned with corruption or lack of capacity among recipient governments often fuel a self-fulfilling prophecy. The best way to build capacity and combat corruption, we have found, is to support the development of systems of accountability and transparency – in a word, accompaniment.

What does accompaniment look like in practice? One example is the General Hospital in Port-au-Prince, Haiti. The hospital is charged with probably the largest patient load in the country, but it has too few resources and medical personnel to keep up with demand. Its staff was small and underpaid even before the January 2010 earthquake; afterward, it was overrun with patients requiring acute medical attention. Though scores of international teams worked on the General Hospital campus, providing acute care and essential surgical services, they sometimes competed for space and control over hospital facilities. Few had much interest in trying to improve the quality of care offered by the struggling public-sector hospital over the long term. When most disaster relief teams packed their bags, the hospital was still overrun, its staff still underpaid.

Our teams tried to bring together a number of international partners interested in traveling the longer road of reconstruction – in this case, helping rebuild the General Hospital. The American Red Cross agreed to send $3.8 million in "performance-based" salary support for the hospital's beleaguered employees. This work has been difficult and slow: Haitian institutions often lack the infrastructure of transparency and platforms for evaluation (electricity, modern bookkeeping, accountants, computers) demanded by western accountability norms. But only an accompaniment approach will help develop such platforms and put them under the control of the intended beneficiaries. The Red Cross collaboration soon bore fruit: today, staff members are better paid and accountability platforms are taking root. We have come to believe that this kind of accompaniment – partnering with Haitian institutions and working through whatever obstacles present themselves – is among the best ways to help address the structural deficits preventing Haiti from rebuilding better.

Accompaniment has, in recent years, gained some traction in the business of official development assistance (ODA). General budget support has been found to reduce transaction costs associated with foreign assistance and to improve coherence of planning and delivery (OECD 2011b). According to a report by the Overseas Development Institute, for example, general budget support to the Tanzanian government enhanced its ability to coordinate ongoing foreign aid initiatives and increased the proportion of new external funds subject to the national budget process (ODI 2005). One analysis by the Organisation for Economic Co-operation and Development (OECD) concludes that even countries with low-quality public financial management systems can make good use of donor funds, so long as partner governments are committed to improving the quality of such systems (OECD 2006). In most cases, budget support has been shown to improve the efficiency and transparency of ministries of finance in managing national budgets and disbursing funds (IDD and Associates 2006: 55–69; DeRenzio *et al.* 2010; Williamson and Dom 2010: 78). As was the case in Port-au-Prince's General Hospital, directing funds through national systems can strengthen the accounting capacity of national institutions, as well as the role of audit institutions (IDD and Associates 2006; Williamson and Dom 2010: 95; OECD 2011c).

Despite the observed effectiveness of direct budget support, there are still challenges to improving public financial management systems, including underdeveloped national capacity, corruption, and lack of political will. Technical assistance, which in an accompaniment framework means helping develop such management systems and train personnel to use them, can increase the efficacy of budget support in settings that lack public financial management capacity (Caputo *et al.* 2011). Corruption is a much-cited concern among donors and foreign aid officials. But donors are, in fact, inconsistent about factoring it into decisions about aid allocation. There is almost no correlation between the quality of a country's public financial management systems and the amount of aid channeled through those systems (OECD 2010a). For example, among five countries with equally low ratings for the quality of public financial management – Guinea-Bissau, Liberia, Madagascar, Nepal, and the Solomon Islands – there is considerable fluctuation in the percentage of aid directed through their country systems (OECD 2011d: 117–25). In 25 countries with only a moderate public financial management rating, donors channeled anywhere from 3% to 79% of aid through those systems (OECD 2011d).

Moreover, two donor-led evaluations have concluded that budget support is subject to comparable losses (to corruption and mismanagement) as other types of "tightly controlled" aid (Wood *et al.* 2011). In fact, a recent evaluation by the UK Department for International Development (DFID) found only marginal inefficiencies among public-sector partnerships: of more than £600 million in budget support in each of the last two fiscal years, it estimated losses of less than 0.016% of total spending (£96,000) (DFID 2011a; House of Commons 2011). This figure pales in comparison to the overhead costs of the great majority of aid contractors and NGOs. For example, in 2010 one international NGO, the British Red Cross, spent more than £40 million – 20% of its annual expenditures – on fundraising alone (British Red Cross 2012).

In addition to strengthening public-sector capacity, channeling development assistance through country systems almost always increases the funding available for state institutions to provide services (Williamson and Dom 2010; Wood *et al.* 2011). In two separate evaluations of direct budget support in a total of 15 countries, 12 of the recipient governments had increased spending in priority social sectors (National Audit Office (UK) 2008: 12; Williamson and Dom 2010). This increase was especially true in the health and education sectors; in one country case of Ethiopia, domestic spending doubled over a two-year timeframe (National Audit Office (UK) 2008). The same evaluation also found that access to social services was twice as likely to increase in countries that received budget support from DFID (National Audit Office (UK) 2008). These results are largely echoed by evaluations conducted by the World Bank, the OECD, and the Overseas Development Institute (Booth *et al.* 2005; IDD and Associates 2006; Lawson *et al.* 2007; de Kemp *et al.* 2011; OECD 2011c).

All that said, in some cases governments simply lack the capacity or will to provide services for their citizens. After the 2010 Haiti earthquake damaged or destroyed 28 out of 29 federal ministries, what was left of the government operated out of makeshift offices and trailers. The government clearly lacked capacity to respond to the enormous need on its own, and the surge of international humanitarian assistance almost exclusively supported NGOs and private relief and rescue efforts. In fact, only 0.9% of the $2.4 billion in post-earthquake humanitarian aid went through government channels (UN OSE 2011). This figure is almost certainly too low. How can international organizations hope to help rebuild public-sector capacity in a place like Haiti if the government is starved of resources? Nonetheless this example highlights how, in certain circumstances, governments may simply be unable to partner with international aid groups. In such circumstances, local NGOs and other private-sector initiatives are often the best available partners for global health work (Case Study 26.2).

Case Study 26.2   Partnering with Local NGOs: An Example in Chiapas, Mexico

In Chiapas, Mexico, indigenous populations have long faced discrimination, political violence, poverty, and poor health conditions. Although Partners In Health usually partners with government ministries of health, in Chiapas they have worked with a group of health promoters, Equipo de Apoyo en Salud y Educación Comunitaria (EAPSEC, Spanish for "Team for the Support of Community Health and Education"). EAPSEC, which serves marginalized communities, was established in 1985 by a group of Mexican health promoters. After first working with Guatemalan refugee communities in the Chiapas border region, EAPSEC later expanded throughout other marginalized communities in the region. This collaboration was suggested by the leaders of the indigenous communities; they asked Partners In Health to work there in 1989. In collaboration with EAPSEC, they have helped develop a network of mobile clinics to provide health education, prevention, and treatment services to some of the poorest communities in Chiapas. They have also supported efforts to use cell phones and other mobile technologies to improve healthcare delivery (Blaya *et al.* 2010). In recent years, EAPSEC and Partners In Health have in fact begun to explore a new partnership with the Ministry of Health. Their experiences working in Mexico underscore that even when working with governments is not initially feasible, it may become so over time. An accompaniment approach entails the flexibility to reassess and adapt programs to a changing context.

Principle 3: Make Job Creation a Benchmark of Success

In all sectors of development – health, education, environment, energy, infrastructure, trade, and finance, to name just a few – donors, policy-makers, and practitioners should prioritize local job creation and transfer of capacity. Lower indices of employment almost always correlate with stagnant poverty, even in fast-growing economies (OECD 2008a). In addition to helping individuals and families achieve autonomy and basic well-being, jobs confer dignity, self-worth, and opportunities to pursue professional development. Job creation can also boost demand and stimulate local economies. As workers earning a living wage spend money on local goods and services, the return on their employment extends from the household to the community to the local and national economy. According to the International Labour Organization, each additional Euro of worker income leads to a multiplier effect of 1.5 to 2.8 in low-income countries (Ellmers 2011). Moreover, job creation expands the national tax base, enabling governments to provide higher quality social services, improve infrastructure, and to create incentives for pro-poor development (OECD 2006). A formal tax structure can also enhance government accountability.

Yet far more people are unemployed now than in recent history (ILO 2010a, 2010b). According to the International Labour Organization, the number of unemployed people globally increased from 185 million in 2008 to over 210 million in 2009 (ILO 2010a). Moreover, among the poor who are employed, an estimated 1.5 billion people – about half the world's workforce – have jobs in the informal sector (ILO 2010b). More than a billion people live on less than $1.25 per day.

Nonetheless, few donor agencies embrace job creation. Based on publicly available online information, the 10 biggest donors in the global development sphere (Canada, the

European Union, France, Germany, Japan, the Netherlands, Spain, the United Kingdom, the United States, and the World Bank) make little reference to jobs as a strategic priority. One example of a donor program that does prioritize job creation is the UN World Food Program's innovative Purchase for Progress (P4P) program, which recognizes the power of food aid to promote employment and broaden access to domestic markets among the world's poorest farmers. A five-year pilot program launched in 2008, Purchase for Progress initiates purchasing contracts with smallholder farmers while also training them in modern farming techniques.

Among the best ways to boost employment in developing countries is to foster a favorable business environment that will attract investment and private enterprise (OECD 2006). But in many developing countries, strict regulations and tax burdens, unfair competition practices, and lack of financial or planning services dampen the vitality of the private sector. In particular, developing world markets often suffer from a lack of competitiveness, without which they rarely serve the interests of the poor. One study found that 16 international cartels overcharged developing countries between $16 billion and $32 billion in 1997; prices fell by 20–40% following the break-up of the cartels (OECD 2006). Donors and foreign aid groups can work with governments and other stakeholders to reduce tax and regulatory burdens, provide financial and business development services, promote fair competition policy, and formulate other policies that are both business-friendly and pro-poor.

Principle 4: Buy and Hire Locally

Almost half of all ODA – which totaled $150 billion in 2010 – is spent on the acquisition of goods and services (Ellmers 2011). The scale of such procurement offers a substantial opportunity to boost aggregate demand, manufacturing capacity, and workforce development of beneficiary countries. Yet most foreign aid projects procure goods and services from donor countries (Wood *et al.* 2011). In a questionnaire on contracts awarded in 2009, OECD donors reported that out of $8.64 billion awarded through 4488 contracts, 58% of funding went to firms in OECD donor countries, 38% to firms in developing countries, and only 4% to firms in least developed countries (OECD 2011a). That same year, 89% of the United States' aid contracts for least developed countries and heavily indebted poor countries were in fact won by US suppliers (OECD 2011e). A year and a half after the 2010 Haiti earthquake, only 2.4% of reconstruction contracts issued by bilateral donors had been awarded to Haitian firms (UN OSE 2011).

At best, failure to buy and hire locally misses an opportunity to stimulate local development; at worst, it can weaken local economies (by importing goods and services at artificially low prices). Some have argued that such "tied" aid – where all goods and services must be procured within the donor country – devalues foreign assistance by one quarter, hinders job creation, and undermines long-term growth (Killick 2004: 20). Alternatively, by buying goods and services within the recipient country, donors can increase the value of every aid dollar by creating jobs and bolstering local economies. Since the Paris Declaration and Accra Agenda, donors have begun to do more in the way of local procurement and hiring.

The P4P program showcases many of the benefits of buying and hiring locally. Instead of distorting (or damaging) agriculture in recipient nations by flooding markets with cheap or free food, P4P's local procurement strategies have boosted demand for the produce of the world's poorest farmers while also providing training in farming techniques, quality control, and post-harvest handling. This approach has also led to a substantial savings: by some estimates, P4P saved $22.6 million in procurement and transportation costs in 2010 (World Food Programme 2011).

A similar initiative has borne fruit in Haiti, where as many as half of school-aged children live with food insecurity. One remedy for acute malnutrition is known as ready-to-use therapeutic food (RUTF), such as nutrient-enriched peanut paste (Defourny 2007). Instead of buying this paste from a company based in France or any other country, Partners In Health has for years made its own RUTF using mostly locally procured ingredients. The paste proved effective in treating moderate and severe malnutrition, and a more reliable market for peanuts helped local farmers. In the last few years, specialists from a US pharmaceutical company and Haitian agronomists have helped to expand this effort by building a larger scale food-processing facility. This initiative will not only provide treatment for all children diagnosed with acute malnutrition in the region, but also provide many jobs and use, whenever possible, locally procured ingredients. It ends up, therefore, being accompaniment not only for malnourished children and their families, but also for local farmers and all those seeking to improve food-processing capacity in rural Haiti.

There are many other examples of the promise of buying and hiring locally. The cost of building a kilometer of road in Ghana or Vietnam is 30–40% less when built by a local company (ActionAid UK 2011: 33). After typhoon Ketsana hit the Philippines in 2009, the American Red Cross – with $500,000 in funding from the US Agency for International Development (USAID) – reportedly doubled the number of emergency sanitation and kitchen kits it distributed among affected families by buying supplies locally (American Red Cross 2010).

In recent years, some donors have adopted new approaches to achieving long-term sustainable development. Their focus has shifted towards increasing their levels of local investments and working with host governments to strengthen internal management and implementation capacity. USAID, for example, has committed, as part of USAID Forward – its agency-wide reform agenda launched in August 2010 – to increasing, from 9.7% in financial year 2010 to 30% in financial year 2015, the share of its program funds that are disbursed directly to national and local partner governments, civil society organizations, and businesses (USAID 2013).

What are the barriers to widespread adoption of similar policies? Donors often point out that issuing more small contracts would likely increase administrative costs. But as untied aid increases the value of every aid dollar; such administrative inefficiencies – equally a product of bureaucracy and dated procedure – are surely worth the multiplier effects associated with buying and hiring locally.

Policies to untie aid, while necessary, are insufficient to boost local procurement. Other policy barriers limit the ability of businesses in beneficiary countries from winning procurement contracts, including donor eligibility criteria (which often demand extensive experience that only established contractors will have), access to credit, and coverage through insurance services. Accompaniment is premised on the accumulation of shared experience and capacity; instead of excluding those that fail to meet these criteria, donors and foreign aid groups can help local businesses gain access to credit and insurance. Small contracts might also better suit startups and young businesses in recipient countries. An analysis by the UN Office of the Special Envoy for Haiti (OSE), for example, found that local businesses have better chances of winning smaller aid contracts. Of the $270 million in contracts awarded by one multilateral donor since the earthquake, Haitian firms were awarded 32.7% (or $88.2 million) of them, including 211 out of 219 contracts valued under $1 million and only one out of seven contracts valued over $5 million (UN OSE 2012).

Principle 5: Co-invest with Governments to Build Strong Workforces and Civil Services

Economic and human development in any country hinges on the strength of its civil service, including frontline service providers who have a direct impact on the health and welfare of the population. Workforce development, whether it is the health workforce or any other, requires platforms of transparent hiring and firing, including performance reviews, continuing training programs for civil servants, and the ability to conduct workforce needs assessments. But there is a severe shortage of civil servants and frontline service providers in most poor countries. A 2006 World Health Organization (WHO) report estimated that there was a shortage of 2.3 million doctors, nurses, and midwives in more than 57 developing countries (WHO 2006); an additional 10.3 million primary teachers are needed to ensure universal primary education (UNESCO Institute for Statistics 2007). Few would dispute that weak human resource capacity is among the most significant factors contributing to the poor quality of services provided by developing-country governments.

The high demand for skilled labor in wealthy countries – and the promise of higher wages – continues to fan the brain drain (when professionals from poor countries seek work in richer ones). Health systems in OECD countries have become especially reliant on professionals from lower income countries. Skilled jobs in the US health sector, for example, outnumber graduates of medical and nursing schools by about 5000 positions each year (Health Resources and Services Administration 2005: 5). Such demand has profound effects on the global supply of skilled labor. Another study estimated that the emigration of doctors (whose training had been publicly subsidized) represented a loss of more than $2 billion in nine sub-Saharan African countries (Mills *et al.* 2011). This loss was, of course, a windfall for wealthier nations, which saved $846 million to $2.7 billion in medical training costs (Mills *et al.* 2011).

Increasing public-sector salaries might help boost retention. In 10 out of 23 developing countries considered in one study, the average salaries of teachers and nurses were not far from the international poverty line (UNICEF 2010). In Haiti, public-sector workers are paid on average 40% less than private-sector workers of comparable skill levels (World Bank 2008: 9). Indeed, the 2011 Paris Declaration survey notes that artificially high wages offered at international organizations functions as a sizeable barrier to maintaining a strong civil service in many developing countries.

In addition to the global shortage of service providers, there are too few skilled civil servants in poor countries (Williamson and Dom 2010). Current aid models do not help. In 2010, only 3.1% of total ODA disbursed ($147.4 billion) was reported as being invested in strengthening civil servants' capacity through education and training (OECD Working Party on Statistics 2011; OECD 2012). Instead, aid programs often erect parallel (if not competing) structures and provide "technical assistance" (usually an "expert" or two from donor nations) without helping develop robust training programs that can build in-country capacity (Bolton 2008). According to the *World Development Report 2011*, a quarter of all aid targeting government capacity in Afghanistan was spent on technical assistance, but the results are mixed (World Bank 2011: 196). Technical assistance is also costly: each full-time expatriate consultant costs about 200 times the average annual salary of an Afghan civil servant (Waldman 2008: 19). In 2002, the cost of 700 international advisors to the Cambodian government was $50–70 million, just shy of the wage bill for the country's entire 160,000-strong civil service (ActionAid International 2005: 22; Waldman 2008).

Investments in health infrastructure are urgently needed but must be matched with investments in training and workforce development in order to take advantage of improved infrastructure. In Mali, the number of community health centers increased from 605 to 993 between 2002 and 2009, yet the country has just 0.08 doctors for every 1000 people (WHO 2006).

Long-term development of the civil service and public-sector service delivery ultimately demands significant internal reform. Donors and foreign aid groups can contribute to this process by prioritizing training and workforce development. Rwanda offers one such example. Using designated international assistance from the World Bank, the Government of Rwanda launched the Public Sector Capacity Building Project. Designed to improve service delivery, the project included a nationwide skills audit and the implementation of new salary scales based on job classifications, equity (including gender equity), and motivation to attract and retain qualified civil servants. In fact, Rwanda has the highest proportion of female civil servants in the world (Devlin and Elgie 2008).

A further example is in Uganda, where the UN supplemented the salaries of all staff in the Ministry of Finance from 1989 to 1996. The total cost of the initiative was "less than a single expatriate technical assistant," yet by the end of it the Ministry was considered one of the strongest in sub-Saharan Africa (Manuel *et al.* 2012: 31).

Principle 6: Work with Governments to Provide Cash to the Poor

A growing body of evidence suggests that cash transfers – giving money directly to the poor – can serve as a complementary tool to reduce poverty, boost demand for goods and services, and thus stimulate local economies (Lagarde *et al.* 2009; Hanlon *et al.* 2010; Arnold *et al.* 2011). While some critics argue that because the transfers are "conditional," they are coercive; in our experience, by letting poor people decide how to use such resources, cash transfers confer upon recipients greater dignity than do most other modalities of foreign assistance.

Such programs are similar to social protection efforts for the poor in high-income countries. In OECD countries, for example, almost 10% of gross domestic product (GDP) is, on average, dedicated to cash-based social assistance; over 80% of the population in these countries receive some form of such support (Farrington *et al.* 2005). Although a subject of debate, most data indicate that the lion's share of such funds are used to buy essentials, such as food, clothing, shelter, and healthcare (Jaspars and Harvey 2007). In Haiti, which has no public cash-transfer program, studies on remittances – comparable to cash transfers – have found similar results: families spend more than three quarters of remittance funds on essentials, including food, utilities, and clothing (Inter-American Development Bank 2007). A feasibility study found that many potential beneficiaries of a cash-transfer initiative intended to use the money to send their children to school (Cohen *et al.* 2007: 17).

The evidence in support of cash transfers in developing countries is impressive and growing. In southern Africa, where the world's worst HIV/AIDS epidemic has disrupted families and caused the death of many caregivers, cash-transfer programs have helped keep many orphaned children in school and families together (in a region where labor migration is, for many of the poorest, the norm) (Jaspars and Harvey 2007). In South Africa, a cash-transfer program has been credited with helping to reduce the poverty gap – the gap between the incomes of the poor and the income required to keep them out of poverty – by 47% (Samson *et al.* 2004). Mexico's conditional cash-transfer program – which requires that, among other things, families bring their children to clinics for a basic package of health interventions – has been credited with improving child health (Gertler 2004; Rivera *et al.* 2004; Frenk 2006). A cash-transfer program in Zambia contributed to an increase in the ownership of goats from 8.5% of households to 41.7% (Scheuring 2008). A similar program in Bangladesh increased the value of household-owned live-stock assets by a factor of 12 (DFID 2011b). DFID's Social Protection Expansion Scheme in Zambia found that the consumption of goods by cash-transfer recipients increased by at least 50% (Scheuring 2008). Another study of a cash-transfer program in Malawi observed a regional multiplier of 2.02 to 2.45 for every program dollar spent; traders, suppliers, services, and other non-recipients in the local economy appear to have benefited from the increase in aggregate demand (EuropeAid 2010; Voipio 2011).

In most developing countries, however, less than 1% of GDP is spent on cash-based social assistance programs; such programs reach less than 10% of the workforce in Africa and Asia (Farrington *et al.* 2005). By supporting cash-transfer programs, donors and aid agencies can help stimulate microenterprise and development while also reinforcing – or at least not undermining – the social contract between the state and its most marginalized citizens.

Cash-transfer programs are no panacea, and can accomplish little without institutions of growth and good governance. But they can give "searchers," to use Bill Easterly's term (Easterly 2006), modest means to improve their lot or even launch small enterprises, and complement efforts to provide healthcare, education, and other forms of social protection seeking to break the cycle of poverty and disease.

Principle 7: Support Regulation of Non-State Service Providers

As discussed, the status quo in foreign assistance often involves contracting local and international NGOs instead of the governments of recipient countries. In many cases, a lack of coordination among NGOs working to provide much needed services prevents foreign aid efforts from adding up to more than the sum of their parts. Even the best intentioned efforts can have unintended and sometimes harmful consequences.

Haiti is a case in point. The Government of Haiti's total revenue pales in comparison to the foreign assistance disbursed on Haitian shores: in 2010, the year of the earthquake, bilateral and multilateral aid roughly equaled 400% of the government's internal revenue (UN OSE 2011). Most NGOs (in Haiti and elsewhere) do valuable work, but without coordination and regulation, they run the risk of being duplicative, inequitable, and unac-countable to the communities they serve. Local organizations, including cash-strapped ministries of health (and the public clinics and hospitals they run), cannot compete with better funded NGOs. Harmonizing foreign aid efforts increases the likelihood that they will help engender lasting improvements for their intended beneficiaries. National gov-ernments are usually in the best position to act as a steward of such efforts.

The Government of Rwanda, for instance, produced a comprehensive development plan, *Vision 2020*, that puts a premium on coordination of foreign aid initiatives to ensure that all providers in the country are working toward the same goals with a unified strat-egy. NGOs that fail to work in accordance with national strategies are often asked to leave the country. This approach, in part, explains why Rwanda is achieving some of the best health and development outcomes on the African continent (Farmer *et al.* 2013). By streamlining procurement systems across the country, for example, the Ministry of Health improved inventory management of HIV/AIDS treatment while bringing down associated costs (Tarrafeta 2007).

Developing-country governments might, of course, need support – accompaniment – in this role as stewards of service provision. Foreign assistance can aid national and local governments through direct support and also through requirements that grantees and contractors align their work with government priorities. This approach respects the regulatory duties of the state and helps ensure that aid does not bypass (or undermine) national accountability structures. Transparent, mutually beneficial partnerships between non-state providers and governments are a precondition of efficient and equitable delivery of basic services on a large scale (OECD and UN Development Programme 2010).

Principle 8: Apply Evidence-Based Standards of Care

Rich and poor settings are almost always separated by different standards of healthcare. Budgets, rather than strategy, too often drive implementation, which usually means paltry healthcare services are available in poor places. But the accompaniment approach, premised on equity, demands raising the standard of care in resource-poor settings to a level that would be acceptable in affluent settings.

Evidence-based practice is fundamental to clinical medicine. A critical feedback loop – service delivery linked with research and training – helps practitioners deliver better care and improves health outcomes among patients. Above all, it establishes standards by which doctors and nurses and other members of the allied health professions can be measured and evaluated. This approach can and should be adopted in the business of foreign assistance.

Food security, for example, is a necessary precondition of effective treatment for many diseases; mortality is two to six times higher in the first months of antiretroviral treatment for individuals who have both AIDS and malnourishment (World Food Programme 2012). But, perhaps due to the stovepiping of foreign aid – AIDS programs funded by one agency, nutrition programs by another – many HIV/AIDS control efforts in resource-poor settings do not include food support as a pillar of HIV/AIDS treatment. Rwanda again offers a model: the Ministry of Health requires that health providers supplement antiretroviral medications with nutritional support (sufficient for a family of six) for the first six months of treatment. After that initial period, providers evaluate the need for further food supplementation on a case-by-case basis while patients continue antiretroviral treatment. Most people who initiate treatment and receive care recover their ability to work after six months.

The application of evidence-based practice should hardly be controversial. Indeed, it has become jargon, and many aid outfits claim evidence-based strategy, even though they lack systems for monitoring and evaluation, not to mention the feedback loop between service delivery, research, and training. A principal barrier to evidence-based practice in foreign assistance is the "socialization for scarcity": a lower standard is reserved for the poor precisely because they are poor. A truly evidence-based strategy seeks to close the delivery gap between rich and poor places, not maintain it in the name of cost-effectiveness. Applying evidence-based standards in rich settings and poor ones is not only humane, it will bring down long-term healthcare costs and promote economic development (see Chapter 7 on evidence-based global health policy).

Conclusions

Accompaniment is not a "quick win" approach to foreign aid. It demands long-term engagement, a commitment to genuine partnership, and flexibility to tackle whatever challenges come along. It can be at odds with process-driven accountability conventions that fetishize short-term cost-effectiveness without asking larger questions about evidence, equity, and sustainable development. We advocate a broadened definition of success in the business of foreign aid.

In recent years, the accompaniment approach has been gaining traction. The World Food Program has highlighted priority areas for "the poorest, most food-insecure people bypassed by conventional development efforts" (World Food Programme 2008). Its programs help the poor engage in education and training programs, preserve assets and gain access to credit, and find more steady employment in the agricultural sector. The US Agency for International Development (USAID) recently announced new commitment to local procurement even when it might counter US laws on competition for bidding on contracts (USAID 2011). The European Commission is seeking to increase direct budget support to national governments. PEPFAR recently made its first sector budget-support grant to fund the Government of Rwanda's Human Resources for Health Initiative, a seven-year program to develop delivery and training capacity through long-term partnerships with a dozen American universities. Efforts such as these suggest a new-found commitment to the Paris Declaration, and green shoots, perhaps, for the world's poorest people.

But a commitment to the principles of accompaniment is not the same as implementation of aid efforts based on these principles. The aid enterprise has historically been resistant to investing in local and national systems directly, citing fears of corruption or lack of absorptive capacity. Such practices, however, can fuel a vicious cycle and miss a chance to strengthen the very systems that donors critique (OECD 2010b). An accompaniment approach guides foreign aid groups to transfer more resources and authority to the national and local institutions of their intended beneficiaries in the form of lasting partnerships. It offers, we contend, a compelling strategy for helping the poor and otherwise vulnerable break the cycle of poverty and disease.

Acknowledgments

We are indebted to Jehane Sedky, Abbey Gardner, Katherine Gilbert, and the United Nations Office of the Special Envoy for Haiti for their research and analysis of aid effectiveness after the 2010 Haiti earthquake, and for an ongoing colloquy that shaped our thinking about an accompaniment approach to development assistance and humanitarian aid. We also would like to thank Claire Wagner, Gretchen Williams, Rosabelle Conover, Kevin Savage, Caroline Craig, and Caleb Murray-Bozeman for their help finalizing this manuscript.

Key Reading

Ellmers B. 2011. *How to Spend It: Smart Procurement for More Effective Aid*. European Network on Debt and Development (Eurodad). http://www.un.org/en/ecosoc/newfunct/pdf/luxembourg_eurodad-how_to_spend_it.pdf (last accessed December 2013).

Farmer P. 2011. Partners in help: assisting the poor over the long term. *Foreign Affairs*. http://www.foreignaffairs.com/articles/68002/paul-farmer/partners-in-help (last accessed December 2013).

High Level Forum on Joint Progress toward Enhanced Aid Effectiveness. 2005. *Paris Declaration on Aid Effectiveness, February 25 to March 2, 2005*. www.oecd.org/dac/effectiveness/secondhighlevelforumonjointprogresstowardenhancedaideffectivenessharmonisationalignmentandresults.htm (last accessed December 2013).

OECD (Organisation for Economic Co-operation and Development). 2006. *Promoting Private Investment for Development: The Role of ODA*. Paris: OECD. http://www.oecd.org/document/55/0,3746,en_2649_34621_46582839_1_1_1_1,00.html (last accessed December 2013).

OECD (Organisation for Economic Co-operation and Development). 2011. *Aid Effectiveness 2005–10: Progress in Implementing the Paris Declaration*. Paris: OECD. http://www.oecd.org/dataoecd/25/30/48742718.pdf (last accessed December 2013).

OECD (Organisation for Economic Co-operation and Development) DAC (Development Assistance Committee). 2010. *Making Aid More Effective through the Strengthening and Use of National Systems*. Policy Brief 1, Paris. www.oecd.org/dac/effectiveness/45497699.pdf (last accessed December 2013).

UN (United Nations) OSE (Office of the Special Envoy for Haiti). 2011. *Has Aid Changed*. New York: OSE.

References

ActionAid International. 2005. *Real Aid: An Agenda for Making Aid Work*. Johannesburg: ActionAid International.

ActionAid UK. 2011. *Real Aid: Ending Aid Dependency*. London: ActionAid UK.

American Red Cross. 2010. *Emergency Response to Typhoon Ketsana in the Philippines: Final Report*. Washington, DC: American Red Cross.

Arnold C, Conway T, Greenslade M. 2011. *DFID Cash Transfers Literature Review*. London: DFID. http://www.dfid.gov.uk/r4d/PDF/Articles/cash-transfers-literature-review.pdf (last accessed December 2013).

Blaya J, Fraser H, Holt B. 2010. E-health technologies show promise in developing countries. *Health Affairs* 29, 244–51.

Bolstad E, Charles J. 2012. Haiti Prime Minister Conille: donor aid needs revision. *Miami Herald* February 7.

Bolton G. 2008. *Africa Doesn't Matter: How the West has Failed the Poorest Continent and What We Can Do About It*. New York, NY: Arcade Publishing.

Booth D, Lawson A, Williamson T, Wangwe S, Msuya M. 2005. *Joint Evaluation of General Budget Support: Tanzania 1995–2004. Revised Final Report*. London and Dar es Salaam: ODI and Daima Associates. www.odi.org.uk/resources/docs/3234.pdf (last accessed December 2013).

British Red Cross. 2012. *Trustees' Report and Account 2012*. http://www.redcross.org.uk/About-us/Who-we-are/Governance-and-annual-reports/Income-and-expenditure (last accessed December 2013).

Caputo E, de Kemp A, Lawson A. 2011. *Assessing the Impacts of Budget Support: Case Studies in Mali, Tunisia, and Zambia*. Evaluation Insights No. 2. Paris: Organisation for Economic Co-operation and Development.

Charumilind S, Jain S, Rhatigan J. 2011. *HIV in Thailand: The 100% Condom Program. Global Health Delivery Online*. HBS No. GHD-001. Boston: Harvard Business School Publishing. http://www.ghdonline.org/cases/ (last accessed December 2013).

Cohen W, Menon R, Smith N. 2007. *Implementing a Conditional Cash Transfer Program in Haiti: Opportunities and Challenges*. Washington, DC: Inter-American Development Bank.

Collier P. 2007. *The Bottom Billion: Why the Poorest Countries are Failing and What Can be Done About It*. Oxford: Oxford University Press.

De Kemp A, Faust J, Leiderer S. 2011. *Between High Expectations and Reality: An Evaluation of Budget Support in Zambia*. The Hague: Ministry of Foreign Affairs of the Kingdom of the Netherlands. www.oecd.org/dataoecd/25/31/49210553.pdf (last accessed December 2013).

De Waal A. 1991. *Evil Days: 30 Years of War and famine in Ethiopia (Africa Watch Report)*. New York: Human Rights Watch.

Defourny I, Seroux G, Abdelkader I, Harczi G. 2007. *Management of Moderate Acute Malnutrition with RUTF in Niger*. MSF Report. http://www.msf.org.au/uploads/media/mod_acc_mal_Niger.pdf (last accessed December 2013).

DeRenzio P, Andrews M, Mills Z. 2010. *Evaluation of Donor Support to Public Financial Management (PFM) Reform in Developing Countries: Analytical Study of Quantitative Cross-country Evidence*. London: Overseas Development Institute.

Devlin C, Elgie R. 2008. The effect of increased women's representation in parliament: the case of Rwanda. *Parliamentary Affairs* 61(2), 237–54.

DFID (Department for International Development). 2011a. *Annual Report and Accounts 2010–11: Volume I*. London: DFID.

DFID (Department for International Development). 2011b. *Transferring Cash and Assets to the Poor*. London: National Audit Office.

Dietrich JW. 2007. The politics of PEPFAR: the President's Emergency Plan for AIDS Relief. *Ethics and International Affairs* 21(3), 277–92

Easterly W. 2006. *The White Man's Burden: Why the West's Efforts to Aid the Rest Have Done So Much Ill and So Little Good*. New York: Penguin.

Easterly W, Pfutze T. 2008. *Where Does the Money Go? Best and Worst Practices in Foreign Aid*. Brookings Global Economy and Development Working Paper No. 21. Washington, DC: Brookings Institute.

Ellmers B. 2011. *How to Spend It: Smart Procurement for More Effective Aid*. European Network on Debt and Development (Eurodad). http://www.un.org/en/ecosoc/newfunct/pdf/luxembourg_eurodad-how_to_spend_it.pdf (last accessed December 2013).

EuropeAid. 2010. *Social Transfers: An Effective Approach to Fight Food Insecurity and Extreme Poverty*. Brussels: Commission Européenne.

Farmer P. 1992. *AIDS and Accusation: Haiti and the Geography of Blame*. Berkeley, CA: University of California Press.

Farmer P. 2008. Challenging orthodoxies: the road ahead for health and human rights. *Health and Human Rights: An International Journal* 10(1), 5–19.

Farmer P. 2011. *Haiti After the Earthquake*. New York: Public Affairs.

Farmer P, Gastineau Campos N. 2003. Partners: discernment and humanitarian efforts in settings of violence. *Journal of Law, Medicine and Ethics* 31(4), 506–15.

Farmer PE, Nutt CT, Wagner CM et al. 2013. Reduced premature mortality in Rwanda: lessons from success. *British Medical Journal* 365, 20–2.

Farrington J, Harvey P, Slater R. 2005. *Cash Transfers in the Context of Pro-Poor Growth*. London: Overseas Development Institute.

Frenk J. 2006. Bridging the divide: global lessons from evidence-based health policy in Mexico. *Lancet* 368, 954–61.

Gertler P. 2004. Do conditional cash transfers improve child health? Evidence from PROGRESA's control randomized experiment. *American Economic Review* 94, 336–41.

Gourevitch P. 2010. Alms dealers: can you provide humanitarian aid without facilitating conflicts? *New Yorker* October 11.

Hanlon J, Barrientos A, Hulme D. 2010. *Just Give Money to the Poor: The Development Revolution from the Global South*. Sterling, VA: Kumarian Press.

Health Resources and Services Administration. 2005. *Physician Workforce Policy Guidelines for the United States, 2000–2020, 16th Report*. Council on Graduate Medical Education, Health Resources and Services Administration. Washington, DC: US Department of Health and Human Services. http://www.hrsa.gov/advisorycommittees/bhpradvisory/cogme/Reports/sixteenthreport.pdf (last accessed December 2013).

High Level Forum on Harmonization. 2003. *Rome Declaration on Harmonization, February 25, 2003*. Rome: World Health Organization.

House of Commons, Public Accounts Committee. 2011. *Fifty-Second Report: DFID Financial Management*. London: Department for International Development.

IDD (International Development Department) and Associates. 2006. *Evaluation of General Budget Support: Synthesis Report*. Birmingham: IDD and Associates.

ILO (International Labour Organization). 2010a. Recovery and growth with decent work. International Labour Conference, 99th session. Geneva: ILO.

ILO (International Labour Organization). 2010b. *Global Employment Trends*. Geneva: ILO.

Inter-American Development Bank. Inter-American Development Bank Haiti remittance survey. Presented in Washington DC, March 6, 2007. http://idbdocs.iadb.org/wsdocs/getdocument.aspx?docnum=916537 (last accessed December 2013).

Jaspars S, Harvey P. 2007. *A Review of UNICEF's Role in Cash Transfers to Emergency Affected Populations*. New York: UNICEF.

Joint UN (United Nations) Programme on HIV/AIDS. 2010. *Global Report: UNAIDS Report on the Global AIDS Epidemic 2010*. Geneva: UNAIDS.

Killick T. 2004. Politics, evidence and the New Aid Agenda. *Development Policy Review* 22(1), 5–29.

Kim JY, Millen JV, Irwin A, Gershman J. 2000. *Dying for Growth: Global Inequality and the Health of the Poor*. Monroe, ME: Common Courage Press.

Krishna A. 2010. *One Illness Away: Why People Become Poor and How They Escape Poverty*. Oxford: Oxford University Press.

Lagarde M, Haines A, Palmer N. 2009. The impact of conditional cash transfers on health outcomes and use of health services in low and middle income countries. *Cochrane Database Systematic Review* 4, CD008137.

Lawson A, Boadi G, Ghartey A *et al.* 2007. *Budget Support to Ghana: A Risk Worth Taking?* Briefing Paper No. 24. London and Legon-Accra: Overseas Development Institute and CDD-Ghana. www.odi.org.uk/resources/download/189.pdf (last accessed December 2013).

Manuel M, McKechnie A, King M, Copping E, Denney L. 2012. *Innovative Aid Instruments and Flexible Financing: Providing Better Support to Fragile States*. London: Overseas Development Institute.

Mills E, Kanters S, Hagopian A *et al.* 2011. The financial cost of doctors emigrating from sub-Saharan Africa: human capital analysis. *BMJ* 343(7031), doi: http://dx.doi.org/10.1136/bmj.d7031.

Ministry of Health. 2011. *Ministry of Health Annual Report 2010–2011*. Kigali: Republic of Rwanda Ministry of Health.

Nampanya-Serpell N. 2000. 2000. Social and economic risk factors for HIV/AIDS-affected families in Zambia. Presented to the AIDS and Economics Symposium, IAEN, Durban, July, 7–8, 2000.

National Audit Office (UK). 2008. *Department for International Development – Providing Budget Support to Developing Countries*. HC 6 Session 2007–2008. www.nao.org.uk/publications/0708/providing_budget_support_to_de.aspx (last accessed December 2013).

OECD (Organisation for Economic Co-operation and Development). 2006. *Promoting Private Investment for Development: The Role of ODA*. Paris: OECD. http://www.oecd.org/document/55/0,3746,en_2649_34621_46582839_1_1_1_1,00.html (last accessed December 2013).

OECD (Organisation for Economic Co-operation and Development). 2008a. *Review of Donors' Policies and Practices Related to Employment and Labour Markets*. OECD Papers, Vol. 7/12. Paris: OECD.

OECD (Organisation for Economic Co-operation and Development). 2008b. *The Paris Declaration on Aid Effectiveness and the Accra Agenda for Action*. Paris: OECD.

OECD (Organisation for Economic Co-operation and Development). 2010a. *What are the Benefits of Using Country Systems?* Paris: OECD.

OECD (Organisation for Economic Co-operation and Development). 2010b. *Making Aid More Effective through the Strengthening and Use of National Systems*. Paris: OECD.

OECD (Organisation for Economic Co-operation and Development). 2011a. *Implementing the 2001 DAC Recommendation on Untying Aid: 2010–2011 Review*. Paris: OECD.

OECD (Organisation for Economic Co-operation and Development). 2011b. *Survey on Monitoring the Paris Declaration: Survey Guidance*. Paris: OECD.

OECD (Organisation for Economic Co-operation and Development). 2011c. Evaluation Conjointe des Opérations d'Aide Budgétaire au Mali, 2003–2009. Paris: OECD. www.oecd.org/dataoecd/30/46/48670047.pdf (last accessed December 2013).

OECD (Organisation for Economic Co-operation and Development). 2011d. *The United States: Development Assistance Committee (DAC) Peer Review*. Paris: OECD.

OECD (Organisation for Economic Co-operation and Development). 2011e. *Aid Effectiveness 2005–2010: Progress in Implementing the Paris Declaration*. Paris: OECD.

OECD (Organisation for Economic Co-operation and Development). 2012. *Creditor Reporting System Database*. Paris: OECD. http://stats.oecd.org/index.aspx?DataSetCode=CRS1 (last accessed December 2013).

OECD (Organisation for Economic Co-operation and Development), UN (United Nations) Development Programme. 2010. *Supporting Haiti's Reconstruction and Development: A New Paradigm for Delivering Social Services*. Paris: Partnership for Democratic Governance.

OECD (Organisation for Economic Co-operation and Development) Working Party on Statistics. 2011. *Guidelines for Reporting in CRS++ Format*. Paris: OECD. www.oecd.org/investment/aidstatistics/39186046.pdf (last accessed December 2013).

ODI (Overseas Development Institute). 2004. "The Challenge of Absorptive Capacity: Will Lack of Absorptive Capacity Prevent Effective Use of Additional Aid Resources in Pursuit of the MDGs?" London: ODI.

ODI (Overseas Development Institute). 2005. *Joint Evaluation of General Budget Support: Tanzania 1995–2004*. London: ODI.

Piot P, Kazatchkine M, Dybul M, Lob-Levyt J. 2009. AIDS: Lessons learnt and myths dispelled. *Lancet* 374(9685), 260–3.

Pogge T. 2005. Human rights and global health: a research program. *Metaphilosophy* 36, 182–209.

Porter ME. 2009. A strategy for health care reform – toward a value-based system. *New England Journal of Medicine* 361, 109–112.

Porter ME. 2010. What is value in health care? *New England Journal of Medicine* 363, 2477–81.

Porter ME, Teisberg EO. 2006. *Redefining Health Care: Creating Value-Based Competition on Results*. Boston, MA: Harvard Business School Press.

Rivera JA, Sotres-Alvarez D, Habicht J-P, Shamah T, Villalpando S. 2004. Impact of the Mexican Program for Education, Health, and Nutrition (Progresa) on rates of growth and anemia in infants and young children: a randomized effectiveness study. *JAMA* 291, 2563–70.

Sachs J. 2005. *The End of Poverty: Economic Possibilities for Our Time*. New York: Penguin.

Samson M, Lee U, Ndlebe A et al. 2004. *The Social and Economic Impact of South Africa's Social Security System*. Cape Town: Economic Policy Research Institute.

Schoepf BG, Schoepf C, Millen JV. 2000. Theoretical therapies, remote remedies: SAPs and the political ecology of poverty and health in Africa. In Kim JV, Millen JV, Irwin A, Gershman J (eds) *Dying for Growth: Global Inequality and the Health of the Poor*, pp. 91–125. Monroe, ME: Common Courage Press.

Schuering E. 2008. Social Cash Transfers in Zambia: A Work in Progress. In Hailu D, Soares FV (eds) *Poverty in Focus: Cash Transfers, Lessons from Africa and Latin America*, pp. 20–1. Brasilia: International Poverty Centre.

Tarrafeta B. 2007. *The Coordinated Procurement and Distribution System in Rwanda: Empowering Local Systems Beyond Supplying ARVs.* Arlington, VA: Management Sciences for Health and USAID.

UN (United Nations). 2008. *Millennium Development Goals Report 2008.* New York: UN.

UN (United Nations) Development Programme. 2002. *UNDP HIV/AIDS Statistical Fact Sheet.* New York: UN Development Programme.

UN (United Nations) Development Programme. 2010. *Beyond the Midpoint: Achieving the Millennium Development Goals.* New York: UN Development Programme.

UN (United Nations) OSE (Office of the Special Envoy for Haiti). 2011. Has Aid Changed? Channeling Assistance to Haiti Before and After the Earthquake. New York: OSE.

UN (United Nations) OSE (Office of the Special Envoy for Haiti). 2012. *Can More Aid Stay in Haiti and Other Fragile Settings.* New York: OSE

UNESCO Institute for Statistics. 2007. *Projecting the Global Demand for Teachers: Meeting the Goal of Universal Primary Education by 2015.* Quebec: UNESCO Institute for Statistics.

UNICEF. 2010. *Protecting Salaries of Frontline Teachers and Health Workers.* Social and Economic Policy Briefs. New York: UNICEF.

USAID (United States Agency for International Development). 2011. *Action Memo for the Administrator: August 30, 2011.* Washington, DC: USAID.

USAID (United States Agency for International Development). 2013. *USAID Forward: Progress Report.* Washington, DC: USAID.

Voipio T. 2011. *Social Protection for All – An Agenda for Pro-Child Growth and Child Rights.* Child Poverty Insights. New York: UNICEF.

Waldman M. 2008. *Falling Short: Aid Effectiveness in Afghanistan.* ACBAR Advocacy Series. Kabul: Oxfam International.

Walton DA., Farmer PE, Lambert W, Léandre F, Koenig SP, Mukherjee SJ. 2004. Integrated HIV prevention and care strengthens primary health care: lessons from rural Haiti. *Journal of Public Health Policy* 25(2), 137–58.

WHO (World Health Organization). 2004. "*Knowledge For Better Health: Strengthening Health Systems.*" Geneva: WHO.

WHO (World Health Organization). 2006. "*Working Together For Health.*" Geneva: WHO.

Williamson T, Dom C. 2010. *Making Sector Budget Support Work for Service Delivery: Good Practice Recommendations.* Project Briefing No. 37. London: ODI. www.odi.org.uk (last accessed December 2013).

Wood B, Betts J, Etta F *et al.* 2011. *Evaluation of the Paris Declaration, Phase II Final Report.* Copenhagen: Danish Institute for International Studies.

World Bank. 2008. *Haiti: Public Expenditure Management and Financial Accountability Review.* Washington, DC: World Bank. www-wds.worldbank.org/external/default/main?menuPK=64187510&pagePK=64193027&piPK=64187937&theSitePK=523679&menuPK=64187510&searchMenuPK=64187283&siteName=WDS&entityID=000333037_20080710023439 (last accessed December 2013).

World Bank. 2011. *World Development Report 2011: Conflict, Security, and Development.* Washington, DC: World Bank.

World Food Programme. 2008. "Consolidated Framework of WFP Policies: An Updated Version (October 2008)." Executive Board, Second Regular Session. Rome: World Food Programme.

World Food Programme. 2011. "Facts Blast: May 2011." Rome: World Food Programme.

World Food Programme. 2012. "World Food Programme: HIV, AIDS, TB, and Nutrition Fact Sheet." Rome: World Food Programme.

Chapter 27

Global Health Partnerships: The Emerging Agenda

Jeremy Youde

Abstract

The globalization of health has led to a tremendous expansion in the number and types of actors and groups taking an active role in addressing global health concerns. The proliferation of government, international organization, private foundation, and non-governmental organization partnerships dedicated to global health issues has significantly increased the amount of resources available and raised the prominence of these issues on the international political agenda. These partnerships show much promise, but their proliferation can also lead to redundancy and create confusion of who is addressing which issues. Without assiduous monitoring and evaluation, it can be difficult to tell which partnerships are successful or whether a partnership is successfully leveraging the strengths and resources of its member organizations. More importantly, the continued global economic downturn poses serious challenges for the ability of these partnerships to maintain operations. This chapter defines global health partnerships, discusses their various forms, analyzes characteristics that promote successful collaborations, and offers suggestions for the future. To provide insight into these issues, the chapter uses the Global Fund to Fight AIDS, Tuberculosis and Malaria as a case study for analyzing the successes, shortcomings, and future challenges faced by global health partnerships in the contemporary international environment.

The Handbook of Global Health Policy, First Edition. Edited by Garrett W. Brown, Gavin Yamey, and Sarah Wamala.
© 2014 John Wiley & Sons, Ltd. Published 2014 by John Wiley & Sons, Ltd.

Key Points

- The globalization of health has led to a proliferation of partnerships among governments, non-governmental organizations, intergovernmental organizations, and the private sector.
- Partnerships can add flexibility and innovation to global responses to health issues.
- Effective global health partnerships need to both address the issue at hand and transform the partners themselves in some way.
- The increase in health partnerships has not necessarily been accompanied by rigorous monitoring and evaluation for effectiveness.
- Economic austerity measures have made global health partnerships attractive as potential cost-saving measures, but effective partnerships still require significant resources.

Key Policy Implications

- Global health partnerships need to improve their coordination with governments.
- The continued global economic downturn significantly challenges the ability of these partnerships to carry out their operations.
- Successful partnerships can give meaningful voice to their members when properly constituted.

Introduction

The globalization of health has led to a tremendous expansion in the number and types of actors taking an active role in addressing health concerns. National governments increasingly partner with international organizations, private foundations, and non-governmental organizations (NGOs) to fund and implement strategies designed to reduce disease burdens. New types of organizations that specifically marry public and private actors have emerged and come to have significant roles. These partnerships have significantly increased the resources available for addressing some key health concerns and increased the visibility of health on political agendas domestically and internationally. They have also introduced confusion and redundancy into disease control programs and raised questions about their long-term viability.

This chapter has four primary aims. First, it seeks to define global health partnerships and why they have achieved prominence in recent years. Second, it describes the various forms that global health partnerships have taken in contemporary global health politics. Third, it details some of the beneficial aspects of global health partnerships and describes how they might be increased more broadly. Finally, it describes some of the potential difficulties global health partnerships present for effective disease management and health promotion strategies. To achieve these aims, this chapter focuses much of its attention on the Global Fund to Fight AIDS, Tuberculosis and Malaria. The Global Fund's experience illustrates both the potential benefits of governments and NGOs working together to address cross-border health concerns, as well as the difficulties they face in achieving and maintaining positive outcomes.

Global Health Partnerships

At their most general level, global health partnerships entail multiple organizations combining human and/or financial resources to work together on a health issue of cross-border concern. This description is technically correct, but greater specificity will provide a more useful definition. Buse and Harmer provide a more detailed definition with a narrower scope, drawing on the global governance idea of public–private partnerships. Their definition of a global health partnership focuses on three primary elements. First, global health partnerships are established specifically to address one or more global health problem. The focus on health is not a spillover from other programs, nor is it incidental to the collaboration. Rather, addressing a global health problem is the partnership's very reason for being. Second, global health partnerships are relatively institutionalized. The exact level of institutionalization will vary from partnership to partnership, but there must exist some sort of formalized agreement to work together and share resources. Third, global health partnerships generally combine public and private organizations and provide both with a voice in decision-making policies and procedures. The collaborative decision-making procedures will, ideally, ensure a greater level of ownership among the various parties. It is this last element, with its emphasis on consensual and collaborative decision-making, that Buse and Harmer identify as being particularly innovative and novel for global health governance (Buse and Harmer 2007).

Thanks to the growing role of global health partnerships, international resources available for health concerns have increased significantly. Between 2002 and 2006, official development assistance for health increased 25% annually, and global health partnerships receive a large portion of these funds (Dodd and Lane 2010). Part of the reason that global health partnerships have had this vital role, Dodd and Lane argue, is that they can provide more sustained and predictable funding for projects over longer periods of time. They also help overcome policy failures by both governments and markets that have prevented a public good, such as health, getting to the poorest and most vulnerable people (Ngoasong 2009).

The connections among organizations in global health partnerships operate at two different levels. *Vertical* linkages are perhaps the most common. In these, international organizations and large private foundations partner with NGOs, the private sector, and national or subnational governments (Magnusson 2010). An example of a vertical global health partnership is the Global Alliance for Vaccines and Immunization (GAVI). GAVI combines the World Health Organization, UNICEF, the Bill & Melinda Gates Foundation, the Norwegian government, the Nicaraguan government, GlaxoSmithKline, and BRAC (formerly the Bangladesh Rehabilitation Assistance Commission), among others, to increase access to vaccinations in developing countries and spur research on new and more effective vaccines. It specifically draws representatives from international, national, and subnational levels to advance its larger goals. *Horizontal* linkages bring together similar types of groups or governments to coordinate activities, pool resources, establish international standards and norms, and report on progress to each other. In these ways, horizontal linkages seek to avoid duplicating services and encourage accountability (Magnusson 2010). An example of a horizontal global health partnership is the Meeting of the Ministers of Health of Pacific Island Countries. First held in Fiji in 1995, the Meeting convenes every two years to develop a shared vision of health in the region based on its unique geographic, economic, political, and health features. This forum allows for the development of shared ideals for regional health and establishes accountability mechanisms for ensuring that governments are living up to their promises.

While populated by different types of organizations, vertical and horizontal linkages have an important symbiotic relationship. Magnusson (2010) argues that horizontal linkages can bring some measure of rationality and order to the proliferating mass of vertical global health partnerships. By bringing together actors at a similar level, horizontal linkages try to avoid the duplication of resources and prevent overwhelming any single country or part of the global health agenda. In other words, horizontal linkages can provide the information and oversight that will allow vertical linkages to operate more efficiently. This function is particularly important, as Ciconne (2010) argues that the efficacy of global health partnerships has been undermined by their lack of public accountability and oversight.

What Makes Global Health Partnerships Work?

Simply bringing organizations together is not enough to create a useful global health partnership. Crafting a successful partnership requires taming a large-scale collective action problem, bringing together a wide variety of actors with their own agendas and interests to achieve a common end. Drawing on a decade's worth of research and interviews with key stakeholders in a wide variety of public–private global health partnerships, Buse and Tanaka (2011) identify seven key elements that contribute to successful arrangements.

First, a partnership must identify a concrete goal that its combination of partner organizations is uniquely qualified to address and exploit that comparative advantage. This requires taking careful stock of the strengths and weaknesses of the member organizations and considering the particular talents or skills this partnership can contribute. Second, partnerships must establish, staff, and adequately fund their secretariats. There exists a tendency to under-resource the organizational secretariat in the name of promoting efficiency and economy, but doing so undermines the partnership's ability to carry out its mission. Third, partnerships must continually engage in internal assessment of their activities and ensure that it remains accountable to all of its members. Fourth, successful partnerships give voice to their stakeholders and allow them to participate in a meaningful manner. They need to formalize these systems to ensure genuine participation, but retain some degree of flexibility to respond to changing situations and needs. Fifth, partnerships must acknowledge and accept that member organizations retain their own interests and perspectives. Groups may come together to work on one particular issue, but that does not mean that the various organizations adopt a shared worldview on all issues. Sixth, partnerships need to avoid having a disruptive presence in countries where they operate by aligning their missions and activities with national health priorities. Failing to do so can lead to duplication of services or introduce processes that inadvertently undermine a country's health services by distracting attention or resources. Finally, effective global health partnerships must continually strive for improvement and introduce procedures that promote continual innovation. Success should breed greater success, not complacency (Buse and Tanaka 2011). At their core, successful global health partnerships succeed on multiple levels. Buse and Tanaka remark, "Effective [global health partnerships] deliver not only health outcomes but are also, in some way, transformative of partners, imbuing the public sector with business skills and encouraging business to operate with social values" (Buse and Tanaka 2011: 9).

To get a better sense of the challenges and opportunities facing global health partnerships, this chapter focuses on one of the most prominent global health partnerships operating today – the Global Fund to Fight AIDS, Tuberculosis and Malaria (GFATM or the Global Fund). The Global Fund embodies many of the basic tenets of global health partnerships and faces many of the same challenges that commonly afflict such collaborations.

The Global Fund to Fight AIDS, Tuberculosis and Malaria

When the Global Fund came into being, it marked something new and novel in the global health governance architecture. It was a wholly new international organization, deliberately created to stand apart from the United Nations or any other international bureaucracy. It had a relatively small staff. Its budget depended wholly on voluntary contributions from both state governments and private sources. Uniquely, the Global Fund explicitly does not conduct programming on its own and instead operates solely as a funding agency. The Global Fund also set itself apart by explicitly recognizing the unique role of civil society organizations and mandating their inclusion in the applications made by national governments. Such innovations offer new opportunities for creating responsive global health structures, but the Global Fund's inability to live up to its promises and aspirations call its ambition into question.

The movement toward creating the Global Fund started at the G8 meeting in 2000 in Okinawa. For the first time, the G8's agenda included health issues. The assembled states acknowledged that poor health threatened international prosperity and development. In their post-conference communiqué, the leaders expressed a commitment to reducing HIV/AIDS, tuberculosis, and malaria rates and involving civil society organizations, industry, and academia in reaching their goals. Furthermore, the G8 countries pledged to hold another conference to agree "on a new strategy to harness our commitments" (Ministry of Foreign Affairs of Japan 2000).

In calling for a new funding mechanism for global health, the G8 countries implicitly acknowledged that existing institutional arrangements fell short in tackling the challenges posed by HIV/AIDS, tuberculosis, and malaria. Though a relatively new disease, HIV/AIDS threatened to overwhelm states with high infection rates and imposed severe strains on national health budgets. Tuberculosis, long thought to be under control, made a dramatic resurgence as it co-infected HIV-positive persons and drug-resistant strains emerged. Malaria rates surged as drug-resistant strains expanded geographically. These new crises overwhelmed the World Health Organization – an institution whose regular budget had remained stagnant since the early 1980s and was generally accorded little respect because health was considered "low politics" (Fidler 2005: 180). With the 2000 G8 summit in Okinawa, the leaders of the world's largest economies acknowledged that health was more significant to international politics than previously assumed. They also acknowledged that additional actors and resources were vital for effectively addressing these crises. Instead of relying on outsiders telling countries how to implement programs, the attendees recognized that states needed to rely on local expertise and take ownership of their health interventions if they were to succeed (Brown 2010). Crafting better interventions would require states to create and implement their own programs, but they would need resources to carry them out. That is where the G8 saw the potential for a new international health organization.

Building on the momentum of the summit in Okinawa, the Organization of African Unity held a special session in Abuja, Nigeria, in April 2001 where member governments pledged to increase their own health spending and requested donor states to "complement our resource mobilization efforts to fight the scourge of HIV/AIDS, tuberculosis, and other related infectious diseases" (Organization of African Unity 2001: 5) by creating a global fund of $5–10 billion for creating and implementing programs targeted toward these diseases.

With this momentum, the creation of the new organization came at a rapid pace. At the United Nations General Assembly's Special Session on HIV/AIDS in June 2001, Member States pledged to create and support a new international funding mechanism for addressing HIV/AIDS. They affirmed their desire to create a fund with $7–10 billion available annually to low- and middle-income states and those with high HIV infection rates, and called on donor states to pledge 0.7% of their gross national product for overseas development assistance and offer debt relief to the most heavily indebted states (United Nations General Assembly 2001: 38–40). This declaration encouraged the international community to create the Global Fund and allowed the United Nations to give its official support for the Fund's creation.

Informal organizational meetings for the new Global Fund began in July 2001 in Geneva. Nearly 40 delegates attended these early planning meetings from a wide range of concerned actors – donor states, recipient states, civil society organizations, the United Nations, and private industry. Drawing on this wide range of interested parties, the Global Fund presented itself as a public–private partnership that could combine the group's collective strengths into a force for good. These meetings set the general framework for the new organization, established its parameters, and put forward the Global Fund's mandate. In January 2002, the Global Fund's Executive Board met for the first time, and the Fund issued its first grants to 36 countries 3 months later (Bartsch 2007). Since that time, the Global Fund has provided more than $19.4 billion for 780 grants in 144 countries. Those funds have allowed 2.82 million people to access antiretroviral treatment to fight HIV, treated 7.11 million people for tuberculosis, and distributed 124 million insecticide-treated nets to stop the spread of malaria (Global Fund 2010b).

Unlike most international organizations, the Global Fund extends beyond states to include non-state actors as active participants with a voice in the policy-making process. It provides explicit roles for donor countries, recipient states, and civil society organizations in an effort to achieve a high degree of deliberative governance and allow as many voices as possible to be heard. It functions as a hybrid, operating between public and private sources of authority and legitimacy. Bartsch describes it as "a new way of doing business in the field of development cooperation and health that goes beyond the state-centered intergovernmental approach of other actors in global health governance" (Bartsch 2007: 147). With its unique structure, the Global Fund has the potential to transcend traditional boundaries, but frequently finds itself unable to fully live up to its stated goals.

The Global Fund's operations are divided into seven key groupings: the Executive Board; the Secretariat; the Technical Review Panel; the Partnership Forum; the Country Coordinating Mechanisms; the Principal Recipients; and the Local Fund Agents. Some work at the organization's headquarters in Geneva, while others work in the member countries (Bartsch 2007: 151). Overseeing the whole organization is the Executive Board, which ultimately makes all the strategy, policy, operational guidelines, and funding decisions. Reflecting the diverse constituencies involved with the Global Fund, the Executive Board's membership includes donor countries, recipient states, and representatives from civil society organizations around the world. The Secretariat handles the Global Fund's daily operations, ensuring compliance with Fund directives, raising additional funds, and reporting the Fund's activities to the Executive Board and the public. The Technical Review Panel (TRP) assesses the feasibility and technical merit of projects and provides recommendations to the Executive Board, which ultimately decides which proposals to fund. Within its membership, the TRP seeks to balance gender, region, and specializations. The panel includes up to 40 members in any given round of proposal evaluations. The Partnership Forum provides an opportunity every two years for all Global Fund stakeholders to come together to discuss strategies and policies. The Partnership Forum's recommendations help to inform the Executive Board in its oversight responsibilities. At the country level, the Country Coordinating Mechanism (CCM) has a vital role in crafting and putting forward proposals. CCMs bring together local stakeholders to develop proposals for funding from the Global Fund, drawing on governmental and non-governmental expertise. CCMs also serve as the vital link between the Global Fund and the recipient country, operating as an informational conduit. Once a country receives a grant, the CCM also oversees the grant's implementation. The Principal Recipient receives the actual grant from the Global Fund and implements programs. Initially, the Principal Recipients tended to be government agencies (particularly Ministries of Health), but NGOs, academic institutions, and faith-based organizations increasingly act as Principal Recipients. Countries may designate multiple organizations to serve jointly as Principal Recipients. Finally, the Local Fund Agent acts as an independent auditor and oversees, verifies, and reports on grant performance to the Global Fund.

Among these seven groups, though, the Executive Board receives the bulk of attention. The Executive Board's composition makes it the key site for bringing together a wide variety of stakeholders and concerns about the relative weight of their influence. The board consists of 25 members (not including the executive director) coming from three different blocs: donors, recipients, and international organizations and the Swiss government (a non-voting bloc). Within these blocs, there exist careful formulas to maintain balance and provide for a higher degree of representation of different constituencies.

Among the donors bloc, eight of the representatives come from donor states (generally selected from the most generous donors). The other two bloc members represent private interests in donor states: one from private industry and one from private foundations. Within the recipient bloc, seven members come from developing countries, one comes from a northern-based civil society organization, one comes from a southern-based civil society organization, and one comes from a civil society organization representing the interests of those affected by HIV/AIDS, tuberculosis, and/or malaria. The non-voting bloc represents the World Health Organization, UNAIDS, World Bank, global partner organizations that work with Global Fund recipients, and the Swiss government.

Despite attempts at balance and providing opportunities for genuine deliberative decision-making, the Executive Board has come under fire for not living up to its promises. The civil society organizations on the Executive Board generally focus on HIV/AIDS, leaving organizations with more direct experience with tuberculosis and malaria without direct representation. Representatives from some developing states have also expressed dismay that they are losing influence relative to donor states. When the board decided to add a seat for an affected community civil society organization, it also added another seat for the donor states to keep the two blocs balanced in size. This raised alarm that the donor states would have an oversized influence on the board and dilute the ability of the recipient states to make their voices heard. Some recipient states also saw this move as an attempt to weaken the influence of national governments in developing countries vis-à-vis civil society organizations, many of which relied on funds from donor states for their operations. They instead envisioned an organizational structure more akin to the World Health Assembly, where each Member State gets a vote and an opportunity to participate in debates regardless of funding (Bartsch 2007).

At a more fundamental level, questions have emerged about whether it is even possible for recipient state interests to get a fair hearing within the structures of the Executive Board. The Global Fund's mandate explicitly recognizes the importance and value of providing a wide range of constituencies with the opportunity to have a genuine influence on policy. The board's structures and mechanisms greatly emphasize the need for deliberative participatory decision-making (Brown 2010). Despite such pledges, interviews with Executive Board members suggest that these deliberative efforts are undermined by the ability of donor states to effectively set the agenda and the terms of debate. Because they have the power of the purse, the donor states can remove or promote certain alternatives, be more or less generous with their pledges, and steer policies in certain directions that will benefit their interests (Brown 2010). One study of the Executive Board's deliberative practices found that some recipient states felt that the interests of the donors, rather than the recipients, were paramount within the organization and that the health experts consulted by the donor states often lacked local legitimacy or accountability (Brown 2009). In other words, some recipients felt that the Global Fund talked a good game about being a deliberative and inclusive partnership, but that the donor states still ran the show.

The Global Fund's Successes and Failures

The Global Fund's creation presented the international community with a new type of international organization – one that focused solely on funding rather than program implementation, sought to empower recipient states, and to incorporate state and non-state actors into all levels of the decision-making process. Buse and Tanaka give the Global Fund high marks for clearly identifying its mission and unique strengths and introducing good governance measures, but they chastise the organization for its relative lack of sustainability, poor country capacity-building measures, and weak organizational effectiveness measures (Buse and Tanaka 2011). Their findings suggest that the Global Fund, while successful in some areas, must address some significant lapses in order to become more useful to the international community and continue its very existence.

First, by creating a primary multilateral source for channeling resources to states in need, the Global Fund has added greater efficiency to the foreign aid process. Bilateral funding, which still makes up the majority of development assistance for health, tends to favor recipients with longstanding or strategic ties to the donor rather than the recipient state's relative need. Bilateral aid flows also do little to promote widespread information sharing and can add administrative costs for recipient countries, meaning that a lower proportion of the aid actually goes to help people (Doyle 2006). Furthermore, existing bilateral and multilateral funding sources proved themselves unable to mobilize enough resources to effectively combat HIV, tuberculosis, and malaria (Bartsch 2007). Since its creation in 2002, the Global Fund has become an increasingly important source of development assistance for health. In its first year of operation, donations to the Global Fund made up less than 1% of all global funds for development assistance for health. By 2007, the Global Fund received 8.3% of the global total of development assistance for health (Ravishankar *et al.* 2009). By 2009, nearly one quarter of all international assistance for HIV/AIDS went through the Global Fund (Kates *et al.* 2010). With these funds, the Global Fund is responsible for providing approximately 25% of all HIV/AIDS funding internationally, 67% of the international funding for tuberculosis, and 75% of international funding for malaria (Global Fund 2010a). It distributes approximately 60% of its annual grants to HIV/AIDS programs, 24% for malaria, 14% for tuberculosis, and 2% for health systems development. Roughly half of the grant money goes toward paying for pharmaceuticals and treatment supplies (Lisk 2010).

The funds available through the Global Fund have added to the overall international resource pool for these three diseases. The Fund's allocation decisions are guided by the "additionality principle" – grants provided by the Global Fund should not subtract from other donors or funding commitments. Instead, Global Fund grants increase the amount of money going to a particular country for work on reducing the effects of these three diseases. They do not replace other funding courses; rather, they fill gaps (Lisk 2010).

Second, the Global Fund's structure and grant application process require a high degree of country ownership that should increase the likelihood of an intervention's success. The Global Fund does not actively seek out grant recipients; it instead employs a "country-defined" or "demand-driven" model. Because the Global Fund cannot implement its own programs, it places the burden on applicants to identify their problems, suggest a solution, and demonstrate the feasibility of their proposal (Kaiser Family Foundation 2009). With such a format, the Global Fund has sought to encourage higher levels of country ownership, bottom-up participation, and opportunities for southern countries to take an active role in global health governance processes. It also empowers the recipient countries to make decisions about potentially sensitive issues, such as the role of generic pharmaceuticals in national treatment strategies and creating prevention strategies that will resonate with local populations (Bartsch 2007). CCMs coordinate a state's application and offer opportunities for a wide variety of actors to take an active role in identifying proper prevention, treatment, and care strategies.

The major problems with the Global Fund tend to focus on the disjuncture between the organization's stated goals and its actual operation. It is one thing to proclaim a new approach to addressing global health needs; it is entirely another thing to put that proclamation into practice. The difficulties faced by the Global Fund implicitly raise questions about the ability to craft and effectively implement a new approach to international organizations given the existing state of the global health governance architecture.

Realizing the new structures and strategies envisioned by its founders continues to bedevil the Global Fund, and the promises of broad participation from a wide variety of stakeholders have largely failed to materialize. Deliberations within the Executive Board are largely seen as favoring the donor states and giving recipient states and civil society organizations a marginalized voice. The promises of accountability and broad participation run into problems when faced with the realities of the distribution of political and economic power in the international arena (Brown 2009, 2010). The problems with a lack of voice go beyond the Executive Board. CCMs, designed to coordinate a country's Global Fund application and draw on a wide range of local expertise, frequently fail to involve non-governmental sources. Government ministries tend to dominate CCMs, and NGOs have little or no input in many cases. Where NGOs have formal representation within CCMs, they often face significant obstacles to meaningful participation, such as a lack of funds to travel to meetings or information deficits that limit their ability to contribution to policy-making (Bartsch 2007).

Complaints about the lack of representation for NGOs have not gone unheeded. Current CCM guidelines from the Global Fund recommend that NGOs make up at least 40% of the membership of a given CCM (Global Fund 2008). Prior to the release of these guidelines, there had been a push to mandate 40% as the minimum level of NGO representation on CCMs. CCMs failing to meet this requirement, according to the proposal, would be ineligible to receive Global Fund grants. Ultimately, the Executive Board decided against requiring a minimum level of representation on the grounds that such a requirement would violate the spirit of country ownership (Bartsch 2007). It is an odd position. The Executive Board wants to encourage widespread participation in CCMs so as to encourage a greater sense of country ownership in their projects, but rejects an attempt to require it because that would violate country ownership. In the place of a formal policy, the Executive Board strongly encourages countries to have their CCMs meet the 40% goal, and a Global Fund study suggests that countries are increasing the participation rates for NGOs on CCMs (Global Fund 2008).

More recently, some donors have raised significant questions about the level of oversight that exist for Global Fund grants. In early 2011, Germany announced that it would suspend its €200 million annual contribution to the Global Fund in light of reports of a high degree of corruption. Germany was the Global Fund's third largest donor, and its decision to withhold payments until it was satisfied that the Global Fund employed sufficient measures to prevent money from going missing, could strike a significant blow to the Global Fund's financial viability (BBC 2011). Two months earlier, the Swedish government, which had contributed $85 million per year for the previous three years, announced that it would not be making pledges to the Global Fund over its concerns about corrupt activities in four African grant recipient states. Sweden's AIDS ambassador, when making the announcement, stated that Global Fund officials failed to adequately investigate the allegations and punish the misdeeds (Usher 2010). Responding to the German and Swedish governments' charges, a spokesperson for the Global Fund states that its investigations found that $34 million – or 0.3% of all of its allocations to that point – had been misallocated. While decrying those instances, the Global Fund representatives argued that the low amount proved that corruption was not endemic among its grant recipients and that it was the Global Fund's own accounting requirements that brought the corruption to international attention (BBC 2011). While some have taken the evidence of misallocated AIDS funds as proof that the Global Fund's systems are inadequate, others have praised the Global Fund for its vigilance. Roger Bate, a fellow at the American Enterprise Institute, praised the Global Fund's transparency. He wrote, "If the Global Fund operated like every other multilateral aid agency, we wouldn't have the information about fraud and other bad behavior that is leading to these funding suspensions. The Fund is admirably open about its failings" (Bate 2011). In November 2011, both countries signaled that they would honor their 2011 financial pledges and would continue to provide funding to the organization during 2012 (IRIN 2011).

Finally, and perhaps most importantly, the global economic downturn has undermined the Global Fund's ability to fund programs. In November 2011, the Global Fund announced that it would stop making new grants until at least 2014 due to a shortfall in fundraising activities. The previous pledge round, completed in October 2010, raised $11.7 billion – $1.3 billion short of the Fund's worst-case-scenario "austerity budget" and far less than the $20 billion the organization hoped to raise. Compounding the problem, a number of countries have failed to fulfill their current pledges, some states have stopped making pledges to the Fund, and pressure within the US Congress has raised doubts about the United States' ability to satisfy its obligations (McNeil 2011). The Fund is establishing a Transitional Funding Mechanism to provide emergency funding to countries to maintain essential services and avoid disruptions in antiretroviral drug access, but it will not permit any expansion of activities (IRIN 2011). The Global Fund is to distribute $10 billion between 2011 and 2013, funding 400 programs in more than 100 countries, but it cannot pay for these programs to add patients or expand services (Brown 2011). As a result, numerous nongovernmental organizations, like South Africa's Treatment Action Campaign, may not have the financing necessary to continue operations (York 2011).

These shortfalls result from the economic pressures being placed on governments. With most developed countries facing austerity budgets, enthusiasm for overseas development assistance has fallen. As a result, the Global Fund faces "the most dire financial situation it has ever seen since its creation," according to a statement from Médecins Sans Frontières (York 2011). The continued viability of global health partnerships like the Global Fund to contribute positively to global health depends crucially on their ability to distribute resources. The global economic downturn has not undermined the underlying logic and intellectual support for global health partnerships, but it has severely compromised the international community's ability to realize their potential. Williams and Rushton (2011) suggest that global health partnerships may weather the economic storm better than governments, but private organizations lack the resources to plug the shortfalls being realized by the Global Fund.

Conclusions

Global health partnerships introduce significant opportunities for public and private entities to collaborate in a mutually beneficial manner to promote good health internationally. When successful, they can leverage the competitive advantages of the partner organizations to produce health outcomes that exceed what each partner could do on its own. Despite such promise, global health partnerships prove incredibly difficult to structure and organize in a manner that will positively contribute to providing necessary services, ensuring some level of sustainability, and incorporating national buy-in from state governments. The successes and failures thus far of the Global Fund demonstrate both how these collaborative arrangements can have a positive effect and how difficult they can be to maintain – even with the best of intentions.

What are the lessons organizers of global health partnerships can draw in order to increase the likelihood of success in the future? The Global Fund's experience emphasizes three important lessons that global health partnerships can draw from in the future. First, global health partnerships must genuinely appreciate and operationalize the notion of "partnership" itself. This has been a particular problem for the Global Fund. It may sound tautological to argue that partnerships require partnership among member organizations, but too many global health partnerships only pay lip service to the roles of stakeholder involvement and genuine dialogue. It is too often the case that certain members of a partnership, particularly NGOs, cannot adequately participate in crafting and implementing the collaboration's mission. Often, these problems arise out of structural imbalances in the partnership's organizational arrangements or informal procedures that remove much of the decision-making from collaborative forums (Buse and Harmer 2007). When this happens, it both undermines the efficacy of the partnership and discourages organizations from entering into other partnerships in which they could have a useful role. Organizations entering into global health partnerships need to ensure that they are willing and actively interested in working with others – even when that means that an organization may not always get its way when designing and implementing programs.

Second, global health partnerships must not forget to work with the governments in whose countries they will be implementing their programs. The Global Fund encourages recipient governments to assume a great deal of ownership, but actual practice sometimes belies these promises. National governments may not formally be part of many partnerships, but ignoring their needs, wishes, and capabilities can seriously imperil the success of a partnership's programs. The multiplicity of global health partnerships can be difficult for national governments to navigate, and onerous reporting requirements can distract from a country's ability to implement health programs (Ciconne 2010). A lack of buy-in and commitment from the recipient country is a problem, as are programs that fail to align with the recipient state's own priorities. This is not to say that national governments should always hold veto power over global health partnership, but such partnerships must recognize that states are not empty vessels into which they can pour their programs. States – even poorly managed ones – retain their autonomy and sovereignty. Working with recipient states in a collaborative manner can thus increase the likelihood that a partnership's programs will achieve a positive outcome.

Finally, global health partnerships, like any other international undertaking, require adequate resources in order to carry out their missions. Increased efficiencies and eliminating corruption can certainly help ensure that more funds go toward programs that help people, but none of these programs can advance if governments starve the partnerships of resources. This is especially important when dealing with an issue like HIV/AIDS, where the interruption of medical services can make a person's health status significantly worse and more difficult to treat. Creating partnerships and then failing to endow them with the resources necessary to carry out their missions both endangers the health of millions around the world and undermines the place of global health on the international agenda.

The future of global health funding looks fairly bleak and the failure of the international community to achieve the health-related Millennium Development Goals may augur the increased importance of global health partnerships (see Chapter 28). By leveraging their combined resources and incorporating both state and non-state actors to work toward common goals, these partnerships may help the international community make meaningful progress toward addressing pressing global health needs. To do this, though, global health partnerships must take proactive efforts to demonstrate their effectiveness, efficiency, and transparency.

Key Reading

Brown GW. 2010. Safeguarding deliberative global governance: the case of the Global Fund to Fight AIDS, Tuberculosis and Malaria. *Review of International Studies* 36(2), 511–30.

Buse K, Harmer AM. 2007. Seven habits of highly effective global public–private health partnerships: practice and potential. *Social Science and Medicine* 64, 259–71.

Buse K, Tanaka S. 2011. Global public–private partnerships: lessons learned from ten years of experience and evaluation. *International Dental Journal* 61(Suppl. 2), 2–10.

Lisk F. 2010. *Global Institutions and the HIV/AIDS Epidemic: Responding to an International Crisis.* London: Routledge.

Reinicke WH, Deng F. 2000. *Critical Choices: The United Nations Networks and the Future of Global Governance.* Ottawa: International Development Research Center.

References

Bartsch S. 2007. The Global Fund to Fight AIDS, Tuberculosis, and Malaria. In Hein W, Bartsch S, Kohlmorgen L (eds) *Global Health Governance and the Fight against HIV/AIDS*, pp. 146–71. New York: Palgrave Macmillan.

Bate R. 2011. Sweden, Germany suspend grants to Global Fund. *The Enterprise Blog* January 27. http://blog.american.com/?p=25795 (last accessed December 2013).

BBC. 2011. Germany halts AIDS fund payment over corruption claims. *BBC News* January 27. http://www.bbc.co.uk/news/world-europe-12294232 (last accessed December 2013).

Brown D. 2011. Fund halts new grants for AIDS, TB and malaria treatment in poor countries. *Washington Post* November 23. http://www.washingtonpost.com/national/health-science/fund-halts-new-grants-for-aidstb-and-malaria-treatment-in-poor-countries/2011/11/23/gIQAPZdspN_story. html (last accessed December 2013).

Brown GW. 2009. Multisectoralism, participation, and stakeholder effectiveness: increasing the role of nonstate actors in the Global Fund to Fight AIDS, Tuberculosis and Malaria. *Global Governance* 15(2), 169–77.

Brown GW. 2010. Safeguarding deliberative global governance: the case of the Global Fund to Fight AIDS, Tuberculosis and Malaria. *Review of International Studies* 36(2), 511–30.

Buse K, Harmer AM. 2007. Seven habits of highly effective global public-private health partnerships: practice and potential. *Social Science and Medicine* 64, 259–71.

Buse K, Tanaka S. 2011. Global public–private partnerships: lessons learned from ten years of experience and evaluation. *International Dental Journal* 61(Suppl. 2), 2–10.

Ciconne DC. 2010. Arguing for a centralized coordinating solution to the public–private partnership explosion in global health. *Global Health Promotion* 17(2), 48–51.

Dodd R, Lane C. 2010. Improving the long-term sustainability of health aid: are global health partnerships the way to go? *Health Policy and Planning* 25(5), 363–71.

Doyle JS. 2006. An international public health crisis: can global institutions respond effectively to HIV/AIDS? *Australian Journal of International Affairs* 60(3), 400–11.

Fidler DP. 2005. Health as foreign policy: between principle and power. *Whitehead Journal of Diplomacy and International Relations* 6(2), 179–94.

Global Fund (Global Fund to Fight AIDS, Tuberculosis and Malaria). 2008. *Country Coordinating Mechanism model: governance and civil society participation.* http://www.theglobalfund.org/documents/ccm/CCMOnePageBrief_GovernanceAndCSPartn_2008_10_en.pdf (last accessed December 2013).

Global Fund (Global Fund to Fight AIDS, Tuberculosis and Malaria). 2010a. *About the Global Fund.* http://www.theglobalfund.org/en/about/?lang=en (last accessed December 2013).

Global Fund (Global Fund to Fight AIDS, Tuberculosis and Malaria). 2010b. *Grant Portfolio.* http://portfolio.theglobalfund.org/?lang=en (last accessed December 2013).

IRIN. 2010. *HIV/AIDS: Global Fund cancels funding.* http://www.irinnews.org/report/94293/hiv-aids-global-fund-cancels-funding (last accessed December 2013).

Kaiser Family Foundation. 2009. *The US and the Global Fund to Fight AIDS, Tuberculosis and Malaria.* http://www.kff.org/globalhealth/upload/8003.pdf (last accessed December 2013).

Kates J, Boortz K, Lief E, Avila C, Gobet B. 2010. *Financing the Response to HIV/AIDS in Low- and Middle-Income Countries: International Assistance from the G8, European Commission, and Other Donor Governments in 2009.* Henry J. Kaiser Family Foundation and UNAIDS. http://www.kff.org/hivaids/upload/7347-06.pdf (last accessed December 2013).

Lisk F. 2010. *Global Institutions and the HIV/AIDS Epidemic: Responding to an International Crisis.* London: Routledge.

Magnusson RS. 2010. Global health governance and the challenge of chronic, non-communicable disease. *Journal of Law, Medicine, and Ethics* 38(3), 490–507.

McNeil DG, Jr. 2011. Global Fund will pause new grants and seek new manager. *New York Times* November 23. http://www.nytimes.com/2011/11/24/health/global-aids-fund-cancels-fund-raising-and-seeks-new-manager.html?_r=1 (last accessed December 2013).

Ministry of Foreign Affairs of Japan. 2000. *G8 Communiqué Okinawa 2000, 23 July 2011.* http://www.mofa.go.jp/policy/economy/summit/2000/communique.html (last accessed December 2013).

Ngoasong MZ. 2009. The emergence of global health partnerships as facilitators of access to medication in Africa: a narrative policy analysis. *Social Science and Medicine* 68(5), 949–56.

Organization of African Unity. 2001. *Abuja Declaration on HIV/AIDS, Tuberculosis, and Other Related Infectious Diseases, 24–27 April 2001.* http://www.un.org/ga/aids/pdf/abuja_declaration.pdf (last accessed December 2013).

Ravishankar N, Gubbins P, Cooley RJ et al. 2009. Financing of global health: tracking development assistance for health from 1990 to 2007. *Lancet* 373(9681), 2113–24.

United Nations General Assembly. 2001. *Declaration of Commitment on HIV/AIDS (A/RES/S-26/2), 27 June 2001.* http://www.un.org/ga/aids/docs/aress262.pdf (last accessed December 2013).

Usher AD. 2010. Defrauding of the Global Fund gives Sweden cold feet. *Lancet* 376(9753), 1631.

Williams OD, Rushton S. 2011. Are the 'good times' over? Looking to the future of global health governance. *Global Health Governance* 5(1), 1–16. http://blogs.shu.edu/ghg/files/2011/11/Williams-and-Rushton_Are-the-%E2%80%98Good-Times%E2%80%99-Over_Fall-2011.pdf (last accessed December 2013).

York G. 2011. Economic crisis hits health aid that has helped millions as donors cut back. *Globe and Mail* November 23. http://www.theglobeandmail.com/news/world/economic-crisis-hits-health-aid-that-has-helped-millions-as-donors-cut-back/article554602/ (last accessed December 2013).

Chapter 28

Partnerships and the Millennium Development Goals: The Challenges of Reforming Global Health Governance

Michael Moran and Michael Stevenson

Abstract

Of the eight Millennium Development Goals (MDGs) that provide a framework for assessing progress toward development, three are directly health-related, while four focus on addressing established determinants of health. The centrality of health to the MDGs has been underpinned by concerted attempts to consolidate a more coherent system of global health governance. New collaborative initiatives, most notably global health partnerships (GHPs) which emerged in the mid-1990s, combined with rising interest in health by a range of public and private actors, has been depicted as representing an important new epoch in the path toward health equity. This chapter unpacks the "partnership moment" by examining GHPs within the context of the MDGs. It then provides commentary on their performance to date and briefly reviews proposals – focused on enhancing state capacity and rights-based approaches – that have been suggested as alternative paths for reform of global health governance.

The Handbook of Global Health Policy, First Edition. Edited by Garrett W. Brown, Gavin Yamey, and Sarah Wamala.
© 2014 John Wiley & Sons, Ltd. Published 2014 by John Wiley & Sons, Ltd.

Key Points

- The Millennium Development Goals (MDGs) provide an important normative framework for those working in development and a means for measuring and tracking progress toward eight broad development goals – three of which are directly health-related.
- The centrality of health to the MDGs shows that health is no longer a "second order element" of "low politics" and is recognized as an important pillar of foreign policy.
- The MDGs have been buttressed by global health partnerships (GHPs), which have led to increased resources for tackling diseases that disproportionately affect low and lower-middle income countries – particularly communicable diseases.
- Progress toward attainment of the MDGs has been uneven and many of the health-related MDGs targets will not be met by 2015.
- The proliferation of GHPs has contributed to fragmentation in the aid architecture, a narrow focus on communicable diseases at the expense of non-communicable diseases, and have exacerbated coordination problems with national health systems.

Key Policy Implications

- The growing number of initiatives and actors in global health governance means that there is a need for greater coordination between GHPs, public and private donors, and national health systems to improve the efficacy and effectiveness of health aid.
- GHPs must move beyond a narrow focus on communicable diseases and begin to tackle non-communicable diseases associated with lifestyle, which are an increasing problem in low and lower-middle income countries.
- A renewed commitment to strengthening state capacity is the key to addressing the social and structural determinants of health inequality: an objective for which partnerships are deemed poorly suited.
- National governments need to be held accountable for ensuring that citizens "rights to health," which are already enshrined in international law, are protected and enforced by rights-based compliance mechanisms.
- A rights-based approach needs to be supported by more coherent and better resourced institutional mechanisms of global health governance than currently available within the existing constellation of GHPs – for example, a Global Social Protection Fund.

Introduction

The past 15 years has seen public health move from the periphery to the center of the global development agenda. Of the eight Millennium Development Goals (MDGs) that provide both a normative framework for those working on development issues and a means of tracking progress, three are directly health-focused, while four others relate to addressing established determinants of health. The centrality of health to the MDGs has been underpinned by concerted attempts to consolidate a more coherent system of global health governance (GHG). New collaborative initiatives, most notably the global health partnerships (GHPs) that first emerged in the mid-1990s, combined with rising interest in health by a range of public and private actors, has been depicted as representing an important epoch in the path toward global health equity. Yet, despite the many tangible contributions GHPs have made toward the attainment of the health MDGs, they have nonetheless been criticized by a range of scholars as being still too narrowly focused, of increasing the complexity of an already fragmented aid architecture, and of failing to reach the world's poorest who are most in need of assistance. This chapter unpacks the "partnership moment," charting the rise of GHPs within the context of the MDGs as the master framework of global development policy. It then provides commentary on their performance to date and briefly reviews proposals – focused on enhancing state capacity and rights-based approaches – that have been forwarded as alternatives paths toward a more genuine "partnership for development."

Partnerships and the "Global Health Revolution"

The end of the Cold War set the stage for the rise of public health in global development in two important ways. First, driven largely by the devastating impact of the HIV/AIDS pandemic, governments increasingly accepted a broadening of the concept of "national security" to include health threats, particularly those posed by communicable disease (Barnes and Brown 2011). Second, the spread of neo-liberal thinking within and across states and multilateral lending institutions ensured a palpable decline in development assistance, a curtailing of public sector expenditures in low and lower-middle income countries (LMICs) and, as a consequence, an increase in the importance of private capital for challenges historically considered the responsibility of governments. In this context, global health began a rapid journey from the margins to the center of foreign policy, and served as a rallying point for private–public collaboration and the impetus for the emergence of novel multisectoral initiatives focused on reversing the effects of global inequality. By 2008, Fidler (2010: 1) notes that it was fair to label this shift a veritable "revolution" in global health.

Origins and Context of Global Health Partnerships

GHPs are both a cause and a manifestation of the changes that have occurred in global health over the past 15 years. Their proliferation at this particular juncture in the history of public health can be explained by five interrelated contextual factors.

First and foremost was illumination in the mid-1990s of LMICs' critical lack of access to essential medicines, which was underpinned by a structural shift in the political economy of pharmaceutical research and development (R&D) away from a state-dominated regime. As high-income countries (HICs) increasingly retreated from the business of producing drugs and vaccines used to safeguard public health, the pharmaceutical firms who took on this role saw little incentive to innovate for those with limited purchasing power and shifted priorities to non-communicable diseases (NCDs) associated with lifestyle (see Chapter 22). The result was a lack of basic research being undertaken into new diagnostic, preventative, and therapeutic options for communicable diseases such as malaria and tuberculosis disproportionately affecting LMICs. Combined with the prohibitive costs of certain treatment options, in particular antiretroviral therapy (ART) used to treat HIV infections, access to health technologies amongst those who needed them most was severely constrained (see Chapter 11). This lack of access laid bare the structural inequalities underlying the maldistribution of the global burden of disease, undermined the legitimacy of the international patent regime, and increased pressure on all parties to develop solutions to the problem of access.

Second, in a reversal of its post-war posture the United Nations (UN), and its organs such as the World Health Organization (WHO), began to actively court the private sector. This created an institutional space for collaboration, predicated on enabling the UN to augment relatively declining resources (Ollila 2005), and the need to engage the innovative capacity of the private sector in the resolution of complex policy problems, perceived as beyond the ability of the state.

Third, in some instances this was reciprocated, particularly by the pharmaceutical industry, within a context of rising pressure for greater corporate social responsibility (CSR) and accountability. At the close of the twentieth century, the private sector was firmly established as both the driver of global health-related R&D and proprietor of the majority of intellectual property (IP) informing essential medicines. Yet industry's use of IP rights to impede LMICs' access to health technologies had made it vulnerable to civil society claims that it acted as an impediment to, rather than an enabler of, global health equity. To showcase its utility, and revitalize its reputation, industry began to embrace the partnership agenda (Buse and Walt 2000).

Fourth, the 1990s marked a transition from market to networked and collaborative modes of governance. This occurred within a context of rising disenchantment with traditional aid delivery mechanisms, questions over the efficacy of multilateral institutions, including the WHO, and a volition on the part of technical experts facing common problems for heightened levels of inter-state and multisectoral collaboration in the resolution of complex policy problems (Slaughter 2004).

Finally, the 1990s also represented a renewed push by private foundations to address health inequalities. Initially this was driven by the Rockefeller Foundation, which provided key seed capital for many of the early partnerships, particularly the first generation of product development partnerships (PDPs) (Moran 2009). However, the Rockefeller Foundation's efforts were quickly overshadowed by the Bill and Melinda Gates Foundation (BMGF), which brought "unprecedented resources" to the challenges facing global heath (Buse and Tanaka 2011: 3) and by the early 2000s had emerged as the principal private benefactor of GHPs (Moran 2011).

Partnership Types and Initiatives

Four broad partnership categories, developed by the United Kingdom's Department for International Development (Carlson 2004), have been widely adopted by UN agencies as well as gaining widespread currency in the global health literature (see Chapter 27):

- *Research and development GHPs* – mostly referred to as PDPs, which are directed at "product discovery and development of new diagnostics, drugs and vaccines," particularly for neglected diseases; for example, the International AIDS Vaccine Initiative (IAVI).

- *Technical assistance/service support GHPs* – "support improved service access, may provide discounted or donated drugs, and give technical assistance" such as in-kind donations by pharmaceutical companies to LMICs; for example, Merck & Co's pioneering donation of Mectizan to treat onchocerciasis (commonly known as "river blindness").
- *Advocacy GHPs* – "which raise the profile of the disease and advocate for increased international and/or national response, and resource mobilization" such as the Roll Back Malaria (RBM) partnership.
- *Financing GHPs* – "which provides funds for specific disease programs" such as the Global Fund to Fight AIDS, Tuberculosis and Malaria (hereafter the Global Fund) and the Global Alliance for Vaccines and Immunization (GAVI or the Alliance).

The MDGs: Aspirational Targets for the Partnership Era

In September 2000 at the UN headquarters in New York City, 147 heads of state converged at the Millennium Summit and committed their governments to a new global development blueprint oriented towards meeting 18 (later increased to 21) numerical targets organized around eight broad goals by 2015. Together, these time-bound targets with 48 (later increased to 60) performance indicators for monitoring progress comprise the MDGs (Box 28.1).

Box 28.1   Millennium Development Goals

Goal 1: Eradicate extreme poverty and hunger (HT)
Goal 2: Promote gender equality and empower women (SD)
Goal 3: Achieve universal primary education (SD)
Goal 4: Reduce child mortality rates (HR)
Goal 5: Improve maternal health (HR)
Goal 6: Combat HIV/AIDS, malaria, and other major diseases (HR)
Goal 7: Ensure environmental sustainability (HT)
Goal 8: Develop a global partnership for development (HT)

HR, health-related MDG; HT, health-related targets and indicators; SD, social determinant of health.

While initially a UN project, ultimately adopted by all 193 member countries, the MDGs have become a universal normative framework for both state and non-state actors working at the intersection of global development and a standard benchmark with which to measure the effectiveness of their efforts. Since their creation, proponents have framed the goals as a novel approach to addressing persistent development challenges. However, as noted by Attaran (2005), the MDGs have effectively served to repackage several pre-existing UN objectives that were never realized, one of which also was explicitly structured around the partnership paradigm. Goal 5: Target 5.A, for example, pledges a 75% reduction in the maternal mortality ratio (the number of pregnancy/delivery-related deaths per 100,000), between 1990 and 2015, which mirrors the goal set in 1994 at the UN Cairo Conference on Population and Development of reducing maternal mortality by 50% by the year 2000, and again by 2015. Moreover, Goal 6: Target 6.C pledges "to have halted and begin to reduce by 2015 the global incidence of malaria"; a tempered version of the target set only 2 years prior in 1998 via the WHO's RBM partnership, of halving the global rate of malaria-associated mortality by 2010, and again by 2015 (Attaran 2005). In sum, in a mere decade the MDGs have become both a universally regarded normative framework spelling out what is most important in global development, and the benchmark used to assess progress. As a result the MDGs have served to reinvigorate interest in issues such as maternal health, which prior to their establishment had been neglected by donor entities.

Health-Related MDGs and the Social Determinants of Health

Putting questions over their originality aside, the implications of the MDGs for global health should not be underestimated. Although the escalation of interest in health among key development actors and subsequent growth in health aid predated the establishment of the MDGs, their institutionalization and wide embrace outside of the UN system have served, in the words of Ong *et al.* (2011: 1), to "elevate the status of health within the development agenda and recognize the two-way, though uneven, link between poverty and health."

Three of the eight MDGs – Goals 4, 5, and 6 – are explicitly health-related. Yet concern for health features prominently in the remaining five MDGs, with the WHO reporting on indicators for Goals 1, 7, and 8, while monitoring a total of eight of the 21 targets and 19 of the 60 indicators. As the WHO Commission on the Social Determinants of Health (CSDH) (2008) has reaffirmed, extreme poverty and hunger, a lack of basic education, gender inequity, and environmental degradation are all both determinants and products of adverse health outcomes in any given population, and especially so in LMICs. Extreme poverty, for example, is closely associated with undernutrition, a key driver of child mortality (Caulfield *et al.* 2004). At the same time, prolonged illness increases poverty and inequality, by reducing the available human, financial, and natural capital that can reverberate from the household to the societal level. Moreover, illness and/or death in a family often means that children, particularly girls who would otherwise be in school, are forced to work. As primary education often includes health education and promotion, a lack of education means that risk avoidance strategies are not conveyed, and that precious opportunities to address stigma or misinformation are missed (Kim *et al.* 2011). Development is thus a polycentric concept with inter-related determinants and effects, and the MDGs represent an attempt to address development as a multidimensional process.

MDGs as Partnerships

Goal 8: Develop a global partnership for development has ultimately emerged as the master ideational concept underpinning the MDGs. The partnership approach acts as an anchor and speaks to the perceived success and political support for GHPs as a governance strategy. It illustrates how the partnership model has spread from a singular, though critical sector, public health, across the entire development spectrum: from agriculture (the Alliance for a Green Revolution in Africa); to gender empowerment (the One Woman Initiative); to environment and climate change (the Clean Development Mechanism); to water resource management (Global Water Partnership). In global health, the major communicable diseases identified within Goal 6: HIV/AIDS, malaria and other diseases were the foci of the first generation of GHPs established in the mid to late 1990s, including the IAVI, the Medicines for Malaria Venture (MMV), and the TB Alliance, with second generation GHPs, embodied by the Global Fund, providing an enormous boost to these efforts. While a range of partnerships contribute toward Goals 4 and 5, the GAVI aligns most closely with reducing child mortality rates.

MDGs and Global Health Governance

While the partnership framework, which had its genesis in global health, is now influencing how global development as a collective enterprise is approached, the implications of the establishment of the MDGs has had more immediate and direct effects on global health for three reasons.

First, the MDGs have been the catalyst for sustaining the *major infusion of funding* into global health-related initiatives that began in the mid-1990s (Ooms *et al.* 2010). From 1990 (the baseline for most of the individual targets) to 2007, development assistance for health (DAH) quadrupled, from approximately US$5.5 billion to $22 billion (Ravishankar *et al.* 2009). Using Raviskankar *et al.*'s (2009) methodology, Murray *et al.* (2011: 9) notes that between 2007 and 2010 DAH "continued to expand" reaching close to $27 billion. From the outset, achieving the MDGs has been largely predicated on what aid skeptic Easterly (2006) has termed the "Big Push" – a massive "influx" of public and private development assistance designed to stimulate development and tackle poverty, with health a major beneficiary due to its perceived centrality in breaking "poverty traps" (Ooms *et al.* 2010: 1–2).

Second, with the establishment of the MDGs, the international community was provided a universal *normative compass* (Barnes and Brown 2011) intended to guide the activities of what Fidler (2010: 4) has described as the "unstructured plurality" of development: the heterogeneous mix of actors, mechanisms, and funding structures that have some role in the fragmentary system of GHG that has evolved against the backdrop of an expansion of health aid. The existence of a shared set of norms informing efforts to strengthen global health and development at a systemic level should not be diminished. As a normative document, the MDGs act as a blueprint to convince a diverse array of actors and agencies, often with very different motivations, to commit to common principles and measurable goals that can assist in bringing greater focus and coherence to the current system. According to Poku and Whitman (2011: 188), "a normative enterprise on the scale of the [MDGs] has an equal only in the human rights regime" with the key distinction being that the MDGs are "performance rather than entitlement" based.

Third, and perhaps most significantly, the MDGs have provided heightened *legitimacy to the logic of endowing private actors with formal agenda-setting power in the governance of global health*. Under the private American foundation inspired GHP model, for-profit entities were for the first time afforded equal levels of responsibility with public sector institutions in the development of strategies to address the adverse health effects of global poverty (Reich 2002). This approach initially attracted criticism from civil society organizations that viewed firms as a barrier to, as opposed to an enabler, of global health equity. However, via the MDGs, and Goal 8 in particular, the UN has signaled its support for the notion that the innovative capacity of the private sector must be tapped if solutions to health challenges affecting the world's poor are to be developed (Mahoney and Maynard 1999), and that the partnership paradigm is the most appropriate means to achieving this (see Chapter 27).

Assessing Effectiveness: Partnerships and the MDGs

There is little doubt that both partnerships and the MDGs have led to a refocusing of efforts toward improving health outcomes. Gains, however, have been uneven. There is large variation in progress within (and between) countries and regions, and across the different MDG targets, with many indicators showing that the health-related targets will not be met by 2015. Similarly, while partnerships and other vertical funding mechanisms have led to clear innovations in aid delivery, product development, and expanded resources for public health, the achievements of the major GHPs have also been mixed. It would be imprudent to conflate partnership performance with the MDGs, given the MDGs are aspirational goals, with no singular organ or institution accountable for achieving the targets. Nonetheless, as noted, the two are underpinned by a shared vision, largely predicated on multisectoral responses to twenty-first century development challenges.

Progress Toward the Health-Related MDGs

The latest WHO figures provide a snapshot of real successes across the health-related MDGs and targets (WHO 2011).

- *MDG 1, Target 1.C* There has been a decrease in the prevalence of underweight children since 1990. The proportion has declined from 25% to approximately 16% in 2010 (WHO 2012).
- *MDG 4* Child mortality has continued to decline, with deaths of children under 5 years of age falling from 12.4 million in 1990 to below 8.1 million in 2009 (WHO 2011). This decline has gathered pace, with rate of decline nearly doubling to 2.7% per year since 2000, compared to 1.3% in the 1990s (WHO 2012). Improved mortality has been underpinned by wider access to basic immunizations, specifically for measles, as per Indicator 4.3. Coverage has increased steadily from 73% in 1990 to 82% in 2009 (WHO 2011), while deaths from measles have decreased by 78% since 2000 (Measles and Rubella Initiative 2012).
- *MDG 5* There have also been clear advances in maternal health. The number of maternal deaths has declined by 34% between 1990 and 2009 from 546,000 to 358,000 (WHO 2012). Attendance at antenatal clinics has increased to "half of all pregnant women," although it remains well below the target of all women, while the "global proportion of births attended by skilled health professional has increased" (WHO 2012).
- *MDG 6* New HIV infections have declined significantly between 2001 and 2009 (17%) (WHO 2011), and in 2009 5 million people in LMICs had access to ARV treatment. Tuberculosis treatments are also more widely available, with a drop from 30 to 20 deaths per 100,000 since 1990 (WHO 2012). It is now expected that 42 countries will meet the MDG target of halting or reversing the incidence of malaria, with the supply of antimalarial drugs and treated nets more widely available (WHO 2011). Approximately "one third of the 108 malarious countries have documented reductions in cases of malaria of 50 percent in 2008 compared to 2000" (WHO 2010b: 2). With continued interventions it is now expected that Target 6.C for malaria and tuberculosis will be achieved.
- *MDG 7, Target 7.C* There has been improved availability of "safe drinking water," with 87% (up from 77% in 1990) of the world's population now with access, meaning that on the current trajectory Progress Indicator 7.8, is likely to be met (WHO 2011).

Role of Global Health Partnerships

While it is not possible to isolate the contribution of partnerships, there is little doubt that GHPs have had an important complementary role in these achievements. GAVI for example, recently recognized at a high-level UN event as a model GHP for its role in helping to advance the MDGs, particularly Goals 4 and 8 (GAVI 2012), has also had a role mainly through the provision of vaccines. By 2015 it aims to have prevented 3.9 million future deaths as part of its "contribution to meeting the" MDGs (GAVI 2010: 12). Moreover, the Global Fund has played a pivotal part in ensuring that people with HIV in developing countries have access to ART, and is the largest provider of treatment in LMICs.

These contributions have been buttressed by the development of "rich pipelines of technologies and [at least] ten product launches" since PDPs first emerged (Grace 2010: 7), indirectly contributing to Goal 8, but directly contributing to a range of other targets. For example, the MMV and Novartis International have developed Coartem, an "artemisinin combination therapy (ACT) formulated" malarial treatment for children, with 100 million treatments delivered to 39 countries (MMV 2012), cutting across a range of targets, for example, Targets 4.A and 6.C. These have largely been developed using "push" mechanisms to incentivize innovation, relying heavily on funds from the BMGF, various public sectors, and in-kind and pro bono support from the pharmaceutical industry to create "virtual pharmaceutical companies" (Grace 2010), which mirror the industry's "portfolio" approach to the product development pipeline (Widdus and White 2004). Consequently, the formation of a range of GHP types, in particular financing and product development, broadly contributes to the spirit of Goal 8.

Will the Health-Related MDG Targets be Met?

Nonetheless, many of the health-related MDG targets will not be met. The macro-level gains in some areas shroud the patchy nature of progress on a regional basis. Moreover, isolating these gains to the MDGs (and indeed GHPs) is a process fraught with danger.

The 10 health-related progress indicators shown in Table 28.1 illustrates the uneven progress being made towards the MDGs, which is further complicated by gaps in data across the seven WHO regions.

While child mortality has declined, the two thirds reduction targeted in MDG 4 is not likely to be met. This can be attributed to the continuing high rate of death associated with pneumonia and diarrheal diseases, "accounting for about 40 percent of all deaths" among children under 5 (WHO 2010b: 2). Similarly, while there have been gains against, for example Indicator 5.1 pertaining to the maternal mortality ratio, MDG 5 as a whole appears to be beyond reach, with "the annual rate of decline of 2.3 percent" being "less than half of the 5.5 percent required" to reduce the ratio by three quarters (WHO 2010b: 2).

Efforts to curb the spread of the "major diseases," has also seen mixed results. For example, despite the increased availability of ART, Target 6.B is off-track. Access to ART currently sits at 36% in LMICs – well below the objective of universal coverage (WHO 2011). This is consistent with the broader problems of access to essential medicines in LMICs as per Target 8.E. Universal access continues to be prohibited by "low availability and high costs" in LMICs (see Chapter 11). WHO surveys indicate that, despite GHPs, "selected generic medicines were available in only 42 percent of health facilities in the public sector and 64 percent of facilities in the private sector," forcing patients to source

Table 28.1   Health Millennium Development Goals scorecard for WHO regions.

	World	Africa	Americas	Eastern Med.	Europe	Southeast Asia	Western Pacific
Under 5 mortality (per 1000 live births)	65	142	18	78	14	63	21
Measles immunization (% coverage)	81	73	93	83	94	75	93
Maternal mortality (per 100,000 live births)	400	900	99	420	27	450	82
Skilled birth attendant (% births)	66	47	92	59	96	49	92
Contraceptive use (% married women 15–49 years)	62	24	71	43	68	58	83
HIV/AIDS prevalence (% adults aged 15–45 years)	0.8	4.9	0.5	0.2	0.5	0.3	0.1
Malaria mortality (per 100,000 population)	17	104	0.5	7.5	–	2.1	0.3
TB treatment (success rate %)	86	79	82	88	67	88	92
Water (% using improved sources)	87	61	96	83	98	86	90
Sanitation (% using improved facilities)	60	34	87	61	94	40	62

☐ On track ☐ Insufficient progress ■ Off track
Source: adapted from WHO (2010a).

medicines elsewhere, with mark-ups, some "630 percent above the international reference price" (WHO 2011: 19). Moreover, while it is probable that the target of "halving tuberculosis prevalence and deaths" is on-track, the decline in the African region will need to accelerate, with multidrug-resistant TB posing a particular problem (WHO 2011: 16).

Impediments to the Realization of the Health-Related MDGs

Two factors stand out as impediments to the realization of the health-related MDGs. First, despite the infusion of capital into global health initiatives over the last decade, health systems across the developing world remain weak. The weakness of national capacity hinders global efforts to assess and compare progress within and across countries while ensuring the poorest segments of LMIC populations will continue to shoulder a disproportionate share of national disease burdens. Second, the fragmented nature of global efforts has led to a lack of coherence regarding the roles, responsibilities, and priorities of participating actors. Duplication is widespread, single-issue and vertical initiatives predominate, while major health threats – most notably NCDs – remain largely unaddressed by GHPs. This combination of a persistence of weak health systems at the country level and ongoing coordination challenges at the global level has diminished confidence in the partnership paradigm as the optimal framework for reducing health inequalities.

Weak National Health Systems

In LMICs, delivery of healthcare is predominantly the domain of the public sector. Whether the result of misplaced domestic priorities (i.e., military expenditures trumping healthcare), or externally imposed constraints on public sector spending (e.g., debt servicing schedules), insufficient financial, material, and human resources work against universal access to healthcare (Asante and Zwi 2007), which in turn gives rise to health inequalities that reverberate beyond national boundaries.

Yet not only do weak health systems hamper government capacity to protect the health of their populations, they also undermine efforts for effective monitoring of population health. Even the most basic data (e.g., mortality rates) informing the MDG indicators, not to mention the causes of such deaths, remain poorly recorded in LMICs (see Chapter 5). Such data limitations are a direct reflection of systems neglect, which have significant ramifications for the validity of the MDGs as measures of progress. As noted by Attaran, "[o]ften the subject matter is so immeasurable, or the measurement so inadequate, that one cannot know the baseline condition, or know if the desired trend of improvement is actually occurring" (Attaran 2005: 955–6). Moreover, because MDG targets are typically meant to reflect aggregate national averages "progress towards the goals can be made" at the country level while health inequalities persist (CDP 2009: 18). They can even increase among particularly marginalized socioeconomic groups who may not have the same access to resources as the "more affluent" who can more easily access resources earmarked for the MDGs (CDP 2009: 18). Gains can therefore accrue to the relatively affluent and can perversely *increase* inequality.

For these reasons doubts have been raised concerning the reliability of the MDGs as a gauge of national and international performance. Moser *et al.* (2005) for example note that because sub-5 mortality is significantly higher within lower socioeconomic divisions in poor countries, the existing child mortality metric is an insufficient indicator of health equity, and to correct for this deficiency, monitoring must target specific socioeconomic levels and incentives created for adopting policies known to address inequalities in population health.

However, the effect of GHPs on health systems is far from clear. Scholars have frequently argued that GHPs have a disruptive impact at the country level, attributed to "high transactions costs on recipient administrations; weakened country ownership of national strategies; and distortion of national priorities, human resource allocations and service delivery structures" (Buse and Tanaka 2011: 7). Yet, while arguments continue to be made that GHPs pay limited attention to health systems strengthening, as Biesma *et al.* (2009: 248) note, there is "a surprisingly thin body of evidence" to support claims that GHPs either strengthen or undermine health systems. Their analysis of three major GHPs – the Global Fund, the World Bank Multi-country AIDS Program, and the US President's Emergency Plan for AIDS Relief – reveals that while the establishment of "parallel bodies and processes" have often initially been poorly "aligned with national systems," GHPs have nonetheless "learned to better utilize" existing national infrastructures, coordinate "financial management and human resource strategies" with governments and support national disease control efforts (Biesma *et al.* 2009: 239).

Poor Coordination and Misplaced Priorities

The inability of bilateral, multilateral, public, and private donors to harmonize initiatives has created unnecessary duplication and direct competition at both the local and international level between service providers. While the MDGs function as an important normative compass, goal attainment is hindered by the poorly coordinated actions of external donors, which adds to burden already strained health systems in LMICs (WHO 2010a).

Undoubtedly, the partnership paradigm upon which the MDGs are based has been integral to bringing increased resources for tackling neglected diseases. In the 1990s, neglected communicable diseases received only 20% of health-related Official Development Assistance (ODA). By 2005–2006 this figure had increased to over 50% (CDP 2009). Buse and Tanaka (2011: 8) rightly note this increase represents "one of the triumphs of global health efforts over the past decade." However, there are now concerns that the pendulum has swung too far in the other direction and that the proliferation of vertical funds focused on individual neglected diseases embodies a siloed approach to addressing a diverse array of health challenges that share many common structural determinants.

More importantly, to date, partnerships and the MDGs have also largely avoided chronic NCDs (Beaglehole and Bonita 2008). This is a concern as NCDs now account for more than half of the burden of disease in LMICs (Buse and Tanaka 2011). Indeed, NCDs such as cardiovascular disease, cancers, tobacco-related illnesses, and diabetes are projected to account for almost 70% of all global deaths by 2030 (Mathers and Loncar 2006). To maintain their legitimacy as the dominant framework informing GHG, GHPs must show the same degree of relevance for addressing NCDs that they have demonstrated in bringing attention and resources to bear on communicable diseases (see Chapters 12 and 16).

Critical Assessments: Partnerships Beyond 2015

The partnership paradigm was never intended to function as a stand-alone model for strengthening global health. While critics of its rapid expansion generally do not doubt the utility of GHPs, their concerns typically center on the diminished role the partnership concept affords to states, international organizations and traditional multilateral processes in the governance of global health. For the MDGs to be achieved, GHG must first be improved, and those who have expressed caution over the current partnership paradigm, four distinctive but interrelated shifts must occur if this general goal is to be realized. First, that public sector capacity across LMICs should be sufficiently strengthened to enable equitable access to health services. Second, that the WHO and other traditional international organizations with mandates relating to health protection (e.g., the World Bank) be afforded greater authority to effectively regulate the health impacting activities of both state and non-state actors. Third, that states be held accountable for the preservation of health as a fundamental right, as per their commitments under the various "rights to health" obligations enshrined within international law through the Universal Declaration on Human Rights and the International Covenant on Economic, Social and Cultural Rights. Fourth, that LMICs might be better served by a single GHP, combining the resources of the Global Fund and GAVI, and specifically designed for achieving the health-related MDGs, rather than a constellation of disease-specific organs (Cometto *et al.* 2009).

First, a renewed commitment to *strengthening state capacity* is deemed key to addressing the social and structural determinants of health inequality: an objective for which partnerships are deemed poorly suited (CDP 2009). From this perspective, arguments that traditional state actors are inefficient, overly bureaucratic, and unable to resolve complex health challenges are fundamentally misguided given the role social policy has historically had in addressing inequity, a key determinant of ill-health in any society. Poor health is thus seen as a product of a multiplicity of factors beyond the biomedical, including a poor socioeconomic environment, insufficient nutrition, housing, and education, much of which states have the capacity to tackle autonomously via informed and appropriate public policy (Lee 2010). The CSDH was created by the WHO in 2008, precisely to map out how such social, economic, and environmental factors informing health affect each other to enable viable policy solutions to health inequalities to be implemented. If the MDGs are to succeed there is a need for a reconfiguration to incorporate CSDH's targets, which focus explicitly on embedding "health equity into global, regional, national and local health policy priorities" (Lee 2010: 6). Neither the MDGs nor the majority of disease-specific GHPs prioritize health equity, instead focusing on achieving narrow measurable targets and indicators or disease-specific goals. Moreover, given the regulatory role that states must have in addressing NCDs (e.g., prohibiting tobacco sales to minors, setting limits for food additives), the state must invariably have a bigger role in public health, "with chronic disease prevention occurring at the *national* level" (Magnusson 2010: 491, emphasis in original).

Second, consistent with the recommendations of the CSDH, the revised template must be global and ensure all countries have an equal voice in the policy process (Lee 2010; Magnusson 2010). There is thus an urgent need for an effective global arbitrator, in the form of stronger public international organizations to help shape, coordinate, and, when necessary, enforce the rules informing global health. The WHO can serve in this role, but to do so it can no longer be starved of resources when national interests conflict with safeguarding global health. Underlying this is the belief that partnerships are neither politically neutral nor divorced from the competitive realm of the global political economy (Magnusson 2010). At best, they are arrangements where responsibilities are not shared equally amongst participants (Moran 2009; Barnes and Brown 2011), and at worst, a mechanism that serves to distract attention from partners' contradictory behaviors, for example pharmaceutical companies challenging LMICs' rights under the TRIPs flexibility provision to circumvent patent law when the protection of public health is deemed threatened (Asante and Zwi 2007).

Third, national governments need to be held accountable for ensuring that citizens "right to health" is protected. While already enshrined in international law, health rights need to be underpinned by a clear rights-based "obligations and compliance mechanisms" (Gostin *et al.* 2011: 3), to ensure, for example, that a minimum of gross domestic product (GDP) is set aside for health spending to guarantee universal access to health services. Moreover, at the international level, if HICs could be accountable for devoting a minimum of ODA (e.g., the 0.7% of GDP agreed to under UN Resolution 2626 in 1970), a collective pool, managed by the WHO, could exist to ensure such coverage exists in LMICs lacking sufficient resources to provide such care autonomously (Gostin *et al.* 2011). The Joint Action and Learning Initiative on National and Global Responsibilities for Health has proposed that such rights and associated "mutual responsibilities" could be enshrined in a new "global agreement, such as a Framework Convention on Global Health, which sets priorities, clarifies national and international responsibilities" for the post-MDG era (Gostin *et al.* 2011: 1).

Fourth, a rights-based approach needs to be supported by more coherent institutional mechanisms of "global governance for health" (Gostin *et al.* 2011: 3). For example, utilizing the pre-existing constellation of partnerships, a "Global Health Fund" (Gostin *et al.* 2011: 1) that united the two major GHPs – the Global Fund and GAVI– for the specific purpose of achieving the MDGs would assist in streamlining the global health architecture (Cometto *et al.* 2009). If such a Fund were "substantially" better resourced it would also be better equipped to act on a broad mandate that incorporated "national health plans, including co-financing non-disease-specific human resources for health" (Cometto *et al.* 2009: 1501). An expanded and more ambitious variation on this proposal is the Global Social Protection Fund (Ooms *et al.* 2010). Similarly rights-based in orientation, this proposal advocates a "permanent system of resource distribution ... similar to – but broader in scope than – the Global Fund" (Ooms *et al.* 2010: 5). Broadly analogous to national systems of social protection, the Protection Fund would utilize a "weighted burden sharing formula" to "assess contributions from member states"; "provide recurrent financing to address persistent threats to health"; and "allocate resources using a needs assessment system so as to harmonize aid with the burden of avoidable and unfair mortality" (Ooms *et al.* 2010: 5). The objective would be a system for "perennial redistribution" between countries preferably through a singular institution that recognizes the centrality of national capacity *and* sustained international funding (Ooms *et al.* 2010: 3–4).

These proposals of reform are predicated on the assumption that the solution to fragmentation is not to tear down the architecture, but rather to consolidate and build on the momentum of the "decade of disease-specific attention" (Cometto *et al.* 2009: 1501), establish a more coherent system of GHG in which national capacity is augmented, international support is expanded, existing human rights to health obligations are met, and external donor's intervention are aligned and harmonized with national systems. These alternatives to the existing aid paradigm may serve as the key to improving health equity post-2015.

Conclusions

We are undoubtedly living through the partnership era, and the successes and failures of the MDGs are representative of this. While GHPs were established to bring new resources and expertise to global health challenges, they were never specifically intended to develop intelligent public policy, confer greater authority to the WHO, or rewrite international law, as these tasks can only be implemented by states. Nevertheless, collective action focused on strengthening global health is now informed by the partnership concept. Given the apparent continued appetite among donors for this model (Buse and Tanaka 2011), it would appear that in the short to medium term, the most feasible means of addressing the aforementioned shortcomings is through commitment among all relevant parties to evidence-based reform, as opposed to abandoning the paradigm with the hope that a superior alterative will be realized.

Key Reading

Barnes A, Brown G. 2011. The idea of partnership within the Millennium Development Goals: context, instrumentality and the normative demands of partnership. *Third World Quarterly* 32, 165–80.

Buse K, Tanaka S. 2011. Global public-private health partnerships: lessons learned from ten years of experience and evaluation. *International Dental Journal* 61, 2–10.

CPD (Committee for Development Policy). 2009. *Implementing the Millennium Development Goals: Health Inequality and the Role of Global Health Partnerships*. New York: United Nations.

DESA (Department of Economic and Social Affairs). 2012. *The MDG Gap Taskforce*. http://www.un.org/en/development/desa/policy/mdg_gap/index.shtml (last accessed December 2013).

Gostin L, Friedman E, Ooms G et al. 2011. The Joint Action and Learning Initiative: towards a global agreement on national and global responsibilities for health. *PLOS Medicine* 8, 1–5.

Ooms G, Stuckler D, Basu S, Mckee M. 2010. Financing the Millennium Development Goals for health and beyond: sustaining the 'Big Push'. *Globalization and Health* 6, 1–8.

WHO (World Health Organization). 2012. *Millennium Development Goals*. http://www.who.int/topics/millennium_development_goals/en/ (last accessed December 2013).

References

Asante A, Zwi A. 2007. Public–private partnerships and global health equity: prospects and challenges. *Indian Journal of Medical Ethics* 4, 176–80.

Attaran A. 2005. An immeasurable crisis? A criticism of the Millennium Development Goals and why they cannot be measured. *PLOS Medicine* 2, 955–61.

Barnes A, Brown G. 2011. The idea of partnership within the Millennium Development Goals: context, instrumentality and the normative demands of partnership. *Third World Quarterly* 32, 165–80.

Beaglehole R, Bonita R. 2008. Global public health: a scorecard. *Lancet* 372, 1988–96.

Biesma RG, Brugha R, Harmer A, Walsh A, Spicer N, Walt G. 2009. The effects of global health initiatives on country health systems: a review of the evidence from HIV/AIDS control. *Health Policy and Planning* 24, 239–52.

Buse K, Walt G. 2000. Global public–private partnerships: Part I. A new development in health? *Bulletin of the World Health Organization* 78, 549–61.

Buse K, Tanaka S. 2011. Global public–private health partnerships: lessons learned from ten years of experience and evaluation. *International Dental Journal* 61, 2–10.

Carlson C. 2004. *Mapping Global Health Partnerships: What They Are, What They Do and Where They Operate*. London: DFID Health Resource Centre.

Caulfield L, de Onis M, Blössner M, Black RE. 2004. Undernutrition as an underlying cause of child deaths associated with diarrhea, pneumonia, malaria, and measles. *American Journal of Clinical Nutrition* 80, 193–8.

Cometto G, Ooms G, Starrs A, Zeitz P. 2009. A global fund for the health MDGs? *Lancet* 373, 1500–2.

CDP (Committee for Development Policy). 2009. *Implementing the Millennium Development Goals: Health Inequality and the Role of Global Health Partnerships*. New York: United Nations.

CSDH (Commission on the Social Determinants of Health). 2008. *Closing the Gap in a Generation: Health Equity through Action on the Social Determinants of Health: Final Report of the Commission on Social Determinants of Health*. Geneva: World Health Organization.

Easterly W. 2006. *The White Man's Burden: Why the West's Efforts to Aid the Rest Have Done so Much Ill and so Little Good*. New York: Penguin.

Fidler D. 2010. *The Challenges of Global Health Governance*. New York: Council on Foreign Relations.

GAVI (Global Alliance for Vaccines and Immunization). 2010. *GAVI Alliance Progress Report 2010*. Geneva: GAVI Alliance.

GAVI (Global Alliance for Vaccines and Immunization). 2012. *GAVI cited as model global development partnership.* http://www.gavialliance.org/library/news/press-releases/2011/gavi-cited-as-model-global-development-partnership/ (last accessed December 2013).

Gostin L, Friedman E, Ooms G et al. 2011. The joint action and learning initiative: towards a global agreement on national and global responsibilities for health. *PLOS Medicine* 8, 1–5.

Grace C. 2010. *Product Development Partnerships: Lessons from PDPs Established to Develop New Health Technologies for Neglected Diseases.* London: DFID Human Development Research Centre.

Kim J, Lutz B, Dhaliwal M, O'Malley J. 2011. The "AIDS and MDGs" approach: what is it, why does it matter, and how do we take it forward? *Third World Quarterly* 32, 141–63.

Lee K. 2010. How do we move forward on the social determinants of health: the global governance challenges. *Critical Public Health* 20, 5–14.

Magnusson R. 2010. Global health governance and the challenge of chronic, non-communicable disease. *Journal of Law, Medicine and Ethics* 38: 490–507.

Mahoney R, Maynard J. 1999. The introduction of new vaccines into developing countries. *Vaccine*, 17, 646–52.

Mathers C, Loncar D. 2006. Projections of global mortality and burden of disease from 2002 to 2030. *PLOS Medicine* 3, 2011–30.

Measles and Rubella Initiative. 2012. *European countries must take action now to prevent continued measles outbreaks in 2012. http://www.measlesrubellainitiative.org/european-countries-must-take-action-now-to-prevent-continued-measles-outbreaks-in-2012/ (last accessed December 2013).*

MMV (Medicines for Malaria Venture). 2012. *Coartem® Dispersable.* http://www.mmv.org/achievements-challenges/achievements/coartem-d (last accessed December 2013).

Moran M. 2009. Philanthropic Foundations and Global Health Partnership Formation: The Rockefeller Foundation and IAVI. In MacLean S, Brown S, Fourie P (eds) *Health for Some: The Political Economy of Global Health Governance*, pp. 118–29. New York: Palgrave Macmillan.

Moran M. 2011. Private foundations and global health partnerships: philanthropists and 'partnership brokerage'. In Rushton S, Williams O (eds) *Partnerships and Foundations in Global Health Governance*, pp. 123–42. New York: Palgrave Macmillan.

Moser K, Leon D, Gwatkin D. 2005. How does progress towards the child mortality Millennium Development Goal affect inequalities between the poorest and least poor? Analysis of demographic and health survey data. *BMJ* 331, 1180–83.

Murray CJL, Anderson B, Burstein R, Leach-Kemon K, Schneider M, Tardif A, Zhang R. 2011. Development assistance for health: trends and prospects. *Lancet* 378, 9–10.

Ollila E. 2005. Global health priorities: priorities of the wealthy? *Globalization and Health* 1, 1–5.

Ong A, Kindhauser M, Smith I, Chan M. 2011. Global health agenda for the twenty-first century. In Detels R (ed.) *Oxford Textbook of Public Health*, pp. 1713–29. Oxford: Oxford University Press.

Ooms G, Stuckler D, Basu S, Mckee M. 2010. Financing the Millennium Development Goals for health and beyond: sustaining the 'Big Push'. *Globalization and Health* 6, 1–8.

Poku NK, Whitman J. 2011. The Millennium Development Goals and development after 2015. *Third World Quarterly* 32, 181–98.

Ravishankar N, Gubbins P, Cooley R, Leach-Kemon K, Michaud C, Jamison D. 2009. Financing of global health: tracking development assistance for health from 1990 to 2007. *Lancet* 373, 2113–24.

Reich M (ed.) 2002. *Public–Private Partnerships for Health.* Cambridge, MA: Harvard University Press.

Slaughter A. 2004. *A New World Order.* Princeton, NJ: Princeton University Press.

WHO (World Health Organization). 2010a. *Accelerating Progress Towards the Health-Related Millennium Development Goals.* Geneva: WHO.

WHO (World Health Organization). 2010b. *Health-Related Millennium Development Goals: Report by the Secretariat.* Geneva: WHO.

WHO (World Health Organization). 2011. *World Health Statistics 2011*. Geneva: WHO.

WHO (World Health Organization). 2012. *Millennium Development Goals: Progress Towards the Health-Related Millennium Development Goals, February 10*. http://www.who.int/mediacentre/factsheets/fs290/en/ (last accessed December 2013).

Widdus R, White K. 2004. *Combating Diseases Associated With Poverty: Financing Strategies for Product Development and the Potential Role of Public–Private Partnerships*. London: Wellcome Trust.

Part VII Beyond Globalization

Chapter 29

Preparing for the Next Pandemic

Adam Kamradt-Scott

Abstract

This chapter aims to provide policy-makers, scholars, and practitioners with a brief overview of the threat of pandemic influenza, the need for developing comprehensive pandemic preparedness plans that adopt a whole-of-government or whole-of-society approach, as well as summarizing the various pharmaceutical (such as influenza vaccines and antiviral medications) and non-pharmaceutical strategies (such as school closures, personal hygiene practices, and the use of facemasks) for responding to the threat.

The Handbook of Global Health Policy, First Edition. Edited by Garrett W. Brown, Gavin Yamey, and Sarah Wamala.
© 2014 John Wiley & Sons, Ltd. Published 2014 by John Wiley & Sons, Ltd.

Key Points

- Influenza pandemics are a regular feature of human existence, but are unlike other natural disasters and crises in that they are non-linear, geographically indistinct events that can cause high morbidity and mortality as well as widespread social and economic disruption.
- Influenza vaccines remain the primary means to protect populations from the threat of influenza; however producing vaccines requires considerable time and resources.
- Antiviral medications are another key strategy actively promoted by leading governance institutions for reducing the severity of influenza-related illness.
- A variety of non-pharmaceutical measures such as social distancing practices (e.g., school and childcare center closures), and personal protective measures (e.g., hand-washing, facemasks, etc.) can assist governments prevent the spread of pandemic influenza, but the evidence base for these interventions is currently limited.
- Influenza pandemics are likely to occur again in the future, and governments are encouraged to develop comprehensive pandemic preparedness plans that will assist in reducing human illness and death.

Key Policy Implications

- The multidimensional nature of an influenza pandemic requires governments to develop comprehensive – or "whole-of-government" – pandemic preparedness plans that minimize economic and social disruption while also protecting human health; such planning entails bringing multiple interest groups such as government, civil society, business, and industry together, and is critical for understanding various roles and responsibilities as well as identifying and addressing vulnerabilities.
- It is highly unlikely that pandemic-specific vaccines will be available for the first months of any new influenza pandemic. Antiviral medications may also be in short supply. Governments therefore need to consider what additional strategies they will implement to: (i) delay the introduction of the virus into their population; and (ii) how to prevent the virus spreading unchecked.
- Various non-pharmaceutical mitigation strategies such as quarantine and isolation, social distancing measures (e.g., school closures, cancellation of mass gatherings, etc.), and public education campaigns to promote personal hygiene practices can be used to help prevent virus transmission.
- Policy-makers need to think through the social, economic, ethical, and practical implications of various mitigation strategies (such as quarantine and isolation, social distancing, etc.) to prevent unintended and unforeseen consequences arising.

Introduction

Influenza pandemics are a regular feature of human existence. Historical records of European epidemics date back to the twelfth century, and the first major pandemic is believed to have occurred around the year 1510 CE. Since that time, influenza pandemics have periodically resurfaced (approximately every 20–30 years). In the twentieth century alone there were three major pandemics – the 1918 Spanish flu pandemic that killed approximately 40 million people worldwide, the 1957 Hong Kong flu pandemic that caused the deaths of approximately 2 million people, and the 1968 Asian flu pandemic that resulted in the deaths of over 1 million people. In 2009, a novel influenza A (H1N1) virus spread globally within a matter of weeks, initiating the first influenza pandemic of the twenty-first century and causing the deaths of over 18,449 people (WHO 2010).

Influenza pandemics occur when two conditions are met: when a novel strain of the virus emerges to which humans have little to no immunity, and when that virus achieves effective human-to-human transmission. Said another way, the influenza virus is an inherently unstable pathogen that mutates frequently. Occasionally a new strain emerges that possesses the ability to infect humans, and because people have not been exposed to the strain before, their immune system does not have the ability to fight off the infection. In the event the virus then mutates further, so that it can spread easily between people, either through close contact or by touching infected objects, an environment is created whereby a pandemic can occur.

Confronted with this reality, governments have been encouraged to develop a range of measures to better protect their populations from the threat of pandemic influenza. These measures, which can be broadly categorized as pharmaceutical and non-pharmaceutical, require significant financial, human, and technological resources – resources that, importantly, many resource-poor countries often struggle to locate or assign. The purpose of this chapter is to examine the wide range of measures and policy options that are currently available to governments of all resource persuasions to strengthen national pandemic preparedness. The chapter commences by discussing the nature of the threat and the need for a whole-of-society (also referred to as "whole-of-government") response prior to identifying the measures that healthcare practitioners and policy-makers may consider appropriate for their particular context and resource setting. In discussing each type of intervention, consideration is given to the existing evidence base of particular measures as well as exploring the various issues, challenges, and policy debates surrounding each type of intervention.

Examining the Threat and the Need for a Whole-of-Society Approach

Influenza pandemics are qualitatively different from every other type of natural disaster. Indeed, unlike floods, fires, earthquakes, tsunamis, and the like, influenza pandemics present a unique challenge to government policy-makers charged with disaster response and recovery. This is principally because influenza pandemics are non-linear, geographically indistinct events. In other words, unlike a flood, fire, or earthquake that occurs as a particular emergency or event in a specific time and place, influenza pandemics have demonstrated that they can extend over two years' duration as successive waves of infection spread globally and reinfect population groups. Moreover, they are widespread, potentially affecting entire countries in contrast to other disasters that are often localized, geographically isolated events.

In the context of the 1918 Spanish flu pandemic, for example, the virus was noted to have spread around the world three to five times over a period of 18 months. Significantly, this was before the advent of commercial air travel. The case fatality rate (the number of deaths divided by the total number of cases) was estimated at only 2.5% (Kolata 1999), and yet conservative estimates place the number of deaths resulting from the novel strain of influenza A (H1N1) around 40 million people worldwide. Admittedly, the Spanish flu pandemic occurred prior to the discovery of the causative agent – an RNA virus – and before influenza vaccines and antiviral medications had been developed. Nonetheless, by comparison, the case fatality rate of the H5N1 avian influenza virus that is now endemic throughout much of Asia and parts of the Middle East is currently estimated at 60%. Fortunately, that virus has not achieved effective human-to-human transmission naturally,[1] but were it to do so, and the case fatality rate remained unchanged at 60%, there is no doubt it would have a devastating effect on the world's population. Even if that fatality rate decreased to an equivalent level as the 1918 pandemic, leading influenza experts have estimated that between 180 and 360 million people would die globally (Osterholm 2005).

Given the infectivity of influenza and its potential to spread rapidly and extensively, influenza pandemics arguably present an imminent and direct threat to not only individual well-being, but also to social functioning (see Chapter 15). A combination of past experience as well as epidemic modeling has revealed, for example, that in the event a new influenza strain emerges that is both highly transmissible and virulent, frontline emergency services such as healthcare workers will often be amongst the first to be adversely affected. This will have a detrimental effect on the healthcare sector, placing it under considerable strain at the precise time when demands for healthcare services will be at their peak. As the virus begins to spread further, it is likely that the effects will spread beyond the healthcare sector as sections of the community start to become sick and/or decide to voluntarily isolate themselves to reduce the risk of infection. If this scenario transpires, the resulting widespread absenteeism would have an adverse impact on not only general business activity, but could also adversely impact essential services such as water, sewerage, and transport, law and order, etc., as employees are unable or unwilling to go to work. National productivity may thus begin to decrease, adversely affecting a country's production outputs and terms of trade.

Added to the widespread societal effects, it is important to remember that in contrast to most disasters the nature of the pandemic threat is also prolonged, conceivably extending over years as opposed to just days or months. What this means in practical terms is that societies can be prevented from entering into a distinct recovery phase, and are instead forced to remain in a constant state of disaster readiness simply because they do not know when, or even if, another wave of infection will strike. This dynamic has subsequently led to the view amongst some policy-makers that if societies can adequately prepare for an influenza pandemic, they are effectively "prepared for anything" (Johnson 2009).

The objective of pandemic preparedness is usually twofold: (i) to save lives; and (ii) to ensure disruption to social functioning is minimized as much as possible. Given the nature of influenza pandemics and the fact that they are, by definition, widespread and can potentially affect every individual, policy-makers need to be cognisant of the wider societal and economic implications of such an event when developing preparedness strategies and plans. This approach has subsequently been termed "whole-of-society" or "whole-of-government" (or "WOG") preparedness, and is intended to incorporate every element of a community that is important to social functioning, from critical infrastructure and emergency responders, to the financial sector, business, and even tourism. In 2009, the World Health Organization (WHO) updated its pandemic preparedness guidelines to reflect a "whole-of-society" approach to planning, and all countries are being subsequently encouraged to adopt this approach (WHO 2009).

Whole-of-society planning operates on the premise that the impacts of an influenza pandemic will be disruptive, pervasive, and sustained, across every level of society. For these reasons, in a similar manner to other crisis management approaches (see McConnell and Drennan 2006), pandemic preparedness planning should ideally be led by officials at the highest level of government and include other government departments, organizations, and agencies beyond the ministry of health. The creation of specific national pandemic planning committees has been demonstrated to be one of the most effective means of progressing preparedness at the country level (Mounier-Jack and Coker 2006). However, it is equally important to acknowledge that once planning is complete, there is no one governance model that has proven to be more effective than another in embedding pandemic preparedness and response within government. In large part, this is because every government administration operates differently, with varying levels of centralization of services, lines of accountability, and departmental structures. Exactly where a national pandemic preparedness and response committee is located will therefore differ.

Yet while the shape and structure of governance arrangements may vary from country to country, the importance of visible political commitment from leaders and senior government officials cannot be understated in ensuring sufficient stakeholder engagement in pandemic planning and response efforts. This is particularly critical given that research has also demonstrated that there is a direct correlation between the comprehensiveness of pandemic preparedness plans (and the mitigation measures they may choose to adopt) and a country's income level and availability of funds (Hanvoravongchai *et al.* 2010). Without political commitment at the highest level, it is likely that pandemic planning will remain incomplete, or attract only minimal buy-in from stakeholders.

Engagement with a wide range of stakeholders, drawn from every sector of society, is critical for developing comprehensive pandemic preparedness plans. In an ideal context, this engagement would occur irrespective of whether services are provided by government departments, non-government organizations, or private enterprise. Government departments involved in the provision of public services and goods should, for instance, be encouraged to examine their activities and staffing levels to determine how they might continue to provide services when confronted with pandemic-related absenteeism and changing work patterns. Likewise, business and industry preferably would be encouraged to review their operations to identify key weaknesses that might prevent them from functioning, and then develop contingency plans to overcome or bypass those limitations. In the event non-government or civil society organizations provide essential services, those organizations would need to consider how they could continue to provide if volunteer workforces are reduced due to illness or absenteeism. As Whitley and Monto (2006) have noted, "The impact of the next influenza pandemic on the world's populations will be influenced, in part, by how well the medical, government, business, and lay communities are prepared."

In an ideal environment, however, consultation will not only occur *within* various groups of actors, but also *between* them. In other words, as much as it is important for each stakeholder group (e.g., government, civil society, business) to examine their own work practices to identify potential inefficiencies and develop remedial strategies to cope when confronted by a pandemic, it is also valuable for these different groups of actors to come together in the planning stages to understand the roles and responsibilities of each other. In so doing, each group of actors learn what to expect from each other and thereby hopefully avoid the risk that the actions and/or decisions taken by one group of actors will adversely affect another group. In fact, facilitating interdisciplinary consultation in the planning process is imperative for addressing expectations and avoiding confusion, particularly when different groups of actors can hold very divergent ideas on the roles, responsibilities, and accountability of stakeholders (Botoseneanu *et al.* 2010).

For example, it is crucial for business and industry to be aware of the mitigation strategies that a government may decide to implement in a pandemic. If policy-makers determine that school closures and shutting down childcare centers will be used to limit community transmission of an influenza virus (given that children are often highly infective due to poor hygiene practices), companies must be encouraged to consider how they would continue to operate in an environment where a percentage of their workforce may be required to remain at home during working hours to care for children. Can a business stagger their working hours to accommodate parents' needs? Can parents use information technology to work remotely from home? If so, does the company have the requisite infrastructure in place to support decentralized work practices? Is there a need for government to strengthen communication technology infrastructure to cope with a surge in activity? If parents are unable to work from home, what financial support and/or compensation will be provided so families can continue to pay their expenses? Is there any obligation on the government or the employer to provide such support? What level or percentage of wages – if any – would be considered appropriate?

Conversely, policy-makers need to be aware of the implications of enacting certain measures such as enforced quarantine for suspected or confirmed cases of influenza to limit transmission of the virus. This is particularly relevant when contemplating the nature of support mechanisms that such a policy would require to ensure compliance. For instance, if stringent measures are adopted whereby all members of a household are prevented from leaving their residence where a suspected or confirmed case of influenza is present, how will those families obtain food and other basic necessities? Would civil society organizations be called upon to assist? If so, what logistic requirements (e.g., food trucks) are necessary to support household quarantine? Would civil society organizations have the personnel to support such a massive undertaking, particularly if the outbreak is countrywide? How would such support be offered to rural and remote areas? If civil society organizations or faith-based groups were unable or unwilling to assist, would the military be drafted in to provide such support? What are the national security and/or law and order implications of reassigning the military to provide food relief? How will government enforce the quarantine if people do not participate voluntarily? Are new laws or regulations required to enact such measures, or do existing legal provisions allow for such measures? If the government is decentralized (i.e., a federal system) are lines of accountability and responsibility between jurisdictions clear and well understood? What are the ethical and/or civil liberty considerations of enforced quarantine? All these factors need to be considered well in advance of an actual pandemic, particularly if social functioning and basic law and order requirements are to be maintained.

Strategies to Mitigate Pandemic Influenza

In short, in order for pandemic planning to be comprehensively addressed, wide-ranging consultation must occur with every sector of society to prevent unforeseen consequences arising at a time of crisis. The focus of the remainder of this chapter is to examine specific measures that policy-makers and practitioners may wish to consider in preparing for an influenza pandemic. Mitigation measures can be broadly categorized into two types, namely, pharmaceutical-based interventions, such as influenza vaccines and antiviral medications, and non-pharmaceutical measures such as quarantine and isolation, social distancing measures (e.g., school and childcare center closures, cancellation of mass gatherings), and personal protective measures (e.g., hand-washing, use of facemasks).

Pharmaceutical Measures (Vaccines and Antivirals)

Since the late 1950s, influenza vaccines have been widely regarded as the "cornerstone" of pandemic preparedness (see, for example, Hota and McGeer 2007). When they were first invented, vaccines were perceived to be of limited utility (Kamradt-Scott 2012), but by 1959, sufficient evidence had been gathered from various clinical trials that led the WHO Expert Committee on Respiratory Virus Diseases to conclude that vaccines were an "efficient" means of protecting human populations, and that, "A reduction in the incidence of the disease of two-thirds or more has repeatedly been observed" (WHO 1959: 15). Over the next decade, emphasis was increasingly placed on refining the vaccines to ensure better efficacy, less toxicity, and greater yield within a shorter timeframe. In 1969, the WHO unambiguously declared that, "Vaccination is the only established procedure for conferring protection against influenza" (WHO 1969: 39). As a result, vaccines have been actively promoted (and increasingly viewed) as the definitive measure for preventing and controlling influenza epidemics and pandemics. All governments have subsequently – and repeatedly – been encouraged by organizations such as the WHO to secure access to vaccines, as they are assessed to be the most effective means of helping to reduce influenza-related morbidity and mortality.

The advent of influenza antiviral medications in the late 1960s added to the pharmacological arsenal for pandemic preparedness, although their widespread use in treating influenza was not promoted until the 1990s. While vaccines had been subject to evaluation for decades, even by the 1990s, few clinical trials had been conducted to demonstrate the efficacy of antivirals against seasonal and pandemic influenza (Hota and McGeer 2007). However, in the wake of the 1997 H5N1 avian influenza outbreak in Hong Kong, the importance of antiviral medications took on new significance. As a result, antiviral medications were soon identified alongside vaccines as "the two most important medical interventions for reducing illness and deaths during a pandemic" (IMF 2006: 12), and by the beginning of the twenty-first century they were being actively promoted by leading governance institutions engaged in strengthening epidemic and pandemic influenza preparedness such as the WHO, United Nations System Influenza Coordination (UNSIC), International Monetary Fund (IMF), and World Bank (WHO 2004; Dutta 2008).

Although scientific consensus maintains that vaccines and antiviral medications are the preferred means of protecting human populations from pandemic influenza, several notable constraints to accessing these vital pharmaceuticals exist. The most significant constraint to date is that the global production capacity of both influenza vaccines and antiviral medications remains limited. In 2002, approximately 292 million does of influenza vaccine were distributed worldwide (Fedson 2005). Although by 2006, production capacity had increased over a third to an estimated 350–425 million doses per year, the majority of the world's manufacturing capacity for influenza vaccines remained based in only nine industrialized countries (Emanuel and Wertheimer 2006; Kieny et al. 2006). Since 2006, the WHO has overseen a project to increase global vaccine production capacity in low- and middle-income countries, but the WHO *Global Action Plan to Increase Pandemic Influenza Vaccine Supply* (GAP) has not been able to secure long-term, sustainable funding, with the corresponding outcome that once the current tranche of funding expires, further increases in global production capacity will likely stall (Kamradt-Scott and Lee 2011).

Likewise, to date, the global manufacturing capacity for two primary antiviral medications – oseltamivir (otherwise known as Tamiflu®) and zanamivir (brand name Relenza®) – has been restricted to a limited number of companies. Unlike vaccines that confer immunity, the two preferred antiviral medications are in a class of drugs known as neuraminidase inhibitors that work by binding to the neuraminidase proteins on the surface structure of the influenza virus, thereby preventing the virus from attaching to and invading a host cell, where it would replicate. Ahead of the 2009 H1N1 influenza pandemic, Roche (the company that produces oseltamivir) and GlaxoSmithKline (who produce zanamivir) had reportedly increased their manufacturing capacity of the neuraminidase inhibitors, but total annual production still remained limited to an estimated 400 million and 190 million treatment courses, respectively (GSK 2009; Reddy 2010). Needless to say, despite the fact these companies have more than doubled their manufacturing capacity of these drugs over the previous decade – usually through sublicensing arrangements with other pharmaceutical companies to produce the drugs – global supplies remain far short of the demand that would be generated by another pandemic (Enserink 2006). As a direct consequence, given that global supply will inevitably not meet demand, governments are forced into deciding on whether they will allocate limited financial resources to establish a national stockpile of antiviral medications – with the related expense of maintaining that stockpile over time as the drugs have a limited shelf-life – for an event that only occurs periodically.

Compounding pharmaceutical production constraints has been the widespread use of advance purchase agreements (APAs). Particularly since 2005, a number of high-income countries have been observed to pre-purchase influenza vaccine and antiviral supplies via APAs. Under these agreements, pharmaceutical manufacturers are contractually obliged to supply governments with APAs ahead of making drug supplies commercially available. This means that countries that do not possess equivalent arrangements are forced to wait until APA drug orders are filled, which may take months or even years (see Chapter 16). Such practices thereby exacerbate the length of time that low-income countries must potentially wait to access these essential, life-saving treatments. Given that influenza vaccines currently take on average between three and six months after a pandemic has begun to be available for community-wide vaccination programs, and that there remains a limited number of pharmaceutical manufacturers authorized to produce antivirals, the WHO has conceded that most low-income countries will not be able to access these drugs for at least the first wave of the pandemic (Fedson and Dunnill 2007).

In recognition of these systemic challenges to access, in 2005 the WHO established a limited stockpile of antiviral medications, with donations from pharmaceutical manufacturers, that low-income countries could access based on demonstrated need. This was followed in late 2006 with the WHO GAP strategy that aims to increase local manufacturing capacity for influenza vaccines amongst low-income countries (Kamradt-Scott and Lee 2011). Critically though, even these measures fail to satisfactorily address the significant shortfall that will arise in the event of a pandemic. Accordingly, many low- and middle-income countries are forced, by necessity, to consider other non-pharmaceutical-based measures to counter the spread and human impacts of an influenza pandemic. Indeed, policy-makers arguably need to consider their ability (or lack thereof) to access pharmaceuticals during a pandemic in the planning and preparation stages. As Oshitani *et al.* (2008: 878–9) have observed, non-pharmaceutical measures "may be the only available interventions" that low-income countries can implement.

Aside from these systemic challenges, however, policy-makers also need to consider the various technical and logistical challenges associated with pharmaceutical-based interventions. For example, if governments do decide to allocate financial resources to purchasing influenza vaccines, additional equipment such as syringes and needles, as well as adequately trained healthcare workers to administer the medications, are essential. A well-developed road network and transport infrastructure to disseminate pharmaceutical supplies is also required, particularly where populations are geographically dispersed. Related to this, policy-makers must take into account whether pharmaceutical supplies, such as vaccines, require refrigeration – both while in storage and in transport – in order for them to remain viable. Needless to say, technical and logistic issues of this nature can present significant challenges to policy-makers in low-income countries, particularly where resources are already limited (Oshitani *et al.* 2008).

Non-Pharmaceutical Measures (Basically, Everything Else)

Although leading governance institutions such as the WHO continue to emphasize the importance of securing access to influenza vaccines and antivirals as the preferred pandemic preparedness strategy (WHO 2004), it is important to recall that pharmaceutical-based interventions are not the only measures available to policy-makers. In fact, there is a wide array of options that policy-makers may choose from in developing national preparedness plans. To date, clinical trials into the effectiveness of some non-pharmaceutical measures have been limited, with the corresponding outcome that the evidence base remains undeveloped. However, a wide range of modeling exercises have been conducted; in the wake of the 2009 H1N1 pandemic, many of these measures have now been extensively tested, generating new data that will facilitate assessing their effectiveness for future pandemics (Halder *et al.* 2010). Even if the 2009 H1N1 pandemic had not occurred though, given that global supplies of influenza vaccines and antiviral medications will remain curtailed for the foreseeable future, no government can afford to rely on a strategy that relies solely on pharmaceutical measures.

At present, non-pharmaceutical measures can be described as falling into three broad categories: quarantine and isolation, social distancing measures, and personal hygiene practices. Since at least the fourteenth century, officials have used various quarantine and isolation practices to limit the spread of infectious diseases. While the methods used may have changed over time, the principle and objective of quarantine has effectively remained the same – namely, to seclude from society an individual who is either suspected or confirmed to have contracted an infectious disease, thereby limiting the opportunity for the disease to spread. The focus of quarantine and isolation practices correspondingly rests on the individual(s) and limiting their opportunity to spread disease. Particularly in the wake of the 2003 SARS outbreak, a number of governments have either passed new or revised existing legislation that allows officials to forcibly quarantine individuals if it is deemed in the public interest and/or safety (Tay *et al.* 2010). However, such practices do raise ethical and cultural concerns, and policy-makers must also take into account the extent such laws may infringe on civil liberties when applying the public interest test (Gostin and Berkman 2007).

By way of contrast, social distancing measures – as the phrase implies – are community-level interventions that aim to limit the amount of close personal interaction between individuals. Social distancing measures have been demonstrated to be effective in some circumstances primarily because, as Bansal *et al.* (2010: 2) have noted, "Influenza spreads during close contacts between susceptible and infected individuals. The likelihood of a person becoming exposed to disease will strongly depend on the number and intensity of his or her interactions." Thus, the rationale is to limit all personal interaction as much as possible, thereby reducing the opportunity for influenza to spread.

In recognition of the fact that children are often the most susceptible to a new strain of influenza and that poor personal hygiene practices often mean that children can serve as effective vectors in spreading influenza (Bansal *et al.* 2010), a number of governments have adopted policies to close schools and childcare centers in a pandemic. Some governments have also chosen to extend this policy to universities. In so doing, the aim is to limit the amount of personal interaction between students, thereby reducing the risk of immediate human-to-human transmission as well as hopefully avoiding the chance of an infected person spreading the disease to other family members. Importantly, however, there are a range of individual and societal risks and consequences associated with school and childcare closures, such as the adverse impact on student learning, which could be extensive and have long-term intergenerational implications if the policy is extended over the duration of a pandemic and additional support mechanisms such as home schooling are not provided. In addition, school and childcare center closures can have an adverse impact on household income if one or more parent is required to stay home and care for the children. As the 2009 H1N1 influenza pandemic revealed, the economic impacts from even short-term application of school and childcare center closures can be significant (Aburto *et al.* 2010). In circumstances where such policies were maintained on a long-term basis (e.g., months or years) it can be anticipated to result in lost productivity and a decrease in national gross domestic product (Sander *et al.* 2009).

In addition to weighing up such factors, policy-makers must also consider how other interventions may support or hinder the objective of limiting the spread of disease. For example, the benefits derived from closing schools may be negated if children are instead able to congregate in locations such as shopping centers or movie theaters. Accordingly, wider social distancing policies such as the cancellation of mass gatherings like sporting events and even church services may be deemed appropriate or necessary. Likewise, if individuals are encouraged under social distancing measures to remain, for example, 1 metre apart at all times, policy-makers need to consider how this can be achieved on public transport or while seeking essential items such as food. It is in this regard that further measures such as extending the trading hours of shopping centers and markets, or increasing the number of buses and trains, may be required to reduce the need for people to gather in large numbers during peak periods. If social distancing principles are applied universally, policy-makers may also need to consult with industry representatives to determine how best to minimize the impact on business productivity. It may be, for example, that manufacturing plants could stagger their work hours or institute shift work for employees to minimize interpersonal contact. Alternatively, if the requisite infrastructure is in place, employees may be able to work from home, thereby limiting their risk of exposure. In short, even from this brief survey it can be seen that there are a variety of factors that policy-makers must consider prior to implementing one particular measure. This importantly includes taking into account the wider societal and/or economic consequences that can arise from a particular policy, as well as considering how policies may further exacerbate or reduce the effectiveness of other public health measures.

The third type of non-pharmaceutical measures that policy-makers can encourage relate to personal hygiene practices. Regular hand-washing has long been considered an important measure in limiting the spread of diseases like influenza (Jefferson *et al.* 2008). Although recent studies have questioned the overall effectiveness of this practice in the context of a pandemic (Oshitani *et al.* 2008), most health professionals continue to maintain that hand-washing remains an important tool for individuals to reduce their risk of exposure (Grayson *et al.* 2009). Similar personal hygiene practices such as cough and sneeze etiquette are also likely to limit the spread of influenza given that the virus is often spread via small airborne droplets (Poalillo *et al.* 2010), and individuals can be encouraged to adhere to such practices through public health campaigns prior to, and throughout, an influenza pandemic.

One intervention where there appears to be considerably less consensus is the use of facemasks in non-clinical settings. Facemasks, when used by trained professionals and fitted correctly with a fine filter (specifically N95), have been demonstrated to be effective in preventing the transmission of influenza in healthcare settings (Loeb *et al.* 2009). Although some governments have subsequently developed pandemic preparedness plans that promote the widespread use of facemasks amongst the general population, evidence of their effectiveness in community or non-clinical environments remains undetermined (MacIntyre *et al.* 2009). Added to this, arguably some policy-makers have been reluctant to promote the use of facemasks because of concerns that it may raise expectations that governments will then be responsible for developing stockpiles of personal protective equipment. In an environment where the evidence on the effectiveness of facemasks in community settings remains poor, it can be appreciated why some governments have chosen to invest their limited resources on other, more proven, means of protecting the public from influenza.

Further, it is important for governments (and by default policy-makers) to plan for the increase in demand for health services that an influenza pandemic will undoubtedly generate. Indeed, it is well recognized that influenza pandemics place additional burdens on healthcare services, both with respect to treating those individuals with genuine illnesses as well as dealing with the "worried well" – namely, those individuals who may not exhibit symptoms but are concerned about their well-being sufficiently that they seek medical assistance (Hanfling and Hick 2009). Due to the nature of the illness, intensive and/or critical care services – both in terms of trained personnel and equipment – are often in high demand (Menon *et al.* 2005), and yet even many high-income countries fail to have sufficient surge capacity to deal with the demand precipitated by an influenza pandemic (McKenna 2006). Influenza pandemics may also require healthcare providers to jettison other non-essential services and/or procedures in order to divert critical resources to dealing with the pandemic. In these circumstances, close collaboration will be required with public (and, if available, private) healthcare providers in order to meet the demand that will be created by a health crisis such as an influenza pandemic. Clear lines of accountability in decision-making, and consistency in decision-making, must also be maintained.

At the global level, considerably more research into assessing the efficacy and effectiveness of non-pharmaceutical measures, and investment in strengthening pandemic response capacity – both in terms of global pharmaceutical production capacity and health system strengthening – will be critical for enhancing preparedness. Indeed, as highlighted above, the evidence base of a number of non-pharmaceutical measures currently remains underdeveloped. Further research and evaluation of non-pharmaceutical measures will therefore be critical in addressing existing knowledge gaps regarding the effectiveness of particular interventions such as school and childcare center closures, public health campaigns that promote regular hand-washing, and the like. This is particularly important for low-income countries that will likely struggle to gain access to influenza-related pharmaceuticals (i.e., vaccines and antivirals) to protect their populations due to supply constraints. It is also in this regard that there is a genuine need for further investment in strengthening global vaccine production capacity – either through direct government investment or via increased funding for collective mechanisms such as the WHO GAP strategy (Kamradt-Scott and Lee 2011). Finally, considerable state-level investment will also be essential for strengthening health systems so they are better prepared to respond to the multiple challenges that influenza pandemics generate. Wide-ranging and long-term investment will be essential in building and strengthening disease surveillance and outbreak response systems, training healthcare personnel, and building the healthcare facilities and laboratories that support an effective pandemic response.

Conclusions

Despite the fact that the 2009 H1N1 influenza pandemic was less severe than many public health officials and policy-makers had initially feared, influenza epidemics and pandemics are a regular feature of human existence. It can be anticipated, therefore, that governments will once again be confronted by this recurrent threat at some point in the future. Accordingly, there is an expectation that governments will be better prepared to respond to such an event, and this chapter has sought to provide a brief overview and examination of the issues and challenges confronting policy-makers in developing "whole-of-government" (or "whole-of-society") pandemic preparedness plans. The chapter commenced with a short summary on the nature of the threat, noting that influenza pandemics are unlike the majority of natural disasters and other crises in that they are non-linear, multidimensional events that are not geographically isolated or limited. Influenza pandemics are caused when a novel strain of the virus emerges to which humans have little to no immunity, and the virus achieves the ability to easily transmit between humans. As a result, pandemics can cause high human morbidity and mortality, and can have profound and far-reaching social and economic impacts. Particularly since 1997, and the resurgence of the H5N1 avian influenza virus, leading governance institutions such as the WHO and the purpose-built UNSIC have been at the forefront in encouraging governments to better prepare to confront this threat. In order to accomplish this objective, policy-makers and officials have been urged to develop pandemic preparedness strategies in consultation with all sectors of society, from business and industry to the voluntary and non-government sector, and to prepare contingency plans to ensure that social and economic disruption is kept to a minimum while also protecting human lives.

Ultimately, influenza pandemics are, unfortunately, events that humanity regularly confronts. There is little doubt that new strains of influenza will continue to emerge, and periodically, a new virus will also achieve effective human-to-human transmission. Societies the world over have developed a reasonable expectation that governments will help to protect them from such threats, and health professionals and policy-makers are at the forefront in developing plans to reduce the impact of such events. In this regard, the 2009 H1N1 influenza pandemic has provided the international community a valuable opportunity to test response mechanisms and further evaluate the effectiveness of various public health measures – information that is essential in developing comprehensive preparedness plans. At the same time, however, further preparation and planning is and will be required to offset and minimize the extent of society-wide, intergenerational impacts.

Note

1. In December 2011 it was revealed that two groups of scientists based in the Netherlands and the United States had successfully manipulated the H5N1 avian influenza virus into a

highly transmissible, airborne strain in ferrets, which have respiratory systems very similar to humans.

Key Reading

Bennett B. 2009. Legal rights during pandemics: federalism, rights and public health laws – a view from Australia. *Public Health* 123, 232–236.

Braunack-Mayer A, Street J, Rogers W, Givney R, Moss J, Hiller J and Flu Views Team. 2010. Including the public in pandemic planning: a deliberative approach. *BMC Public Health* 10, 501.

Fauci A. 2006. Seasonal and pandemic influenza preparedness: science and countermeasures. *Journal of Infectious Diseases* 194(Suppl 2), S73–S76.

Fedson D. 2009. Meeting the challenge of influenza pandemic preparedness in developing countries. *Emerging Infectious Diseases* 15(3), 365–71.

Lee K, Fidler D. 2007. Avian and pandemic influenza: progress and problems with global health governance. *Global Public Health* 2(3), 215–34.

Thompson A, Faith K, Gibson J, Upshur R. 2006. Pandemic influenza preparedness: an ethical framework to guide decision-making. *BMC Medical Ethics* 7, 12.

WHO (World Health Organization). 2012. *Influenza.* http://www.who.int/topics/influenza/en/ (last accessed December 2013).

References

Aburto N, Pevzner E, Lopez-Ridaura R *et al*. 2010. Knowledge and adoption of community mitigation efforts in Mexico during the 2009 H1N1 pandemic. *American Journal of Preventive Medicine* 39(5), 395–402.

Bansal S, Pourbohlol B, Hupert N, Grenfell B, Meyers L. 2010. The shifting demographic landscape of pandemic influenza. *PLOS One* 5(2), e9360.

Botoseneanu A, Wu H, Wasserman J, Jacobson P. 2010. Achieving public health legal preparedness: how dissonant views on public health law threaten emergency preparedness and response. *Journal of Public Health* 33(3), 361–8.

Dutta A. 2008. *The Effectiveness of Policies to Control a Human Influenza Pandemic: A Literature Review.* Policy Research Working Paper No. 4524. Washington, DC: World Bank.

Emanuel E, Wertheimer A. 2006. Who should get influenza vaccine when not all can? *Science* 312(5775), 854–5.

Enserink M. 2006. Oseltamivir becomes plentiful – but still not cheap. *Science* 312(5772), 382–3.

Fedson D. 2005. Preparing for pandemic vaccination: an international policy agenda for vaccine development. *Journal of Public Health Policy* 26, 4–29.

Fedson D, Dunnill P. 2007. From scarcity to abundance: pandemic vaccines and other agents for "have not" countries. *Journal of Public Health Policy* 28(3), 322–40.

Gostin L, Berkman B. 2007. Pandemic influenza: ethics, law, and the public's health. *Administrative Law Review* 59, 121–75.

Grayson M, Melvani S, Druce J *et al*. 2009. Efficacy of soap and water and alcohol-based handrub preparations against live H1N1 influenza virus on the hands of human volunteers. *Clinical Infectious Diseases* 48(3), 285–91.

GSK (GlaxoSmithKline). 2009. *Pandemic (H1N1) 2009 influenza FAQ.* http://www.gsk.com/media/flu_faq.htm#%3Cem%3ERelenza%3C/em%3E (last accessed February 2012).

Halder N, Kelso J, Milne G. 2010. Analysis of the effectiveness of interventions used during the 2009 A/H1N1 influenza pandemic. *BMC Public Health* 10, 168.

Hanfling D, Hick J. 2009. Hospitals and the novel H1N1 outbreak: the mouse that roared? *Disaster Medicine and Public Health Preparedness* 3(Suppl 2), s100–s106.

Hanvoravongchai P, Adisasmito W, Chau P *et al.* 2010. Pandemic influenza preparedness and health systems challenges in Asia: results from rapid analyses in 6 Asian countries. *BMC Public Health* 10, 322.

Hota S, McGeer A, 2007. Antivirals and the control of influenza outbreaks. *Clinical Infectious Diseases* 45(10), 1362–8.

IMF (International Monetary Fund). 2006. *The Global Economic and Financial Impact of an Avian Flu Pandemic and the Role of the IMF*. Washington, DC: IMF.

Jefferson T, Foxlee R, Del Mar C *et al.* 2008. Physical interventions to interrupt or reduce the spread of respiratory viruses: systematic review. *BMJ* 336(7635), 77–80.

Johnson T. 2009. Arizona affiliate helping state's employers prepare for H1N1 flu. *Nation's Health* 39(8), 13.

Kamradt-Scott A. 2012. The politics of medicine and the global governance of pandemic influenza. *International Journal of Health Services* 43, 105–21.

Kamradt-Scott A, Lee K. 2011. The pandemic influenza preparedness framework: global health secured or a missed opportunity? *Political Studies* 59(4), 831–47.

Kieny M, Costa A, Hombach J, Carrasco P, Pervikov Y and the WHO (World Health Organization). 2006. A global pandemic influenza action plan. *Vaccine* 24(40–41), 6367–70.

Kolata G. 1999. *Flu: The Story of the Great Influenza Pandemic of 1918 and the Search for the Virus that Caused It*. New York: Farrar, Straus, and Giroux.

Loeb M, Dafoe N, Mahony J *et al.* 2009. Surgical mask vs N95 respirator for preventing influenza among health care workers. *JAMA* 302(17), 1865–71.

MacIntyre C, Cauchemez S, Dwyer D *et al.* 2009. Face mask use and control of respiratory virus transmission in households. *Emerging Infectious Diseases* 15(2), 233–41.

McConnell A, Drennan L. 2006. Mission impossible? Planning and preparing for crisis. *Journal of Contingencies and Crisis Management* 14(2), 59–70.

McKenna M. 2006. Anatomy of a pandemic: emergency departments woefully unprepared for bird flu outbreak. *Annals of Emergency Medicine* 48(3), 312–14.

Menon D, Taylor B, Ridley S. 2005. Modelling the impact of an influenza pandemic on critical care services in England. *Anaesthesia* 60(10), 952–4.

Mounier-Jack S, Coker R. 2006. How prepared is Europe for pandemic influenza? Analysis of national plans. *Lancet* 367(9520), 1405–11.

Oshitani H, Kamigaki T, Suzuki A. 2008. Major issues and challenges of influenza pandemic preparedness in developing countries. *Emerging Infectious Diseases* 14(6), 875–80.

Osterholm M. 2005. Preparing for the next pandemic. *New England Journal of Medicine* 352(18), 1839–42.

Poalillo F, Geiling J, Jimenez E. 2010. Healthcare personnel and nosocomial transmission of pandemic 2009 influenza. *Critical Care Medicine* 38(Suppl), e98–e102.

Reddy D. 2010. Responding to pandemic (H1N1) 2009 influenza: the role of oseltamivir. *Journal of Antimicrobial Chemotherapy* 65(Suppl 2), ii35–ii40.

Sander B, Nizam A, Garrison L, Postma M, Halloran E, Longini R. 2009. Economic evaluation of influenza pandemic mitigation strategies in the United States using a stochastic microsimulation transmission model. *Value in Health* 12(2), 226–33.

Tay J, Ng Y, Cutter J, James L. 2010. Influenza A (H1N1-2009) pandemic in Singapore – public health control measures implemented and lessons learnt. *Annals Academy of Medicine* 39(4), 313–24.

Whitley R, Monto A. 2006. Seasonal and pandemic influenza preparedness: a global threat. *Journal of Infectious Diseases* 194(Suppl 2), S65–S69.

WHO (World Health Organization). 1959. *Expert Committee on Respiratory Viruses: First Report*. Technical Report Series No. 170. Geneva: WHO.

WHO (World Health Organization). 1969. *Respiratory Viruses: Report of a WHO Scientific Group*. Technical Report Series No. 408. Geneva: WHO.

WHO (World Health Organization). 2004. *WHO Influenza Pandemic Preparedness Check-list*. Geneva: WHO. http://www.wpro.who.int/internet/resources.ashx/CSR/Publications/WHO+Influenza+Pandemic+Preparedness+Checklist.pdf (last accessed February 2011).

WHO (World Health Organization). 2009. *Pandemic Influenza Preparedness and Response: A WHO Guidance Document*. Geneva: WHO.

WHO (World Health Organization). 2010. *Pandemic (H1N1) 2009 – update 112*. http://www.who.int/csr/don/2010_08_06/en/index.html (last accessed December 2013).

Chapter 30

Globalization and Global Health

Matt X. Richardson, Mike M. Callaghan, and Sarah Wamala

Abstract

Globalization is a multifocal multivariate process that affects health through increasing interconnectedness in global economic, political, and cultural realms. Its modern engines and agendas are different from in the past, but its effects on capital flows, and on our subsistence, nutrition, and living environments have been consistently pervasive and powerful. This has contributed greatly to improved human health and development, but not for all – and there are clear risks where the negative aspects of globalization amplify continued imbalances in the future. This chapter presents the role that international policy has in globalization and health over time, and the complications for global health that may arise when various sectors collide. Greater policy coherence in the future, with health as the foundation for decision-making, may ensure that greater global interconnectedness is to the benefit of all.

The Handbook of Global Health Policy, First Edition. Edited by Garrett W. Brown, Gavin Yamey, and Sarah Wamala.
© 2014 John Wiley & Sons, Ltd. Published 2014 by John Wiley & Sons, Ltd.

Key Points

- Information and knowledge access and exchange has increased exponentially, while governments' ability to control and influence information flows has diminished.
- Increased access to global markets has intensified trade between countries and regions, as well as competition between sectors and individual tasks.
- Urbanization continues to occur on a massive scale, while the influence of rural and agricultural sectors continues to diminish. Nutritional production and supply is increasingly uniform and large-scale, but global shortages and rapid price fluctuations are still prevalent.
- Non-communicable diseases have become the greatest cause of mortality in developing countries (as developed countries' living and consumption patterns spread globally), but globalization has also raised the risk for the re-emergence of infectious disease.

Key Policy Implications

- Increased global competition makes it more essential, but also more difficult, to respond with appropriate macro-level policies to ensure trade fairness, healthy working conditions, and employment.
- Trade and market policies should aim to increase access for smaller players in both rural and urban environments as well as increase the variety of healthier products and services globally.
- Policy-makers must urgently work toward globally coordinated monitoring, reporting, and response to disease outbreaks and a rationalized global accord on the use of antibiotics in humans and animals.
- Overall, policies must focus on protecting the health of those on the periphery of globalization and most likely to fall ill of it; and on fine-tuning global integration such that the benefits are more evenly spread amongst populations, and within and between countries.

Introduction

Globalization is everywhere and nowhere: a pervasive, powerful force that shapes the trivial and transcontinental alike, but remains elusive and complex – a process whose precise definition is fleeting and whose causes and effects defy easy explanation. Objectively, developments in technology – especially communications and transport – have clearly created unprecedented global interconnectedness, particularly in the economic realm. Critically, this process is often seen to serve the interests of market capitalism by perpetually subsuming the local and reproducing itself in new spheres (Mácha and Drobík 2011). Philosophically, the core of globalization may be a massive new flow of ideas that are appropriated in new places and in new ways (Romer 2010) and bind disparate communities together in new social relations (Giddens 1990). We do not belabor the definition of globalization, but treat it as a multifocal multivariate process with different engines and agendas in different places and times – economically, politically, and culturally (Brown and Labonté 2011).

In this chapter, we take for granted the reality of globalization, however complex it may be. We also take for granted that the most important effects of globalization are its impacts on human health and well-being. Health should be the ultimate "downstream variable" in the assessment of globalization, an "index" of the lived, human-level consequences of the reshaping of our world. In short, if globalization is not making us healthier, it is not working. Finally, as the overarching theme of the chapter, we ask what role policy-makers can have in globalization and health. There are few explicit "globalization policies" among governments and international organizations that encompass the many sectors that contribute to integration in global society. There is therefore substantial risk that these various sectors may contradict or collide with each other, complicating their effects on health.

Below, we offer a longitudinal analysis of globalization's past, present, and future. In keeping with our treatment of globalization as a multifaceted process, we examine five key sectors with clear implications for health: communication, capital, subsistence, the lived environment, and disease. We illustrate this discussion with references to policy, peer-reviewed literature, and examples from the ethnographic record.

History of Globalization and Health

Our consideration of globalization begins with a look at the past. The historical record, and ethnographic evidence from preliterate societies, can inform our understanding of globalization. Below, we examine past trends in our five key areas, which will run through our assessment of the present and our predictions for the future.

Information and Knowledge Access and Exchange

In preliterate hunting and gathering societies, abstract knowledge was (and is) shared orally, prioritizing depth of transmission at the cost of speed and breadth. This remained essentially unchanged for thousands of years, despite myriad changes in other aspects of life associated with the transformation from nomadic foraging to settled agrarianism. Knowledge about subsistence is a shared concern; among the !Kung San, for instance, there is so little division and specialization of labor that most adults can produce everything needed for their family's survival (Lee 1979). Medical knowledge in such societies is often arcane and conflated with ritual and spiritual knowledge, frequently concerning the dangerously powerful or liminal (Douglas 2002). Acquisition of healing knowledge therefore usually involves long periods of apprenticeship and transition through ceremonial rites of passage (Van Gennep 1960).

The extraordinary rate at which these communication forms have changed for the majority of the world's population over a relatively short period of time has had enormous consequences for human health and progress. Each step in the development of "modern" systems of communicating information resulted in a massive increase in information availability, the means to exchange it, and the speed of that exchange (Willmore 2001). Government restriction generally followed closely thereafter – albeit often with limited success. The invention of the printing press in the fifteenth century dramatically increased printed volumes and literacy rates in Europe, but also prompted a government-backed Catholic Church decree strictly regulating print and banning many titles. Postal systems, telegraph and telephone services, and radio and television were, or still are, subject to government monopolization. The health effects of this kind of information control are debatable. Historically, government control over the flow of information has afforded a good opportunity to deliver public health messaging; the durability of that control, however, has been poor. While information sources were more discernible, they were also heavily subject to the political wills of the day, which may not always have been concerned with the well-being of the average citizen.

Ironically, the precursor to the modern-day Internet was a government military project, ARPANET. Although relatively easy to regulate, it grew remarkably quickly into a largely uncontrolled form of private communication, with the highest rate and volume of information exchange seen yet.

Formal and Informal Flows of Capital

Trade and markets   The increase in global trade is considered to be one of the defining characteristics of globalization. For centuries, merchandise trade has grown faster than output. In 1820, merchandise exports as a share of global gross domestic product (GDP) was 1%, growing to 5% in 1870 and 8% in 1913 (1990 prices; Maddison 2001). The last few decades have seen a dramatic increase, however, with exports rising from 19% of global GDP in 1979 to 26% by 2004 (Sandri *et al.* 2007). A brief history of the globalization of trade helps contextualize its significance for health.

The Western European mercantilism that dominated much of the sixteenth to eighteenth centuries placed the welfare of the individual behind that of the state, but as the inexpensive movement of bulk commodities between continents increased, commodity prices between countries converged, affecting resource allocation within nations and improving overall living standards. These processes were well established by the nineteenth century (O'Rourke and Williamson 2002), leading many to describe globalization as a 200-year-old phenomenon.

International trade had a large impact on domestic politics in the nineteenth century, especially during the Industrial Revolution, increasing urban economic activity by promoting the placement of large factories in cities, by developing roads, rails, and canals, and through legislation that weakened urban craft guilds to the advantage of the mercantile class. This engendered major changes known as the "first great unbundling" of globalization (Baldwin 2006): goods could now be produced further from their intended markets, and urban centers offered larger denser markets, higher real wages, and greater capital. The growth gap that resulted between the northern and southern regions of the globe during the unbundling remains today (Baldwin *et al.* 2001; also see Chapter 21).

The nature of labor and competition during this period also made it relatively easier to predict "winners and losers" and in global competition, a theme to which we return.

The General Agreement on Tariffs and Trade (GATT) negotiations signed in 1947 further reduced trade barriers established by industrialized countries in response to high unemployment during the Depression and the World Wars. The GATT prescribed reciprocity between developed countries, while allowing developing countries greater freedoms to control tariffs and imports to protect their growth. This "differential and more favorable treatment" allowed developed nations to more easily promote imports in their own markets.

A general exception to these trends was agriculture, where price fluctuations on the international market were promoted by a combination of protectionist policies in developed countries and anti-agricultural policies in developing countries (Anderson 2010). Global agricultural trade decreased from more than 30% in the 1960s to less than 9% on average since 2000 (Sandri *et al.* 2007). Governmental policies were a major contributor to this drop: the rate of assistance for farmers in developed countries grew from around 20% in the 1950s to 50% in the 1980s, and fell to approximately 30% at the turn of the millennium; over the same period the average rate of assistance for developing countries rose more continually, but from a starting level of around −25% to +5%. The resulting overproduction in developed countries and underproduction in developing countries has been implicated in global poverty (and its related health effects) as the majority of the world's poor are heavily reliant on agricultural incomes (Anderson 2010).

Human capital   Human capital is another form of capital whose flows are affected by globalization and, in turn, have an impact on health. The concept traces back to Sir William Petty's work in the late seventeenth century on the cash value of human beings, and by extension the costs to England of war, disease, and migration (Kiker 1966). A person whose "production cost" is offset by substantial future earnings might be said to embody a great deal of human capital, and therefore merit substantial investments of education, healthcare, national defense, and legal protection. Globalization has had important effects on the movements of human beings and the investments governments make on their behalf.

While contemporary hunter–gatherer societies are highly mobile and have fluid territorial boundaries (Devore and Lee 1968), they generally move as an entire community and on foot, at approximately 4–5 kilometers per hour (Lee 1979). Pack animals and boats expanded human range and speed in the agricultural age, but large-scale and long-distance migrations remained limited, particularly by morbidity and mortality. Like today, much mobility during this period was economically motivated, such as commodities exploration during the Middle Ages, but loss of human capital was often great: of the approximately 2400 Portugese sailors who left annually in the spice trade, fully half did not return (Fleming 2004). Ultimately, migration and long-distance trade during this period was risky, slow, and usually unidirectional, making investments in human resources conservative, local, and static.

The involuntary and unethical movement of human resources was also a powerful cause and effect of globalization, with major implications for health. Over 12 million Africans were shipped to the Americas in the transatlantic slave trade of the sixteenth to nineteenth centuries, with enormous human losses due to disease, abuse, and executions. Government policies started this horrendous period and also largely put an end to it, with the enactment of British Slave Trade Act (1807), Abolition (1837), and the American Emancipation Proclamation (1863) and Constitutional Amendment (1865).

This altered human capital flows immensely, as many firms employed migrants moving between Europe and the colonies. Globalization during this period was driven by mass migration, with roughly 60 million people fleeing the labor oversupply in Europe. This resulted in income gaps in many of these countries, further promoting migration. In many cases these countries established government immigration infrastructure to promote and manage the influx and promote continued economic development, although this did not occur without social turmoil.

Nourishment and Subsistence

Human subsistence for 99% of our time on Earth has been based on some combination of hunting and gathering. About 12,000 years ago, the Neolithic Revolution saw most humans move from food foraging to food production. This move had mixed effects on health: agriculture reduces the energy costs of collecting food, but decreases dietary diversity and resilience in the face of crop failures and extreme weather. Food surpluses went hand-in-hand with higher birth rates, technological development, and the emergence of civilization. The osteological record, however, almost universally shows that the switch to agriculture brings with it decreased height, increased chronic nutritional stress, and generally ill-health (Cohen and Armelagos 1984). In comparison, contemporary hunter–gatherers like the !Kung San spend roughly 20 hours per week meeting all of their subsistence needs, leaving a large amount of time for leisure. Tasks were unspecialized and labor shared; before hunts, men would exchange arrows randomly so that no single hunter could take full credit for a kill. Because they have no need for surplus, production never outstrips subsistence except perhaps to feed pets and provide food for visitors and ceremonies. !Kung San calorie intake is estimated at roughly 2355 kcal/day, suggesting their subsistence does not require taxing physical effort; for this reason foragers were once dubbed "the original affluent society" (Sahlins 1972). Importantly, no obesity is reported among the !Kung San, nor any other contemporary hunter–gatherer groups (Lee 1979).

Agricultural production has improved dramatically since the Neolithic Revolution, with successive "Green Revolutions" massively increasing global yield. Technological advances in the agricultural sector are a large part of what made rapid migration from rural to urban environments sustainable, especially as rural manpower decreased. But the initial shift to agricultural subsistence and especially more modern industrial trends such as monocropping have inherent risks for food security. Alarm bells have rung out over imminent food shortage several times in the twentieth century, even in affluent cities, as witnessed during the New York food riots of 1917 (Webb 2010). There were many contributors to this crisis, including crop failures linked to droughts and limited use of fertilizer, but also a number of globalization-related factors such as rising demand, commodity and currency speculation, inflation, trade constraints, low productivity due to widespread lack of credit, and scarce investments in the seeds and technology used by developing country smallholders.

Urbanization   The transition from agrarian to urbanized industrial societies has historically been considered essential for economic growth, demographic change, and the development of modern nation states (Fields 1999). However, the non-agricultural populations' demand for food in the West became unsustainable by the seventeenth century, requiring trade in bulk from further afield, contributing to a positive feedback cycle of population growth and the establishment of capital cities. These capitals centralized political capital and became symbols of power, both catalyzing and giving a face to nation states.

The standards of living in Industrial Revolution Europe are widely debated, although growth in per capita terms was likely slower than often imagined, and with real wages growing less than 20% from 1780 to 1830 (Feinstein 1998). Sanitary conditions and housing environments during this period were substandard for most working class urbanites; child labor was common and, by 1750, England's average work week was 65 hours; in Germany and France it was over 70 hours (Voth 2003). Although real wages did increase, personal consumption did not keep pace, and food consumption may actually have fallen. Height data from the time (Nicholas and Steckel 1991) indicate restrictions in growth development, suggesting hardship associated with living standards. Urban–rural variations in height also suggest that workers in the cities had poorer living standards than their country-based counterparts. At the same time, agricultural employment dropped from one in two to one in four between 1750 and 1850 in Britain (Voth 2003).

Halfway through the twentieth century, there were eight cities with over 5 million inhabitants. Rapid urbanization began in the in the late nineteenth century and continues apace, while many Asian centers expanded even more rapidly during the latter half of the twentieth century.

Disease and Mortality

Generally, the period before the Neolithic transition was marked by an almost complete absence of chronic disease, dental carries, chronic allergies, and other "diseases of civilization." Small foraging groups lack the population density to efficiently transmit many common pathogens; upper respiratory tract infections, for instance, disappear in isolated communities. Hunter–gatherer societies generally live in good health well into old age (Gurven and Kaplan 2007), but their senescence is undercut by extremely high rates of accidental, maternal, infant and child mortality, and violence (Hill 2007). Anemia and other markers of dietary insufficiency were traditionally very rare among the !Kung (Bronte-Stewart 1960), but rates increased substantially as they were moved to settlement camps and adopted a more western lifestyle (Coetzee 1994).

Along with agriculture and urbanization, increases in human mobility as globalization took hold are implicated in the spread of infectious disease (see Chapters 15 and 29): in the "Columbian Exchange," explorers brought plague, smallpox, and influenza to the New World, and returned to the Old World carrying syphilis (Harper 2008); the disastrous effects of novel pathogens in immunologically naïve populations are well documented (Crosby 1976). Eventually, the long shift from foraging to industrial production also involved an "epidemiologic transition" (Omran 1971) from high fertility and mortality marked by a preponderance of infectious disease and infant mortality, to the urbanized industrial context of low fertility and mortality, driven primarily by chronic disease.

The rapid rise of these chronic non-communicable diseases (NCDs) – including cancer and diabetes – grew particularly rapidly in relation to communicable diseases in the final decades of the twentieth century. This was particularly true in developed countries, where by 1990 they accounted for 86% of all deaths. NCDs were historically problems of wealthy developed nations, but spread throughout the developing world with industrial agriculture and the worldwide profusion of tobacco, alcohol, and certain foods. This trend in the latter half of the twentieth century largely escaped policy attention, in part because of global health organizations' focus on communicable disease, and in part because of the speed at which it developed (see Chapter 12).

Globalization and Health Now

Having explored some of the past of globalization and health, we turn our attention to the present: what are the current trends in each of our five focus areas? Most contemporary analyses of globalization rely on overarching quantitative indicators (of both health and economics), though establishing causality remains very difficult. Underneath these grossly aggregated statistics lie the everyday experiences of different populations (Brown and Labonté 2011), where daily life can be equally influenced by global trends and macroeconomic policy (see Chapter 14). The clear picture emerging is that it is increasingly difficult to pick the "winners" and "losers" in the game of globalization. Today, policy decisions are taken more rapidly and are more informed by extra-national or extra-regional influences. At the same time there are far more changes happening on the ground, below the radar of government policy-makers, who thus have less ability to influence populations and their health.

Information and Knowledge Access and Exchange

The newest forms of information transmission are essentially immediate, with millions of instantaneous search results and the ability to send entire volumes of books around the world in seconds. What does this development mean for health? Widespread access to modern information and communication technologies (ICTs) is described in the Millennium Development Goals as a means of improving health by promoting social inclusion and participation. However, there is a difference between access to ICTs and their meaningful use.

Globally, 34.7 inhabitants out of 100 used the Internet in 2011. There are disparities between regions, with Asia (27.2), Africa (12.8), and the Arab States (29.1) lagging behind Europe (74.4) and the Americas (56.3). Access method is increasingly difficult to identify, as access via mobile broadband and smartphones is more than double that of computer-based fixed lines. At the same time, most Organisation for Economic Co-operation and Development (OECD) countries face declining print news readership due to competition from online sources (OECD 2010). Recent trends in national newspaper websites show an increasing proportion of readers is from abroad and in many cases larger than domestic readership (Thurman 2007).

Perhaps most remarkable has been the rise of the mobile phone, where subscriptions per 100 inhabitants increased from 15.5 to 86.7 globally between 2001 and 2011, in virtually all regions and with little difference between developed and developing countries (ITU 2012). In Africa, land-line penetration never exceeded 2%; the continent essentially skipped fixed line development and moved straight to mobile. That the first cellular phone network became operational in 1978 underlines the staggering adoption rate of this technology.

The overarching trend is of an increased volume and availability of information, but a decreased use (especially among youth) of conventional news or public sources of information (OECD 2010) and concomitant difficulty in critically assessing sources. There is a greater risk today that public sector policy, and in some cases private sector practices, cannot keep up with trends in information access and exchange. Furthermore, freedom of information laws laudably promote transparency but often exempt private sector actors.

However, trends in information access and use have health implications. For example, scientific literature is increasingly controlled by international publishing corporations which target rich users. Furthermore, the dominance of European languages on the Internet (both its content and architecture) may exacerbate the digital divide, excluding poorer populations from information that is valuable to economic welfare and health.

There is also much left to be explained in our understanding of information knowledge and access on aspects of social development important for health. Studies have not established a clear link between public access to ICTs and socioeconomic development, and there is only sparse evidence associating ICT access with particular development goals such as governance, civic engagement, gender empowerment, and social equity (Sey and Fellows 2011).

Regulation of information flows has changed dramatically with globalization. The World Summit on the Information Society (WSIS) Declaration of Principles, adopted in 2003, coupled freedom of opinion and expression without interference (as outlined in the Universal Declaration of Human Rights) to new media forms. Nonetheless, organizations such as ICANN (Internet Corporation for Assigned Names and Numbers), which administers global domain assignment and networks, and the Internet Engineering task Force (IETF), which coordinates Internet standards, are generally autonomous, but not publicly held. Regulation of new ICTs and people's access to them is, in other words, out of public control in the globalized world.

The public sector has thus largely been reduced to monitoring trends in access and usage, rather than regulating them – with a few exceptions in authoritarian regimes or national providers monopolizing markets. But there are other, softer regulatory roles for governments, such as those that regulate cultural content in ether-based media. Canada, Australia, the Philippines, Mexico, Nigeria, and Israel require broadcasters to air a certain percentage of domestically produced cultural and creative content. UNESCO's Universal Declaration of Cultural Diversity, with 148 countries signed up, addresses protection of local customs and languages in the face of global communications. Government-facilitated access to public cultural and heritage content is increasing through new ICTs, and may increase social cohesion and even socioeconomic benefits (OECD 2006). However, Internet-based information channels remain difficult to regulate in this manner. To reduce disparities in access to health research, initiatives such as the World Health Organization's HINARI (Health InterNetwork Access to Research Initiative), AGORA (sister program for agriculture), and OARE (environment) provide free or reduced-fee access to medical journals and scientific literature in developing nations.

New communications technologies have also been co-opted for medical use. In sub-Saharan Africa, where mobile phone uptake is high and rising, text messages are an effective means of improving adherence to – and outcomes on – medication for HIV (Lester et al. 2010). Phone–managed care uses locally accepted technology to deliver care that is both high quality and cost-effective. Public health initiatives such as oral rehydration therapy and water purification methods are non-rival goods whose gains are made increasingly available globally via new communication channels (Romer 2010). This flow of medical knowledge may be a major explanation for the closing gap in life expectancies between rich and poor countries over the last century even as per capita income gaps increased (Bourguignon and Morrisson 2002). It also has important effects on local knowledge about health, healthcare demand and delivery, often leading to a diversity of medical approaches rather than a medical monoculture. The globally exposed Sherpas, for instance, now utilize a large and growing number of distinct healing systems, including Shamanism, Tibetan medicine, Ayurveda, and western medicine (Adams 1988; Callaghan 2006).

Formal and Informal Flows of Capital

Trade and markets While previous advances in manufacturing allowed goods to be produced far from the consumer, modern manufacturing has allowed the various stages in a given manufacturing process to also occur far from each other. This development, known as the "second unbundling" of globalization (Baldwin 2006) introduced off-shoring. This complexity in trade in both tasks and ideas makes it increasingly difficult to determine who will benefit from globalized processes – it was easier to predict outcomes when competition was on a sector-to-sector or firm-to-firm scale. The speed at which producers can be out-competed in the globalized economy is also increasing, bringing competition down to the individual level and making the formation of policy – which still occurs on much larger scales – considerably less accurate. This situation makes new demands on individuals, who must be rapidly reposition themselves in dynamic markets, and on governments, who find large portions of their workforce or infrastructure quickly made redundant. This can strain established welfare states that may have more difficulty responding with nimble policies; for states with weaker welfare systems it makes the health outcomes of unemployment all the more dire (see Chapter 21).

International trade is also undergoing rapid fragmentation. The long and fraught negotiations in the current World Trade Organization (WTO)-launched Doha Round illustrate how weak multilateral trade has become. Instead, the number of bilateral and regional agreements is increasingly making it difficult for the WTO and other multinational organizations to ensure internationally "fair" arrangements. The depth of these regional trade agreements is also on an unprecedented level, moving beyond tariffs and into health-related realms such as labor rules, environmental agreements, and safeguard provisions – again often under the radar of international monitoring.

Financial globalization also revealed its darker side during the contagion of the 2008 financial crisis across equity markets in virtually all economies. Financial market crises in one country may have only "infected" other countries to a small extent, but this in turn triggered larger domestic crises that amplified the initial foreign "contagion," causing domestic capital from affected countries to take flight abroad and leading to further domestic impoverishment (see Chapter 21). Such effects have been seen previously, including Mexico in 1994–1995 and Asia in 1997–1998.

The dramatic increase in the mobility of capital fostered by globalization also facilitates offshore tax sheltering. Recent estimates from 139 low to middle income countries, accounting for 85% of the world's population, show that between US$21 and $32 trillion are likely sheltered offshore (Henry 2012) – a sum equal to the GDP of the United States and Japan combined. This not only constitutes a massive loss of potential health-development funding, but also a source of frustration for developing countries which may have to resort to private investment to fund their own poverty-reduction or service-provision strategies (Labonté 2004; also see Chapter 14).

Despite these concerns, there appears to be a positive relationship between economic globalization and life expectancy that is not solely driven by rich countries (Owen and Wu 2007; Nilsson 2009), even when controlling for nutrition, literacy, income, and number of physicians per capita (Nilsson 2009). However, these statistics may hide the negative effects on certain groups. The OECD states that economic globalization and technological change raises income equality within countries among full-time workers, mostly if unions or employment protection is weak and especially among medium-skilled workers whose jobs can be readily automated (OECD 2012a). Research also suggests that trade openness increases average within-country income equality at higher income levels but not lower-income contexts, largely attributable to credit and labor-market deregulation (Nilsson 2009). Domestic government policy can reduce the negative health effects of financial crises and tax sheltering both by creating more stable macroeconomic fundamentals and institutions (Bekaert *et al.* 2011) as well as by implementing protective policies such as active labor market programs (Stuckler *et al.* 2009). Policies that lead to smaller gaps in employment protection between temporary and full-time contracts also lead to narrower income distribution.

Human capital   Developments in transportation and communications technology have facilitated massive increases in migration, and roughly 3% of the world's population has left their country of origin to work elsewhere (Page and Plaza 2006). There are currently at least 80 million labor migrants worldwide and possibly 200 million migrants altogether, and their training, skill, and knowledge now circle the globe more readily than ever. This also allows business to access larger and more skilled labor pools, as well as increased access to foreign labor markets for individuals. This may provide individuals with a legitimate buffer against offshoring for specific jobs, albeit one that is still subject to immigration laws, qualification assessment procedures, and language barriers. There is evidence that foreign-born workers often earn significantly less than natives in their new country of employment, particularly in the EU, even with similar levels of education (OECD 2012b). Some countries, however, including Brazil, Chile, Australia, Germany, Norway, Portugal, and Switzerland, have managed to greatly reduce these gaps, through policies including language training and recognition of foreign qualifications.

Labor migration also exacts a steep toll on family life, development, and health. Migration often results in decreased economic opportunities for women as "trailing spouses" in the developed world (Boyle 2001), and has been shown to increase infant mortality in villages experiencing substantial out-migration (though this effect can be mitigated by remittances) (Kanaiaupuni and Donato 1999). Qualitatively, ethnographic studies demonstrate the extent to which labor migration powerfully and detrimentally rearranges the social order (Gordon 1981).

In some cases, movement to cosmopolitan urban areas facilitates access to more varied and sophisticated healthcare; in Africa, for instance, the persistence of significant disparities in rural versus urban healthcare is well documented (Booysen 2003). Conversely, urban life and the removal of traditional support systems brings with it extra threats: HIV rates were observed to have increased among the !Kung San only with the arrival of transport routes; distance to a major road and HIV prevalence are powerfully correlated in many parts of Africa (Tanser 2000). As with many aspects of globalization, increased mobility may be a double-edged sword, with the dramatic improvements in earning power and access to services offset by real (if nebulous) social impacts and the exposure to new threats far from home.

Perhaps the greatest socioeconomic consequence of increased human capital movement between countries is the flow of remittances. Remittances are transfers of money from migrant workers to dependents in their home country. The value of global remittances is massive and growing rapidly; the World Bank (2012) estimates the total value for 2010 at roughly $440 billion. The exact figure is difficult to calculate, and some feel that official data underestimate total flows by 10–50% (Ratha 2009). Remittances now make up over 25% of GDP in Moldova, Tonga, and Guyana, and over 20% of GDP in several other countries (Ratha 2007). Remittances are spent primarily on household consumption, including healthcare (Page and Plaza 2006) and have direct consequences for health. In Sri Lanka, for instance, birth weight is positively correlated with receipt of remittances (Ratha 2009).

While mobility may be positive for individuals and families, and for receiving countries, the associated "brain-drain" can have severe economic and social consequences, and amplify inequalities (see Chapter 10). New EU members such as Hungary and Romania, for instance, have state-financed medical training but suffer a net loss of qualified doctors which appears to be increasing. High-skill migration from poor to rich countries is the dominant pattern. Although the motivations for migration are complex, institutional corruption, poverty, discrimination, and political repression are emerging as clear drivers (Docquier and Rapoport 2011). Economic shocks can also drive high-skill emigration, something that may become more common. Incentives such as corporate tax rates can also influence migration, although a "race to the bottom" in this regard is not guaranteed to generate economic benefits unless it produces a substantial movement of individuals, as the largest benefits for states come from increases in personal income tax revenues (Ekholm 2008). The countries being "drained" are not entirely the helpless victims of these trends, nor are receiving countries passive beneficiaries; policy on both sides of the exchange drives the process and shapes its outcomes.

Nourishment and Subsistence

The world currently faces a dietary dichotomy unprecedented in human history: 1 billion people are undernourished, while roughly 2 billion are overweight or obese. While those in the former category are still largely found in developing countries, the latter category is becoming evenly spread. Food delivery systems have changed the food industry, where multinational corporations control an ever-increasing proportion of all food consumed: the 10 largest account over 15% of world food sales, with virtually all growth in developing countries (Stuckler and Nestle 2012). Governments have been slow catching up with this development, and are only now starting to engage the major private sector players in partnership and responsibility pacts, although the benefits are unclear. The profit motive is often, according to critics, at odds with government health promotion.

The period of financial turmoil in 2007–2009 was also a period of unique global fuel and food price increases. Levels of undernutrition in absolute numbers reached record levels despite increasing global yields during this period (Webb 2010), suggesting supply problems did not drive prices. This may be partially due to the increasing share of food crops used for biofuels and feedstock, as meat consumption increases globally. Regardless, gains in food supply do not appear to be reaching the areas that need it most, with production per capita flat or falling developing regions. This creates reliance on imports, which are predicted to increase (FAO 2002), with subsequent risks for market-dictated food consumption patterns, including more volatile prices, food insecurity, and ultimately malnutrition. For instance, small-scale Ugandan coffee exporters now have increased access to global markets, but find that their income is vulnerable to global market pressures. As a result, farmers' food security is precarious, and opportunities to change crops and production or export methods limited.

Case studies from Africa illustrate the complexity of food security in the globalized world. Structural Adjustment Programs, which promote privatization and liberalization, especially in sites such as Export Processing Zones (EPZs) in developing countries, have led to higher salaries but often poorer health for women. As women are responsible for 80% of food production in Africa, this impacts entire households. In urban Tanzania, female EPZ workers earn higher wages, but time constraints associated with longer working hours reduce their dietary diversity and nourishment (Kamuzora *et al.* 2011). Monoculture production, targeted at large-scale export markets, has also reduced the variety of crops that were once used to sustain local populations. On the other hand, many of the problems facing small-scale farmers are related to local infrastructure, government regulations, and other domestic policy issues. Lack of working animals and modern machinery can limit access to foreign markets, while in some cases economic liberalization can stimulate yields and facilitate export by providing intermediate products such as fertilizers and pesticides (Bardhan 2006).

Among groups on the periphery of the globalizing world, those who appear most successful are those who have been able to manage a partial integration process while maintaining traditionally useful and valuable politicoeconomic strategies and sociocultural values. The Sherpas are again instructive in this regard: perhaps because of their geographic isolation, development projects and foreign influences have arrived relatively slowly. Schools were built first, bridging the modern and the traditional, and offering a buffer before the full-speed onset of globalization (Fisher 1997). Their ability to selectively engage with globalization without subsuming their identity has been a successful strategy for the Sherpas for decades (Adams 1996); in food production as in many other areas, drawing benefits from globalization while buffering locally against its risks appears to offer the best of both worlds.

Urbanization In 2000 there were 42 cities with 5 million or more residents, 20 of which are in Asia. There was also an estimated "slum" population of around 924 million people in 2001 – almost 43% of all urban dwellers worldwide. In the least developed countries, this figure was 78.2% (UN 2003). Today, the largest rural-to-urban migration in history is occurring, with more than half of the global population living in cities that cover only 0.5% of the world's land mass (Schneider *et al.* 2009). China is particularly active, with rural-to-urban migration tripling over the past 30 years and continuing to accelerate (Gong *et al.* 2012).

Urbanization has an "organic" bottom-up component, but is also clearly driven by policy. China's national policy openly promote urbanization to drive domestic demand and transform national development models (Xiaoji 2010). Many other countries may also do so, perhaps inadvertently: urbanization often results from sectoral shifts as economies develop (Henderson 2003), but may be a cause rather than an effect of growth. Depending on the size of the country and its level of development, there are clear advantages in pooling talent densely in cities; however, there may be an optimal degree of urbanization outside of which productivity is stalled or even damaged (Henderson 2003). This may be due to the necessary rerouting of resources to maintain living standards in very large cities. Such a drain from rural communities may also increase inequality and catylze further urbanization. Indeed, the "urbanization of poverty" is already underway, where an increasing percentage of the world's poor are found in urban environments instead of rural ones. Attempts to attract international investment may exacerbate this process. Paradoxically, those major cities that are most excluded from global trade systems today also appear to have poorer social welfare and increased slum size and population (UN 2003), while also having less financial ability to change this situation (see Chapter 14).

Disease and Mortality

Communicable diseases In the middle of the last century, as the burden of chronic disease grew, many observers declared the problem of infectious disease solved (Pier 2008).

But while the 1900s did indeed witness major victories against infectious disease, primarily through basic sanitation infrastructure, mass vaccination campaigns, and pharmacology, recent trends instead suggest a resurgence of infectious disease related to three situations: novel diseases such as HIV/AIDS (Zhu *et al.* 1998) and SARS (Li *et al.* 2005); existing disease moving to new environments, such as West Nile virus (Rappole *et al.* 2000); and newly virulent or drug-resistant strains of old diseases, such as methicillin-resistant *Staphylococcus aureus* (MRSA; Enright *et al.* 2002). Globalization is implicated in this process, in positive and negative ways (see Chapter 15). Theoretically, globalization should reduce immune naivety, increasing global herd immunity. It also allows for outbreak monitoring and the sharing of knowledge and training, all of which are crucial in containing infectious disease. On the other hand, globalization also reduces physical and political sources of epidemiological friction, allowing pathogens to cross the world faster than ever and exploit new environments almost instantly (see Chapters 15 and 16).

Non-communicable diseases   Non-communicable diseases (NCDs), which now kill more people worldwide than communicable diseases, are also powerfully associated with globalization (see Chapter 12). Chronic conditions like cancer, diabetes, and obstructive lung disorders, have physical inactivity, poor diet, tobacco use, and harmful alcohol consumption as major risk factors, which in turn have ties with urbanization and its nutrition and exercise-poor environments, the establishment of global food trade, and worldwide marketing of tobacco and alcohol products. The burden of these diseases today is borne equally by rich and poor nations; over 80% of deaths from NCDs occur in low and middle-income countries (Abegunde *et al.* 2007). Developing countries also carry a "double burden" in that undernutrition is also present (Swinburn *et al.* 2011), but the trends are clear: the nutritional transition is occurring in poor countries with far fewer publically financed health resources to mitigate the process. In India for example, out-of-pocket expenses for NCD-related medical care has increased catastrophically in comparison to communicable disease treatment (Mahala *et al.* 2010).

The recent refocusing of global health policy on NCDs has been dramatic. At the beginning of the millennium the World Health Assembly set a global agenda for combatting NCDs in the non-healthcare sector, emphasizing the role for trade, agriculture, urban development, and allied policies in shaping health. Interventions at the level of the family and community were deemed essential for successful prevention strategies as many of the causal risk factors of NCDs are deeply entrenched in the social and cultural framework of the society (see Chapter 14). The assembly subsequently passed resolutions on tobacco control, health promotion, diet and exercise, and alcohol abuse. In 2011, for only the second time in history, the United Nations General Assembly held a high-level meeting on a health issue. The result was a political declaration regarding prevention and control of NCDs, with the WHO receiving a subsequent assignment to set global voluntary targets and indicators for monitoring.

Possible Futures of Globalization and Health

Making predictions about globalization and health is extremely difficult. However, some of threads we have identified in the past and present support projections into the future. In particular, two paradoxical trends that have emerged from globalization are likely to continue. One is the degree to which individuals are exposed to both positive and negative aspects of global integration. We have discussed the myriad benefits of this process, including the wider faster sharing of knowledge and economic opportunities. On the other hand, increasing global competition makes it harder to respond with appropriate macro-level policies to ensure trade fairness, healthy working conditions, and employment.

The second trend is at odds with the first: the (often insidious) reduction of choice that is developing with global consolidation. Here, urbanization and subsistence are particularly good examples. With improved ICT access and the spread of knowledge, it should be easier to remain in remote areas and be able to obtain an education, remain employed, and enjoy many of the trappings of modern life without having to relocate to urban centers. Yet an increasingly concentrated number of corporations continue to gain control over agricultural and industrial production. This is contrary to the commonly understood promises of globalization: increased opportunities for smaller players to access larger markets, and thus an increase in marketplace variety, as well as improved selection for the individual. Considering the development of NCDs in recent decades and the resurgence of infectious disease, something has gone wrong here. Partnerships and policies may reduce health impacts (see Chapters 27 and 28), but the root of the problem can only be assessed by policies that put health first (see Chapter 4). This will not be an easy sell.

Information and Knowledge Access and Exchange

Information will continue to move at faster speeds in greater volumes, and with wider accessibility worldwide. Although gaps will persist for those on the periphery (whether due to age, income, lifestyle, or political isolation), the "digital divide" between countries and regions will continue to close – and continue to solve global health problems. The real challenge for health in terms of globalized information flow is threefold: reliability, relevance, and impact. The first challenge involves the ability of individuals to find information from reliable transparent sources grounded in real evidence. The second is to tailor knowledge and information that can improve health to the user's circumstances. The final challenge will be to provide knowledge in a manner that encourages application and achieves lasting health benefits, something that is increasingly difficult as the total volume and flow increases almost exponentially with each passing year. Policy-makers should be well-positioned to respond to the first two, but the latter will require nimble thinking.

Medical consultation by distance, as well as online therapy and robotic surgery, should continue to develop, facilitating better training and care in remote and developing regions. The risk of privatization or "trade" in these services is significant, however. Public health campaigns that use ICTs and social media are already well established in some spheres, although they can still be refined, improved, and scaled up for larger populations. Perhaps most important will be improved international cooperation and compatibility for access to health data for migrants, as well as population disease and health development databases and statistics (see Chapters 5 and 6). This will further improve international coordination as both communicable and non-communicable diseases spread across borders at ever-faster rates.

Formal and Informal Flows of Capital

Trade and markets   An increased specialization in trade and a greater prevalence of bilateral and regional trade agreements is likely. This would allow countries to reduce the risks of unwanted technology transfer and competition, increase control over tariffs, and priviledge strategic or regional partners. At the same time, this might decrease transparency in global trade and establish tariffs and rules that prove detrimental to the health of many. While a great deal of anti-WTO sentiment exists, the undermining of its authority by failing to establish a multilateral trade agreement in the Doha Round might exacerbate this decreased transparency. Depending on the severity of the scenario that develops after a failed round, potential tariff adjustments and subsequent global reductions in trade estimated at 3.2–7.7% (Bouet and Debucquet 2009) would hit agricultural exports of developing countries particularly hard.

Human capital   In so far as humans are expected to continue to flow to areas with greater resources and opportunities, globalization may facilitate the rise of a sort of neo-nomadism, both for the freelancing jet-setter and the developing-world laborer. In the short to medium term, sectors and skill groups will quickly become redundant, and it is difficult to identify which groups will be affected. Many technology and knowledge-based jobs from developed countries may rapidly be lost to newer developing nations with built-in wage advantages. These wage gaps will decrease with time, but in the interim we may assume that a global redistribution of employment will continue. Aside from the health gains and losses attributed to employment status in "winning" and "losing" countries (see Chapter 10), there may be unpredictable global economic consequences. Educational and employment training schemes to "push" workers into specific skill sets may often be in vain, as governments fail to predict correctly which sectors will bear fruit. While the most highly trained skill sets may remain "safe," low-skill labor that will almost always be required locally may also thrive. The specificity with which demand for certain skills or sectors shift internationally will punch holes in traditional relationships between training and economic security. "Flexicurity" may be a successful government policy solution in these unpredictable circumstances, providing a high level of economic support and retraining during the periods between jobs. While such programs are expensive and require a well-established administrative structure, they also likely produce savings in the medium to long term by reducing the ill effects of income loss and insecurity.

Over the longer term we may see a reduction in the flow of migrants. As skills are rapidly shared worldwide through communications technology, the need for individuals to bring their own labor to a fixed production site will gradually decrease. Migration and labor policies are still reactive, local, and disorganized in much of the world. In the long term, policy-makers should harmonize policies and target negative drivers of migration, including global and regional inequality and political instability (Castles 2004). Ideally, this process brings health benefits: a population that can both profit from the international labor market and the support structures inherent in traditional communities.

As with most globalizing processes, predicting the future of remittance flows is difficult but two potential trends seem worth watching. First, some governments may soon find remittances a tempting source of revenue. Some nations already have *de facto* tax structures in place. Money sent from the United States to Cuba, for instance, must be changed from dollars into pesos and subsequently taxed, providing the government with not only revenue but hard currency after the end of Soviet trade and aid (Eckstein 2010). Several other countries achieve similar results by requiring conversion to local currency at official (but uncompetitive) rates. Over the longer term, however, remittances seem likely to slow as growth in developed countries slows and the developing world catches up. Taking remittances for granted – and using their value as an excuse to reduce foreign direct investment or domestic investment in health – would be a mistake. Unlike direct investment and, to a lesser extent, trade, remittances are not predictable from one year to the next, nor is their spending particularly responsive to policy. In the medium term, remittances clearly represent a powerful force for health development. Policy-makers should encourage the efficient, safe, and free flow of remittances to the developing world to leverage their potential to improve health in tandem with government investment.

Nourishment and Subsistence

Agriculture   While the trend of overall lower food prices may resume globally after recent turbulence, periods of food price volatility are likely to become more frequent and the Food and Agricultural Organization (FAO) and OECD predict 40–80% higher prices for wheat, maize, and vegetable oils in the decade from 2010 compared with the previous decade. A still-growing world population may drive this, as well as cultural globalization; a growing global middle class adopting a western taste for meat, for instance, would require massive increases in livestocking feed crops. Climate change and severe weather are also likely to affect key crops more often as the human impact on global climate continues to increase. Fuel prices will affect farming costs and in turn consumer prices. Policies promoting land use change and biofuel production may also contribute to volatility in prices. Interconnected markets' hedging on food and fuel futures will have more far-reaching global effects during periods of uncertainty. Finally, the level of government complacency during high crop yields and inaction during failures will affect national and regional health outcomes. The share of the global population meeting minimum nutritional needs will likely increase regardless as distribution chains become more efficient, but the absolute number of undernourished will likely increase with price volatility. The poorer populations in developing countries that lack the capacity to absorb domestic shocks will again be most affected. The nutrition status of pregnant women, children, and those affected by long-term diseases in particular will also see their capacity to purchase education, healthcare, or other basic needs compromised when food prices are high. Small-scale farms can be a key buffer against food price volatility, but only where they are primarily engaged in producing for local consumption. In order for such farms to offer local relief from disordered global markets, they must have flexibility, access to credit, and appropriate agricultural technology.

Processed food sales are also likely to remain dominated by a handful of major multinational corporations in the future. Public–private agreements and partnerships with these corporations to promote healthy food consumption are likely to fail unless profit margins can be guaranteed. To achieve this, a wide consumer consensus on healthy foods is necessary. Failing this, the most likely alternative is for public authorities to increase regulation and taxation on unhealthy products. Future policy should follow this order, and create definitive consequences at each step. This is a relatively new battleground, but the stakes for public health are already massive.

Urbanization   By 2015 the world will have 61 cities of over 5 million inhabitants. As natural population growth slows around the world, the majority of this urban expansion will be explained by rural-to-urban migration. Poverty will also urbanize, with the majority of the poor likely to be located in urban areas instead of rural in the relatively near future. Urban poverty is different from rural poverty: cash flows are higher but property ownership is rare, the environment is less healthy, and access to basic services often compromised. Those governments that have attempted to stop migration to cities through strict regulation or restricted access to public services have generally failed: such policies tend to increase the economic strain on migrants without affecting their flow into cities. Governments must accept that urbanization cannot be stopped in the short-to-medium term, and focus on spreading populations evenly throughout several urban regions. Globalization also creates the possibility for increasing cross-border migration between large cities, which may also help even out populations. For existing cities, progressively achieving adequate housing, ensuring proper zoning and building regulations, engaging public and private sectors as well as civil society, and improving participation in urban policy-making would all improve health for urban residents. Low-cost rental housing must increase, allowing mobility for casual workers. For slum regions, the best practices will involve participatory improvement, whereby formalized government-led facilitation involves occupants from the outset of improvement work, and requires investments from the occupants themselves. Governments will have to strengthen their role here if the increase in slum areas is to be halted or reversed.

Disease and Mortality

Communicable diseases The problem of "re-emerging infectious disease" in the developed world may be indicated by trends in the last two decades of the twentieth century, where infectious disease mortality in affluent countries increased for the first time since the Industrial Revolution (Pinner *et al.* 1996). It is possible that we are now on the cusp of a third epidemiological transition, which after the changes of the Neolithic and Industrial Revolutions, will see us return to a high burden of infectious disease (Barrett 1998). This scenario is made more likely not only by increases in novel pathogens, but the increased frequency and speed with which pathogens – assisted by climate change and human mobility – "spill out" of traditional reservoirs (see Chapters 15 and 29). Perhaps most alarming of all is our inability to treat many of these diseases because of the rapid evolution of drug resistance. The factors that facilitate their spread – socioeconomic and ecological disruption, human movement, and drug resistance (Jones *et al.* 2008) – are closely tied to accelerating globalization. Two immediate internationally coordinated policy courses of action would yield great returns. First, policy-makers must urgently work toward globally coordinated monitoring, reporting, and response to disease outbreaks. Second, a rationalized global accord on the use of antibiotics – in humans and animals.

Non-communicable diseases NCDs are projected to account for 69% of global deaths by 2030. Tobacco-related deaths will rise to 6.4 million in 2015 – 10% of all deaths globally – and to 8.3 million in 2030. The shift in global health policy focus to NCDs will continue in parallel. Tobacco policy is still in its infancy, with China, India, the Middle East, and Africa only just beginning to show interest in tackling rapidly growing smoking rates. Obesity has leveled off in many developed countries, albeit at record levels, but this does not mean that developing countries must follow the same curve. Preventative policies and market regulation must be implemented now in developing countries at the same level and with the same urgency as in developed countries to alter current projections.

Conclusions

In the past, globalization was driven by macro-level policy, and its effects on health, though substantial, were a haphazard afterthought. In the future, globalization will continue in spite of macro-level policy, through individuals who are more integrated in a globalized society. This does not mean that national and international policies will be irrelevant in the future, nor do we suggest that globalization need be reversed by policy-makers – on the contrary, globalization has offered unprecedented benefits. Instead, policies must focus on protecting the health of those on the periphery of globalization and most likely to fall ill of it, and on fine-tuning global integration such that the benefits are more evenly spread amongst populations, within and between countries. The future of globalization is not the global village but the global network: a web of relations that individuals and states can access selectively to their greatest benefit. Globalization will certainly produce winners and losers, and predicting outcomes will be increasingly difficult. It does seem clear, though, that more than anything globalization offers unprecedented potential, and unprecedented risk. The winners will be those engaged in a maturing globalization – not a free-for-all of expansion and acceleration, but a refining of connections; drawing unique benefit from an ever-shrinking world while maintaining local risk sinks to buffer against shocks elsewhere in the global network. This potential applies also to policy-makers: globalization has been among the most powerful forces shaping health across all human history. The right policies will leverage the forces of globalization to improve health, worldwide.

Key Reading

Brown GW, Labonté R. 2011. Globalization and its methodological discontents: contextualizing globalizations through the study of HIV/AIDS. *Globalization and Health* 7, 29.

Cockerham G, Cockerham W. 2010. *Health and Globalization*. Cambridge: Polity Press.

Kawachi I, Wamala, S (eds). 2006. *Globalization and Health*. New York: Oxford University Press.

Labonté R, Schrecker R, Packer C, Rummels V (eds). 2012. *Globalization and Health: Pathways, Evidence and Policy*. London: Routledge.

Woodward D, Drager N, Beaglehole R, Lipson D. 2001. Globalization and health: framework for analysis and action. *Bulletin of the World Health Organization* 79, 876.

References

Abegunde DO, Mathers CD, Adam T *et al.* 2007. The burden and costs of chronic diseases in low-income and middle-income countries. *Lancet* 370(9603), 1929–38.

Adams V. 1988. Modes of production and medicine: an examination of the theory in light of Sherpa medical traditionalism. *Social Science and Medicine* 27(5), 505–13.

Adams V. 1996. *Tigers of the Snow and Other Virtual Sherpas*. Princeton: Princeton University Press.

Anderson K. 2010. Globalization's effects on world agricultural trade, 1960–2050. *Philosophical Transactions of the Royal Society of London Series B Biological Sciences* 365(1554), 3007–21.

Baldwin, R. 2006. *Globalization: the great unbundling(s)*. http://appli8.hec.fr/map/files/globalisationthegreatunbundling(s).pdf (last accessed December 2013).

Baldwin R, Martin P, Ottaviano GIP. 2001. Global income divergence, trade, and industrialization: the geography of growth take-offs. *Journal of Economic Growth* 6(1), 5–37.

Bardhan, P. 2006. *Globalization, Inequality and Poverty: An Overview*. http://emlab.berkeley.edu/users/webfac/bardhan/papers/BardhanGlobalOverview.pdf (last accessed December 2013).

Barrett R, Kuzawa CW, McDade T, Armelados GJ. 1998. Emerging and re-emerging infectious diseases: the third epidemiologic transition. *Annual Reviews of Anthropology* 27, 247–71.

Bekaert G, Ehrmann M, Fratzscher M, Arnaud M. 2011. *Global crises and Equity Market Contagion*. Working Paper Series. Frankfurt am Main: European Central Bank.

Booysen F. 2003. Urban–rural inequalities in health care delivery in South Africa. *Development Southern Africa* 20(5), 659–73.

Bouet A, Debucquet D. 2009. *The Potential Cost of a Failed Doha Round*. IFPRI Discussion Paper No. 00886. Washington, DC: International Food Policy Research Institute.

Bourguignon F, Morrisson C. 2002. Inequality among world citizens: 1820–1992. *American Economic Review* 92(4), 727–44.

Boyle P, Cooke TJ, Halfacree K, Smith D. 2001. A cross-national comparison of the impact of family migration on women's employment status. *Demography* 38(2), 201–13.

Bronte-Stewart B, Budtz-Olsen OE, Hickley JM, Brock JF. 1960. the health and nutritional status of the Kung Bushmen of South West Africa. *South African Journal of Laboratory and Clinical Medicine* 6, 187–216.

Brown GW, Labonté R. 2011. Globalization and its methodological discontents: contextualizing globalizations through the study of HIV/AIDS. *Globalization and Health* 7, 29.

Callaghan M. 2006. *Medical Pluralism on Mount Everest*. Edmonton: University of Alberta Press.

Castles S. 2004. Why migration policies fail. *Ethnic and Racial Studies* 27(4), 205–27.

Coetzee M, Badenhorst PN, de Wet JI, Joubert G. 1994. Haematological condition of Bushmen relocation from Namibia to South Africa: a three-year follow-up. *Revista de Investigacion Clinica* April (Suppl), 227.

Cohen M, Armelagos G (eds). 1984. *Paleopathology at the Origins of Agriculture*. New York: Academic Press.

Crosby A. 1976. Virgin soil epidemics as a factor in the Aboriginal depopulation in America. *William and Mary Quarterly* 33(2), 289–99.

Devore I, Lee R. 1968. *Man the Hunter*. New Jersey: Aldine Press.

Docquier F, Rapoport H. 2011. *Globalization, Brain Drain and Development*. Discussion Paper Series. Bonn: Institute for the Study of Labor.

Douglas M. 2002. *Purity and Danger: An Analysis of Concepts of Pollution and Taboo*. London: Routledge.

Eckstein S. 2010. Remittances and their unintended consequences in Cuba. *World Development* 38(7), 1047–55.

Ekholm K. 2008. [*Globalisation's Driving Forces and Socioeconomic Consequences*. Report No. 9 for the Swedish Globalisation Council.] Västerås: Swedish Globalisation Council.

Enright MC, Robinson DA, Randle G, Feil EJ, Grundmann H, Spratt BG. 2002. The evolutionary history of methicillin-resistant *Staphylococcus aureus* (MRSA). *Proceedings of the National Academy of Sciences of the United States of America* 99(11), 7687–92.

FAO (Food and Agricultural Organization). 2002. *World Agriculture: Towards 2015/2030*. Rome: FAO.

Feinstein CH. 1998. Pessimism perpetuated: real wages and the standard of living in Britain during and after the Industrial Revolution. *Journal of Economic History* 58(3), 625–58.

Fields G. 1999. City systems, urban history and economic modernity: urbanization and the transition from agrarian to industrial society. *Berkeley Planning Journal* 13, 102–28.

Fisher JF. 1997. *Sherpas: Reflections on Change in Himalayan Nepal*. Delhi: Oxford University Press.

Fleming F. 2004. *Tales of Endurance*. London: Phoenix.

Giddens A. 1990. *The Consequences of Modernity*. Stanford, CA: Stanford University Press.

Gong P, Liang S, Carlton EJ, Jiang Q, Wu J, Wang L, Remais JV. 2012. Urbanisation and health in China. *Lancet* 379(9818), 843–52.

Gordon E. 1981. An analysis of the impact of labour migration on the lives of women in Lesotho. *Journal of Development Studies* 17(3), 59–76.

Gurven M, Kaplan H. 2007. Longevity among hunter-gatherers: a cross-cultural examination. *Population and Development Review* 33(2), 321–65.

Harper K, Ocampo PS, Steiner BM, *et al.* 2008. On the origin of the treponematoses: a phylogenetic approach. *PLOS Neglected Tropical Diseases* 2(1), 148.

Henderson V. 2003. The urbanization process and economic growth: the so-what question. *Journal of Economic Growth* 8(1), 47–71.

Henry J. 2012. *The price of offshore revisited: new estimates for "missing" global private wealth, income, inequality and lost taxes.* http://www.taxjustice.net/cms/upload/pdf/Price_of_Offshore_Revisited_120722.pdf (last accessed January 2014).

Hill K, Hurtado AM, Walker RS. 2007. High adult mortality among Hiwi hunter-gatherers: implications for human evolution. *Journal of Human Evolution* 52(4), 443–54.

ITU (International Telecommunications Union). 2012. *World telecommunications/ICT indicators database.* Geneva: ITU.

Jones KE, Patel NG, Levy MA *et al.* 2008. Global trends in emerging infectious diseases. *Nature* 451(7181), 990–3.

Kamuzora P, Loewenson R *et al.* 2011. The effects of women's employment in export processing zones on household food security and dietary patterns in urban Tanzania. In *Effects of Globalisation on Women's Occupational Roles and Health in Sub-Saharan Africa through a Food Security and Nutrition Lens.* Stockholm: Swedish International Development Agency.

Kanaiaupuni S, Donato K. 1999. Migradollars and mortality: the effects of migration on infant mortality in Mexico. *Demography* 36(3), 339–53.

Kiker B. 1966. The historical roots of human capital. *Journal of Political Economy* 74(5), 481–99.

Labonté R. 2004. Globalization, health and the free trade regime: assessing the links. *Perspectives on Global Development and Technology* 3(1–2), 47–72.

Lee R. 1979. *The !Kung San: Men, Women and Work in a Foraging Society.* Cambridge: Cambridge University.

Lester RT, Ritvo P, Mills EJ *et al.* 2010. Effects of a mobile phone short message service on antiretroviral treatment adherence in Kenya (WelTel Kenya1): a randomised trial. *Lancet* 376(9755), 1838–45.

Li W, Shi Z, Yu M *et al.* 2005. Bats are natural reservoirs of SARS-like coronaviruses. *Science* 310(5748), 676–9.

Mácha P, Drobík T. 2011. Introduction: the scales of globalizations. *The Scale of Globalization: Think Globally, Act Locally, Change Individually in the 21st Century.* Ostrava, Czech Republic: University of Ostrava.

Maddison A. 2001. *The World Economy: A Millennial Perspective.* Paris: OECD.

Mahala A, Karanb A, Engelgau M. 2010. *The Economic Implications of Non-Communicable Diseases for India.* Health, Nutrition and Population (HNP) Discussion Papers. Washington, DC: World Bank.

Nicholas S, Steckel R. 1991. Heights and living standards of English workers during the early years of industrialization, 1770–1815. *Journal of Economic History* 51(4), 937–57.

Nilsson T. 2009. *Inequality, globalization and health.* PhD thesis, Lund University, Lund.

OECD (Organisation for Economic Co-operation and Development). 2006. *Digital Broadband Content: Public Sector Information and Content.* Paris: Working Party on the Information Economy, OECD.

OECD (Organisation for Economic Co-operation and Development). 2010. *The Evolution of News and the Internet.* Paris: Working Party on the Information Economy, OECD.

OECD (Organisation for Economic Co-operation and Development). 2012a. *Inequality in Labour Income: What are Its Drivers and How can It be Reduced?* OECD Economics Department Policy Notes 8. Paris: OECD.

OECD (Organisation for Economic Co-operation and Development). 2012b. *Reducing Income Inequality while Boosting Economic Growth: Can It be Done? Economic Policy Reforms 2012: Going for growth,* pp. 181–202. Paris: OECD.

Omran A. 1971. The epidemiological transition: a theory of the epidemiology of population change. *Milbank Memorial Fund Quarterly* 49, 509–38.

O'Rourke K, Williamson J. 2002. When did globalization begin? *European Review of Economic History* 6(1), 23–50.

Owen A, Wu S. 2007. Is trade good for your health? *Review of International Economics* 15, 660–82.

Page J, Plaza S. 2006. Migration remittances and development: a review of global evidence. *Journal of African Economies* 15(Suppl 2): 245–336.

Pier G. 2008. On the greatly exaggerated reports of the death of infectious diseases. *Clinical Infectious Diseases* 47(8), 1113–4.

Pinner RW, Teutsch SM, Simonsen L *et al.* 1996. Trends in infectious diseases mortality in the United States. *Journal of the American Medicical Association* 275(3), 189–93.

Rappole JH, Derrickson SR, Hubálek Z. 2000. Migratory birds and spread of West Nile virus in the Western Hemisphere. *Emerging Infectious Diseases* 6(4), 319–28.

Ratha D. 2007. Leveraging remittances for development. Second Plenary Meeting of the Leading Group on Solidarity Levies to Fund Development, Oslo.

Ratha D. 2009. Dollars without borders. *Foreign Affairs* October 16. http://www.foreign affairs.com/articles/65448/dilip-ratha/dollars-without-borders (last accessed December 2013).

Romer P. 2010. *Which Parts of Globalization Matter for Catch-Up Growth?* NBER Working Paper Series. Cambridge, MA: National Bureau of Economic Research.

Sahlins M. 1972. *Stone Age Economics*. New Jersey: Transaction Press.

Sandri D, Valenzuela E, Anderson K. 2007. *Economic and Trade Indicators, 1960 to 2004*. Agricultural Distortions Working Paper No. 02. Washington, DC: World Bank.

Schneider A, Friedl M, Potere D. 2009. A new map of global urban extent from MODIS satellite data. *Environmental Research Letters* 4, 1–11.

Sey A, Fellows M. 2011. *Loose Strands: Searching for Evidence of Public Access ICT Impact on Development*. iConference, pp. 189–94. Seattle, WA: ACM.

Stuckler D, Basu S, Suhrcke M, Coutts A, McKee M. 2009. The public health effect of economic crises and alternative policy responses in Europe: an empirical analysis. *Lancet* 374(9686), 315–23.

Stuckler D, Nestle M. 2012. Big food, food systems, and global health. *PLOS Medicine* 9(6), e1001242.

Swinburn BA, Sacks G, Hall KD *et al.* 2011. The global obesity pandemic: shaped by global drivers and local environments. *Lancet* 378(9793), 804–14.

Tanser F, Lesueur D, Solarsh G, Wilkinson D. 2000. HIV heterogeneity and proximity of homestead to roads in rural South Africa: an exploration using a geographical information system. *Tropical Medicine and International Health* 5(1), 40–6.

Thurman N. 2007. The globalization of journalism online. *Journalism* 8(3), 285–307.

UN-Habitat. 2003. *The Challenge of Slums: Global Report on Human Settlements 2003*. http://www.unhabitat.org/pmss/listItemDetails.aspx?publicationID=1156 (last accessed January 2014).

Van Gennep A. 1960. *The Rites of Passage*. London: Routledge.

Voth HJ. 2003. Living standards during the Industrial Revolution: an economist's guide. *AEA Papers and Proceedings* 93(2), 221–6.

Webb P. 2010. Medium- to long-run implications of high food prices for global nutrition. *Journal of Nutrition* 140(1), 143S–7S.

Willmore L. 2001. *Government Policies Toward Information and Communication Technologies: A Historical Perspective*. DESA Discussion Paper. New York: United Nations.

World Bank. 2012. *Remittance market outlook*. http://go.worldbank.org/NPD63OTRR0 (last accessed December 2013).

Xiaoji Q. 2010. *Urbanization policies to help boost domestic demands*. http://www.chinadaily .com.cn/bizchina/2010–03/08/content_9554671.htm (last accessed December 2013).

Zhu T, Korber BT, Nahmias AJ, Hooper E, Sharp PM, Ho DD. 1998. An African HIV-1 sequence from 1959 and implications for the origin of the epidemic. *Nature* 391(6667), 594–7.

Index

Figures and tables are indexed as, for example, 268f and 269t; notes are indexed as, for example, 222n.

The Handbook of Global Health Policy, First Edition. Edited by Garrett W. Brown, Gavin Yamey, and Sarah Wamala.
© 2014 John Wiley & Sons, Ltd. Published 2014 by John Wiley & Sons, Ltd.

CPSIA information can be obtained
at www.ICGtesting.com
Printed in the USA
BVOW04*1814130917

494154BV00013B/11/P